Praeger Handbook of
Black American Health

Praeger Handbook of Black American Health

2nd Edition

Policies and Issues Behind Disparities in Health, Volume I

Edited by IVOR LENSWORTH LIVINGSTON

Foreword by David Satcher

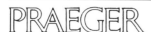

Westport, Connecticut
London

Library of Congress Cataloging-in-Publication Data

Praeger handbook of Black American health : policies and issues behind disparities in health / edited
by Ivor Lensworth Livingston ; foreword by David Satcher.—2nd ed.
   p. cm.
  First ed. published under : Handbook of Black American health.
  Includes bibliographical references and index.
  ISBN 0–313–32477–8 (set: alk. paper)—ISBN 0–313–33220–7 (vol. 1: alk. paper)—ISBN 0–313–33221–5
(vol. 2: alk. paper)
  1. African Americans—Health and hygiene—Handbooks, manuals, etc. 2. African
Americans—Medical care—Handbooks, manuals, etc. I. Title: Handbook of Black
American health. II. Livingston, Ivor Lensworth.
  RA448.5.N4H364 2004
  362.1'089'96073—dc22   2003069010

British Library Cataloguing in Publication Data is available.

Library of Congress Catalog Card Number: 2003069010
ISBN: 0–313–32477–8 (set)
        0–313–33220–7 (vol. 1)
        0–313–33221–5 (vol. 2)

First published in 2004

Praeger Publishers, 88 Post Road West, Westport, CT 06881
An imprint of Greenwood Publishing Group, Inc.
www.praeger.com

Printed in the United States of America

The paper used in this book complies with the
Permanent Paper Standard issued by the National
Information Standards Organization (Z39.48–1984).

10 9 8 7 6 5 4 3 2 1

To my parents, who gave me the opportunity to have "conscious" unlimited dreams and, by their actions, to better understand the importance of resiliency, tolerance, tenacity, introspection, self-awareness, and courage in the pursuit of these dreams.

To my wife, Shaffarian ("Toy"), who has been my coworker, confidante, "objective" critic, and principal supporter of my ideas and "audience to the world;" my daughter, Litonya Selima, and son, Stefan Lensworth, who, for all of my professional life, have always been very helpful, supportive, and tolerant of my evolutionary insights, as well as my atypical, and other, pursuits.

To the millions of African Americans and other people of color, who by virtue of the color of their skin, continue to disproportionately experience the ill-effects of a morally unjust and unequal society but who will, in the near future, have an abundance of opportunity and the increased quality and quantity of life that they truly deserve.

Contents

VOLUME II

PART IV: SOCIOPOLITICAL, ENVIRONMENTAL, AND STRUCTURAL
            CHALLENGES

Illustrations

TABLES

FIGURES

Abbreviations

AA	African Americans
AA	Alcoholics Anonymous
AAASPS	African American Antiplatelet Stroke Prevention Study
AACN	American Association of Colleges of Nursing
AACTG	Adult Aids Clinical Trials Group
AADM	African American diabetes mellitus
AAHPC	African American hereditary prostate cancer
AAP	American Academy of Pediatrics
AAP	American Academy of Periodontology
AASK	African American Study of Kidney Diseases and Hypertension
ACAS	Asymptomatic Carotid Atherosclerosis Study
ACCESS	A Case Control Etiologic Study of Sarcoidosis
ACE	Angiotensin converting enzyme
ACEHSA	Accrediting Commission on Education for Health Services Administration
ACEI	Angiotensin converting enzymes inhibitors
ACIP	Advisory Committee on Immunization Practices
ACOG	American College of Obstetricians and Gynecologists
ACS	American Cancer Society
ACT	American Council on Testing
AD	Alzheimer's disease
ADA	American Diabetes Association
ADC	Aid to Dependent Children
ADN	Associated degree in nursing
ADPKD	Autosomal dominant polycystic kidney disease
ADR	Annual Data Report

AF	Atrial fibrillation
AFCAPS/TexCAPS	Air Force/Texas Coronary Artery Prevention Study
AFDC	Aid to Families with Dependent Children
AHA	The American Heart Association
AIDS	Acquired immunodeficiency syndrome
ALL	Acute lymphoblastic leukemia
ALLHAT	Antihypertensive and Lipid-Lowering Trial to Prevent Heart Attacks
AMFRREHD	Action Model for Reducing Racial and Ethnic Health Disparities
AMI	Acute myocardial infarction
ARBs	Angiotensin receptor blockers
ARC-PA	Accreditation Review Commission on Education for Physician Assistant
ARIC	Atherosclerosis Risk in Communities Study
ASI	Addiction Severity Index
AUPHA	Association of University Programs in Health Administration
AVEG	AIDS vaccines evaluation group
AZT	Zidovudine
BB	Beta blocker
BBA	Balanced Budget Act
BF	Black female
BM	Black male
BMI	Body mass index
BRFSS	Behavioral Risk Factor Surveillance System
BSN	Science degree in nursing
CABG	Coronary artery bypass graft
CAD	Coronary artery disease
CALGB	Cancer and Leukemia Group B
CAM	Complementary and alternative medicine
CAPD	Chronic ambulatory peritoneal dialysis
CARDIA	Coronary Artery Risk Development in Young Adults
CAS	Chronic antigenic stimulation
CASI	Computer-assisted self-interviewing
CASS	Coronary artery surgery study
CBOs	Community-based organization
CBRR	Consumer Bill of Rights and Responsibilities
CCB	Calcium channel blocker
CCE	Chiropractic education
CCPD	Continuous cycling peritoneal dialysis
CD	Cadaver donor
CDC	Centers for Disease Control and Prevention
CEN	Certified emergency nurse
CEPH	Council of Education for Public Health
CHC	Community Health Center

CHD	Coronary heart disease
CHIP	Children's Health Insurance Program
CKD	Chronic kidney disease
CMS	Center for Medicare and Medicaid Services
CMV	Cytomegalovirus
CNS	Clinical nurse specialist
COHS	Cherishing Our Hearts and Souls
COPD	Chronic obstructive pulmonary disease
CORN	Council of Regional Networks for Genetic Services
CPCRA	Community Programs for Clinical Research on AIDS
CPR	Cardiopulmonary resuscitation
CPSC	Consumer Product Safety Commission
CRESPAR	Center for Research on Education of Students Placed at Risk
CRH	Corticotropin-releasing hormone
CRJ	Commission for Racial Justice
CRNA	Certified Registered Nurse Anesthetist
CSFII	Continuing Survey of Food Intake of Individuals
CT	Computed tomography
CTM	Community Transformation Model
CVA	Cerebrovascular accidents
CVD	Cardiovascular disease
CYP450	Cytochrome P450
DAPRO	Disadvantaged Area Support PRO
DAT	Dementia of Alzheimer's type
DAT	Dental Admission Test
DATRI	Division of AIDS Treatment Research Initiative
DAWN	Drug Abuse Warning Network
DC	Doctor of chiropractor
DDS	Doctor of dental survey
DFS	Disease-free survival
DHHS	Department of Health and Human Services
DIS	Diagnostic Interview Schedule
DMD	Doctor of dental medicine
DNA	Deoxyribonucleic acid
DO	Osteopathic physician
DOA	Dead on arrival
DOE	Department of Energy
DPP	Diabetes Prevention Program
DRE	Digital rectal exam
DSM III	Diagnostics and Statistical Manual of Mental Disorders (3rd Edition)
DSM-IV	Diagnostic and Statistical Manual (4th Edition)
EAF	European American females

EAM	European American males
EC	Enterprise communities
ECA	Epidemiologic Catchment Area Study
ECC	Early childhood caries
ECFMG	Educational Commission for Foreign Medical Graduates
ECG	Electrocardiogram
ED	Emergency Department
EF	Etiological fraction
E-I-I	Environment-institutions-individuals
ELSI	Ethical, legal, and social issues
EMTALA	Emergency Medical Treatment and Labor Act
EPA	Environment Protection Agency
EPO	Erythro-poietin
EPSDT	Early periodic screening detection and treatment
ER	Emergency room
ESLD	End-stage liver disease
ESRD	End-stage renal disease
EZ	Empowerment zones
FDA	Food and Drug Administration
FEV_1	Forced expiratory volume in one second
FLP	Front-Line providers
FMPV	Female-to-male partner violence
FPL	Federal poverty level
FRC	Family Resource Center
FRCS	Filter Resource Capability System
FSGS	Focal and segmental glomerulosclerosis
GAO	General Accounting Office
GBC	Group B streptococcal infection
GDM	Gestational diabetes mellitus
GIS	Geographic Information System
GME	U.S. Graduate Medical Education
GRAD	Genomic Research in African Diaspora
GSS	General social survey
H. pylori	Helicobacter pylori
HAART	Highly active antiretroviral therapy
HAD	HIV-associated dementia complex
HAV	Hepatitis A virus
HBCU	Historically Black college or university
HBM	Health belief model
HBV	Hepatitis B virus
HCC	Hepatocellula carcinoma
HCFA	Health Care Financing Administration

HCV	Hepatitis C virus
HDL	High-Density Lipoprotein
HDV	Hepatitis D virus
HEI	Healthy Eating Index
HER	Health education-risk reduction
HEV	Hepatitis E virus
HFC	Health field concept
Hgb F	Fetal hemoglobin
HGP	Human Genome Project
HIV	Human immunodeficiency virus
HIVD	Human immunodeficiency virus-dementia
HLA	Human leukocyte antigens
HPA	Hypothalamic-pituitary-adrenocortical
HPA-axis	Hypothalalamic pituitary adrenal axis
HPC	Heredity prostate cancer
HPEA	Health Profession Educational Assistance
HPTN	HIV Prevention Trials Network
HR	Hazard ratio
HRSA	Health Resources and Service Administration
HRT	Hormone replacement therapy
HTN	Hypertension
HU	Hydroxyurea
HVTN	HIV vaccine trials network
IARC	International Agency for Research on Cancer
ICD-9	Ninth Revision of the International Classification of Diseases
ICH	Intragency Counsel of the Homeless
IDDM	Insulin-dependent diabetes mellitus
IDU	Injecting drug user
IFG	Impaired fasting glucose
IgE	Immunoglobulin E
IGT	Impaired glucose tolerance
IHD	Ischemic heart disease
IMG	International medical graduates
IMR	Infant mortality rate
IOM	Institute of Medicine
IPV	Intimate partner violence
IR	Institutionalized racism
IUD	Injection drug use
JNC	Joint National Committee
K/DOQI	Kidney Disease Outcomes Quality Initiative
LBW	Low birth weight
LDL-C	Low density lipoprotein cholesterol

LE	Life expectancy
LIP	Licensed independent practitioners
LPN	Licensed practical nurse
LRD	Living related donor
LURD	Living unrelated donor
LVH	Left ventricular hypertrophy
LVN	Licensed vocational nurse
MAC	Mycobacterium avium complex
MAST	Michigan Alcoholism Screening Test
M.B.A.	Master of business administration
MCHC	Mattapan Community Health Center
MD	Allopathic physician
MDIUS	Midlife development in the United States
METs	Metabolic equivalence
MHA	Master of health administration
MHC	Major histocompatibility complex
MHSA	Master of health services administration
MI	Myocardial ischemia
MICRO-HOPE	Microalbuminuria, cardiovascular and renal outcomes—Heart Outcome Prevention Evaluation
MID	Multiple infarct dementia
MM	Multiple myloma
MMF	Mycophenalate Mofetil
MMWR	Morbidity and Mortality Weekly Report
MODOPP-C	Medicine, osteopathy, dentistry, optometry, pharmacy, podiatry, and chiropractic
MOTTEP	Minority Organ Tissue Transplantation Education Program
M.P.A.	Master of public administration
M.P.H.	Master of public health
MSM	Men who have sex with men
MST	Multisystemic therapy
NAACP	National Association for the Advancement of Colored People
NAEP	National Assessment of Educational Progress
NASCET	North American Symptomatic Carotid Endarterectomy Trial
NCCAM	National Center on Complementary and Alternative Medicine
NCEP	National Cholesterol Education Program
NCHS	National Center for Health Statistics
NCI	National Cancer Institute
NCIPC	National Center for Injury Prevention and Control
NCLEX-RN	National Council Licensure Examination for RN
NCMHD	National Center for Minority Health Disparities
NCS	National Comorbidity Study
NEISS	National Electronic Injury Surveillance System

NHAMCS   National Hospital Ambulatory Medicare Care Survey
NHANES   National Health and Nutrition Examination Survey
NHANES II   Second National Health and Nutrition Examination Survey
NHANES III   Third National Health and Nutrition Examination Survey
NHBPEP   National High Blood Pressure Education Program
NHDS   National Hospital Discharge Survey
NHGC   National Human Genome Center
NHGRI   National Human Genome Research Institute
NHIS   National Health Interview Survey
NHSC   National Health Service Corps
NHSDA   National Household Survey on Drug Abuse
NIAAA   National Institute of Alcohol Abuse and Alcohol
NIAID   National Institute of Allergy and Infectious Diseases
NICHD   National Institute of Child Health and Development
NIDA   National Institute of Drug Abuse
NIDCD   National Institute on Deafness and Other Communication Disorders
NIDCR   National Institute of Dental and Craniofacial Research
NIDDK   National Institute of Diabetes and Digestive and Kidney Diseases
NIDDM   Non-insulin-dependent diabetes mellitus
NIH   National Institutes of Health
NIHSS   National Institutes of Health Stroke Scale
NINDS   National Institute of Neurological Disorders and Stroke
NKDEP   National Kidney Disease Education Program
NMR   Neonatal mortality rate
NMW   Nurse midwife
NP   Nurse practitioner
NRC   Nuclear Regulatory Commission
NSAL   National Survey of American Life
NSBA   National Survey of Black Americans
NSDUH   National Survey of Drug Use and Health
NSHAPC   National Survey of Homeless Assistance Providers and Clients
NUL   National Urban League
OAS   Office of Applied Studies
OC   Oral contraceptives
O.D.   Optometry degree
ODM   Organ donors per million
OEO   Office of Economic Opportunity
OGTT   Oral glucose tolerance test
OMB   Office of Management and Budget
OPTN   Organ Procurement and Transplantation Network
OR   Odds ratio
ORMH   Office of Research and Minority Health

ORWH	Office of Research on Women's Health
PA	Physician assistant
PACTG	Pediatrics AIDS Clinical Trials Group
PCP	Pneumocystis carinii pneumonia
P.C.P.	Primary care providers
PDR	Proliferative diabetic retinopathy
PEHD	Program to Eliminate Health Disparity
PIR	Poverty income ratio
PNMR	Postneonatal mortality rate
PRAISE	Partnership to Reach African Americans to Increase Smart Eating
PRO	Peer review organization
PSA	Prostate specific antigen
PSR	Proliferative sickle-cell retinopathy
PSS	Progressive systemic sclerosis
PTCA	Percutaneous transluminal coronary angioplasty
PTDM	Posttransplant diabetes mellitus
RBC	Red blood cells
RCT	Randomized clinical trial
REACH	Racial and Ethnic Approaches to Community Health
RFA	Request for applications
R.N.	Registered nurse
RRT	Renal replacement therapy
RSV	Respiratory syncytial virus
RTOG	Radiation Therapy Oncology Group
SA	Sympatho-adrenomedullary
SADR	Social and Demographic Research Institute
SADS-RDC	Schedule for Affective Disorders and Schizophrenia Research Diagnostic Criteria
SAMHSA	Substance and Mental Health Services Administration
SAPAC	Self-administered Physical Activity Check
SBE	Service-based enumeration
SCD	Sickle-cell disease
SCD	Sudden cardiac death
SCOR	Specialized Centers for Research
SEER	Surveillance Epidemiology and End Results
SES	Socioeconomic status
SFU	Size of a small family unit
SI	Special intervention
SIDS	Sudden infant death syndrome
SPPM	Sociopsychophysiological model
SRC	Sociopsychophysiological Resource Center
SSI	Supplemental Security Income
STDs	Sexually transmitted diseases

TBI	Traumatic brain injury
TC	Total cholesterol
TCA	Trycyclic antidepressant
TNFa	Tissue necrosis factor alpha
TPA	Tissue plasminogen activator
TSDF	Treatment, storage, and disposal facilities
UAP	Unlicensed Assistive Personnel
UC	Usual care
UGT	Glucuronosvitransferase
UNOS	United Network for Organ Sharing
USCM	United States Conference of Mayors
USDHHS	U.S. Department of Health and Human Services
USM	U.S. medical schools
USPHS	U.S. Public Health Service
USRDS	U.S. Renal Data System
VAST	Veterans Administration Symptomatic Trial
VCV	Varicella-Zoster viral encephalitis
VFC	Vaccines for children
VISIONS	Vigorous Interventions in Ongoing Natural Settings
VLBW	Very low birth weight
VPS	Vaccine Preparedness Study
WF	White female
WHO	World Health Organization
WM	White male
YE	Yersinia enterocolitica
YLL	Years of life lost
YMC	Youth Mediation Corps
YPLL-75	Years of potential life lost before the age of 75
YRBSS	Youth Risk Behavior Surveillance System

Foreword

The publication in 2004 of these books on health and health-related issues is both timely and urgently needed to add fresh, invigorating, and comprehensive insights to ongoing national, regional and local discussions concerning the unequal distribution of "good" health and "desirable" services in America. Eliminating disparities in health care and health status between racial/ethnic groups in the United States has become perhaps the most serious challenge facing the nation. Although various ethnic groups can be singled out for special consideration, no group comes to the national attention more vividly than African Americans, who trail their White counterparts on just about all major indicators of morbidity and mortality.

Since the publication of the Secretary's Task Force Report on the health of Blacks and other minorities over 18 years ago, which officially brought the issue of ethnic disparities in health to national consciousness, a great deal of activity has occurred to underscore this national problem. For example, in the past few years the U.S. Department of Health and Human Services has introduced major initiatives in the area, (1) the Healthy People 2010 goal of eliminating health disparities among various segments of the population and (2) activities at the National Institutes of Health (NIH) and the Centers for Disease Control and Prevention (CDC) supporting research to better understand racial/ethnic disparities in health.

Although major progress has been made in reducing morbidity and mortality, as well as increasing the life expectancy among vulnerable and at-risk populations, such as African Americans, the ethnic divide continues to widen. As a matter of fact, in some cases it has even gotten worse! Because we are essentially dealing with the inherent complexities of human behavior on the micro or individual level, which are inextricably tied to ongoing factors and conditions at the macro or societal level, the reasons for the lack of more substantial improvements over the ensuing years are complex.

To suffice, however, it can be reasoned that increased vulnerability to adverse health among African Americans is differentially mediated by various environmental factors and conditions. All of these factors and conditions serve to influence individuals' personal choices concerning healthy lifestyle choices; availability, accessibility, and acceptability of services; and, ultimately, impact negatively on their physiologic functioning, hence the current health disparities dilemma. At the risk of oversimplifying a complex situation, what is desperately needed at the macro level is health-care reform to guide the nation's policies and research agenda. Such reform should also serve to underscore the fact that health care is a right and not a privilege. At the micro level, self-care actions must be fueled by greater feelings of efficacy and empowerment. Such feelings can be expressed and sustained only by the acquisition of health and lifestyle alteration information and resources, for example, through federal, state, and local educational campaigns.

Even with the eventual advent of health-care reform, African Americans and their advocates must continue looking to, and dealing with, various challenges. Some of these challenges are associated with (a) attitude and lifestyle modification and (b) prevention of disease and disability in the context of an ever-changing, dynamic, unpredictable, and, sometimes, "racially unsympathetic" social and political environments. One way to begin, or continue on this difficult journey, is to be more fully aware of the "information puzzle" associated with the variety of conditions that affect the lives and health status of African Americans.

This two-volume, *Praeger Handbook of Black American Health: Policies and Issues Behind Disparities in Health* greatly expands on the first edition by Ivor Livingston that was published in 1994. This widely expanded treatment, which has 20 new chapters (i.e., from 27 to 47), attests to the comprehensive nature of the text. The additional topical areas (e.g., oral health, physical activity, reproductive health, emergency room medicine, complementary health, geographic information systems, human genome, clinical trials) further attest to the wide range of areas that have to be addressed because of their individual and collective contribution to the debate on disparities in health in the twenty-first century.

The volumes are clearly multidisciplinary, and their 47 chapters reflect this perspective. The editor, Dr. Livingston, who is a trained medical sociologist and social epidemiologist, was successful in bringing together a team of known experts in their respective areas from a variety of institutions across the country. Where applicable, the common public health theme throughout the volumes includes the importance of (primary) prevention, the etiology of the problem being addressed, detection and diagnosis of the problem, and the need to successfully intervene. The voluminous information that resonates through all of the chapters and the sequencing of the chapters are deliberately orchestrated to give the reader the opportunity to contribute valuable information to the race/ethnicity–health disparities relationship.

The perspective of Livingston, an eclectically trained editor, is reflected in the vast, comprehensive, and unique topics covered in these books, which make them ideal reference texts. The books are unique in that they include a variety of very current topical areas (e.g., oral health, emergency room medicine, rural America, prisons, human genome, geographic information systems) not previously covered in a single work. The content of these books argues strongly that they will make significant and timely contributions in the increasingly crowded field of health disparities publications. Not to be deterred by the vast array of information, the chapters are sequentially presented under five major sections. Moving from cardiovascular and general conditions through lifestyle and sociopolitical and structural challenges, the second volume ends with an examination of ethics, research, technology, and social policy issues.

As a former surgeon general of the United States, I am uniquely aware of the multidisciplinary focus needed to understand, and ultimately successfully resolve, the complex issues that contribute to African Americans' trailing their White counterparts on just about all recognizable health status indicators. I am encouraged to see that the chapters included reflect the basic four determinants of health and illness as defined by the Office of the Surgeon General, as well as others (i.e., lifestyle, environment, genetics/biology, and access to medical care). The 10 leading health indicators in Healthy People 2010 further explicate these determinates.

The careful selection of chapters in the book reflects an appreciation by Dr. Livingston of the interaction of all the four determinants of health, as well as a greater appreciation that over 50 percent of health-care risks can be explained in terms of lifestyle factors. The data are increasingly suggesting that lifestyle conditions—for example, stress, exercise, spirituality, nutrition, mental health, pharmacological therapy, and reproductive activities—may have either a direct or indirect impact on other more physiological health outcomes, for example, heart disease, cancer, immunological functioning, HIV/AIDS, and diabetes. Again, all of these topical areas are represented by chapters in the books. Because the final action resides with individuals, whether to engage in preventive and/or protective health behaviors, they have to become empowered to realize and accept this responsibility for their health. This being the case, a chapter on "Transforming Structural Barriers to Improve the Health of African Americans" addresses this issue quite clearly in discussing how African Americans can become more empowered, in the context of available structural realities (e.g., access and availability of health care), to improve their health.

The second edition of Dr. Livingston's comprehensive *Praeger Handbook of Black American Health* deserves to be on the bookshelf. For years to come, it will serve as an invaluable resource for policymakers, health-care practitioners, teachers, researchers, and students, in both the medical and behavioral sciences, who are seriously concerned about understanding and, subsequently, reducing the numerous health disparities between African Americans and their White counterparts. As we move forward as a nation to resolve issues relating to health disparities, whether they be at the societal or individual levels, this book will be an invaluable resource that will assuredly move us in that direction.

David Satcher, M.D., Ph.D., F.A.A.A.P.,
F.A.C.P.M., F.A.C.P.
Director
National Center for Primary Health Care
Morehouse School of Medicine

Preface

The *Praeger Handbook of Black American Health: Policies and Issues Behind Disparities in Health* is a two-volume, 47-chapter collection of original scholarly presentations covering a variety of areas relating to the health of Blacks or African Americans. The terms Black and African American are used interchangeably throughout the book. Because of the varying views expressed by certain authors, the decision was made to include both terms; however, an attempt was made to have consistency within a chapter when either term was used. Regarding the use of "Black" versus "African American" in the title of the book, it is my view that the former best encompasses the growing variability of non-American Blacks (e.g., from Africa and the Caribbean) that currently live in the United States.

Initial thoughts that led to the first edition, which in turn contributed to this much-expanded edition, began over two decades ago, when I was pursuing postgraduate work in public health at the Harvard School of Public Health (HSPH). During this period, I was responsible for coordinating a conference entitled "Selected Health Care Issues in the Black American Community," sponsored, in part, by the minority students at the HSPH. Apart from this conference, the class discussions at the HSPH and later experiences I had while pursuing postdoctoral studies in the Department of Behavioral Sciences and Health Education, at the then Johns Hopkins School of Hygiene and Public Health (now called the Johns Hopkins Bloomberg School of Public Health), helped to stimulate my initial ideas for the first edition of the book. These experiences also formulated my professional research agenda relating to my two-decade-long pursuit of the social epidemiology of cardiovascular and immunological disease in Black populations in America, Africa, and the English-speaking Caribbean. These initial experiences, as well as my subsequent research over the years in the area of Black and minority health, uncategorically suggested a void in the comprehensive illumination of "salient" health problems and issues in Black America and, hence, the need for the first volume, its scope, and its timely importance.

It is a sad testimony of the times that just about the same reasons that motivated me to edit the first volume also motivated me to edit this set. Although the earlier edition addressed issues related to racial and ethnic disparities, because of the greater need and attention paid to health disparities today, it became more of a direct theme of these books and throughout their 47 chapters.

As I labored over the scope and the ultimate direction these volumes would take, I came to two inescapable conclusions. First, they must be more expansive to include issues and conditions that were not visibly important 20 years ago, so this second project was expanded from 27 to 47 chapters; second, when completed, the volume must make a significant contribution to the area of racial and ethnic disparities in health. This need for these volumes to make a contribution led in turn to the purpose of the books, which is twofold: (1) to go beyond the traditional areas covered in past publications on health of Blacks (i.e., cardiovascular and cerebrovascular diseases and cancer) and adopt a multidisciplinary focus on a variety of other conditions and issues (e.g., rural America, human genome, complementary/alternative health); (2) apart from presenting representative selections of conditions and issues that contributed to poorer morbidity and mortality rates for Blacks, to provide an illuminating forum to provoke dialogue for academicians, clinicians, researchers, and politicians alike to debate and discuss the urgency of the Black health crisis and, it is hoped, how best to intervene now and in the future to reduce racial disparities in health.

While Blacks in this country have made improvements to their health, a multitude of racial disparities still exists. A major reason is that, although legislation may have made health care relatively more available and affordable, the fundamental and unequal structure of American society, which is primarily responsible for racial disparities in health, did not change and has not changed over the years.

The Report of the Secretary's Task Force on Black and Minority Health (1985), a landmark clarion call for change, was revealing, showing, for example, that there is an excess of 60,000 Black deaths annually compared with White Americans. However, since its publication, much has changed for the worse and little has changed for the better. Not only do Black babies die earlier than White babies, but in recent years reports suggest that a continued reduction and leveling off in life expectancy for Blacks have occurred while there has been, in contrast, an extension for Whites.

Understanding health in general is a difficult undertaking, and understanding Black health in particular is perhaps even more difficult. The complexities associated with understanding Black health are compounded by several factors, for example, *intra*racial variations, socioeconomic status or poverty, racial admixture, health practices, and the compelling realities of an unequal, unjust, insensitive, and institutionally racist American society. Many changes over the last 25 years in the geopolitical, sociopolitical, and technological arenas, both in this country and overseas, while ushering in many new opportunities, have also brought new miseries or exacerbated old ones, especially for minority communities.

These volumes are not intended to provide exhaustive coverage of all major conditions and issues affecting the health of Blacks. Instead, the 47 chapters, divided into five parts, provide a mosaic of salient conditions, issues, and policies that are behind disparities in health related to Black American health, heretofore not covered under a single text. This multidisciplinary approach to health adopted in these volumes is one of their major advantages. The 44 contributing authors, drawn from institutions across America, are premier scholars in their respective fields. The scope and multidisciplinary nature of the volumes are, in part, reflected in areas from which these authors came: clinical medicine, epidemiology, health-care administration, medical sociology, nursing, nutritional sciences, political science, physiology, and public health. These varied backgrounds lent not only an illuminating presentation of epidemiologic data, where applicable, but also facilitated the discussion of designated problems from preventive and internventionist points of view. The guidelines given to authors also supported the discussions of how best to intervene to address a problem, thereby allowing authors to discuss prospects and suggest recommendations. By way of a summary, two questions need to be answered about this handbook: Who is the intended audience? What is its significance?

Because of the multidisciplinary focus of this two-volume handbook, it can be used by a variety of professionals and disciplines in the behavioral sciences, allied sciences, and clinical sciences. Whether the volumes are used as a reference text, a main text, or a supplementary text from which selected readings are taken, they provide a cross-section of readers with a wealth of current information pertaining to the disproportionate incidence of morbidity and mortality in the Black American population.

Additionally, these volumes are significant because of (a) their timely presentation of crucial issues pertaining to the health of Black Americans, especially now when the U.S. Congress and administration, policymakers, and others are debating the need and direction of health-care form; (b) their multidisciplinary and public health foci; (c) their ability to stimulate and provoke serious and difficult debates affecting policy decisions in a variety of forums involving crucial areas influencing the health of Blacks living in America; and (d) the variety of models and recommendations suggested by knowledgeable scholars, all within a framework for social action and change, during the twenty-first century. While racial parity in health will not be achieved by Blacks overnight, it is very important that any future improvements made be progressive, relevant, significant, and perhaps most important, sustainable. Therefore, as we work toward a brighter twenty-first century, which involves racial parity in health, it is further hoped that these books will help to make a brighter future out of the darkness of the past.

Acknowledgments

The writing and completion of these great volumes are undoubtedly the work and effort of a collective number of individuals. Although many of these individuals did not know each other, they were all bonded in different ways to a common purpose. This common purpose was to be a part of a group of individuals who contributed their time, effort, and expertise in making this second edition of the *Praeger Handbook of Black American Health* an unparalleled success. Writing and compiling a "first-of-its-kind," 47-chapter, two-volume set requires a level of dedication and passion on everyone's part to see the project through to its successful conclusion. The passion that everyone shared was the need to make a difference, based on respective areas of expertise, in contributing vitally important information that will make a positive contribution in the effort to eliminate racial and ethnic health disparities in America. I am forever grateful for the level of dedication and professionalism displayed by these many colleagues, who come from various universities, organizations, and institutions across the United States.

Although the list seems endless, I would particularly like to thank certain individuals who did indeed make a difference. Thanks first of all go to my family, who fully supported me throughout the year-and-a-half duration of the project. My wife's unyielding support and encouragement were particularly helpful, not only from a clinical sense regarding the verification and clarification of information but from a "partner's" sense, supporting me through those difficult "aching-back" and muscle-aching hours late at night and in the early morning. Approximately ten years ago, when I edited the first edition of the book, which had 27 chapters, my children were too young to render anything other than words of encouragement that were limited by their relatively young ages (8 and 11 years). However, this second time around, because they are older and more mature and possess appreciable amounts of expertise for their young adult years, their support was more tangible and very gratifying. My daughter Litonya's encouraging comments from college, in addition to her assistance when she came home on visits, were very helpful and supportive. My son Stefan's expertise with computers, along with his encouraging remarks during his senior year in high school and freshman year in college, were particularly helpful, especially during the last phases of the project.

Many colleagues across the United States, who are too numerous to mention, were helpful, especially during the prewriting phase of these books. During this period in the summer of 2001 I was busy contemplating the pros and cons of doing a second edition of my book. The constructive advice and support I received were very encouraging. Directions and support for particular sections, as well as for the overall book, were well received from my colleagues at different institutions, as well as in the Department of Sociology and Anthropology, where I have been on faculty for over 20 years. For the initial planning phase of the project, as well as during the writing phase and period spent allocating authors for designated chapters, I received a great deal of help from colleagues at Howard University and across the United States. Some of these individuals who are at other institutions include Drs. Christine Branche, B. Waine Kong, Aloysius Cuyjet, Richard Gillum, Eugene Tull, Marian McDonald, Keith Norris, Hector Myers, and Jane Otado. Within the department, as well as from the greater Howard University community, I received invaluable insights, feedback, and encouragement from the following colleagues: Drs. Ralph C. Gomes (my former advisor), Ron Manuel, Johnnie Daniel, Rebecca Reviere, Sue Taylor, and Jacqueline Smith. My former classmates at the Harvard School of Public Health, Drs. J. Jacques Carter and Deborah Blocker, who also contributed chapters to the volume, were helpful with different phases of the project. My colleagues associated with the Historically Black Colleges and Universities Network, Drs. Eleanor Walker and Ivis Forrester-Anderson, as well as Dr. Richard Bragg of the Centers for Medicare and Medicaid Services (CMS) were very helpful at crucial junctions of the project.

My home institution, Howard University, and the Department of Sociology and Anthropology provided me with leave time at the onset of the project that was helpful in the writing and submitting of the prospectus. The chairperson, Dr. Florence Bonner, and associate chairperson, Dr. Ralph C. Gomes, were especially supportive of my involvement with the project and gave me "full access" to all available resources of the department. Other colleagues, such as Drs. Johnnie Daniel, Ron Manuel, Charles Jarmon, Vernetta Young, and Rebecca Reviere, some of whom contributed chapters, were also very supportive during the process. I would like to thank the secretarial staff of the department, Ms. Odette Godwin-Davis and Ms. Joan King, for the help and assistance rendered, especially involving the sending and receiving of numerous faxes to contributing authors throughout the United States. This phase was extremely important for the success of the project. The checking and verification of references, as well as other activities related to the project, were ably conducted by graduate assistants Ms. Feven Negga and Mr. Sheldon Applewhite and my former student Ms. Carmen Warren.

Finally, I want to directly thank the many (more than one hundred) contributing authors who first of all consented to be a part of the project, knowing full well the obligations that follow such an agreement. These authors worked diligently to produce outlines, drafts, and final chapters. For some authors, the pressing deadlines were very difficult to accomplish given their other competing professional responsibilities. Some of these authors when they submitted chapters in the first volume ten years ago were junior members at their respective institutions. Although today many of these same authors are now senior members at their institutions, they unflaggingly consented to be part of the project, for yet another time. I am very grateful for such commitments! I was very deliberate in choosing a number of junior faculty to coauthor certain designated chapters. Like their more seasoned and older colleagues, being the true professionals that they are, they came through and delivered their respective chapters in a timely fashion. Without this kind of professional dedication and commitment, this important second edition of the *Praeger Handbook of Black American Health* would have remained just an idea without coming to fruition.

I would be very remiss if I did not express my appreciation to the publisher, Greenwood Publishing Group, Inc., first, to the staff members who were very diligent and professional in conducting their duties and especially to my assigned editor, Debora Carvalko, who responded to my many requests in an extremely timely and proficient manner. I also want to express my appreciation to Dr. James Sabin, who, as executive vice president when the first edition was published, was very helpful and accessible. He, along with various other individuals, helped to provide the opportunity for publishing the valuable information concerning "health disparities associated with Black Americans" contained in the first edition that led to this very expanded second edition of the book.

Introduction

IVOR LENSWORTH LIVINGSTON

On the international front, the twenty-first century has ushered in many of the same occurrences of the previous century, economic strife, famines, military conflicts, sociopolitical turmoil, ill health, and various diseases. In terms of health conditions, the world is more interconnected today than it was before, hence, from a public health perspective, the potential is greater for the rapid spread of infectious diseases like severe acute respiratory syndrome (SARS). What is spreading equally fast throughout the world, as well as in countries like the United States, which is the focus of these volumes, is the further dichotomizing of people into the "haves" and the "have-nots." Although the focus of the volumes disallows any full elaboration on the reasons (e.g., slavery, racism, war, poverty) for this accelerated dichotomy, given the topic of interest covered in the volumes, this division has enormous implications for the growing racial and ethnic divide in terms of health disparities seen in the United States today.

This higher burden of disease and mortality among minorities has profound implications for all Americans, as it results in a less healthy nation and higher costs for health and rehabilitative care. All members of a community are affected by the poor status of its least healthy members. (Smedley et al., 2003, p. 31)

THE IMPORTANCE OF THE SOCIOECONOMIC-HEALTH RELATIONSHIP

A relationship that has stood the test of time is the inverse relationship between socioeconomic status (SES) and ill health and disease. Low-SES individuals (i.e., those who are relatively poor) have other attending social, psychological, and physiological problems that serve to further confound and exacerbate the realities of the SES–health outcome relationship.

Whether the SES–health relationship is examined in the United States or elsewhere, the outcomes are the same: people who are poor and occupy the lower strata of the SES continuum are more at risk to get prematurely sick or infirmed, require more medical care, and, ultimately, have a disproportionately higher premature mortality rate than their counterparts who occupy middle and upper levels on the SES continuum. Sustained improvements in the SES–health relationship can be attained only through a multilevel approach involving the government, private sector communities, neighborhood/community agencies, and impacted individuals.

A Public Health War on Poverty

One possible solution to the problem of inequities in health along racial and ethnic lines is to literally wage a credible and lasting "war" on poverty. Basically, because of the extreme, long-lasting, and destructive health-related effects of poverty, it should be defined in terms of a public health problem. This being the case, the warlike effort that is suggested will include the application of all necessary resources to its eradication. Such a war would have great implications for the health of minority populations, especially Black or African Americans, given their disproportionate representation at lower levels on the SES continuum. However, for such a war to be successful, there would have to be unprecedented agreements and cooperation on various fronts, including issues dealing with politics, economics, health, race, culture, mutual respect for each other, and the belief that adequate health care is a fundamental right, not a privilege, for all Americans. Without such far-reaching agreements and commitments from leaders at the federal, state, and local levels, as well as from the private sector, any successes achieved regarding the war on poverty will not be sustained, and the racial and ethnic disparities in health will get progressively worse.

For the United States to successfully win its war on poverty, which involves a complex series of conditions, it has to address a fundamental issue that is undeniably linked, in part, to poverty. This problem is institutional racism, where minorities, especially people of color, like Black Americans, have been systematically and insidiously denied basic rights and opportunities. Therefore, the denial of these rights and opportunities, which in turn have contributed to their overall relatively dismal economic standings (i.e., compared to their White counterparts), have played a large role in the conditions that are, then, responsible for the need for these volumes to be written with the ensuing theme "Eliminating Racial and Ethnic Health Disparities."

Although a "war" of sorts is being waged in the United States, for example, at the level of the federal government with the Healthy People 2010 initiative, there still exists vast disparities in SES, ill health, and disease outcomes, especially for minority populations in general and Black Americans in particular. This being the case, the question that needs asking is as follows: *Is there a deep and genuine commitment by those in power to rectify the ills of the past, thereby allowing racial equality, among other things, to be achieved?* Only with time can an accurate answer to this question be achieved.

Essentially, Healthy People 2010 presents a comprehensive, nationwide health promotion and disease prevention agenda. It is designed to serve as a "road map" for improving the health of all people in the United States during the first and second decade of the twenty-first century. Healthy People 2010 is committed to a single, overarching purpose—*promoting health and preventing illness, disability, and premature death.*

Known Disparities in Health

The existence of significant racial and ethnic disparities in health care have been widely reported and documented in various government reports, including *Healthy People 2010* (USDHHS, 2000b) and *A Public Health Action Plan to Prevent Heart Disease and Stroke* (USDHHS, 2003). Most striking are the differences between the incidence and prevalence of many diseases affecting Black Americans when compared to the U.S. population as a whole. Although life expectancy and overall health for most Americans have improved tremendously over the past two decades, there continue to be major disparities in the burden of disease/illness and death experienced by Blacks living in America.

The three leading causes of death in the United States in 2000 were heart disease, cancer, and stroke. In each of these categories, the Black American death rate was significantly greater than the White rate (National Center for Health Statistics [NCHS], 2002). In fact, when one looks at the ten leading causes of mortality in this country, the Black American rate exceeds the White rate in every category except chronic obstructive lung disease, suicide, and Alzheimer's disease. The ten leading causes of death in the United States in 2000 for Black Americans were heart disease, cancer, stroke, unintentional injuries, diabetes, homicide, HIV/AIDS, chronic lower respiratory disease, kidney disease, and influenza and pneumonia (National Center for Health Statistics [NCHS], 2002).

The plight of Black Americans is particularly devastating and urgent because, as a group, they experience a disproportionate burden of poverty, sickness, and death. By way of summary statistics, one-third of Blacks live in poverty, a rate three times that of the White population (U.S. Bureau of the Census, 2000). Over half live in central cities, areas characterized by poverty, urban congestion, poor schools, a pervasive drug culture, unemployment, and stress. Additionally, diabetes is three times that of Whites; heart disease is more than 40 percent higher than Whites; prostate cancer is more than double that of Whites; HIV/AIDS is more than seven times that of Whites; breast cancer is higher than it is for Whites, even though Black American women are more likely to receive mammography screening than are White women; and infant mortality is twice that of Whites (National Center for Health Statistics [NCHS], 2002). However, the best cumulative statistic that underscores the racial disparities in health is life expectancy, especially for Black males (68.3), who trail White males (74.8), Black females (75.0), and White females (80.0) (Minino & Smith, 2001). Again, the question begs asking, *Why do Black Americans continue to manifest these vast disparities in morbidity and mortality rates?*

PURPOSE OF THE BOOK

These volumes are not intended to examine exhaustively all critical areas affecting the health of Black Americans. However, as a call for action, the 47 chapters represent a variety of conditions and issues, all of which need serious examination in any attempt to achieve racial parity in health. For some skeptics who look beyond the posturing of program bureaucrats and technocrats and other like-minded persons, the belief is that the needed "seeds" have not been adequately sown to reap the intended harvest, especially as it relates to sustained improvements in the health conditions of Blacks living in the United States. The *Praeger Handbook of Black American Health: Policies and Issues Behind Disparities in Health* provides authoritative, factual, and insightful information and guidelines about a variety of "seeds" and how these seeds can, and should, be sown to reap the intended harvest of eventual racial parity in health for Black Americans.

This 47-chapter book is intended to show the complexity and scope of conditions and issues that contribute to racial and ethnic disparities in health. In the book's comprehensive view, these conditions and issues include, but are not limited to, the leading causes of morbidity and mortality (e.g., cardiovascular disease, stroke, cancer). In keeping with the comprehensive view that needs to be taken in addressing the very complex problems associated with eliminating racial and ethnic health disparities, some previously infrequently addressed areas are included, such as ophthalmology (especially the problem of glaucoma), the politics of health and health care, unintentional injuries, homelessness, environmental racism, rural America, organ transplantation, and the human genome.

ORGANIZATION OF THE BOOK

As a marked departure from the first edition written a decade ago, this edition includes a variety of new (e.g., human genome, complementary/alternative health, rural health) topical areas (20 in all). Although not directly contributing to morbidity and mortality rates for African Americans, these do, in the long run, contribute vital information that could lower these rates over time. The volumes are divided into five parts. For an overview of the five major parts of the book and a selection of topics that fall under each of these parts, see Figure I.1. Chapters are grouped under each of the parts

Figure I.1
Selected interrelated conditions* that need addressing in attempting to eliminate racial and ethnic disparities

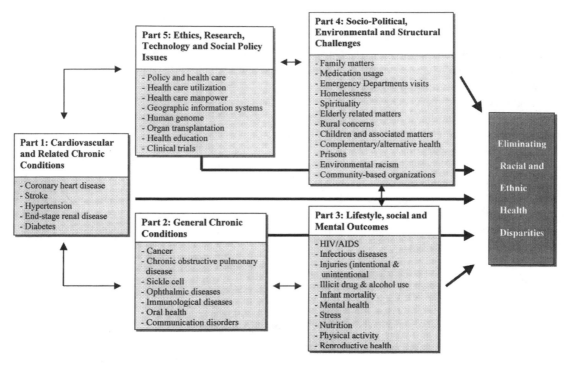

*These conditions represent selected chapters in the books: ↔ = The interrelated nature of the conditions

according to one or more commonalities. What follows is a brief overview of the chapters that fall under each of the five parts of the books. Volume I consists of Parts I, II, and III, and Volume II consists of Parts IV and V.

Part I (Volume I), "Cardiovascular and Related Chronic Conditions," comprises six chapters. This section holds priority status, because cardiovascular diseases are the number one killer of all Americans. In Chapter 1, Richard Gillum introduces the area with an overview of cardiovascular diseases. In Chapter 2, Ivor Livingston and colleagues look at coronary heart disease from a social epidemiologic perspective, emphasizing salient risk factors and the need for lifestyle change in modifying these risk factors. In Chapter 3, Gary Friday and Edgar Kenton III examine cerebrovascular disease in Blacks, which is the number three killer of all Americans. Certain types of strokes are discussed, along with treatment modalities and risk factors. In Chapter 4, Keith Norris and David Martins discuss hypertension in Blacks. They look at risk factors and discuss primary, secondary, and tertiary ways of intervening to reduce its incidence. Community education is emphasized as an important mode of prevention. In Chapter 5, Lawrence Agodoa examines the issue of end-stage renal disease, discussing its causes, distribution, and treatment in the Black population as well as in the general population. In Chapter 6, Eugene Tull and Earle Chambers look at diabetes mellitus in the African American community, considering the different types of diabetes, the etiology of diabetes, and its risk factors and treatment modalities.

Part II (Volume I), "General Chronic Conditions," contains seven chapters. These chapters, with the possible exception of one (cancer), while not contributing as directly to overall mortality as the chapters in Part I, have an enormous impact on the long-term racial and ethnic disparities in health. In Chapter 7, Ki Moon Bang, looks at cancer among Blacks, examining its epidemiology and risk factors. In Chapter 8, Ki Moon Bang looks at chronic obstructive (COPD) disease and asthma in Blacks, examining their etiologies, risk factors, and treatment modalities. In Chapter 9, Joseph Telfair looks at sickle-cell anemia and uses a biopsychosocial model to suggest better ways to understand the disease and to intervene when it becomes necessary. In Chapter 10, Shaffdeen Amuwo and colleagues look at ophthalmology in Blacks, with an emphasis on selected entities. Some of these entities, which present differently and are sometimes disproportionately seen in Blacks, include cataract, glaucoma, and diabetic retinopathy. The distribution of these entities is discussed, as are their risk factors and treatment. In Chapter 11, Marguerite Neita and Lateef Olopoenia discuss the epidemiology of immunologic disorders in Blacks (e.g., sarcoidosis), immune sensitivity reactions, and risk factors contributing to the outcomes. In Chapter 12, Yolanda Slaughter and Joan Gluch discuss racial disparities in oral health and disease, at-risk behaviors for these diseases, and public health strategies to reduce these disparities. In Chapter 13, Carolyn Stroman and Joan Payne present a discussion on communications disorders in Blacks and issues in speech, language, and hearing for African Americans.

In Part III (Volume I), "Lifestyle, Social, and Mental Outcomes," there are 13 chapters. In Chapter 14, Donald Ware and Ivor Livingston present information as to why the Black male is oftentimes referred to as the "endangered species." Racial disparities in the morbidity and mortality of selected diseases are discussed, and prevention strategies are presented. In Chapter 15, John McNeil and Kim Williams present an array of information on the social epidemiology and clinical aspects of HIV/ AIDS and sexually transmitted diseases (STDs) afflicting African Americans. Prevention strategies are presented, as well as future trends in the area. In Chapter 16, Marian McDonald and colleagues present an expanded discussion and epidemiology on racial differences in selected infectious health outcomes (e.g., viral hepatitis, influenza), as well as various prevention strategies to adopt. In Chapter 17, LeRoy Reese and colleagues present the epidemiology of racial differences in various forms of intentional violence (e.g., homicide), where they normally occur, possible reasons for their occurrence, and suggested prevention strategies. In Chapter 18, Christine Branche and colleagues discuss evidence as to racial disparities in various forms of unintentional injuries (e.g., drowning, falls, motor vehicle injuries). Risk factors are discussed along with prevention strategies.

In Chapter 19, Howard Chilcoat and James Anthony present epidemiologic evidence of racial disparities in the use of illicit drugs and drug-related activities, comorbidities, and outcomes (e.g., arrests, HIV/AIDS). In Chapter 20, Frederick Harper and colleagues look at the racial differences in alcohol use and abuse, what groups are more at risk, patterns of use/abuse and diagnoses, and therapeutic intervention modalities. In Chapter 21, Jane Otado and colleagues look at risk factors for infant mortality and strategies for improvement. In Chapter 22, Colwick Wilson and David Williams present a brief history of mental health in America and provide information on the multiple indicators of mental health for Black Americans. In Chapter 23, Ivor Livingston and colleagues look at the relationship between social status and stress and examine the implications for Black Americans using a conceptual model. In Chapter 24, Deborah Blocker and Ivis Forrester-Anderson look at nutrition concerns of African Americans, how their dietary habits predispose them to unnecessary sickness and disease, and ways to intervene. In Chapter 25, Carlos Crespo and Ross Andersen use national data sets to show how African Americans are disproportionately inactive and how this fact relates to higher racial and ethnic morbidity and mortality rates concerning their health. In Chapter 26, Diane Rowley and Yvonne Fry look on the epidemiology of selected reproductive health problems for African American women, the risk factors involved, and ways of reducing these risk factors.

In Part IV (Volume II), "Sociopolitical, Environmental, and Structural Challenges," there are 12 chapters. The topics covered by these chapters deal with events and conditions in the social and physical environment, as well as macro-level challenges that urgently need addressing. In Chapter

27, Hector Myers and colleagues address the very important and support role the Black family plays in the health of the African American community. In Chapter 28, Akima Howard and colleagues address the complexities associated with disparities in medication use, action, and prescribing for African Americans and the implications for disparities in health. In Chapter 29, Reynold Trowers looks at the dynamics associated with the use of the Emergency Department (ED), the procedures that need following, and the implications for African Americans' health. In Chapter 30, Richard English and colleagues compare empirical data in assessing the plight of the African American homeless and the implications for their health. In Chapter 31, Martha Crowther and colleagues examine the role spirituality and religion play in the lives of African Americans and the implications for their health. In Chapter 32, Ron Manuel and Jacqueline Smith, using empirical data, address health disparity issues between Blacks and Whites and within Blacks themselves. In Chapter 33, Mark Eberhardt examines the sometimes forgotten subject of rural health and African Americans and the ensuing implications.

In Chapter 34, A. Wade Boykin and Robert Jagers use a program they are affiliated with to show the important relationship between African Americans' readiness to attend school, their academic achievements, and the relationship to their overall health, more so when they become adults. In Chapter 35, Eric Bailey and Jacqueline Watson examine current practices and trends regarding complementary and alternative health in the Black community. In Chapter 36, Vernetta Young and colleagues not only speak about the disproportionate numbers of African Americans in prisons, but also address the experience behind bars and its relationship to ill health and disease. In Chapter 37, Sheila Foster addresses the issue of environmental racism by reporting instances of its occurrence over the years, as well as its implications for poor health in minority communities. In Chapter 38, Brian Gibbs and Deborah Prothrow-Stith show the importance of a working relationship between universities and people in the community to study and contain a variety of health-related problems.

In Part V (Volume II), "Ethics, Research, Technology, and Social Policy Issues," there are nine chapters that deal with issues surrounding ethics, research, technology, and social policy. In Chapter 39, Samuel Brown provides information on the evolution of American society, landmark social and political achievements, and ways of closing the gap, thereby reducing racial and ethnic disparities. In Chapter 40, Llewellyn Cornelius addresses the conditions that impact utilization and the implications for African Americans' health. In Chapter 41, Sterling King Jr. and Richard Enochs show how staffing, hiring, and having adequate numbers of personnel in medical and related programs contribute to health disparities. In Chapter 42, Joseph Oppong and Sara Garcia use geographic information system's technology to identify and assess selected areas of disease disparities in the United States with an emphasis on Texas. In Chapter 43, Georgia Dunston and Charmaine Royal explore how knowledge of the human genome can have beneficial consequences for diseases associated with African Americans. They also explore the ethical, legal, and social ramifications of genomic research. The National Health Genome Center (NHGC) at Howard University is used as the focal point of the discussions. In Chapter 44, Clive Callender and his colleagues discuss issues related to African Americans' need to have organ transplantation. They also discuss the problems associated with the transplantation process and ways of intervening to reduce risk factors associated with both the need for surgery as well as the transplantation process itself. In Chapter 45, Collins Airhihenbuwa and colleagues speak about the structural and other barriers that contribute to health disparities and identify strategies to successfully intervene. In Chapter 46, Oscar Streeter Jr., along with his colleagues, discusses the complex issues surrounding clinical trials focusing on four selected conditions that have a high incidence in the African American community: heart disease, cancer, end-stage renal disease (ESRD), and HIV/AIDS. In Chapter 47, Ivor Livingston and J. Jacques Carter provide wrap-up information pertaining to the previous chapters and provide some insights, along with a conceptual framework/model, as to where we go in the future in addressing the complex issues surrounding the elimination of racial and ethnic health disparities.

A Call for Action

This volume identifies a wide variety of conditions, issues, and policies that both directly and indirectly influence the health of African Americans or all Blacks living in the United States. It also offers prospects for the future. Consistent with the theme of the book, most of the chapters not only discuss the respective conditions, issues, and policies that are detrimental to the health of African Americans, but also offer information, guidelines, and/or recommendations to remedy the problem. In many of the chapters (e.g., Chapters 2, 9, 14, 17, 23, 27, 40, 47) original models are introduced as frameworks for action. The deaths of more than sixty thousand African Americans a year is an excessive, unjust, and immoral price to pay, especially when, as the richest nation on the earth, the "tools" exist to prevent this problem from occurring. Therefore, it is hoped that the vast array of information presented in this second edition will serve to further inform and reawaken the need to use these "tools" to achieve parity in health for all people of color in the United States, especially Black Americans.

REFERENCES

Minino, A.M., & Smith, B.L. (2001). Deaths: Preliminary data for 2000. National Center for Health Statistics, *National Vital Statistics Reports*, 49(12).

National Center for Health Statistics (NCHS). (2002). *Health, United States with Chartbook on Trends in the Health of Americans*. Hyattsville, MD: Department of Health and Human Services.

Smedley, B.D., Stith, A.Y., & Nelson, A.R. (Eds.). (2002). *Unequal Treatment: Confronting Racial and Ethnic Disparities in Health Care*. Washington, DC: National Academy Press.

U.S. Bureau of the Census. (2000). Available at http://www.census.gov (Accessed March 15, 2003).

U.S. Department of Health and Human Services (USDHHS). (2000a). *Healthy People 2010: With Understanding and Improving Health and Objectives for Improving Health* 2nd ed. 2 vols. Washington, DC: U.S. Government Printing Office, November.

U.S. Department of Health and Human Services (USDHHS). (2000b). *Understanding and Improving Health* (2nd ed.). Washington, DC: U.S. Government Printing Office.

U.S. Department of Health and Human Services (USDHHS). (2003). *A Public Health Action Plan to Prevent Heart Disease and Stroke*. Atlanta, GA: U.S. Department of Health and Human Services, Centers for Disease Control and Prevention.

PART I

Cardiovascular and Related Chronic Conditions

CHAPTER 1

Trends in Cardiovascular Diseases: An Overview of Evolving Disparities

RICHARD F. GILLUM

INTRODUCTION

Rates of death from major cardiovascular diseases declined throughout the second half of the twentieth century but still were the cause of 950,314 deaths, including 104,693 African Americans (AA), in the United States in 1999 (Hoyert et al., 2001; Gillum, 1994). Worldwide the toll in 1990 was 3,028,000 men and 2,201,000 women, including 183,000 men and 211,000 women in sub-Saharan Africa (Yusuf et al., 2001a). As in 1950, diseases of the heart remained the leading cause of death and cerebrovascular diseases, the third leading cause of death in the United States (Hoyert et al., 2001; National Center for Health Statistics, 2001). Of the 2,391,399 total deaths, diseases of the heart [International Classification of Diseases,10th Revision (ICD-10) I00-I09, I11, I13, I20-I51] accounted for 725,192 (30.3 percent) and cerebrovascular diseases for 167,366 (7.0 percent).

As more developing countries pass through the epidemiologic transition, atherothrombotic cardiovascular disease, a man-made disease of relative affluence and European culture, has become the leading cause of death globally (Yusuf et al., 2001a; Yusuf et al., 2001b). The patterns and trends of mortality and morbidity from these and other cardiovascular diseases generally display strong associations with socioeconomic status, ethnicity, culture, ancestral geographic origin, age, and gender.

Using data from the National Center for Health Statistics (NCHS), this chapter highlights selected aspects of these trends and patterns, focusing particular attention on evolving disparities adversely affecting Americans with one or more ancestors from sub-Saharan Africa (i.e. African Americans, Afro-Americans, Black Americans, Blacks, Negroes, etc.). An overview is presented on disease entities, including coronary heart disease, cerebrovascular disease, and hypertensive disease, which are treated at length in Chapters 2, 3, and 4, respectively.

Important Trends

Trends in health disparities among ethnic groups are an important topic of study, despite the fact that many authors have criticized that historical practice of classifying human beings into a few so-called races, which are assumed to carry meaningful information about traits of population groups as widely varied as health status and intelligence and to imply genetic determination of apparent variation among categories (Zuberi, 2001; Graves, 2001). Indeed, the very concept of "race" in the biological sense of "subspecies" has largely been invalidated by current research in population genetics and evolutionary biology (Jackson, 1993; Cavalli-Sforza et al., 1994; Bowman & Murray, 1990; Wade, 2001; Evans, 1999). However, the reality of "race" as a social and political concept in Eurocentric societies is unquestioned. The standards of the U.S. Office of Management and Budget for use by federal agencies are clear on this (Durch & Madans, 2001).

Because American social and political consensus has evolved to embrace the premise that major health disparities among the historical categories of this social and political variable are no longer acceptable, the importance becomes clear of quantifying the magnitude of disparities and trends in disparities over time. Further, the organizational, social, economic, and cultural bases for these disparities must be understood to develop effective interventions to reduce their magnitude. It is hoped that this chapter aids in this effort.

DISEASES OF THE HEART

Between 1950 and 1998, the last year when ICD-9 was used, age-adjusted death rates of diseases of the heart (ICD-9 390-398, 402, 404-429) declined from 586.7 to 340.6 deaths per 100,000 in African Americans and from 584.8 to 268.1 in European Americans (see Table 1.1) (Hoyert et al., 2001). Compared to 1950, rates in 1998 were 42.0 percent lower in African Americans and 54.2 percent lower in European Americans. In 1950 age-adjusted death rates for diseases of the heart were 0.3 percent higher in African than European American men, compared to 21.3 percent higher in 1999 (Hoyert et al., 2001). Thus, despite declines in both groups, a marked disparity in death rates developed since 1950 due to the more rapid decline in Europeans than African Americans between 1960 and 1998. Data from the 1999 National Hospital Discharge Survey (NHDS) indicate an estimated 4.465 million discharges with a first-listed diagnosis of heart disease (ICD-9 Clinical Modification 391-392.0, 393-398, 402, 404, 410-416, 420-429) (see Table 1.2) (Popovic & Hall, 2001).

Coronary Heart Disease

Because Chapter 2 is devoted to coronary heart disease, this overview need only indicate that over half the U.S. deaths due to diseases of the heart in 1999 were attributed to coronary heart disease (CHD), termed ischemic heart disease by the ICD for purposes of mortality analyses (ICD-10 I20-I25). In sub-Saharan Africa, an estimated 117,000 women and 92,000 men died of CHD in 1990, projected to increase to 263,000 and 92,000 men by 2020. In the United States, CHD is also a leading cause of morbidity and health expenditures. In addition to the excellent review to be found in Chapter 2 of the present volume, numerous reports and reviews are available in the literature (Gillum, 1982, 1987c, 1987d, 1989a; Sempos et al., 1988; Roig et al., 1987; Ford et al., 1989; Ries, 1990; Collins, 1988; LaCroix et al., Leaverton et al., 1990; Gillum et al., 1991; Gillum & Makuc, 1992; Otten et al., 1990; Gillum & Grant, 1982; Ford & Jones, 1991.

Sudden Cardiac Death

The importance of prevention of heart disease is made clear by the fact that about 450,000 persons annually suffer sudden cardiac death (SCD). Although detailed study of cardiac arrest and SCD requires special methodology, routinely collected vital statistics can provide valuable indicators of the epidemiology of this problem. A useful indicator of SCD is defined as heart disease deaths

Table 1.1
Age-adjusted death rates per 100,000 for diseases of the heart according to gender and ethnicity: United States, selected years 1950–1999

Year	EAM	AAM	EAF	AAF	MR	FR
1950	700	639	478	537	0.91	1.12
1960	695	615	442	489	0.88	1.11
1970	640	607	378	436	0.95	1.15
1980	540	561	316	379	1.04	1.19
1990	409	485	251	328	1.19	1.31
1995	368	449	234	309	1.22	1.32
1998	333	408	218	292	1.23	1.34
1998*	329	402	215	288	1.22	1.34
1999	325	399	216	291	1.23	1.35

Data are based on the National Vital Statistics System with adjustment using Year 2000 U.S. Population Standard.

*ICD-10/ICD-9 Comparability modified for comparison with 1999
EAM, European American males
AAM, African American males
EAF, European American females
AAF, African American females
MR, male rate ratio
FR, female rate ratio

occurring out of hospital or in emergency room (ER) (includes "dead on arrival," DOA). Since its development in the 1980s by the author (Gillum, 1989b), the CDC has adopted this technique for routine reporting and research. For heart disease as defined above plus congenital malformations of the heart (ICD-10 Q20-Q24) in 1999, 462,340 (63.4 percent) of total cardiac deaths were SCD, including 16.5 percent ER or DOA and 46.9 percent out of hospital (Zheng et al., 2001). The percent was similar in men and women, though women had a higher percent out of hospital and men a

Table 1.2
Number and rate of discharges from short-stay hospitals for first-listed diagnosis of heart disease by year, sex, age, and race: NHDS, United States

				Discharges in thousands					
Year	Total	Male	Female	Under 15	15-44	45-64	Over 65	White	Black
1998	4,335	2,242	2,093	17	241	1,248	2,829	2,975	395
1999	4,465	2,302	2,163	15	263	1,299	2,889	3,055	411
2000	4,385	2,243	2,142	16	244	1,271	2,854	2,784	388
				Discharge rate per 10,000 population					
1998	158.7	168.1	149.8	2.9	19.8	218.6	829.5	132.6	110.8
1999	162.0	170.9	153.5	2.4	21.5	220.1	843.7	135.2	133.9
2000	157.7	165.0	150.7	2.6	20.0	208.6	827.8	122.3	106.3

Source: National Center for Health Statistics, *National Hospital Discharge Survey* (NHDS) 2000.

Note: Heart Disease is a category of the following CD-9-CM codes: 391–392.0, 393–398, 402, 404, 410–416, 420–429, 391–392.0, 393–398, 402, 404, 410–416, 420–429

higher percent of ER/DOA. The percent was highest at age 35–44 and declined with age. The percents were 63.7 in Whites and 62.3 in African Americans (AA). AA had a higher percent ER/DOA and a lower percent out of hospital. AA had the highest age-adjusted SCD rates.

Tables 1.3–1.5 show detailed statistics for the subgroup of heart disease deaths attributed to coronary heart disease (ICD-9 410-414, 429.2). Table 1.3 shows the percentage dying of coronary heart disease by place of death, race, age, and sex. Unlike previously reported data for 40 states in 1980–1985 (Gillum, 1989b), the percentage of AA dying of coronary heart disease out of hospital or in emergency rooms was not consistently greater than that among Whites. The percentage dying in emergency rooms was slightly lower in AA than White men at each age below 65–74 and slightly higher in AA than White women above age 55–64. The percentage dying out of hospital or in emergency rooms decreased with increasing age except for a slight increase in the oldest group. This may represent increased numbers of deaths in institutionalized persons aged 85 and over.

Sixty-seven percent of deaths out of hospital or in emergency rooms occurred under age 75 in AA men compared to 52 percent in White men. A greater percentage of men than women died out of hospital or in emergency rooms at each age except 85 and over (Table 1.3). The difference between AA men and women was due to a much higher percentage of men coded as dying out of hospital (e.g. in AA aged 55–64, 44.4 percent of deaths in men and 35.6 percent in women were coded out of hospital). Tables 1.4 and 1.5 show the absolute and percentage declines in death rates by age, sex, and race. Coronary heart disease death rates declined relatively more rapidly in AA out of hospital or in emergency rooms but more rapidly in Whites in hospital, with declines in sudden death accounting for more of the total decline in AA.

A recent report examined pathological findings and risk factors for SCD in an autopsy series of U.S. AA (Burke et al., 2002). Estimated rates of SCD were higher in AA than in Whites at each age in men and women. The rate of SCD with stable plaque was higher in AA while the rate with with acute thrombus was similar to Whites. Among SCD cases, the heart weight, plaque burden, and prevalence of healed infarcts were similar in AA and Whites. Patterns of association between conventional risk factors and SCD were similar by race. Stable plaque was associated with hypertension and diabetes, acute thrombus with smoking, and plaque rupture with low HDL-C and high total cholesterol (TC). Compared to non-SCD deaths, SCD with stable plaque was most strongly associated with left ventricular hypertrophy in AA and diabetes in Whites. TC and diabetes were

Table 1.3
Death from coronary heart disease by place of death, race, sex, and age:
United States, 1992

Age	Out of hospital Deaths*	Percent+	In ER Deaths	Percent	Out or in ER Deaths	Percent	In hospital Deaths	Percent
Black men								
25-34	80	41.2	76	39.2	156	80.4	38	19.6
35-44	432	44.4	360	37.0	792	81.4	181	18.6
45-54	1071	43.4	841	34.1	1912	77.5	554	22.5
55-64	2096	44.4	1269	26.9	3365	71.3	1354	28.7
65-74	3058	43.4	1539	21.8	4597	65.2	2456	34.8
75-84	2590	43.1	951	15.8	3541	58.9	2469	41.1
85+	1546	49.8	360	11.6	1906	61.4	1200	38.6
Black women								
25-34	22	27.8	29	36.7	51	64.6	28	35.4
35-44	182	38.5	158	33.4	340	71.9	133	28.1
45-54	473	37.3	349	27.5	822	64.8	446	35.2
55-64	1105	35.6	758	24.4	1863	60.0	1240	40.0
65-74	2248	38.3	1093	18.6	3341	56.9	2533	43.1
75-84	3238	42.7	1100	14.5	4338	57.2	3252	42.8
85+	3414	49.8	779	11.4	4193	61.1	2667	38.9
White men								
25-34	293	41.2	307	43.1	600	84.3	112	15.7
35-44	1945	39.4	2101	42.6	4046	82.0	889	18.0
45-54	5627	38.0	5736	38.7	11363	76.7	3454	23.3
55-64	12666	37.6	10250	30.4	22916	68.1	10749	31.9
65-74	23787	35.1	15458	22.8	39245	57.9	28584	42.1
75-84	31690	39.7	12252	15.3	43942	55.0	35943	45.0
85+	24578	53.1	4023	8.7	28601	61.7	17719	38.3
White women								
25-34	82	36.3	85	37.6	167	73.9	59	26.1
35-44	390	36.5	356	33.3	746	69.8	323	30.2
45-54	1265	34.9	1012	27.9	2277	62.8	1349	37.2
55-64	4280	34.6	2667	21.6	6947	56.2	5414	43.8
65-74	14040	36.8	5990	15.7	20030	52.5	18152	47.5
75-84	35307	45.0	8437	10.7	43744	55.7	34791	44.3
85+	63839	62.4	6002	5.9	69841	68.3	32475	31.7

ER, emergency rooms
*49 states and DC.
+Percent of total coronary heart disease deaths in age group
(ICD 410–414, 429.2)

also related to SCD with stable plaque in AA. Plaque rupture was most strongly associated with elevated TC in both groups. Thus, excess SCD in AA is largely due to deaths with stable plaque associated with left ventricular hypertrophy and hypertension.

Rates of survival to hospital discharge following cardiac arrest are very low (<5%) in inner cities

Table 1.4
Coronary heart disease* deaths per 100,000 occurring out of hospital or in emergency rooms by age: United States, 1989 and 1992

Race, sex

Age	1989 Deaths	Rate	1992 Deaths	Rate	Absolute change	Percent change
Black men						
25-34	167	7	156	6	-0.5	-7.6
35-44	750	40	792	36	-3.7	-9.1
45-54	1976	172	1912	152	-20.2	-11.7
55-64	3722	425	3365	381	-44.8	-10.5
65-74	4593	760	4597	720	-39.8	-5.2
75-84	3654	1341	3541	1247	-93.6	-7.0
85+	1822	2792	1906	2764	-28.3	-1.0
Black women						
25-34	54	2	51	2	-0.1	-6.0
35-44	283	13	340	14	0.6	4.7
45-54	803	58	822	54	-3.8	-6.6
55-64	2005	178	1863	163	-15.6	-8.7
65-74	3486	401	3341	367	-33.4	-8.3
75-84	4557	946	4338	854	-92.5	-9.8
85+	3855	2546	4193	2530	-16.8	-0.7
White men						
25-34	609	3	600	3	0.0	1.2
35-44	3826	25	4046	24	-0.7	-2.7
45-54	10740	104	11363	99	-5.1	-4.9
55-64	24663	282	22916	266	-15.7	-5.6
65-74	40583	583	39245	545	-37.4	-6.4
75-84	43750	1331	43942	1223	-107.4	-8.1
85+	26959	3649	28601	3536	-113.0	-3.1
White women						
25-34	132	1	167	1	0.2	30.2
35-44	611	4	746	5	0.5	13.0
45-54	2154	20	2277	19	-0.9	-4.6
55-64	7831	81	6947	74	-6.9	-8.6
65-74	20655	233	20030	221	-12.2	-5.2
75-84	44977	814	43744	747	-67.2	-8.3
85+	66792	3457	69841	3294	-162.6	-4.7

*ICD9 410–414, 429.2

and rural areas where most AA live. Further, recent studies have documented that AA are less likely than Whites to receive an intracardiac defibrillator if they survive to hospital admission (Alexander et al., 2002). Therefore, increased efforts to prevent cardiac arrest and SCD are urgently needed (Gillum, 2000). Research and programs for prevention of new or recurrent acute cardiac ischemic

Table 1.5

Coronary heart disease* deaths per 100,000 occurring in hospital by race, sex, and age: United States, 1989 and 1992

Race, sex Age	1989 Deaths	Rate	1992 Deaths	Rate	Absolute change	Percent change
Black men						
25-34	33	1	38	1	0.2	13.8
35-44	204	11	181	8	-2.6	-23.6
45-54	627	55	554	44	-10.6	-19.4
55-64	1549	177	1354	153	-23.9	-13.5
65-74	2603	431	2456	385	-45.9	-10.7
75-84	2520	925	2469	870	-55.1	-6.0
85+	1156	1772	1200	1740	-31.4	-1.8
Black women						
25-34	43	1	28	1	-0.5	-35.2
35-44	114	5	133	5	0.1	1.7
45-54	394	28	446	29	0.9	3.2
55-64	1361	121	1240	108	-12.7	-10.5
65-74	2747	316	2533	279	-37.3	-11.8
75-84	3403	706	3252	640	-66.6	-9.4
85+	2501	1652	2667	1609	-43.0	-2.6
White men						
25-34	136	1	112	1	-0.1	-15.4
35-44	1014	7	889	5	-1.3	-19.3
45-54	3933	38	3454	30	-8.0	-21.1
55-64	13647	156	10749	125	31.1	-20.0
65-74	32105	461	28584	397	-63.8	-13.8
75-84	38061	1158	35943	1001	-157.1	-13.6
85+	18237	2468	17719	2190	-277.8	-11.3
White women						
25-34	67	0	59	0	0.0	-9.3
35-44	318	2	323	2	-0.1	-6.0
45-54	1446	14	1349	11	-2.2	-15.8
55-64	6280	65	5414	58	-7.2	-11.1
65-74	20447	231	18152	200	-30.6	-13.2
75-84	38869	704	34791	594	-109.6	-15.6
85+	34110	1765	32475	1532	-233.6	-13.2

*ICD 410–414, 429.2

events and rapid access to emergency care through the 911 system are most important (e.g., the REACT Study and the PULSE Initiative) (Becker et al., 2002; Hedges et al., 2000).

Congestive Heart Failure

In the United States, death rates for congestive heart failure (CHF, ICD-9 428) have been higher in older than younger, males than females, and AA than White persons (Haldeman et al., 1999; Gillum, 1987a, 1993; Ni et al., 1999; Philbin et al., 2000; McCullough et al., 2002). Again in 1999, a similar pattern was seen for death and hospital discharge rates. From 1976–1980 to 1988–1991, estimated prevalence of CHF increased to nearly 4.8 million, with 1.4 million under age 60 (NIH 96). Prevalence rose with age from 2 percent at 40–59 to 10 percent at 70 and over. Prevalence was at least 25 percent greater in AA than in Whites. Rate of hospitalization tripled between 1970 and 1994, but the percentage of discharged dead decreased from 11.3 percent in 1981 to 6.3 percent in 1993. The death rate increased from 1968 to 1993 despite declines in CHD death. This may reflect an increased population at risk due to increased survival following acute myocardial infraction (AMI) and increasing prevalence of risk factors such as diabetes. In 1999, data from the National Health Interview Study (NHIS) on 30,801 respondents (response rate 70 percent) yielded an estimate of four million adults aged 18 and over in the United States noninstitutionalized population who reported having been told by a doctor or health professional that they had CHF, for a crude prevalence of 1.2 percent.

Atrial Fibrillation

Heart disease, especially atrial fibrillation (AF), is an established risk factor for ischemic stroke in populations (Gillum, 2002a). The epidemiology of atrial fibrillation has been reviewed elsewhere (Gillum, 2002b). Prevalence of AF increases with age. Among 244 AA aged 65 and over in the Cardiovascular Health Study, 1.5 percent of men and 3.6 percent of women had ever been told by a doctor they had AF. Among 4,926 Whites, rates were 6.0 percent in men and 4.8 percent in women. AF by electrocardiogram (ECG) was reported in 1.1 percent of AA men and 0.7 percent of AA women compared to 4.0 percent and 2.7 percent, respectively, in Whites (nonsignificant racial difference).

Prevalence of abnormal left atrial size ranged from 13.9 percent of AA women to 21.4 percent of White men. In one large U.S. study, Whites were more likely than AA to have AF at ages over 50 years (prevalence in Whites 2.2 percent, in AA 1.5 percent, $p < 0.001$). Among patients with AMI in a clinical trial, the frequency of atrial fibrillation prior to randomization was 1.8 percent in AA and 6.7 percent in Whites. Thus, AF prevalence is higher in Whites than AA, and higher in older than younger persons.

In the United States in 1998, there were 2,101,000 hospital discharges with any diagnosis of atrial fibrillation (Gillum, 2002a). One report of AF incidence is from the Cardiovascular Health Study. In persons 65 and over, incidence was higher with advancing age, in males, among Whites, those with history of cardiac disease, those using diuretics, those not using beta blockers, and those with higher systolic blood pressure, fasting glucose, ECG cardiac injury score, and left atrial size. Thus, in the United States, the number of elderly persons with AF is large and increasing, perhaps contributing to the slowdown in the decline of stroke mortality and morbidity (Gillum, 2002a).

Other Heart Diseases

Nearly half the deaths from diseases of the heart were attributed to causes other than coronary heart disease among AA. Data from NCHS have been used to examine epidemiologic patterns of several other heart diseases. In 1982, age-adjusted death rates for acute rheumatic fever and rheumatic heart disease combined (ICD-9 390-398) were higher in women than in men and slightly lower in AA than Whites (Gillum, 1986a). Cardiomyopathy (ICD-9 425) death rates were higher in older than younger, males than females, and non-White or AA than White persons (Gillum, 1989a). AA had age-adjusted hospital discharge rates 2.2 times higher than Whites aged 35–74. Pulmonary embolism (ICD-9 415) death and hospital discharge rates were also higher in AA than Whites (Gillum, 1987b). Due to relatively small numbers of deaths and discharges, trends in numbers and rates of these conditions are rarely reported. Analyses of Medicare data for the U.S. population over 65 may be able to provide useful trend data for some of these conditions.

STROKE

Since Chapter 3 is devoted to cerebrovascular disease, this overview need only indicate that in 1999, cerebrovascular diseases (ICD-10 I60-I69) was the third leading cause of death in Black females (BF) and White females (WF) and the fourth leading cause in Black males (BM) and White males (WM). Cerebrovascular diseases accounted for the following age-adjusted rates (numbers of deaths): European American males (EAM) 60.0 (54,867), European American females (EAF) 58.7 (89,960), African American males (AAM) 87.4 (7,894), African American females (AAF) 78.1 (10,990) (Hoyert et al., 2001). In 1999, 48 percent occurred pretransport, 0.7 percent DOA, 3.3 percent in emergency department, 48.0 percent in hospital (CDC, 2002b). In sub-Saharan Africa, an estimated 231,000 women and 152,000 men died from stroke in 1990, projected to increase to 521,000 and 356,000, respectively, in 2020 (Yusuf et al., 2001a).

In the United States, stroke is also a leading cause of morbidity, disability, and costly health expenditures. Between 1980 and 1999, the hospital discharge and in-hospital mortality rates decreased both for AA and Whites, but hospital discharge rates were 70 percent higher for AA (Kennedy et al., 2002). In addition to the excellent review to be found in Chapter 3 of the present volume, numerous reports and reviews are available in the literature (Yusuf et al., 2001a; Rocella & Lenfant, 1989; Klag et al., 1989; Gillum, 1986c, 1988; Cooper et. al., 1990; Iso et al., 1989; White et al., 1990; Kittner et al., 1990; Ayala et al., 2001, 2002; CDC, 2002a, 2002b; Worral et al., 2002; Willich et al., 1999).

HYPERTENSIVE AND PERIPHERAL ARTERIAL DISEASE

Hypertension acting in concert with other risk factors determines many patterns of cardiovascular mortality and morbidity. In addition to considering its contribution to mortality and morbidity from cerebrovascular diseases and diseases of heart, it is useful to examine deaths and illness attributed to hypertensive disease (ICD-10 I10, I12) and hypertensive heart disease (ICD-10 I11, I13). Surveys of the NCHS also provide extensive data on the prevalence of hypertension and elevated blood pressure as well as hypertension awareness, treatment, and control in the United States.

Since Chapter 4 is devoted to hypertension, this overview need only indicate that in 1999 there were 16,968 deaths with the underlying cause coded as hypertensive disease and that data on underlying cause of death underestimate the impact of hypertension. This is illustrated by the following: essential hypertension not specified as malignant or benign (ICD-9 401.9) was listed as the underlying cause of death 3,581 times but as a secondary cause 74,026 times. In addition to the excellent review to be found in Chapter 4 of the present volume, numerous reports and reviews are available in the literature (Tu, 1987; Ries, 1990; Collins, 1988; Dannenberg et al., 1987; Ayala, 2002b, Ford, 1991; Rautaharju et al., 1988).

Few epidemiologic data are available on aortic aneurysm and dissection and peripheral arterial disease in African Americans (Gillum, 1995). Aortic aneurysm and dissection (ICD-10 I71) was listed as the underlying cause for 15,807 deaths in 1999. For 1999, average annual age-adjusted death rates per 100,000 were 6.3 in AA males, 9.0 in European American males, 4.0 in AA females, and 3.8 in EA females. Rates were higher in EAM than in other groups at each age.

Few epidemiologic data are available on peripheral arterial disease in AA. Atherosclerosis was listed as the underlying cause for 14,979 deaths, including 1,069 AA, in 1999. Chronic peripheral arterial disease of the extremities (ICD9-CM 440.2, 443.9, or 447.1) was listed as the underlying cause for fewer than 4,000 deaths in 1985 (Gillum, 1990). For 1979–1985, average annual age-adjusted death rates per 100,000 were 1.3 in non-White males, 0.8 in White males, 0.9 in non-White females, and 0.5 in White females. Rates were higher in non-Whites than in Whites at each age. Rates at age 75–84 were non-White males (M) 20.1, EA(M) 15.8, non-White females (F) 17.2, and EA(F) 9.0.

In 1985–1987 an average of 332,000 Whites and 44,000 AA were discharged from U.S. hospitals with peripheral arterial, disease and up to seven diagnoses coded per discharge. Average annual diagnosis rates at ages 65 and over were 891 per 100,000 for Whites and 1,192 for AA. About three million days of care for Whites and 605,000 for AA were associated with a mention of these diagnoses. However, a peripheral arterial disease was the first-listed diagnosis (or principal diagnosis) in only about 99,000 discharges for all ages and races combined (Gillum, 1990). Further, these estimates must be viewed with caution since about 23,000 discharges with any diagnosis had unknown race, and a single patient might have multiple diagnoses and discharges and hence be counted more than once. Despite these severe limitations, the data suggest peripheral vascular disease is a significant problem among AA.

UTILIZATION OF CARE

Since an early report in 1982 (Gillum, 1982), a large number of studies have confirmed a marked disparity among ethnic groups in the utilization of coronary revascularization procedures. A review of published studies showed lower utilization of coronary artery bypass grafts (CABG) in AA than Whites (odds ratios 0.23–0.68) (Kressin & Petersen, 2001). Among Medicare-aged beneficiaries of all races, the number of discharges from short-stay hospital with CABG increased steadily from 95,168 in 1990 to 154,054 in 1996, then declined slightly to 150,048 in 1997. Percutaneous transluminal coronary angioplasty (PTCA) rates increased steadily over the period. A review of published studies showed lower utilization in AA than Whites for PTCA (odds ratios 0.32–0.80), little different than for CABG (Kressin & Petersen, 2001).

The ethnic gap may indicate underutilization by AA, overutilization by EA, or both. Reasons for underutilization by AA are depicted in Figure 1.1 (Gillum, 1997). They include the following barriers: lack of insurance and wealth, lack of access to specialists, failure of providers to refer patients for diagnostic procedures or revascularization, lack of patient education and information, patient misunderstanding and fear of surgery, and lack of caregivers and savings to cope with loss of earnings and uncovered costs associated with surgery (see Figure 1.1). It may be hoped that a shift in utilization away from CABG in favor of PTCA, which has lower initial costs and shorter recovery, may favor more frequent revascularization in AA patients. However, continued monitoring is needed to determine whether such a long-term trend of declining disparity develops.

GOALS FOR THE YEAR 2010

Given the growing burden of disease due to stroke, national research and stroke control efforts are vital. Through an extensive consultative process in the late 1980s, the U.S. Department of Health and Human Services set a target goal for age-adjusted stroke mortality in AA for the year 2000 of a nearly 50 percent decline from the 1987 level (Healthy People, 1991). The 1996 rate for AA was

Figure 1.1
Barriers on the road to bypass

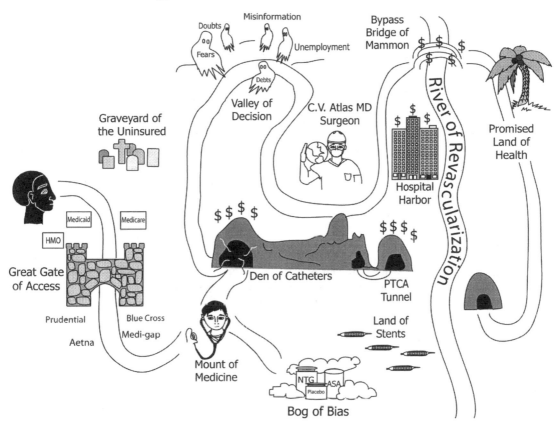

well short of the goal for 2000. A similar process has set goals for health promotion and disease prevention for the year 2010 (USDHHS, 2000).

Increasing the years and quality of healthy life and eliminating (not merely reducing) health disparities among population groups are the two overarching goals. In moving toward these two goals in the United States, several health objectives relating to stroke were established for the year 2010. The target for age-adjusted stroke mortality rate is 48 per 100,000 for all Americans, White and AA, a 20 percent improvement from the baseline of 60 per 100,000 in 1998 (Objective 12-7 Reduce stroke deaths). Regarding eliminating disparities, the effects of the year 2000 age standard on the age-adjusted rates of cerebrovascular disease deaths in AA and Whites and on mortality race ratios are of particular concern. Use of the year 2000 age standard reduces the apparent racial disparity in age-adjusted rates. Even using the year 2000 standard, it seems unlikely that the AA White disparity in age-adjusted rates can be eliminated by 2010 (1997 age-adjusted rates AA 82, Whites 60 per 100,000). However, it will be important to continue to emphasize the large disparities in age-specific rates at younger ages and to target programs accordingly. For example, the rate of years of life lost (YLL) before age 75 due to stroke in AA was triple that of Whites in 1995. National guidelines for control of the major cardiovascular risk factors (ATPIII, JNCVI) and excellent reviews of CHD and stroke prevention have been published (Kromhout et al., 2002; Gorelick, 2002). It is hoped that the present volume contributes to this effort.

CONCLUSIONS AND SUMMARY

In 1999 heart disease was the leading cause of death, and cerebrovascular disease was the third leading cause of death for both AA and Whites in the United States. Despite improvements in hypertension control and declines in mortality rates for all groups, AA continue to experience excess mortality compared to Whites from all heart disease, from coronary heart disease in younger men and in women, from stroke, and from hypertensive disease. Data are needed on peripheral arterial disease in AA. Epidemiologic monitoring of several indicators of disease over time can assist in guiding research and prevention efforts. Longitudinal studies including sizable numbers of AA are needed to enhance understanding of factors influencing cardiovascular risk. Ambitious yet achievable goals for cardiovascular prevention and health promotion have been set forth for the year 2010 to guide the efforts of health care providers and policymakers. Despite declines of cardiovascular disease outcomes in both Whites and AA, a marked disparity in heart disease death rates developed since 1950. This fact was due mainly to a more rapid decline in heart disease in European than in African Americans between 1960 and 1998.

ACKNOWLEDGMENTS

The author acknowledges the staff and contractors of the National Center for Health Statistics, Centers for Disease Control and Prevention, who conducted the surveys and prepared the data for analysis, F. M. Gillum of the Division of Data Services for assistance with the illustration, and S. Wahi of the Division of Health Care Statistics for assistance with Table 1.2.

REFERENCES

Advance Report of Final Mortality Statistics, 1989. (1991). National Center for Health Statistics. *Monthly Vital Statistics Report, 40*, (8 Suppl) 1–52.

Alexander, M., et al. (2002). Management of ventricular arrythmias in diverse populations in California. *American Heart Journal, 144*, 431–439.

Ayala, C., Croft, J.B., Greenlund, K.J., Keenan, N.L., Donehoo, R.S., Malarcher, A.M., & Mensah, G.A. (2001). Racial/ethnic disparities in mortality by stroke subtype in the United States, 1995–1999. *Am J Epidemiol 200, 154*, 1057–1063.

Ayala, C., et al. (2002). Sex differences in U.S. mortality rates for stroke and stroke subtypes by race/ethnicity and age, 1995–1998. *Stroke, 33*, 1197–1201.

Becker, L.B., et al. (2002). The PULSE Initiative: Scientific priorities and strategic planning for resuscitation research and life saving therapies. *Circulation, 10*, 2562–2570.

Bowman, J.E. & Murray, R.F. (1990). *Genetic variation and disorders in peoples of African origin.* Baltimore: Johns Hopkins University Press (76–77).

Burke, A.P., et al. (2002). Traditional risk factors and the incidence of sudden coronary death with and without coronary thrombosis in blacks. *Circulation, 105*, 419–424.

Cann, R.L., Stoneking, M., & Wilson, A.C. (1999). Mitochondrial DNA and human evolution. *Nature, 325*, 31–36.

Cavalli-Sforza, L., Menozzi, P., & Piazzi, A. (1994). *The history and geography of human genes.* Princeton: Princeton University Press (19).

Centers for Disease Control and Prevention. (2002a). State-specific trends in self-reported blood pressure screening and high blood pressure in the United States, 1991–1999. *MMWR, 51*, 456–460.

Centers for Disease Control and Prevention. (2002b). Sudden cardiac death in the United States, 1999. *MMWR, 51*, 23–126.

Collins, J.G. (1988). Prevalence of selected chronic conditions, United States, 1983–85. *Advance Data From*

Vital and Health Statistics (No. 155. DHHS Publication No. PHS 88–1250). Hyattsville, MD: Public Health Service.

Cooper, R.S., & Ford, E. (1990). Coronary heart disease among Blacks and Whites in the NHANES-I Epidemiologic Follow-up Study: Incidence of new events and risk factor prediction. *Circulation, 81*, 723.

Cooper, R., Sempos, C., Hsieh, S.C., & Kovar, M.G. (1990). The slowdown in the decline of stroke mortality in the United States, 1978–1986. *Stroke, 21*, 1274–1279.

Cornoni-Huntley, J., LaCroix, A.Z., & Havlik, R.J. (1989). Race and sex differentials in the impact of hypertension in the United States. The National Health and Nutrition Examination Survey I Epidemiologic Follow-up Study. *Archives of Internal Medicine, 149*, 780–788.

Coughlin, S., Szklo, M., Baughman, K., & Pearson, T. (1990). The epidemiology of idiopathic dilated cardiomyopathy in a biracial community. *American Journal of Epidemiology, 13*, 48–56.

Dannenberg, A.L., Drizd, T., Horan, M.J., Haynes, S.G., & Leaverton, P.E. (1987). Progress in the battle against hypertension. Changes in blood pressure levels in the United States from 1960 to 1980. *Hypertension, 10*, 226–233.

Durch, J.S., & Madans, J.H. (2001). Methodological issues for vital rates and population estimates: 1997 OMB standards for data on race and ethnicity. *Vital Health Statistics, 4* (31):1–30.

Evans, W.E., & Relling, M.V. (1999). Pharmacogenetics: Translating functional genomics into rational therapeutics. *Science, 286*, 487–491.

Executive Summary of the Third Report of the National Cholesterol Education Program. (NCEP) (2001). Expert Panel on Detection Evaluation and Treatment of High Blood Cholesterol in Adults (Adult Treatment Panel III). *JAMA, 285*, 2486–2497.

Ford, E., Cooper, R., Castaner, A., Simmons, B., & Mar, M. (1989). Coronary arteriography and coronary bypass survey among Whites and other racial groups relative to hospital-based incidence rates for coronary artery disease: Findings from NHDS. *American Journal of Public Health, 79*, 437–440.

Ford, E.S., & Cooper, R.S. (1991). Risk factors for hypertension in a national cohort study. *Hypertension, 18*, 598–606.

Ford, E.S., & Jones, D.H. (1991). Cardiovascular health knowledge in the United States: Findings from the National Health Interview Study, 1985. *Preventive Medicine, 20*, 725–736.

Gillum, R.F. (1979). Pathophysiology of hypertension in blacks and whites. A review of the basis of racial blood pressure differences. *Hypertension, 1*, 468–75.

Gillum, R.F. (1982). Coronary heart disease in black populations. I. Mortality and morbidity. *American Heart Journal, 104*, 839–851.

Gillum, R.F. (1986a). Trends in acute rheumatic fever and chronic rheumatic heart disease—a national perspective. *American Heart Journal, 111*, 430–432.

Gillum, R.F. (1986b). Idiopathic cardiomyopathy in the United States, 1970–1982. *American Heart Journal, 111*, 752–755.

Gillum, R.F. (1986c). Cerebrovascular disease morbidity in the United States, 1970–1983. Age, sex, region, and vascular surgery. *Stroke, 17*, 656–661.

Gillum, R.F. (1987a). Heart failure in the United States 1970–1985. *American Heart Journal, 113*, 1043–1045.

Gillum, R.F. (1987b). Pulmonary embolism and thrombophlebitis in the United States, 1970–1983. *American Heart Journal, 114*, 1262–1264.

Gillum, R.F. (1987c). Acute myocardial infarction in the United States, 1970–1983. *American Heart Journal, 113*, 804–811.

Gillum, R.F. (1987d). Coronary artery bypass surgery and coronary angiography in the United States, 1979–1983. *American Heart Journal, 113*, 1255–1260.

Gillum, R.F. (1988). Stroke in Blacks. *Stroke, 19*, 1–9.

Gillum, R.F. (1989a). The epidemiology of cardiomyopathy in the United States. *Progress in Cardiology, 2*, 11–21.

Gillum, R.F. (1989b). Sudden coronary death in the United States: 1980–1985. *Circulation, 79*, 756–765.

Gillum, R.F. (1990). Peripheral arterial occlusive disease of the extremities in the United States: Hospitalization and mortality. *American Heart Journal, 120*, 1414–1418.

Gillum, R.F. (1993). Heart failure in the United States. *American Heart Journal, 126*, 1042–1047.

Gillum, R.F. (1994) The epidemiology of cardiovascular diseases: An American overview. In I.L. Livingston (Ed.), *Handbook of Black American Health*. Westport, CT: Greenwood Press, 3–23.

Gillum, R.F. (1995) Epidemiology of aortic aneurysm in the United States. *Journal of Clinical Epidemiology, 48*, 1289–1298.

Gillum, R.F. (1996). The epidemiology of cardiovascular disease in Black Americans. *New England Journal of Medicine, 335*, 1597–1599.

Gillum, R.F. (1997). Sudden cardiac death in Hispanic Americans and African Americans. *Am Journal Public Health, 87*, 1461–1466.

Gillum, R.F. (2000). Epidemiology of stroke in Blacks. In R.F. Gillum, P.B. Gorelick, & E.S. Cooper (Eds.), *Stroke in Blacks: A guide to management and prevention*. Basel: S. Karger AG, 83–93.

Gillum, R.F. (2002a). Cardiac disease and risk of ischemic stroke. In P.B. Gorelick & M. Alter (Eds.), *Stroke prevention*. New York: Parthenon Publishing.

Gillum, R.F. (2002b). Emergency department and hospital preventive care of elderly next of kin of victims of sudden cardiac death and fatal acute myocardial infarction. *Circulation, 105*, e191.

Gillum, R.F., Gillum, B.S., & Francis, C.K. (1997). Coronary revascularization and cardiac catheterization in the United States: Trends in racial differences. *Journal of the American College of Cardiology, 29*, 1557–1562.

Gillum, R.F., & Grant, C.T. (1982). Coronary heart disease in black populations. II. Risk factors. *American Heart Journal, 104*, 852–864.

Gillum, R.F., & Makuc, D.M. (1992). Serum albumin, coronary heart disease, and death. *American Heart Journal, 123*, 507–513.

Gillum, R.F., Makuc, D.M., & Feldman, J.J. (1991). Pulse rate, coronary heart disease, and death: The NHANESI Epidemiologic Follow-up Study. *American Heart Journal, 121*, 172–177.

Gillum, R.F., Thomas, J., & Curry, C.L. (2000). Atrial fibrillation heart disease, and ischemic stroke in Blacks. In R.F. Gillum, P.B. Gorelick, & E.S. Cooper (Eds.), *Stroke in Blacks: A guide to management and prevention*. Basel: S. Karger AG, 129–141.

Gordon, T., & Garst, C.C. (1965). Coronary heart disease in adults, United States, 1960–62. Vital and Health Statistics. (Series 11, No. 10, PHS Publication No. 1000). Washington, DC: U.S. Government Printing Office.

Gorelick, P.B. (2002). Stroke prevention therapy beyond antithrombotics: Unifying mechanisms in ischemic stroke pathogenesis and implication for therapy. *Stroke, 33*, 862–875.

Graves, J.L., Jr. (2001). The emperor's new clothes: Biological theories of race at the millennium. New Brunswick, NJ: Rutgers University Press.

Haldeman, G., Croft, J., Giles, W., & Rashidee, A. (1999). Hospitalization of patients with heart failure: National Hospital Discharge Survey, 1985–1995. *American Heart Journal, 137*, 352–360.

Healthy People 2000: National health promotion and disease prevention objectives. (1991). U.S. Department of Health and Human Services, Public Health Service, DHHS Publication No. PHS 91-50212.

Hedges, J.R., Feldman, H.A., Bittner, V., Goldbery, R.J., Zapka, J., & Osganian, S.K., et al. (2000). Impact of community intervention to reduce patient delay time on use of reperfusion therapy for acute myocardial infarction: Rapid early action for coronary treatment (REACT) trial: REACT Study Group. *Acad Emerg Med, 7*, 862–872.

Hoyert, D.L., Arias, E., Smith, B.L., Murphy, S.L., & Kochanek, K.D. (2001). Deaths: final data for 1999. National Center for Health Statistics. National Vital Statistics Reports; vol. 49 no 8, Hyattsville, MD, 2001.

Iso, H., Jacobs, D.R., Wentworth, D., Neaton, J.D., & Cohen, J.D. (1989). Serum cholesterol levels and six-year mortality from stroke in 350,977 men screened for the Multiple Risk Factor Intervention Trial. *New England Journal of Medicine, 320*, 904–910.

Jackson, F.L.C. (1993). Evolutionary and political economic influences on biological diversity in African Americans. *J Black Studies, 23*, 539–560.

Kennedy, B.S., Kasl, S.V., Brass, L.M., & Vaccarino, V. (2002). Trends in hospitalized stroke for Blacks and Whites in the United States, 1980–1999. *Neuroepidemiology, 21*:131–141.

Kittner, S.J., White, L.R., Losonczy, K.G., Wolf, P.A., & Hebel, R. (1990). Black–White differences in stroke incidence in a national sample: The contribution of hypertension and diabetes mellitus. *JAMA, 264*, 1267–1270.

Klag, M.J., Whelton, P.K., & Seidler, A.J. (1989). Decline in U.S. stroke mortality: Demographic trends and antihypertensive treatment. *Stroke, 20*, 14–21.

Kressin, N.R., & Petersen, L.A. (2001). Racial differences in the use of invasive cardiovascular procedures: Review of the literature and prescription for future research. *Ann Intern Med, 135*, 352–366.

Kromhout, D., Menotti, A., Kesteloot, H., & Sans, S. (2002). Prevention of coronary heart disease by diet and lifestyle: Evidence from prospective cross-cultural, cohort, and intervention studies. *Circulation, 105*, 893–898.

LaCroix, A.Z., Haynes, S.G., Savage, D.D., & Havlik, R.J. (1989). Rose Questionnaire angina among United States Black, White, and Mexican-American women and men. Prevalence and correlates from the Second National and Hispanic Health and Nutrition Examination Surveys. *American Journal of Epidemiology, 129*, 669–686.

Leaverton, P.E., Havlik, R.J., Ingster-Moore, L.M., LaCroix, A.Z., & Cornoni-Huntley, J.C. (1990). Coronary heart disease and hypertension. In J.C. Cornoni-Huntley, R.R. Huntley, & J.J. Feldman (Eds.), *Health status and well-being of the elderly*. New York: Oxford University Press, 53–70.

McCullough, P.A., Philbin, E.F., Spertus, J.A., Kaatz, S., Sandberg, K.R., & Weaver, W.D. (2002). Confirmation of a heart failure epidemic: Findings from the resource utilization among congestive heart failure (REACH) study. *J Am Coll Cardiol, 39*, 60–69.

National Center for Health Statistics. (1989). Vital statistics of the United States, 1986, Vol. II. Mortality, Part A. (DHHS Publication No. PHS 89-1101). Washington, DC: U.S. Government Printing Office.

National Center for Health Statistics. (2000). *National Hospital Discharge Survey*. Hyattsville, MD: U.S. Department of Health and Human Services, Centers For Disease control and Prevention.

National Center for Health Statistics. (2001). Health, United States, 2001. DHHS Pub. No. (PHS)01-1232. Public Health Service. Washington, DC: U.S. Government Printing Office.

National Institutes of Health. (1996). Congestive heart failure in the United States: A new epidemic. USDHHS, PHS, NHLBI.

Ni, H., Nauman, D., & Hershberger, R. (1999). Analysis of trend in hospitalizations for heart failure. *Journal of Cardiac Failure, 5*, 79–84.

Otten, M.W., Teutsch, S.M., Williamson, D.F., & Marks, J.S. (1990). The effect of known risk factors on the excess mortality of Black adults in the United States. *Journal of the American Medical Association, 263*, 845–850.

Philbin, E., Weil, H., & Francis, C. (2000). Race-related differences among patients with left ventricular dysfunction: Observations from a biracial angiographic cohort. Harlem-Bassett Lp(a) Investigators. *Journal of Cardiac Failure, 6*, 187–193.

Popovic, J.R., & Hall, M.J. (2001). 1999 National Hospital Discharge Survey. Advance data from vital and health statistics; no. 319. Hyattsville, MD: National Center for Health Statistics.

Rautaharju, P.M., et al. (1988). Electrocardiographic estimate of left ventricular mass versus radiographic cardiac size and the risk of cardiovascular disease mortality in the epidemiologic follow-up study of the First National Health and Nutrition Examination Survey. *American Journal of Cardiology, 62*, 59–66.

Ries, P. (1990). Health of Black and White Americans, 1985–187. Vital and Health Statistics. (Series 10, No. 171, DHHS Publication No. PHS 90-1599). Washington, DC: U.S. Government Printing Office.

Rocella, E.F., & Lenfant, C. (1989). Regional and racial differences among stroke victims in the United States. *Clinical Cardiology, 12*, IV, 18–22.

Roig, E., Castaner, A., Simmons, B., Patel, R., Ford, E., & Cooper R. (1987). In-hospital mortality rates from acute myocardial infarction by race in U.S. hospitals: Findings from the National Hospital Discharge Survey. *Circulation, 76*, 280–288.

Sempos, C., Cooper, R., Kovar, M.G., & McMillen, M. (1988). Divergence of the recent trends in coronary mortality for the four major race-sex groups in the United States. *American Journal of Public Health, 78*, 1422–1427.

Tu, E.J. (1987). Multiple cause-of-death analysis of hypertension-related mortality in New York state. *Public Health Reports, 102*, 329–335.

U.S. Department of Health and Human Services. (2000a). *Healthy People 2010: Understanding and improving health*. Washington, DC: U.S. Department of Health and Human Services, U.S. Government Printing Office.

U.S. Department of Health and Human Services. (2000b). *Health People 2010: Objectives for improving health*. Washington, DC: U.S. Department of Health and Human Services, U.S. Government Printing Office.

Wade, N. (2001). *Lifescript*. New York: Simon and Schuster, 85–118.

White, L.R., Losonczy, K.G., & Wolf, P.A. (1990). Cerebrovascular disease. In J.C. Cornoni-Huntley, R.R. Huntley, & J.J. Feldman (Eds.), *Health status and well-being of the elderly*. New York: Oxford University Press, 115–135.

Willich, S.N., Lowel, H., Mey, W., & Trautner, C. (1999). Regionale unterschiede der Herz-kreislauf-mortalitat in Deutschland. *Deutsches Artzteblatt, 96*, A-483-488.

Worrall, B.B., Johnston, K.C., Kongable, G., Hung, E., Richardson, D., & Gorelick, P.B., (2002). Stroke risk factor profiles in African American women: An interim report from the African-American Antiplatelet Stroke Prevention Study. *Stroke, 33*, 913–919.

Yusuf, S., Reddy, S., Ounpuu, S., & Anand, S. (2001a). Global burden of cardiovascular diseases. Part I: General consideration, the epidemiologic transition, risk factors, and impact of urbanization. *Circulation, 104*, 2746–2753.

Yusuf, S., Reddy, S., Ounpuu, S., & Anand, S. (2001b). Global burden of cardiovascular diseases. Part II: Variations in cardiovascular disease by specific ethnic groups and geographic regions and prevention strategies. *Circulation, 104*, 2855–2864.

Zheng, Z.J., et al. (2002). Sudden cardiac death: United States, 1999 *MMWR, 51*, 123–126.

Zheng, Z.J., Croft, J.B., Giles, W.H., & Mensah, G.A. (2001). Sudden cardiac death in the United States, 1989 to 1998. *Circulation, 104*, 2158–2163.

Zuberi, T. (2001). *Thicker than blood: How racial statistics lie*. Minneapolis: University of Minnesota Press, 58–122.

CHAPTER 2

The Social Epidemiology of Coronary Heart Disease in African Americans

IVOR LENSWORTH LIVINGSTON, J. JACQUES CARTER, TROYE MCCARTHY, AND SHAFFIRAN LIVINGSTON

INTRODUCTION

Coronary heart disease (CHD) accounts for the largest proportion of heart disease, affecting twelve million people in the United States (NHLBI, 1998a). Every 29 seconds someone suffers a coronary event in the United States. Every 60 seconds, someone dies from such an event (USDHHS, 2003). Although many factors contribute to racial health disparities, CHD is increasingly seen as an important and salient contributing factor. Therefore, any attempts to address and, ultimately, reduce health disparities have to take into consideration the racial differences in CHD. Furthermore, it is equally important to understand the epidemiological distribution of known risk factors across the focal minority group—African Americans. This knowledge is very important in ongoing efforts to develop successful interventions to reduce CHD among at-risk African Americans and, subsequently, overall health disparities. This chapter reviews and presents information in both of those areas.

CHD is the leading cause of death in the United States, and not unexpectedly, CHD maintains this dubious distinction in almost every racial and ethnic group in the United States (Lillie-Blanton et al., 2002; USDHHS, 2003). Overall, deaths from heart disease accounted for 31.7 percent of all deaths in 1996 (NCHS, 1998) and were responsible for 15.8 percent of the years of potential life lost before age 75 (NCHS, 1998). CHD, which accounts for two-thirds of all heart disease deaths, alone accounted for more than 2 million hospital stays in 1995, with an average stay of 5.3 days, and almost 10 million physician visits (NHLBI, 1998b).

Reports suggest that CHD remains the most common cause of mortality among African Americans, and the difference in CHD mortality between Blacks and Whites is growing. These trends may be due, in part, to the higher prevalence of CHD risk factors among Blacks (Willems & Saunders, 1997). However, despite recent impressive declines in overall CHD mortality, these declines are more rapid in the White population than in the African American or Black population (USDHHS, 2000).

Given the disproportionate incidence of CHD in the African American population, and given the fact that CHD is a major killer of all Americans, it is reasonable to argue that any meaningful attempt to reduce racial health disparities must include a reduction in CHD and its associated risk factors. However, even within the group of CHD risk factors, there are racial differences. The prevalence of selected CHD risk factors (e.g., hypertension, diabetes mellitus, obesity, cigarette smoking, physical inactivity) is greater in African Americans than in the general population (Gillum et al., 1997; Hutchinson et al., 1997; Willems & Saunders, 1997). This adds another level of complexity to any effort to reduce the incidence of CHD among African Americans.

The main objective of this chapter is to present a social epidemiologic view of selected risk factors for CHD in African Americans. It is hoped that the information presented will achieve the following results: (a) underscore the importance of CHD in race-related health differentials; (b) underscore the need to reduce CHD as efforts are made to comprehensively address factors that contribute to racial disparities in health; and (c) focus attention on salient CHD-risk and other related factors for African Americans, especially those that are lifestyle-related and, therefore, modifiable through appropriate interventions. To achieve these and other objectives, the chapter takes a more social epidemiologic focus (i.e., with an emphasis on social, psychological lifestyle determinants of CHD) in addressing CHD. The assumption is that the risk factors that are more related to lifestyle (i.e., social, psychological, and behavioral conditions) are more easily modified in ongoing attempts to reduce race-related CHD morbidity and mortality.

CARDIOVASCULAR DISEASE

Cardiovascular disease (CVD), which includes coronary heart disease, hypertension, and stroke, is the main cause of morbidity and mortality in the United States. The annual cost of CVD to the nation is projected to exceed $351 billion in 2003. This costs exceeds comparable costs for all cancers ($202 billion) and for immunodeficiency virus (HIV) infections ($28.9) reported in 2002 (AHA, 2003). CVD claimed 39.4 percent of all deaths or 1 of every 2.5 deaths in the United States in 2000. CVD was approximately 60 percent of the "total mention mortality." Basically, it meant that of over 2,400,000 deaths from all causes, CVD was recognized as a primary or contributing cause on about 1,415,000 death certificates (AHA, 2002). The importance of CVD is underscored by the following facts:

- Since 1900, CVD has been the number one killer in the United States every year but 1918.
- In 2004 the estimated direct and indirect cost of CVD is 362.4 billion.
- Nearly 2,600 Americans die of CVD each day, an average of one death every 33 seconds.
- Almost 150,000 Americans killed by CVD each year are under age 65. In 2001, 32 percent of deaths from CVD occurred prematurely (i.e., before age 75).
- CVD claims more lives each year than the next five leading causes of death combined, which are cancer, chronic lower respiratory diseases, accidents, diabetes mellitus, and influenza and pneumonia.
- Almost 150,000 Americans killed by CVD each year are under 65.
- The 2001 overall death rate from CVD was 329.6. The rates were 384.3 for White males and 510.5 for Black males; 273.6 for White females and 376.6 for Black females. (AHA, 2003, pp. 1–7)

Despite major steps gained in the fight against CVD, there is compelling evidence that in the United States there is a disconnect between effectively translating and disseminating scientific advances to improving CVD outcomes in our society as a whole. Essentially, the full potential of scientific discoveries for improvements in cardiovascular health has not been realized (Bonow et al., 2002).

A recent Institute of Medicine (IOM) report (Committee on Quality of Health Care in America, 2001) underscored this dilemma by suggesting that between the care that exists and the care that could have existed lie not only a gap but also a chasm. Because of this chasm, efforts to achieve the Healthy People 2010 Objectives for the U.S. population, as established by the Department of

Figure 2.1
Percentage breakdown of deaths from cardiovascular diseases: United States, 2001

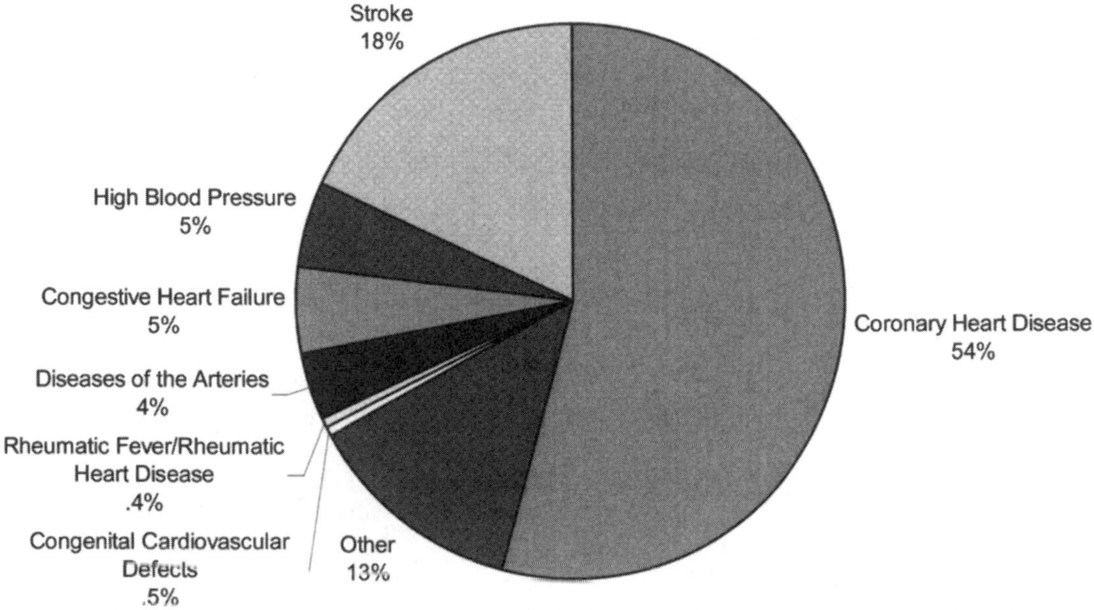

Source: Taken with permission from AHA (2002a), *Heart Disease and Stroke Statistics—2004 Update.*

Health and Human Services, may be severely impeded (USDHHS, 2000). As seen in Figure 2.1, of the various conditions that constitute cardiovascular diseases, CHD is the largest contributor at approximately 54 percent. It is primarily for this and related reasons that CHD is the focus of this chapter.

THE EPIDEMIOLOGY OF RACIAL DISPARITIES IN CORONARY HEART DISEASE

Definition of CHD

Any attempt at interpreting the risk estimates for CHD requires a precise definition of CHD. One such definition comes from the Framingham Heart Study estimates, which are traditionally used to predict total CHD. This includes angina pectoris, recognized and unrecognized myocardial infarction, coronary insufficiency (unstable angina), and CHD deaths (Grundy, Benjamin et al., 1999a). In contrast, many clinical trials (e.g., Sacks et al., 1996; LIPID, 1998) that have evaluated specific risk-reducing therapies have specified major coronary events (i.e., recognized acute myocardial infarction and CHD deaths) as the primary coronary end points. A recent clinical trial, the Air Force/Texas Coronary Artery Prevention Study (AFCAPS/TexCAPS) (Downs et al., 1998), specified acute myocardial infarction, and coronary death, as the primary end point. According to Grundy, Pasternak, et al. (1999), "this combined end point probably corresponds closely to the Framingham study's definition of hard CHD. Definitions of coronary end points assume critical importance when risk cut points are defined to select patients for specific therapies" (p. 1482).

Other related views have been expressed regarding CHD. According to Curry (1994), "Atherosclerosis is a condition marked by loss of elasticity and thickening of the intima of blood vessels.

This condition may progress until the lumen of the affected blood vessel is partially occluded, leading to diminished blood flow through the affected vessel." Curry went on to say that "the development of this process in the coronary arteries is called coronary artery disease. When there is cardiac malfunction as a result of the ischemia-induced atherosclerosis, the process is called atherosclerotic heart disease (CHD). CHD may manifest itself as myocardial infarction, angina pectoris, cardiac dysrhythmias, congestive heart failure and sudden death. CHD is frequently (erroneously) used synonymously with ischemic heart disease (IHD)" (p. 25).

Coronary Heart Disease and African Americans

Generally speaking, the CHD rate has been consistently higher in males than in females and higher in the African American population than in the White population. Furthermore, in the last 30 years, the CHD mortality rate has declined unevenly by gender and race. However, the steep decline leveled off in the 1980s, when the rates of decline for White males and females exceeded those for African American males and females, and African females had the lowest rate of decline (AHA, 2001).

It has been said (Clark et al., 2001) that "CHD is the leading cause of death in the United States for Americans of African and all other ancestries" (p. 97). African Americans have the highest overall mortality rate, as well as the highest out-of-hospital coronary death rate of any ethnic group in the United States, especially at younger ages (Traven et al., 1996; Gillum et al., 1997; Gillum, 1997). The earlier onset of CHD in African Americans highlights the striking racial differences in years of potential life lost (NCHS, 1998). Put differently, Blacks experience twice the number of years of potential life lost before age 75 compared to their White counterparts (USDHHS, 2003).

Sudden cardiac death, which is the most serious initial clinical manifestation of CHD, is considerably higher in African Americans than in Whites (Williams, 2000; Traven et al., 1996). Sudden cardiac rates have been seen to be as much as three times higher in Black men than in White men, even after adjusting for socioeconomic status, age, and access to care (Clark et al., 2001). The magnitude of the racial difference in CHD mortality is greater in women than in men and higher in middle age, so that CHD deaths tend to occur in African American men approximately five years earlier than in Whites (Sempos et al., 1999).

Congenital heart defects are diagnosed in 1 in 100–150 newborns (Botto et al., 2001). Mortality from congenital defects is higher and decline more slowly among Blacks than among Whites. In 1995–1997, for example, infant mortality was 19 percent higher among Blacks than among Whites (68.4 and 55.5 per 100,000, respectively) and declined more slowly (by 2.1 percent versus 2.7 percent per year, respectively). For a number of defects (e.g., transposition of the great arteries, tetralogy of Fallot, ventricular septal defects), Blacks died at a younger age, which in many cases was approximately half the age of Whites (Boneva et al., 2001).

As seen in Table 2.1, the age-adjusted death rate among persons aged ≥35 years in 1998 was higher among men than women. CHD death rates were highest among White men (440.0) and second highest among Black men (421.6). AMI deaths were similar among both groups (196.7 and 198.7 for White and Black men, respectively). Black women had the highest death rates for CHD (301.9) and AMI (140.4), followed by White (263.8 and 113.2 for CHD and AMI, respectively). Compared with Black and White men and women, Hispanics had lower death rates for CHD (285.4 and 189.8 for men and women, respectively) and AMI (121.6 and 76.7 for men and women, respectively).

Relatively few data are available on risk for, or survival with, CHD in African Americans. In order to determine whether the incidence of CHD, rate of survival with the disease, and rate of coronary surgery differ between ethnic groups, Gillum et al. (1997) analyzed data from the National Health and Nutrition Examination Survey (NHANES) I Epidemiologic Follow-up Survey. The summarized results were that compared with Whites, the age-adjusted risk for CHD was higher in African

Table 2.1

Age adjusted death rates* for coronary heart disease† and acute myocardial‡ infarction for persons aged GE 35 years, by sex and race/ethnicity: United States, 1998

Sex	Coronary heart disease		Acute myocardial infarction	
	No	Rate	No	Rate
Men				
White	209,457	440.0	95,617	196.7
Black	19,138	421.6	9,185	198.7
Hispanic	8,431	285.4	3,735	121.6
Asian/Pacific Islander	3,247	258.3	1,417	109.1
American Indian/Alaska Native	750	247.7	377	120.9
Women				
White	202,056	263.8	85,248	113.2
Black	21,202	301.9	9,873	140.4
Hispanic	7,602	189.8	3,102	76.7
Asian/Pacific Islander	2,259	148.1	607	62.2
American Indian/Alaska Native	617	160.2	268	69.3

Source: Taken from Mortality from coronary heart disease and acute myocardial infarction—United States, *Morbidity and Mortality Weekly Report*, February 16, 2001/ 50(06), 90–93.

*Per 100,000 population. Standardized to the 2000 U.S. Bureau of the Census population of persons aged GE 35 years.
†International Classification of Diseases, Ninth Revision, codes 410.0–414.9.
‡Code 410.

American women aged 25–54 years (relative risk, 1.76 [95 percent CI (Confidence Interval), 1.36 to 2.29]), but was lower in African American men within each subgroup. The age-adjusted risk was lower in African American men for all ages combined (25–74 years) (relative risk, 0.78 [CI, 0.65 to 0.93] for all CHD and 0.62 [CI, 0.42-0.92] for acute myocardial infarction. Ethnic groups did not differ significantly in survival after the first hospitalization for CHD. However, it was reported that the incidence of coronary procedures after hospitalization for CHD was markedly lower in African Americans than in Whites (age- and sex-adjusted relative risk, 0.40 [CI, 0.16-0.99]).

CONTROLLING CHD BY KNOWING SALIENT RISK FACTORS

Major progress has been made in the prevention of CHD through modifications of its causes. According to Grundy, Pasternak et al. (1999), the most dramatic progress has been the demonstration

Figure 2.2
Risk factors and other conditions associated with CHD

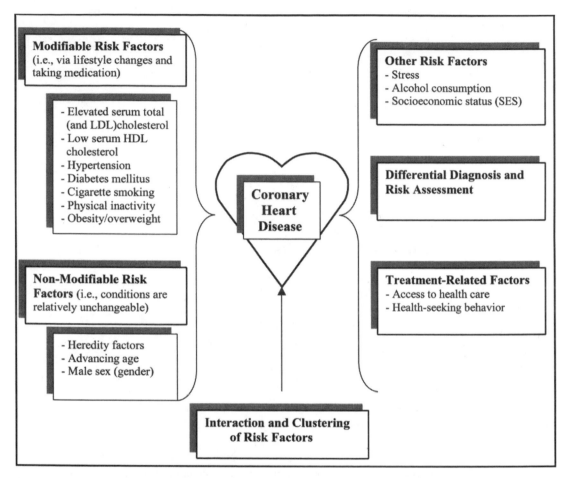

Source: Figure drawn specifically for this chapter by Ivor Lensworth Livingston.

that aggressive medical therapy substantially reduces the likelihood of recurrent major coronary syndromes in patients with established CHD (secondary prevention). The American Heart Association (AHA) and the American College of Cardiology (ACC) have published joint recommendations for medical intervention in patients with CHD and other forms of atherosclerotic disease (Smith et al., 1995).

There are certain risk factors for CHD that are nonmodifiable, such as age, gender, family history, and some possible genetic determinants. However, there are many modifiable risk factors that, if adequately controlled or eliminated, can increase the likelihood of surviving CHD, or ideally evading its onset completely. Since African Americans are 1½ times more likely to possess multiple risk factors for CHD than Whites (Clark et al., 2001), it is key that they take measures to decrease the impact of as many of these modifiable factors and behaviors as possible (see Figure 2.2).

Modifiable Risk Factors

It is clear that to prevent and control CHD in the general population, as well as more specifically in the African American population, knowledge has to be ascertained concerning salient risk factors.

Figure 2.3
Risk and other factors associated with CHD

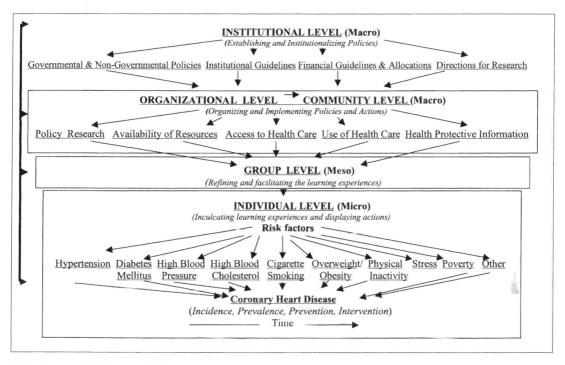

© Ivor Lensworth Livingston (2004).

However, as illustrated in Figure 2.3, the vast majority of modifiable risk factors, which occur at the "micro"-individual level, over time, are in turn impacted by conditions at the intermediate "meso"-group level and at the larger "macro"-institutional and organizational levels. Figure 2.3 illustrates the important connection between macro-level institutions and organizations, meso-level groups and micro-level individuals, where any comprehensive effort aimed at controlling CHD, especially in the African American population, has to appreciate the "embededness" of individual lifestyles and, hence, CHD risk factors.

As seen in Figure 2.3, at the institutional level policies are established and institutionalized; at the level of organizations and communities, policies are further organized and implemented through desired actions; at the meso-level of groups, the learning process is refined and channeled into more easily acceptable means and structures (e.g., families). In total, individuals at the micro-level are socialized in acquiring a variety of experiences from their environments with the assistance of other people around them.

For purposes of this chapter, it is reasoned that certain lifestyle attitudes and behaviors acquired over time contribute to a variety of risk factors that lead to increased vulnerability of some persons to experience CHD. Therefore, any comprehensive effort to prevent and control CHD must, of necessity, appreciate the dynamic interaction between the macro factors (i.e., institutions, organizations, and communities), meso factors (i.e., groups) and micro factors (i.e., individual behaviors). Due to space limitations, this chapter addresses selected risk factors only at the micro-individual level. As a result of the ultimate need to intervene to reduce CHD, the emphasis of the chapter, with some exceptions, is on these micro-level factors, especially those that are modifiable. Figure 2.3 illustrates and lists the salient modifiable and non-modifiable factors and their collective relationship to CHD.

Recent data suggest that mortality rates among African Americans now exceed those for Whites among old and young women, and among men less than 65 years of age (Gillum, 1991). While the reasons for these different rates are unclear, factors that contribute to the higher coronary risk in African Americans (versus Whites) are higher rates of diabetes, obesity, and tobacco use (Otten et al., 1990). Additionally, less extensive use of advanced treatment for CHD in the African American population may also contribute to the differences in racial risk outcomes. This latter point is demonstrated, for example, in the rate of revascularization procedures (Whittle et al., 2002). More is said about this in a later section of the chapter. An additional reason is the disproportionate distribution of individual and multiple CHD risk factors across ethnic and racial groups (e.g., African Americans).

The presence of multiple risk factors has contributed to the racial disparities of mortality rates for CHD (Willems & Saunders, 1997). Clark et al. (2001) found that in addition to the prevalence of coronary risk factors, the delay in identifying and treating those persons at a high risk for developing CHD and limited access to cardiovascular care also contribute greatly to the ethnic differences in rates of CHD. These researchers found the following actions key to reducing the risks for CHD: (1) controlling hypertension; (2) treating dyslipidemia; (3) regressing left ventricular hypertrophy (LVH); and (4) discontinuing smoking.

In terms of salient risk factors for CHD, Grundy, Pasternak, et al. (1999) mentioned that the main independent risk factors include cigarette smoking, elevated blood pressure, elevated serum total cholesterol and low-density lipoprotein cholesterol (LDL-C), low serum high-density lipoprotein cholesterol (HDL-C), diabetes mellitus, and advancing age. A further distinction was made between conditional and predisposing risk factors, where the former are associated with increased risk for CHD and the latter worsen the independent risk factors (see Table 2.2). Two such factors are obesity and physical inactivity, which have been designated as major risk factors by the AHA (Eckel, 1997; Fletcher et al., 1996). It has been reported that the adverse effects of obesity are more problematic when obesity is expressed as abdominal obesity (NHLBI, 1988b), an indicator of insulin resistance (Grundy, Pasternak et al., 1999).

Serum Cholesterol—Total and Low-density Lipoprotein (LDL).   Elevated LDL levels are established risk factors for CHD. Reductions in LDL cholesterol have been associated with corresponding reductions in the incidence of CHD in large clinical studies (e.g., Sacks et al., 1996; LIPID, 1998). Also, population-based studies report that African Americans have lower total serum cholesterol levels than Whites and also a lower prevalence of hypercholesterolemia (Hutchinson et al., 1997; Johnson et al., 1993). It was reported (Clarke et al., 2001), however, that in young middle-aged adults in the Coronary Artery Risk Development in Young Adults (CARDIA) Study, the prevalence of LDL cholesterol levels of 160 mg/dL or more was 5 percent in African American women, 4 percent in White women, 10 percent in African American men, and 9 percent in White men (Gidding et al., 1996).

Elevated serum cholesterol is one of the most modifiable risk factors for CHD and treating hypercholesterolemia lowers the risk of developing disease (Manninen et al., 1988). Based on the strength of this evidence, the National Cholesterol Education Program recommends measuring the serum cholesterol in all adults older than 20 years at least once every five years (Summary of the NCEP, 1993). Data analyzed from the Third National Health and Nutrition Examination Survey showed that among individuals with high cholesterol who were instructed to take medication, African Americans (P<.001) were less likely than Whites to be taking a cholesterol-lowering agent (Nelson et al., 2002).

Serum Cholesterol—High-density Lipoprotein (HDL).   According to Clarke et al. (2001), low HDL cholesterol levels increase the risk for development of CHD independent of LDL levels and other risk factors. Elevated levels of HDL cholesterol are viewed as protective, hence reducing the risk of CHD. It has been reported that increasing HDL cholesterol without corresponding reductions in LDL cholesterol reduces the risk for CHD events (Rubins et al., 1999). Although the reasons are not fully known, HDL cholesterol levels are higher in African Americans, especially in African American men, than in their White counterparts (Hutchinson et al., 1997). Speculations are that these racial differences may relate to a genetically lower activity of hepatic lipase (Vega et al., 1998).

High Blood Pressure or Hypertension.   The number of existing cases of hypertension is approximately 40 percent higher in African Americans than in Whites (an estimated 6.4 million African Americans have high blood pressure (Burt et al., 1995), and its effects are more frequent and severe in the African American population (Livingston, 1991; Livingston et al., 1991; USDHHS, 2000). The National Health and Nutrition Examination Survey I (NHANES I) Epidemiologic Follow-up Study (Gillum et al., 1998) found that for African American women, the significant, independent risk factors for CHD were elevated systolic blood pressure and smoking. In African American men, the study found elevated systolic blood pressure and serum cholesterol as key risk factors for the disease.

While both systolic and diastolic hypertension are established risk factors for CHD, some evidence suggests that systolic blood pressure is a better predictor than diastolic blood pressure of CHD, heart failure, stroke, end-stage renal disease, and overall mortality (Kannel, 1999). Hypertension increases CHD risk by predisposing to left ventricular hypertrophy (LVH) and by causing endothelial dysfunction and injury, thereby increasing the risk for atherosclerosis (Walsh et al., 1995). In the CARDIA Study, systolic blood pressure correlated more with left ventricular mass than did diastolic blood pressure (Flack et al., 1999).

For African Americans, not only is hypertension more prevalent, but also it develops at younger ages and is associated with a three to five times higher cardiovascular mortality rate than in Whites (Livingston, 1993a; Cooper et al., 1996). In a related manner, young to middle-aged African Americans also manifest greater left ventricular wall thickness/chamber ratios across a broad spectrum of mostly normal blood pressures (Flack et al., 1999).

It is suggested that higher mortality rates in hypertensive African Americans reflect greater disease severity with more LVH (Liao et al., 1995). Both electrocardiographic LVH and echocardiographic measurements of increased left ventricular mass have been reported to be more prevalent in African American than in Whites (Cooper et al., 1996; Liao et al., 1995). In the African American population, LVH is very predictive of ischemic heart disease morbidity and mortality, and it is also a stronger risk factor than cigarette smoking, hypertension, or hypercholesterolemia (Thomas et al., 1997).

Diabetes Mellitus.   Diabetes and CHD are two of the most prevalent epidemic diseases of the twenty-first century. As the mortality rate of CHD is declining, there is an increase in the incidence rate for diabetes (Mann, 2002). Research finds that diabetes-related morbidity and mortality are mainly attributed to cardiovascular complications. It was reported that the aging of the American population, along with the increase in prevalence of obesity and physical inactivity, aids in the increase of diabetes cases (Grundy, Benjamin, et al., 1999a). The burden of diabetes and its vascular complications are higher in the African American versus the White population (Brancati et al., 2000).

The most common form of diabetes mellitus is type 2 diabetes (formerly called non-insulin-dependent diabetes), which usually occurs later in life. Type 1 diabetes mellitus (formerly called insulin-dependent) is the other type of diabetes. Insulin resistance develops from obesity and physical inactivity, acting on a substrate of genetic susceptibility (Gerick, 1998). Insulin secretion declines with advancing age (Dechenes et al., 1998), and this decline may be accelerated by genetic factors (Humphriss et al., 1997).

The prevalence of type 2 diabetes is two to three times higher in African Americans than in Whites (Brancati et al., 2000). The relative number of persons with diabetes in African American, Hispanic, and American Indian communities is one to five times greater than in the White population (Flegal et al., 1991). Also, deaths from diabetes are two times greater in the African American population than in the White population, and diabetes-associated renal failure is 2.5 times greater in the African American population than in the Hispanic population (CDC, 1997; 1999). Persons with diabetes who develop a CHD have a lesser chance of survival than those with CHD, but no diabetes (Grundy, Benjamin et al., 1999).

Cigarette Smoking.   According to the U.S. Department of Health and Human Services (HHS), cigarette smoking increases the risk of lung cancer, emphysema, and heart disease. In 2000, 25 percent of men and 21 percent of women were smokers. Smoking is viewed as the leading cause of death and diseases that are preventable in the United States (USDHHS, 2002). Approximately 30 percent of all CHD deaths in the United States each year are attributable to cigarette smoking, with the risk being dose-related (USDHHS, 1990). Smoking acts synergistically with other risk factors to noticeably increase the risk of CHD (Anderson et al., 1991).

Compared with nonsmokers, the risk of heart attack for smokers is more than double, and cigarette smoking is found to be the leading risk factor for sudden cardiac death. Cigarette smoking also acts with other risk factors to greatly increase the risk for coronary heart disease. (www.americanheart. org, 2002). Studies find that nearly 30 percent of CHD deaths are due to the smoking of cigarettes. The risk of developing CHD for smokers increases drastically when one or more additional risk factors are present. When people diagnosed with CHD quit smoking, they can possibly experience a 50 percent reduction in their risk of developing complications (up to and including death) from the disease (Ockene & Miller, 1997).

In an analysis of data obtained by the Sample Adult Core component of the 1997–2002 National Health Interview Surveys (NCHS Web site, 2003), it was found that the rate of smoking among U.S. adults is steadily declining. The rates declined from 24.7 percent in 1997 to 24.1 percent in 1998, 23.5 percent in 1999, 23.3 percent in 2000, and 22.0 percent in 2001. This same report also revealed that in the first quarter of 2002, the prevalence of smoking for Hispanics was 15.3 percent, 22.0 percent for Whites, and 23.1 percent for Blacks (non-Hispanic). While more African American men smoke than White men, they consume fewer cigarettes per day (Clark et al., 2001). However, African American and White women smoke at comparable rates (Taylor et al., 1997).

Physical Inactivity.   An inactive lifestyle is now recognized as an independent risk factor for CHD. Research finds that regular, moderate-to-vigorous physical activity helps to prevent diseases of the heart and blood vessels. Exercising can have the following effects on certain people: control of blood cholesterol levels, diabetes, and obesity; increase of cardiovascular functional capacity; and the lowering of blood pressure (Fletcher et al., 1996). It is reported that regular, physical activity reduces mortality, lessens the risk of developing certain diseases, and enhances one's total physical functioning (Fletcher et al., 1996). In NHANES III, which has a national representative sample of African Americans (as well as other racial and ethnic groups), it was reported that the highest prevalence of physical inactivity was observed among African Americans and Mexican Americans (Crespo et al., 2000) (see Figure 2.4).

Overweight and Obesity.   People who have excess body fat, especially concentrated in the waist area, are more likely to develop heart disease, even when no other risk factors are present. This excess of weight increases the amount of strain on the heart; raises blood pressure, blood cholesterol, and triglyceride levels; and lowers HDL cholesterol levels (www.americanheart.org, 2002). When weight is concentrated in the abdominal area, this increases the risk of CHD (Grundy, Benjamin, et al., 1999). Only recently has the relationship between obesity and CHD been viewed as direct. Studies now indicate that obesity can be an independent predictor of CHD. Although heredity explains 30 percent to 70 percent of cases of obesity, environmental contributions to the increasing prevalence of obesity must be sought (Eckel, 1997).

It is common for obese patients to have other risk factors for CHD. The presence of these multiple factors increases the likelihood of developing CHD or responding negatively to treatment. Obese people are found to be three times more likely to develop hypertension than those of normal weight ranges (Eckel, 1997). Medical research shows that the major cause of the increase in rates of diabetes

Table 2.2
Risk factors for coronary heart disease

Major independent risk factors

. Cigarette smoking
. Elevated blood pressure
. Elevated serum total (and LDL) cholesterol
. Low serum HDL cholesterol
. Diabetes mellitus
. Advancing age

Other risk factors – Predisposing risk factors

. Obesity*†
. Abdominal obesity†
. Physical inactivity*
. Family history of premature coronary heart disease
. Ethnic characteristics
. Psychosocial factors

Other risk factors – Conditional risk factors

. Elevated serum triglycerides
. Small LDL particles
. Elevated serum homocysteine
. Elevated scrum lipoprotein(a)
. Prothrombotic factors (e.g., fibrinogen)
. Inflammatory markers (e.g., C-reactive protein)

Source: Adapted with permission from Grundy, Pasternak et al. (1999). Assessment of cardiovascular risk by use of multiple-risk factor assessment equations. Circulation, 100, 1481–1492.

*The risk factors are defined as major risk factors by the AHA. Eckel, 1997; Fletcher et al., 1996.
†Body weights are currently defined according to BMI as follows: normal weight 18.5–24.9 kg/m²; overweight 25–29 kg/m²; obesity > 30.0 kg/m²; (obesity class I 30.0–34.9, class II 35.9–39.9, class III GE 50 kg/m²). Abdominal obesity is defined according to waist circumference: men >102 cm (>40 in) and women >88 cm (35 in). NHLBI, 1998.

is obesity. The fatty acid intake through one's diet is a major cause in the development of Type 2 diabetes. Over the past ten years, the rates of obesity have doubled, resulting also in an increase in the onset of diabetes (Mann, 2002).

The NHLBI Obesity Education Initiative, in cooperation with the National Institute of Diabetes and Digestive and Kidney Diseases, released in 1998 the first federal guidelines on the identification, evaluation, and treatment of overweight and obesity in adults (Clinical Guidelines on the Identification, Evaluation and Treatment of Overweight and Obesity in Adults, 1998). According to the guidelines, the assessment of overweight involves three basic factors: the body mass index (BMI),

Figure 2.4
Age-sex-adjusted percent of adults aged 18 years and over who engaged in regular leisure-time physical activity, by race/ethnicity in the United States, quarter one, 2002

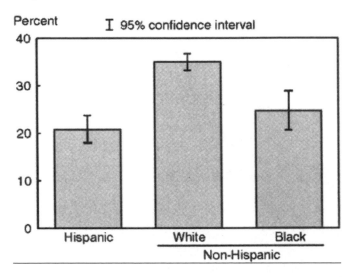

Notes: This measure reflects the new definition being used for the physical activity leading health indicator (Healthy People 2010). Regular leisure-time physical activity was defined as engaging in light-moderate leisure-time physical activity for greater than or equal to 30 minutes greater than or equal to five times per week or engaging in vigorous leisure-time physical activity for greater than or equal to 20 minutes greater than or equal to three times per week. The analysis excluded 200 persons with unknown physical activity participation. Estimates are age-sex-adjusted to the projected year 2000 standard population using five age groups: 18–24 years, 25–44 years, 45–64 years, 65–74 years, and 75 years and over.

Source: Based on data collected from January through March in the Sample Adult Core component of the 2002 National Health Interview Survey.

waist circumference, and risk factors for diseases and conditions associated with obesity. Overweight is defined as a BMI of 25 to 29.9 and obesity as a BMI of 30 and above (Clinical Guidelines on the Identification, Evaluation and Treatment of Overweight and Obesity in Adults, 1998). It has been reported that the waist circumference is an excellent surrogate for visceral adipose tissue and correlates better with cardiovascular disease than does the customarily used BMI, or waist/hip ratio (Okosum et al., 1999).

The prevalence of obesity among African American men is similar to that of White men; however, in African American women, obesity is twice as prevalent and the abdominal pattern of obesity is more common than in their White counterparts (Kumanyika, 1995; Stevens et al., 1994). See Figure 2.5 for the prevalence of obesity in the United States in the first quarter of 2002.

Nonmodifiable Risk Factors

There are additional risk factors for CHD that are considered nonmodifiable. They are increasing age, gender, and heredity. The aging of the population brings with it an increased incidence of chronic diseases, including CHD, heart failure, and stroke (Bonow et al., 2002). At older ages,

Figure 2.5
Age-adjusted prevalence of obesity among adults aged
20 years and over, by sex and race/ethnicity in the
United States, quarter one, 2002

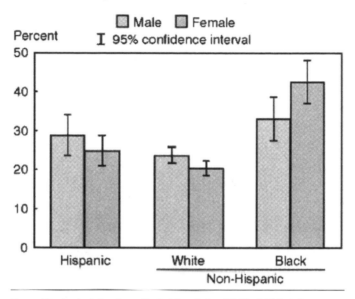

Notes: Obesity is defined as a Body Mass Index (BMI) of 30 kg/m2 or more. The analysis excluded 322 people with unknown height or weight. Estimates are age-adjusted to the projected year 2000 standard population using three age groups: 20–39 years, 40–59 years, and 60 years and over

Source: Based on data collected from January through March in the Sample Adult Core component of the 2002 National Health Interview Survey.

females who have a heart attack are twice as likely as males to die within weeks (Gillum et al., 1997). These differences are, in part, explained by the presence of a variety of coexisting conditions (e.g., diabetes, hypertension, and congestive heart failure) (USDHHS, 2000). Also, the usual view was that differences in behavior were more important determinants of the higher male mortality than inherent sex differences in physiology (Waldron, 1976). However, recent studies, after adjusting for unhealthy behaviors, show that while they contribute to the gender-related CHD differences, they do not fully explain the increased risk of CHD in men (Wingard et al., 1983).

Those persons with a family history of heart disease are likely to develop the condition as well. Those with a family history of CHD are also likely to possess other risk factors for the disease. In regard to race, African Americans are more likely to develop CHD due to higher rates of high blood pressure, diabetes, and obesity (www.americanheart.org, 2002). Regarding the issue of race/ethnicity, the incidence of existing cases of hypertension is approximately 40 percent higher in African Americans than in Whites. An estimated 6.4 million African Americans have hypertension, and its effects are usually more frequent and severe in this population (Burt et al., 1995).

The following age, race, gender-specific rates were recently reported, serving to underscore the importance of the nonmodifiable risk factors. The annual rates per 1,000 population of new and recurrent heart attacks in non-Black men are 26.3 for ages 65–74, 39.7 for ages 75–84, and 53.6 for age 85 and older. For non-Black women in the same age groups, the rates are the 7.8, 21.0 and 24.2, respectively. For Black men the rates are 16.3, 54.9 and 40.8, and for Black women the rates are 13.3, 18.3 and 14.1, respectively (AHA, 2003).

Other Risk Factors

Stress.   The AHA finds that the way individuals respond to life stressors may be a contributing factor to the onset of CHD. The added stress in one's life may have negative effects on possible risk factors already present in one's life to include diet and smoking habits (AHA, 2002). Persons with atherosclerosis and increased reactivity to laboratory-induced mental stress may demonstrate a generalized exaggerated response to everyday life stresses (Fredrikson et al., 1990). In a related manner, the relationship of stress to cardiac reactivity and elevated high blood pressure in African Americans has been reported in the past (Livingston & Marshall, 1991).

In patients with manifest clinical CHD events, mental stress is associated with both silent and symptomatic myocardial ischemia (Legault et al., 1995). Patients with known CHD who develop ischemia during mental stress have greater increases in heart rate, blood pressure, and systemic vascular resistance, all of which are suggestive of a greater sympathetic response (Goldberg et al., 1996). Furthermore, stress initiated by mental arithmetic exercises have been shown to produce coronary artery constriction in patients with documented CHD rather that dilation, as was reported in normal individuals (Yeung et al., 1991). Given the reported connection of stress to CVD in the Black population (Livingston, 1985, 1988, 1991, 1993b), the importance of the stress–CHD relationship is further underscored for African Americans.

Alcohol Consumption.   The alcohol–CHD relationship can, at times, appear very complexing, where at one point alcohol consumption appears to be beneficial, while at another it appears to be harmful. What is apparent in trying to understand this relationship, however, is the rate at which a person drinks, what he or she is drinking, and the gender and overall health of the person who is drinking. For example, light-to-moderate drinking can have beneficial effects on the heart, especially among those at greatest risk for heart attacks, such as men over age 45 years and women after menopause (Zakhari, 1997). However, long-term heavy drinking increases the risk for high blood pressure, heart rhythm irregularities (arrhythmias), heart muscle disorders (cardiomyopathy), and stroke (USDHHS, 2000).

The AHA, while not recommending alcohol use, finds that the consumption of one or two drinks per day leads to a reduction in risk of total mortality. It finds that not consuming any alcohol actually leads to a higher total mortality rate than having the one to two drinks a day (Pearson, 1996). However, recent evidence indicates that approximately 50 percent of the protective effect of alcohol is mediated through increased levels of HDL cholesterol (Gordon et al., 1981). Although African Americans tend to have similar rates of alcohol consumption within the wider population (excepting Asians), reports suggest that they have higher rates of alcohol-related health and social problems compared with a national sample of the U.S. population (Caetano & Clark, 1998).

Socioeconomic Status (SES).   A large and consistent body of evidence demonstrates that SES, which is usually measured by one or a combination of a person's education, income, and occupational classification, is positively associated with a variety of health outcomes. The strongest data on this association come from studies of CVD, in which SES has consistently predicted morbidity and mortality (Kaplan & Keil, 1993; Woodward et al., 1992). Although not fully known, it is suggested that the SES–CVD relationship may operate through the pathways of other risk factors, such as smoking, diet, alcohol consumption, and physical inactivity (Lynch et al., 1995).

Reports also suggest that SES is inversely related to CHD and is also predictive of other risk factors as well (e.g., Smith et al., 1998; Harrell & Gore, 1998). Also, some of the racial differences in health problems are attenuated by adjustment for SES (Potts & Thomas, 1999). In all ethnic groups, including African Americans, there is a positive correlation between SES and the prevalence of CHD risk factors, including hypertension, cigarette smoking, diabetes, and obesity, as well as other related factors (e.g., lower utilization of cardiac-related procedures) (Ferguson et al., 1997;

Harris, Andrews & Elixhauser, 1997; Clark et al., 2001). It has been reported that notwithstanding the relationship between CHD risk factors and SES being somewhat comparable for both African Americans and Whites, a lower SES may have a more enormous impact on the health of African Americans (Keil et al., 1997; Escobedo et al., 1997). One contributing reason for this could be the disproportionate prevalence of the CHD risk factors in the African American compared to the White populations.

Interaction and Clustering of Risk Factors

It was mentioned before that one of the reasons that African Americans are disproportionately affected by CHD compared to their White counterparts has to do with the fact that they tend to have a higher prevalence of most of the salient CHD risk factors (Hutchinson et al., 1997). A very important related point is that the presence of multiple risk factors increases the CHD risk synergistically (Clark et al., 2001). An equally related point is the possible interactive effect of both genetic and environmental factors that contribute to the kind and extent of some of these CHD risk factors. Insulin resistance and hyperinsulinemia appear important to risk factor clustering and contribute to the pathogenesis of coexistent hypertension, diabetes, dyslipidemia, and atherosclerosis (Reaven, 1994).

DIFFERENTIAL DIAGNOSIS AND RISK ASSESSMENT

Selected Racial Differences

Before any successful treatment can be made of African Americans with CHD, they first have to be successfully diagnosed, which could also involve doing risk assessments of the individuals. Both of these activities are certainly not accurate all the time and can present some resident challenges. For example, many frequently accepted diagnostic modalities used for risk assessment have not been sufficiently validated with African Americans. This is a very important point given that some non-invasive tests appear to show a lower predictive value in African Americans. Furthermore, African Americans referred for coronary angiography more often have angiographically normal coronary arteries or less obstructive coronary artery disease (Diver et al., 1994; Stone et al., 1996). It has been said, however, that the total burden of atherosclerotic disease may in fact be higher in African Americans (Strong et al., 1997).

Presentation of Myocardial Ischemia

The majority of African Americans having symptomatic myocardial ischemia and acute myocardial infarction have typical chest pain symptoms (Strong et al., 1997; Summers et al., 1999). However, silent ischemic episodes and atypical symptoms occur more frequently in African Americans than in Whites. According to Clark et al. (2001), this may be due, in part, to the high prevalences associated with hypertension and diabetes, both of which are associated with an increased frequency of atypical ischemic symptoms.

Non-Invasive Diagnostic Studies

Many customary accepted diagnostic modalities used for risk assessment have not been validated in African Americans. According to Clark et al. (2001), nondiagnostic ST- and T-wave changes, early repolarization changes, and increased QRS-wave voltage on electrocardiography are more common in African American men than in White men. Furthermore, these electrocardiographic abnormalities are frequently interpreted as "normal variants;" however, their role as markers of increased CHD risk for African Americans has not been fully evaluated. (For a more thorough review of diagnosis of CHD and risk assessment associated with African Americans, see Clark et al. [2001].)

TREATMENT-RELATED FACTORS

Each year approximately 1.1 million persons experience a new or recurrent heart attack (defined as acute myocardial infarction or fatal CHD). About 650,000 of these will be first attacks and 450,000 will be recurrent attacks.[1] Over 40 percent of the people who experience a coronary event in a given year will die of it (AHA, 2001). Also, approximately 50 percent of these coronary deaths occurred suddenly, within one hour of symptom onset, outside the hospital (NHLBI, 1998). Early treatment of heart attack patients reduces heart-muscle damage, improves heart muscle function, and lowers heart attack death rate (Ryan et al., 1996). Early access to emergency health care services is an additional determinant of outcome for victims of out-of-hospital cardiac arrest. Adequate control of risk factors in the vulnerable population (e.g., African Americans) can reduce the overall rate of heart attacks and CHD mortality in the United States by over 20 percent. However, many CHD patients are not receiving the aggressive risk factor management they require (USDHHS, 2000).

Access to Health Care

Access to health care plays a very important role in the ultimate presence of CHD. Evidence exists that African Americans have less access to cardiovascular care and that those with CVD are treated less aggressively than their White counterparts, even when access is not a direct issue (Leape et al., 1999; Gillum, Gillum, et al., 1997). Compared with their White counterparts, African Americans made fewer physician office visits, were more likely to be seen in emergency rooms and clinics, were less likely to be seen by a cardiovascular specialist, and were less likely to undergo a series of important cardiovascular-related procedures (e.g., coronary arteriography and coronary bypass surgery) (Lillie-Blanton et al., 2002). Revascularization procedures, such as percutaneous transluminal coronary angioplasty (PTCA) and coronary artery bypass grafting (CABG), are known to provide relief of symptoms (Hultgreen et al., 1985) and, in some groups of patients, prolong life (Alderman et al., 1990).

An individual's ability to access and use modern, available cardiac therapy is very much related to precision in diagnosis, relieving symptoms, and deducing premature CHD morbidity and mortality. A recent review of strong studies provide credible evidence that African Americans are less likely than White Americans to receive diagnostic procedures, revascularization procedures, and thrombolytic therapy, even when patient characteristics are controlled (Lillie-Blanton et al., 2002). Others have also underscored these points by reporting that, compared with their White counterparts, African Americans receive less often adequate treatment for risk factors, receive cardioprotective drugs less frequently, and undergo coronary catheterization, coronary angioplasty, and bypass surgery less frequently (Clark et al., 2001).

A study involving cholesterol screening practices in an office-based family medicine residency program over an 18-month period showed that African Americans and Hispanics were 16 percent less likely to be screened. This occurred even after controlling for insurance coverage, socioeconomic status, and number of visits (Naumburg et al., 1993). In one of the earlier studies (Maynard et al., 1997), it was reported that 58 percent of Whites in the Coronary Artery Surgery Study were recommended for surgery, compared to 38 percent of African Americans, even after adjusting for clinical characteristics and diagnostic findings. Since those earlier years, such disparities to access to quality

Figure 2.6
Evidence of racial/ethnic differences in cardiac care, 1984–2001

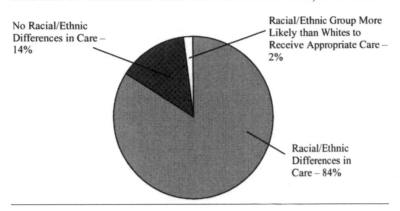

Source: Taken with permission from the Kaiser Family Foundation, *Racial/Ethnic Differences in Cardiac Care: The Weight of the Evidence*, Summary Report, October 2002.

health care have been replicated by others. These studies have found African Americans to be 13 to 40 percent less likely to receive coronary angioplasty and 32 to 70 percent less likely to receive bypass surgery than their White counterparts (Peterson et al., 1997; Weitzman et al., 1997).

Studies have shown that when both African Americans and Whites receive comparable care for coronary artery disease, that outcomes are similar (Clark et al., 2001). However, disparities in care exist for many reasons. Behaviorally, African Americans are more likely to delay in receiving medical care, in general. As found by Clark et al. (2001), and by the Henry J. Kaiser Family Foundation (Lillie-Blanton et al., 2002), African Americans are sometimes treated less aggressively for cardiovascular disease than are Whites. It was concluded that "African Americans are less likely than Whites to receive diagnostic procedures, revascularization procedures, and thrombolytic therapy, even when patient characteristics are similar" (Lillie-Blanton et al., 2002, p. 1). Figure 2.6 illustrates these disparities in access to care.

Health Care–Seeking Behaviors

It is reported that African Americans delay seeking medical care for myocardial infarctions for periods up to three times longer that Whites (Dracup et al., 1995). Although the reasons for these delays are varied, a contributing factor could be a lower level of symptom recognition and less belief in the treatability of the disease (Clark et al., 1992). Given that early access to emergency health care services is an important determinant for patients with CHD, especially those experiencing out-of-hospital cardiac arrests (USDHHS, 2000), delays in seeking medical care restricts the benefits patients can receive from the advances made in the treatment of myocardial infarction.

CALL FOR ACTION

Any major effort directed at reducing racial health disparities has to focus a great deal of attention on reducing CHD, given that it contributes to the majority of deaths in the number one killer of all Americans—cardiovascular disease. Additionally, because African Americans are disproportionately afflicted with CHD, as well as its risk factors, a push for increased resources (i.e., through research funding and health education activities) must be directed to this area.

The following areas represent a renewed call for action that will help reduce racial disparities in CHD:

1. Since a majority of the modifiable risk factors shown in Figure 2.2 are associated with "habits" that are learned and influenced by various institutions, organizations, communities, and groups (see Figure 2.3), over time, which makes them lifestyle-related, they are essentially modifiable (see Figure 2.2 and Table 2.2). Screening and early risk factor detection, especially in poor African American communities, are key to preventing the onset and exacerbation of CHD risk factors and CHD itself.

2. Given the importance of successfully applying needed and available technology and expertise to efforts to control CHD, especially in the at-risk African American population, measurements must be put in place among medical professionals to help evaluate their success rate in identifying and treating patients at high risk for CHD. Since revascularization procedures, such as coronary artery bypass grafting (CABG) and percutaneous transluminal coronary angioplasty (PTCA), are proven to prolong the life of patients suffering from cardiovascular disease (Garg et al., 2000), these options must be not only communicated to African American patients, but also made more accessible to them by the medical community.

3. Because knowledge can change attitudes and attitudes in turn are related, in part, to behaviors (or lifestyles), some attempt must be made to recapture the earlier successes of national educational campaigns and programs (e.g., National High Blood Pressure Education Program, or NHBPEP, in 1972; the National Cholesterol Education Program, or NCEP, in 1985). These campaigns and programs were reasonably successful in reinvigorating and reeducating vulnerable segments of the African American population about CHD risk factors and the important benefits of (a) early detection through screening, (b) compliance with any prescribed (e.g., antihypertensive medication), (c) adhering to recommended dietary guidelines, (d) engaging in regular physical exercise, (e) practicing stress reduction activities, and (f) being empowered by monitoring one's own health.

CONCLUSION

The intervention of multiple risk factors is key to decreasing the risk of developing coronary heart disease. Also, the complexity and the dynamics associated with any meaningful attempts at reducing racial and ethnic health disparities can be readily seen in the various figures presented in the chapter. Figure 2.3 is especially important as a guide for future efforts directed at reducing and eliminating CHD disparities. All of these efforts are especially directed at African Americans, who are more likely to die from CHD, as well as its risk factors, compared to Whites. Those facing the highest risks for developing CHD—African Americans—after they are educated about CHD risk factors (both modifiable and nonmodifiable) must become empowered, along with medical personnel, in engaging in behaviors to prevent and/or reduce their experiences with CHD-risk factors. Positive health protective behaviors, such as weight control, physical activity, balanced diet, avoidance of tobacco, reduced stress, and control of the physical conditions of cholesterol (LDL), diabetes, hypertension, etc. will help to increase both the quality and quantity of their lives.

African Americans who are male and older should be informed about the nonmodifiable CHD-risk factors of race/ethnicity, gender, and age and the need, therefore, to have regular and frequent physical examinations with qualified medical personnel. These medical personnel will be able to monitor, evaluate, and advise individuals of their CHD-risk factor condition and what, if any, appropriate action is needed. Therefore, if African Americans, as well as the medical community, work in a complementary manner, the outcome will, over time, contribute to a reduction in racial and ethnic health disparities through improvements in the incidence of CHD in the at-risk African American population.

NOTE

1. Based on data from the Atherosclerotic Risk in Communities (ARIC) study of the National Heart, Lung, and Blood Institute (NHLBI), 1987–1994. These data represent Americans hospitalized with definite or probable myocardial infarction, not including MIs (AHA, 2001).

REFERENCES

Alderman, F.L., et al. (1990). Ten-year follow-up of survival and myocardial infarction in the randomized Coronary Artery Surgery Study. *Circulation, 82*, 1629–1646.

American Diabetes Association. (2002). Retrieved November 26, 2002. www.diabetes.org.

American Heart Association. (1996). *Heart and stroke facts*. Dallas, TX: American Heart Association.

American Heart Association. (2001). *Heart and stroke statistical update*. Dallas, TX: American Heart Association.

American Heart Association. (2002a). *Heart disease and stroke statistics—2004 Update*. Dallas, TX: American Heart Association.

American Heart Association. (2002b). Retrieved December 2, 2002. www.americanheart.org.

American Heart Association. (2003). *Coronary heart disease and angina pectoris*. Heart disease and stroke statistics update. Dallas, TX: American Heart Association.

Anderson, K.M., Wilson, P.W., Odell, P.M., & Kannel, W.D. (1991). An updated coronary risk profile: A statement for health professionals. *Circulation, 83*, 356–362.

Boneva, R.S., Botto, L.D., Moore, C.A., Yang, Q., Correa, A., & Erickson, J.D. (2001). Mortality associated with congenital heart defects in the United States—Trends and racial disparities, 1979–1997.

Bonow, R.O., Smaha, L.A., Smith S.C., Jr., Mensah, G.A., & Lenfant, C.L. (2002). The international burden of cardiovascular disease: Responding to the emerging global epidemic. *Circulation, 106*, 1602–1605.

Botto, L.D., Correa, A., & Erickson, J.D. (2001). Racial and temporal variations in the prevalence of heart defects. *Pediatrics, 107*, E32.

Brancati, F.L., et al. (2000). Incident type 2 diabetes mellitus in African American and White adults. The Atherosclerosis Risk in Communities study. *Journal of the American Medical Association, 283*, 2253–2259.

Burt, V., Whelton, P., & Roccella, E.J. (1995). Prevalence of hypertension in the U.S. adult population. *Hypertension, 25*, 305–313.

Caetano, R., & Clark, C.L. (1998). Trends in alcohol-related problems among Whites, Blacks and Hispanics: 1984–1995. *Alcoholism: Clinical and Experimental Research, 22*, 534–538.

Centers for Disease Control and Prevention (CDC). (1997). Diabetes Surveillance. Atlanta, GA: HHS.

Centers for Disease Control and Prevention (CDC). (1999). National diabetes fact sheet: National estimates and general information on diabetes in the United States. Atlanta, GA: USDHHS (HHS), CDC.

Clark, L., et al. (2001). Coronary heart disease in African Americans. *Heart Disease, 3*, 97–108.

Clinical Guidelines on the Identification, Evaluation and Treatment of Overweight and Obesity in Adults. (1998). Evidence Report. *Journal of Obesity Research* (Suppl. 2), 51S–204S.

Committee on Quality of Health Care in America. (2001). Institute of Medicine. Crossing the quality chasm: A new health system for the 21st century. Washington, DC: National Academy Press.

Cooper, R.S., Liao, Y., & Rotimi, C. (1996). Is hypertension more severe among U.S. blacks, or is severe hypertension more common? *Annuals Epidemiology, 6*, 173–180.

Crespo, C.J., Smit, E., Andersen, R.E., Carter-Pokras, O. & Ainsworth, B.E. (2000). Race/ethnicity, social class and their relation to physical inactivity during leisure time: Results for the Third National Health Nutrition Examination Survey, 1988–1994. *American Journal of Preventive Medicine, 18*, 46–53.

Curry, C. (1994). Coronary artery disease in blacks. In I.L. Livingston (Ed.), *Handbook of black American Health* (pp. 24–32). Westport, CT: Greenwood Press.

Dechenes, C.J., Verchere, C.B., Andrikopoulos, S., & Kahn, S.E. (1998). Human aging is associated with parallel reductions in insulin and amylin release. *American Journal of Physiology, 275*, E785–E791.

Diabetes Mellitus: A major risk factor for cardiovascular disease. (1999). *Circulation, 100*, 1132–1133.

Diver, D.J., et al. (1994). Clinical and arteriographic characterization of patients with unstable angina without critical coronary arterial narrowing. *American Journal of Cardiology, 74*, 531–537.

Downs, J.R., et al. (1998). [For the AFCAPS/TexCAPS Research Group] Primary prevention of acute coronary events with lovastatin in men and women with average cholesterol levels: Results of AFCAPS/TexCAPS. *Journal of the American Medical Association, 279*, 1615–1622.

Dracup, K., et al. (1995). Causes in delay in seeking treatment for heart attack symptoms. *Social Science and Medicine, 40*, 379–392.

Eckel, R. (1997). Obesity and heart disease: A statement for health care professionals from the Nutrition Committee, American Heart Association. *Circulation 96*, 3248–3250.

Escobedo, L.G., Giles, W.H., & Anda, R.F. (1997). Socioeconomic status, race and death from coronary heart disease. *American Journal of Preventive Medicine, 13*, 123–130.

Ferguson, J.A., et al. (1997). Examination of racial differences in management of cardiovascular disease. *Journal of the American College of Cardiology, 30*, 1707–1713.

Flack, J.M., et al. (1999). Statis and pulsatile blood pressure correlates of left ventricular structure and function in Black and White young adults: The CARDIA study. *American Heart Journal, 138*, 856–864.

Flegal, K., et al. (1991). Prevalence of diabetes in Mexican Americans, Cubans and Puerto Ricans for the Hispanic Health and Nutrition Examination Survey, 1982–1984. *Diabetes Care, 14*, 628–638.

Fletcher, G.F., et al. (1996). Statement on exercise: Benefits and recommendations for physical activity programs for all Americans: A statement for health professionals by the Committee on Exercise and Cardiac Rehabilitation of the Council on Clinical Cardiology, American Heart Association. *Circulation, 94*, 857–862.

Fredrikson, M., Tuomisto, M., & Melin, B. (1990). Blood pressure in healthy men and women under laboratory and naturalistic conditions. *Journal Psychosomatic Research, 34*, 675–686.

Garg, M., Vacek, J., & Hallas, D. (2000, December). Coronary angioplasty in Black and White patients: Demographic characteristics and outcomes. *Southern Medical Journal, 93, 12*, 1187–1191.

Gerick, J.E. (1998). The genetic basis of type 2 diabetes mellitus: impaired insulin secretion versus impaired insulin sensitivity. *Endocrine Review, 9*, 491–503.

Gidding, S.S., et al. (1996). Prevalence and identification of abnormal lipoprotein levels in a biracial population aged 23 to 35 years (the CARDIA Study). The Coronary Risk Development in Young Adults Study. *American Journal of Cardiology, 78*, 304–308.

Gillum, R.F. (1991). Cardiovascular disease in the United States: An epidemiologic overview (pp. 3–16). In E. Saunders (Ed.), *Cardiovascular disease in Blacks*. Philadelphia: F.A. Davis.

Gillum, R.F. (1997). Sudden cardiac death in Hispanic Americans and African Americans. *American Journal of Public Health, 87*, 1461–1466.

Gillum, R.F., Gillum, B.S., & Francis, C.K. (1997). Coronary revascularization and cardiac catheterization in the United States: Trends in racial differences. *Journal of the American College of Cardiology, 29*, 1557–1562.

Gillum, R.F., Mussolino, M.E., & Madans, J.H. (1997). Coronary heart disease incidence and survival in African American women and men. *Annals of Internal Medicine, 127*, 111–118.

Gillum, R., Muscolino, M., & Madans, J. (1998). Coronary heart disease risk factors and attributable risks in African-American women and men: NHANES I Epidemiologic follow-up study. *American Journal of Public Health, 88, 6*, 913–917.

Goldberg, A.D., et al. (1996). Ischemic, hemodynamic and neurohormone responses to mental stress: Experience from the Psychophysiological Investigations of Myocardial Ischemia (PIMI). *Circulation, 94*, 2402–2409.

Gordon, T., Ernst, N., Fisher, M. & Rifkind, B.M. (1981). Alcohol and high-density lipoprotein cholesterol. *Circulation, 64* (Suppl III): III-63–III-67.

Grundy, S., Benjamin, I., et al. (1999). Diabetes and cardiovascular disease. *Circulation, 100*, 1134–1146.

Grundy, S., Pasternak, R., Greenland, P., Smith, S., Fuster, V. (1999). Assessment of cardiovascular risk by use of multiple risk factor assessment equations. *Circulation, 100, 1481–1492*.

Harrell, J.S., & Gore, S.V. (1998). Cardiovascular risk factors and socioeconomic status in African American and Caucasian women. *Res Nur Health, 21*, 285–295.

Harris, D.R., Andrews, R., & Elixhauser, A. (1997). Racial and gender differences in use of procedures for Black and White hospitalized adults. *Ethnicity Disease, 7*, 91–105.

Hultgreen, H., et al. (1985). The 5-year effect of bypass surgery on relief of angina: Predictors of survival benefits and strategies for patient selection. *Annals of Internal Medicine, 114*, 1035–1049.

Humphriss, D.B., et al. (1997). Multiple metabolic abnormalities in normal glucose tolerant relatives of NIDDM families. *Diabetologia, 40*, 1185–1190.

Hutchinson, R.G., et al. (1997). Racial differences in risk factors for atherosclerosis. The ARIC Study. *Angiology, 48*, 279–290.

Johnson, C.L., et al. (1993). Declining serum total cholesterol levels among U.S. adults. The National Health and Nutrition Examination Surveys. *Journal of the American Medical Association, 269*, 3002–3008.

Kannel, W.B. (1999). Historic perspectives on the relative contributions of diastolic and systolic blood pressure elevation to cardiovascular risk profile. *American Heart Journal, 138*, 205–210.

Kaplan, G.A., & Keil, J.E. (1993). Socioeconomic factors and cardiovascular disease: A review of the literature. *Circulation, 88*, 1973–1998.

Keil, J.E., et al. (1997). Hypertension; effects of social class and racial admixture: The results of a cohort study in the Black population of Charleston, South Carolina. *American Journal of Public Health, 67*, 634–639.

Kumanyika, S. (1995). Searching for the association of obesity with coronary artery disease. (Editorial). *Annals Internal Medicine, 3*, 273–275.

Leape, L.L., et al. (1999). Underuse of cardiac procedures: Do women, ethnic minorities and the uninsured fail to receive needed revascularization? *Annals of Internal Medicine, 130*, 183–192.

Legault, S.E., Freeman, M.R., Langer, A., & Armstrong, P.W. (1995). Path physiology and time course of silent myocardial ischemia during mental stress: Clinical, anatomical and physiological correlates. *British Heart Journal, 73*, 242–249.

Liao, Y., et al. (1995). The relative effects of left ventricular hypertrophy, coronary artery disease, and ventricular dysfunction on survival among Black adults. *Journal of the American Medical Association, 273*, 1592–1597.

Lillie-Blanton, M, Rushing, O., Ruiz, S., Mayberry, R., & Boone, L. (2002, October). Racial/ethnic differences in cardiac care: The weight of the evidence. The Henry J. Kaiser Foundation, Manlo Park, California.

Livingston, I.L. (1985). The importance of stress in the interpretation of the race–hypertension association. *Humanity and Society, 9(2)*, 168–181.

Livingston, I.L. (1988). Stress and health dysfunctions: The importance of health education. *Stress and Medicine, 4(3)*, 155–161.

Livingston, I.L. (1991). Stress, hypertension and renal disease in Black Americans: A review with implications. *National Journal of Sociology, 5(2)*, 143–181.

Livingston, I.L. (1993a). Renal disease and Black Americans: Selected issues. *Social Science and Medicine, 37(5)*, 613–621.

Livingston, I.L. (1993b). Stress, hypertension and young Black Americans: The importance of counseling. *Journal of Multicultural Counseling, 2(3)*, 132–142.

Livingston, I.L., Levine, D.M., & Moore, R. (1991). Social integration and Black intraracial blood pressure variation. *Ethnicity and Disease, 1(2)*, 135–149.

Livingston, I.L., & Marshall, R. (1991). Cardiac reactivity and elevated blood pressure levels among young African Americans: The importance of stress. In D.J. Jones (Ed.), *Prescriptions and policies: The social well-being of African Americans in the 1990* (pp. 77–91). New Brunswick, NJ: Transaction.

Long-term Intervention with Pravastatin in Ischaemic Disease (LIPID) Study Group. (1998). Prevention of cardiovascular events and death with pravastatin in patients with coronary heart disease and a broad range of initial cholesterol levels. *New England Journal of Medicine, 339*, 1349–1357.

Lynch, J., Kaplan, G.A., Salonen, R., Cohen, R.D., & Salonen, J.T. (1995). Socioeconomic status and carotid atherosclerosis. *Circulation, 92*, 1786–1792.

Mann, J.I. (2002). Diet and risk of coronary heart disease and Type 2 diabetes. *Lancet 360, 9335*, 783–790.

Manninen, V., et al. (1988). Lipid alterations and decline in the incidence of coronary heart disease in the Helsinki Heart Study. *JAMA, 260*, 641–651.

Maynard, C., et al. (1997). Causes of chest pain and symptoms suggestive of acute cardiac ischemia in African American patients presenting to the emergency department: A multicenter study. *Journal of the National Medical Association, 89*, 665–671.

Morbidity Mortality Weekly Report. (1998, November 27). Coronary heart disease mortality trends among Whites and Blacks Appalachia and United States, 1980–1993. *MMWR Weekly 47 (46)*, 1005–1008, 1015.

Morbidity and Mortality Weekly Report. (2001, February 16). Mortality from coronary heart disease and acute myocardial infarction—United States. *MMWR Weekly, 50 (6)*, 90–93.

National Center for Health Statistics (NCHS). (1998). Health, United States, 1998 with socioeconomic status and health chartbook. Hyattsville, MD: NCHS.

National Center for Health Statistics (NCHS). (2003). Retrieved February 15, 2003. www.cdc.gov/nchs/nhis. htm.

National Center for Health Statistics, Division of Health Interview Statistics (2002). *National health interview survey.* Maryland: U.S. Department of Health and Human Services.

National Heart, Lung and Blood Institute (NHLBI). (1998a). Morbidity and Mortality: 1998 Chartbook on cardiovascular, lung and blood diseases. Bethesda, MD: Public Health Service (PHS), national Institutes of Health (NIH), NHLBI, October.

National Heart, Lung and Blood Institute (NHLBI), Obesity Education Initiative Expert Panel (1998b). *Clinical guidelines on identification, evaluation, and treatment and obesity in adults: The evidence report.* Bethesda, MD: National Institutes of Health, National Heart, Lung and Blood Institute.

Naumburg, E.H., Franks, P., Bell, B., Gold, M., & Engerman, J. (1993). Racial differences in the identification of hypercholesterolemia. *Journal of Family Practice, 36,* 425–430.

Nelson, K., Norris, K., & Mangione, C.M. (2002). Disparities in the diagnosis and pharmologic treatment of high serum cholesterol by race and ethnicity. *Archives of Internal Medicine, 162,* 929–935.

Ockene, I., & Miller, N. (1997). Cigarette smoking, cardiovascular disease, and stroke. *Circulation, 96,* 3243–3247.

Okosun, I.S., et al. (1999). The relation of central adiposity to components of the insulin resistance syndrome in a biracial U.S. population. *Ethnicity and Disease, 2,* 219–229.

Otten, M.W., Jr., Teutsch, S.M. Williamson, D.F., & Marks, J.S. (1990). The effect of known risk factors on the excess mortality on Black adults in the United States. *JAMA, 263,* 845–850.

Pearson, T. (1996). Alcohol and heart disease. *Circulation, 94,* 3023–3025.

Peterson, E.D., Shaw, L.K., DeLong, E.R., Pryor, D.B., Califf, R.M., & Mark, D.B. (1997). Racial variation in the use of coronary-revascularization procedures. Are the differences real? Do they matter? *New England Journal of Medicine, 336,* 480–486.

Potts, J.L., & Thomas, J. (1999). Traditional coronary risk factors in African Americans. *American Journal of the Medical Sciences, 317,* 189–192.

Reaven, G.M. (1994). Syndrome X: 6 years later. *Journal Internal Medicine, 736* (Suppl), 13–22.

Rubins, H.B., et al. (1999). Department of Veterans Affairs High-density Lipoprotein Cholesterol Intervention Trial Study Group, gemfibrozil for the secondary prevention of coronary heart disease in men with low levels of high-density lipoprotein cholesterol. *New England Journal of Medicine, 341,* 410–418.

Ryan, T.J., et al. (1996). ACC/AHA Guidelines for the Management of Patients with Acute Myocardial Infarction: A Report of the American College of Cardiology/American Heart Association Task Force on Practice Guidelines (Committee on Management of Acute Myocardinal Infarction). *Journal American College of Cardiology, 28,* 1328–428.

Sacks, F.M., et al. (1996). The effect of pravastatin on coronary events after myocardial infarction in patients with average cholesterol levels.: Cholesterol and Recurrent Events Trial Investigators. *New England Journal of Medicine, 335,* 1001–1009.

Sempos, C.T., Bild, D.E., & Manolio, T.A. (1999). Overview of the Jackson Heart Study: A study of cardiovascular diseases in African American men and women. *American Journal of Medical Sciences, 317* (3), 142–146.

Smith, G.D., Neaton, J.D., Wentworth, D., Stamler, R., & Stamler, J. (1998). Mortality differences between Black and White men in the USA: Contribution of income and other risk factors among men screened for the MRFIT. *Lancet, 351,* 934–939.

Smith, S.C. Jr., et al. (1995). Secondary prevention panel. Preventing heart attack and death in patients with coronary disease. *Circulation, 92,* 2–4.

Stevens, J., Kumanyika, S.K., & Keil, J.E. (1994). Attitudes toward body size and dieting: Differences between elderly Black and White women. *American Journal of Public Health, 84,* 1322–1325.

Stone, P.H., et al. (1996). Registry Study Group. Influence of race, sex and age, on management of unstable angina and non-Q-wave myocardial I infarction. *Journal of the American Medical Association, 275,* 1104–1112.

Strong, J.P., et al. (1997). The PDAY study: Natural history, risk factors and pathobiology. Pathobiological determinants of atherosclerosis in youth. *Annals of the New York Academy of Sciences, 811,* 226–235.

Summary of the Report of the National Cholesterol Education Program (NCEP) Expert Panel on Detection,

Evaluation and Treatment of High Blood Cholesterol in Adults (Adult Treatment Panel II). 1993. *Journal of the American Medical Association, 269,* 3015–3023.

Summers, R.L., et al. (1999). Prevalence of atypical chest pain descriptions in a population from the southern United States. *American Journal of Medical Sciences, 318,* 142–145.

Taylor, H.A., et al. (1997). Long-term survival of African Americans in the Coronary Artery Study (CASS). *Journal American College of Cardiology, 29,* 358–364.

Thomas, J., et al. (1997). Cardiovascular disease in African and White physicians: The Meharry Cohort-Hopkins Cohort Studies. *Journal Health Care Poor and Underserved, 8,* 270–283.

Traven, N.D., et al. (1996). Coronary heart disease mortality and sudden death among the 35–44 age group in Allegheny County, Pennsylvania. *Annals of Epidemiology, 6,* 130–136.

U.S. Department of Health and Human Services. (USDHHS). (1990). The health benefits of smoking and health: A report of the surgeon general. DHHS Publication (CDC) 90-8416.

U.S. Department of Health and Human Services (USDHHS). (2000). Healthy People 2010 (2nd Ed.). With understanding and improving health and objectives for improving health. 2 vols. Washington, DC.: U.S. Government Printing Office, November.

U.S. Department of Health and Human Services (USDHHS). (2003). A public health action plan to prevent heart disease and stroke. Atlanta, GA: USDHHS, CDC and Prevention.

Vega, G.L., et al. (1998). Hepatic lipase activity is lower in African American men than in White American men: Effects of 5' flanking polymorphism in the hepatic lipase gene (LIPC). *Journal of Lipid Research, 39,* 228–232.

Waldron, I. (1976). Why do women live longer than men? *Social Science and Medicine, 10,* 349–362.

Walsh, M.F., Dominguez, L.J., & Sowers, J.R. (1995). Metabolic abnormalities in cardiac ischemia. *Cardiology Clinics, 13,* 529–538.

Weitzman, S., et al. (1997). Gender, racial and geographic differences in the performance of cardiac diagnostic and therapeutic procedures for hospitalized acute myocardial infarction in four states. *American Journal of Cardiology, 79,* 722–726.

Whittle, J., Conigliaro, J., Good, C., Hanusa, B., & Macpherson, D. (2002). Black–White differences in severity of coronary artery disease among individuals with acute coronary syndromes. *Journal of General Internal Medicine, 17,* 867–873.

Willems, J.P., & Saunders, T. (1997). The prevalence of coronary heart disease risk factors among rural Blacks. A community based study. *Southern Medical Journal, 90, 8,* 814.

Williams, R.A. (2000). Race and gender considerations in sudden death in the athlete. In R.A. Williams (Ed.), the athlete and heart disease (pp. 285–296). Philadelphia: F.A. Davis.

Wingard, D.L., Suarez, L., & Barrett-Connor, E. (1983). The sex differential in mortality from all causes and ischemic heart disease. *American Journal of Epidemiology, 117,* 165–172.

Woodward, M., Shewry, M.C., Smith, W.C., & Tunstall-Pedoe, H. (1992). Social status and coronary heart disease: Results from the Scottish Heart Health Study. *Preventive Study, 21,* 136–148.

Yeung, A.C., et al. (1991). The effect of atherosclerosis on the vasomotor response of coronary arteries to mental stress. *New England Journal of Medicine, 325,* (22), 1551–1556.

Zakhari, S. (1997). Alcohol and the cardiovascular system: Molecular mechanisms for beneficial and harmful action. *Alcohol Health & Research World, 21,* (1), 21–29.

CHAPTER 3

Cerebrovascular Disease in Black Americans: Disparities in Burden and Care

GARY H. FRIDAY AND
EDGAR JACKSON KENTON III

EPIDEMIOLOGY

Mortality Rates

In the United States, stroke is the third leading cause of death, after heart disease and cancer. However, the disparity in the ratio of Black to White mortality is greatest for stroke (Gillum & Feinleib, 1993). African American men and women have almost twice the rate of death due to stroke as Whites. This disparity is most prominent at relatively younger ages (Friday, 1994). Stroke was the third leading cause of death in Black women (after heart disease and cancer) and the sixth in Black men (after heart disease, cancer, HIV, unintentional injuries, and homicide) in the United States in 1996 (Gillum, 1999). Stroke mortality has been declining since 1900 with an acceleration in the decline since about 1970. However, since the early 1980s a marked slowdown has occurred in the decline in U.S. stroke mortality in Black and White Americans (Cooper et al., 1990). The number of stroke deaths in Blacks actually increased by >8 percent between 1992 and 1996 (Gillum, 1999).

The reason for the slowing of the decline in stroke mortality may be an increase in the prevalence of chronic ischemic heart disease, heart failure, atrial fibrillation, diabetes mellitus, and obesity or a drop-off in control of hypertension (Gillum & Sempos, 1997; National High Blood Pressure Education Program, 1997). Within regions, Blacks in nonmetropolitan areas had higher stroke death rates than those in metropolitan areas (Gillum, 1997). In 1996 Blacks had almost twice the rate of stroke deaths as Whites (Figure 3.1). The age adjusted Black to White ratio for stroke mortality was 1.4 in 2000 (Minino et al., 2002). This lower ratio is partially due to the higher average age in 2000 compared to earlier years, with the racial disparity in stroke mortality being more pronounced in the younger age groups. As shown in Table 3.1 in 2000 the rate of stroke mortality in Blacks remained quite high in the younger age groups (<75 year of age) ranging from about two to four times that of Whites.

Incidence Rates

The incidence of stroke has been found to be approximately twice as high for African American men and women when compared with White Americans (Broderick et al., 1998; Friday et al., 1989).

Figure 3.1
1996 U.S. stroke mortality rates by race and sex

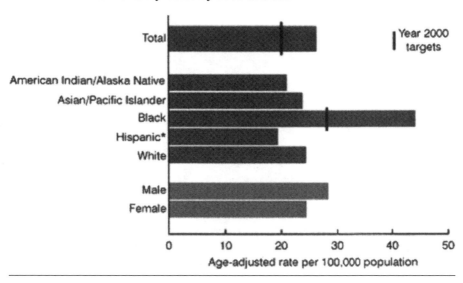

Death rates are age adjusted to the 1940 U.S. standard population.
* Persons of Hispanic origin may be of any race.

Source: COC-NCHS National Vital Statistics System 1996.

In a study conducted to identify all cases of first stroke occurring in northern Manhattan, New York City, between July 1, 1993, and June 30, 1996, the average annual age-adjusted stroke incidence rate at age > or =20 years, per 100,000 population, was 223 for Blacks, 196 for Hispanics, and 93 for Whites. Blacks had a 2.4-fold and Hispanics a 2-fold increase in stroke incidence compared with Whites (Sacco et al., for the Northern Manhattan Stroke Study Collaborators, 1998). This disparity is most pronounced at younger ages. These data suggest that part of the reported excess stroke mortality among Blacks in the United States may be a reflection of racial differences in stroke incidence.

Risk Factors

It is proposed that the excess stroke mortality and risk in African Americans is due to higher prevalence of cardiovascular risk factors such as hypertension, diabetes mellitus, and smoking and greater severity of risk factors or greater sensitivity to the risk factors in African Americans (Gaines & Burke, for the SECORDS Investigators, 1995). However, there has been little research on cardiovascular risk factors for stroke in this group. In a population-based incident case-control study of stroke risk factors among White, Blacks, and Caribbean Hispanics living in the same urban community of northern Manhattan, hypertension was an independent risk factor for Whites (odds ratio [OR] 1.8, etiological fraction [EF] 25 percent), Blacks (OR 2.0, EF 37 percent), and Caribbean Hispanics (OR 2.1, EF 32 percent), but greater prevalence led to elevated EFs among Blacks and Caribbean Hispanics. Greater prevalence rates of diabetes increased stroke risk in Blacks (OR 1.8, EF 14 percent) and Caribbean Hispanics (OR 2.1 $P<0.05$, EF 10 percent) compared with Whites (OR 1.0, EF 0 percent), whereas atrial fibrillation had a greater prevalence and EF for Whites (OR 4.4, EF 20 percent) compared with Blacks (OR 1.7, EF 3 percent) and Caribbean Hispanics (OR 3.0, EF 2 percent). Coronary artery disease was most important for Whites (OR 1.3, EF 16 percent),

Table 3.1

Death rates (per 100,000) for cerebrovascular diseases according to age, sex, and race: United States, 2000

	White Men	Black Men	White Women	Black Women
All Ages, Age adjusted	58.6	87.1	57.8	78.1
45-54	13.8	51.6	11.2	38.5
55-64	40.2	120.5	30.4	75.5
65-74	135.9	256.6	108.8	188.7
75-84	472.0	640.1	441.0	575.4
85+	1,471.8	1,346.2	1,653.1	1,612.4

Source: Department of Health and Human Services. (2002). *Health, United States, 2002*, 144–146. Hyattsville, MD: U.S. Government Printing Office. DHHS Pub. No. (PHS) 2000–1232.

followed by Caribbean Hispanics (OR 1.5, EF 6 percent) and then Blacks (OR 1.1, EF 2 percent). Prevalence of physical inactivity was greater in Caribbean Hispanics, but an elevated EF was found in all groups (Sacco et al., 2001). These results indicate that modifiable cardiovascular risk factors may not have a uniform impact among different ethnic groups and therefore would affect the design and implementation of stroke prevention programs across ethnic groups.

TREATMENT

Acute Treatment

In 1996 the U.S. Food and Drug Administration (FDA) approved the use of recombinant tissue plasminogen activator (tPA) in the treatment of acute ischemic stroke. This is currently the only medication approved for the acute treatment of stroke. This approval was based on the results of a two-part study conducted by the National Institute of Neurological Disorders and Stroke (NINDS) (National Institute of Neurological Disorders and Stroke rt-PA Stroke Study Group, 1995). A total of 624 patients were enrolled, of whom approximately 30 percent were African American. Recovery was based on the National Institutes of Health Stroke Scale (NIHSS, a measure of neurological deficit), the Barthel Index (a measure of activities of daily living), the Rankin Scale (a global measure of disability), and the Glasgow Outcome Scale (a measure of handicap). Complete or near complete recovery was seen in 11 percent to 13 percent more patients treated with tPA than with placebo across all outcome measures.

An inclusion criterion for the study was treatment with intravenous tPA or placebo within 3 hours of stroke onset. Patients with a risk for bleeding were excluded as well as patients with hard-to-control blood pressure (BP >185 mm Hg systolic or >110 diastolic on repeated measures). The complication of intracerebral hemorrhage is a major concern with thrombolytic treatment. Such hemorrhage occurred within 36 hours of treatment in 6.4 percent of the patients treated with tPA as compared with 0.6 percent of the patients given placebo. Deaths due to hemorrhage occurred in 2.9 percent and 0.3 percent of tPA and placebo treated patients, respectively. However, the mortality rate at three months was not significantly different between the two groups (17 percent for tPA and 21 percent for placebo).

In a post hoc subgroup analysis, which included race, a beneficial effect of tPA was found in all subgroups studied (NINDS and Stroke tPA Stroke Study Group, 1997). Also, in a prospective open-label study involving 30 patients treated with tPA (at a university and two community hospitals) in Houston, Texas, 11 of 30 patients were Black (Chiu et al.,1998). Patient outcomes were similar to those in the NINDS tPA study. Race was found to have no significant effect on outcome in that study.

In another study of the clinical use of tPA for acute treatment of stroke between June and December 1999 at 42 academic medical centers in the United States, rates of tPA use were compared for African Americans and Whites in univariate analysis and after adjustment for age, gender, stroke severity, and type of medical insurance with multivariable logistic regression (Johnston et al., 2001). Of the 1,195 ischemic stroke patients in the study, 788 were Whites and 285 were African Americans. Overall, 49 patients (4.1 percent) received tPA. African Americans were one-fifth as likely to receive tPA as Whites (1.1 percent African Americans versus 5.3 percent; $P = 0.001$), and the difference persisted after adjustment for other factors as noted above (OR 0.21, 95 percent CI 0.06 to 0.68; $P = 0.01$). When comparison was restricted to those without a documented contraindication to tPA, the difference remained significant (OR 0.24, 95 percent CI 0.06 to 0.93; $P = 0.04$). The authors concluded that tPA is used infrequently for ischemic stroke at U.S. academic medical centers and that African Americans are significantly less likely to receive tPA. Contraindications to treatment did not appear to account for the difference.

A study was conducted of tPA treatment for ischemic stroke in 137 community hospitals in the United States from 1998 to 1999 involving 23,058 patients (Reed et al., 2001). It was found that African Americans were only approximately one-half as likely to be treated with tPA (OR 0.54, 95 percent CI 0.31 to 0.95). Taken together, these studies point to a nationwide racial disparity in tPA treatment of acute stroke.

Rehabilitation

Stroke units are helpful in improving outcome after stroke. For example, randomized clinical trials have shown that care of patients in stroke units reduces mortality, institutionalization and dependency (Stroke Unit Trialists' Collaboration, 1997). A meta-analysis of data from 19 randomized trials showed a reduction of death within a median follow-up of one year with an odds ratio of 0.83 (95 percent CI 0.69-0.98), combined outcome of death or dependency (odds ratio 0.69 [95 percent CI 0.59-0.82]) and death or institutionalization (odds ratio of 0.75 [95 percent CI 0.65-0.87]).

The definition of a stroke unit in the 19 studies mentioned above was variable and included acute care stroke units, rehabilitation stroke units to which patients were sent after acute care, and a combination of the latter two. It is felt by some of the investigators from this meta-analysis that the beneficial effect of a stroke unit is due to the rehabilitation component since the benefit in mortality is seen after one to two weeks. Only 2 of the 19 randomized trials were conducted in the United States, one in Chicago (Gordon & Kohn, 1966) and one in New York City (Feldman et al., 1962). Neither of these studies mentioned the race of the participants. Also these two studies compared rehabilitation units with regular medical care and did not assess the results from acute care stroke units. In one U.S. study comparing outcome following stroke in relation to characteristics of academic medical centers, they did not find a decrease in mortality for hospitals with acute care stroke units (Gillum & Johnston, 2001).

PREVENTION

Carotid Endarterectomy

Two large randomized studies, the North American Symptomatic Carotid Endarterectomy Trial (NASCET) and the Veterans Administration Symptomatic Trial (VAST), have shown the benefit of carotid endarterectomy in symptomatic patients with carotid stenosis treated surgically compared with medical management. The NASCET study enrolled patients with carotid artery stenosis and ipsilateral recent hemispheric or retinal TIA or nondisabling stroke. Patients with major strokes were not enrolled in these studies. In patients with 70–99 percent stenosis, risk of stroke over two years was 26 percent in medically treated patients and 9 percent in surgical patients. Major or fatal stroke occurrence was 13.1 percent in the former group and 2.5 percent in the latter. Of the 659 patients enrolled only about 3 percent were Black. The difference between surgical and medical treated patients in two years survival free of ipsilateral stroke declined with declining degree of stenosis. Patients with 90–99 percent stenosis showed a difference of 26 percent, while a difference of 18 percent was observed in those with 80–89 percent stenosis and only 12 percent in those with stenosis of 70–79 percent. There was a modest perioperative increase in risk of major stroke or death of 1.2 percent (North American Symptomatic Carotid Endarterectomy Trial Collaborators, 1991).

In the VAST study with a mean follow-up of 12 months, the risk of stroke or crescendo TIA was 19.4 percent with medical treatment and 7.7 percent with surgical treatment. This study was conducted at Veterans Administration hospitals and included 193 men with symptomatic stenosis of 50 percent or greater. The percentage of African Americans in the study was not reported (Mayberg et al., for the Veterans Affairs Cooperative Studies Program 309 Trialist Group, 1991). Based on the NASCET, VAST, and also the European Carotid Surgery Trial, carotid endarterectomy is strongly recommended in patients who have TIA and mild stroke within a six-month interval and stenosis of 70 percent or greater and who are good candidates for surgery (Moore et al., 1995).

Since benefit of carotid endarterectomy is dependent on a low rate of peri- and postoperative surgical complication, it is important to consider surgical experience. The AHA guidelines for carotid endarterectomy set a 5 percent surgical complication rate (i.e., combined death and /or stroke associated with the procedure) as a maximum acceptable risk in symptomatic patients. In a retrospective meta-analysis of surgical risk for endarterectomy at 12 academic medical centers which included 36 non-White patients out of a total of 697 patients, race was not associated with increased surgical risk (Goldstein et al., 1994). However, a complication rate of 7.3 percent for death and stroke was reported in that study. In a study of carotid endarterectomy among Medicare beneficiaries in Georgia in 1993, an outcome of severe stroke or death within 30 days postoperatively occurred in 3.3 percent of 184 non-White patients, of whom half were classified as African American. This compared with a rate of 2.9 percent in 1,761 White patients (Karp et al., 1998).

In the Asymptomatic Carotid Atherosclerosis Study (ACAS) the incidence of cerebral infarction was compared in patients with asymptomatic carotid artery stenosis receiving carotid endarterectomy versus medical management alone (Executive Committee for the Asymptomatic Carotid Atherosclerosis Study, 1995). In this study 1,662 patients were enrolled, of whom 3 percent were African American. In patients with 70 percent or more stenosis, the results showed a reduction in five-year risk of stroke from 11.0 percent to 5.1 percent in surgical compared to medical management alone. Women did not show the same level of positive response as men possibly due to a higher perioperative complication rate in women. There was a perioperative morbidity and mortality of less than 3 percent. Also, arteriography was not required for determination of degree of stenosis.

The small numbers of African Americans in the NASCET and ACAS studies may be due to more than one factor. African Americans may have a lower incidence of TIAs, which was one of the inclusion criteria for the study (Friday et al., 1989). In addition, African Americans in general have been underrepresented in clinical trials (Harris et al., 1996). It is believed, based on a number of case series, that African Americans have a lower percentage of extracranial carotid disease, which was a requirement for inclusion in the study (Wityk et al., 1996). However, in a population-based study, African Americans hospitalized for acute ischemic stroke were found to have a similar rate of extracranial atherosclerotic stroke as Whites and Hispanics (Sacco et al., 1995). Generally, it has also been found that African Americans receive endarterectomy at a lower rate than Whites. In 1985 and 1986, 188,000 carotid endarterectomies were performed in the United States, and only 2.7 percent of the patients were African American compared with 12 percent of hospital discharges and 12 percent of the population being African American (Maxwell et al., 1989).

In a study of carotid endarterectomy among Medicare beneficiaries in Georgia in 1993, it was found that only 4.8 percent of the patients were African American, while the racial distribution of all Medicare beneficiaries was approximately 22 percent African American (Karp et al., 1998). Possible explanations for this, in addition to those already mentioned, could include differences in access or financing of medical care, bias on the part of physicians in offering this option to the patient, or differences in patient willingness to undergo the procedure (Horner et al., 1995).

Based on a study of patient perceptions, it was found that among patients hospitalized with stroke or TIA, African American patients expressed more aversion to carotid endarterectomy than Whites (Oddone et al., 1998). It is likely that rapport is not established as readily in minority patients by majority health workers, especially when there is no personal physician advocate to intercede on the behalf of the patient.

In the secondary prevention of stroke, carotid endarterectomy has been shown to be effective in symptomatic patients with moderate and severe stenosis (>50 percent) as well as in asymptomatic patients with severe stenosis (>70 percent) on arteriography. African Americans in both clinical studies and clinical practice have been underrepresented in receiving this procedure. The risk of surgical complications does not appear to be greater in African Americans based on the small number of studies looking at risk and race, but more information is needed. Whether a benefit can be seen in African Americans with endarterectomy has not been clearly demonstrated in controlled clinical trials. It is unlikely that randomized trials will be performed in African Americans in the future, and therefore, information from other clinical trials will have to suffice.

STROKE OUTCOMES

Disability

African Americans may be more seriously ill initially after stroke (Heyman et al., 1972; Becker et al., 1986). They have been found to suffer more functional impairment according to the Barthel index, which measures daily activities of living such as walking, eating, and bathing. Their initial scores were only one-half of those of White patients. There was also slower improvement for Black patients. The investigators felt that delayed health care and a "worse risk profile" may have been reasons for greater initial impairment in Blacks (Horner et al., 1991). Additional study in this area is needed.

Access to Care

Traditionally, African Americans have had less access to medical care. This may be due to differences in the distribution of health-care insurance, discrimination against minorities in various aspects of medicine (e.g., utilization of procedures, treatments, and surgery), and lower rates of participation in clinical trials. Such inequalities have led to a deep mistrust of health institutions on the part of African Americans. In addition, African Americans face other barriers to health-care participation such as economic factors; social isolation; lack of awareness of disease risk factors, warning signs, and treatment programs; and communication barriers (Gorelick, 1998).

FUTURE DIRECTIONS AND NEEDS

Research

There has been increasing awareness that clinical research has historically not included sufficient numbers of minorities. This has been apparent for stroke research. Elijah Saunders (1995), in comments on the Antihypertensive and Lipid-lowering Trial to Prevent Heart Attack (ALLHAT) study, emphasized the importance of recruiting African American patients into clinical trials and the short-falls of extrapolating conclusions of studies in other populations to African Americans. Although he was referring to a study of hypertension and heart disease, this comment can also be applied to other diseases including stroke.

As an example of the problems that occur when performing research that excludes populations, the recommendations for aspirin in secondary prevention of stroke were based on studies that included few women and minorities. This resulted in uncertainty about indication of this therapy in women and minorities (McAnally et al., 1992).

National Institutes of Health (NIH) Research

The NIH has recognized the need to fund research that benefits all people (Healy, 1992). In 1986 the NIH issued guidelines for inclusion of women in clinical studies and in 1987 issued a policy encouraging inclusion of minorities in clinical studies. However, a 1990 GAO investigation found implementation of guidelines for women and minorities lacking (National Institutes of Health, NIH Tracking/Inclusion Committee, 2000). In 1990 the Office of Research on Women's Health (ORWH) was established with a mandate to ensure that minorities and women are included in NIH-supported clinical research (Pinn, 1994). In 1993 the NIH Revitalization Act was passed (National Institutes of Health Revitalization Act of 1993 [Public Law 103-43], 107, Stat.22 [codified at 42 U.S.C. 289.a-1], June 10, 1993, at 486[d] [4] [D]). This included provisions to ensure that women and minorities and their subpopulations were included in all human subject research, that women and minorities and their subpopulations were included in Phase III clinical trials in numbers adequate to allow for valid analyses of differences in intervention effect, that cost is not allowed as an acceptable reason for excluding these groups, and that the NIH initiate programs and support for outreach efforts to recruit and retain women and minorities and their subpopulations as volunteers in clinical studies. In 1994 new NIH guidelines for inclusion of women and minorities as subjects in clinical research were published in the *Federal Register* and went into effect in fiscal year 1995.

Selected examples of NIH-supported stroke clinical research over the past decade years show the effect of these measures on enrollment of minorities in NIH-supported stroke research. The North American Symptomatic Endarterectomy Trial (NASET) and the Asymptomatic Carotid Endarterectomy Study (ACAS) (both started in 1988) showed decreased risk of stroke in surgical versus medically treated patients with carotid artery stenosis (North American Symptomatic Carotid Endarterectomy Trial Collaborators, 1991; Executive Committee for the Asymptomatic Carotid Atherosclerosis Study, 1995). Only 3 percent of patients in these studies were African American. In 1996 tissue plasminogen activator was approved for treatment of acute ischemic stroke based on results of a NIH study of 624 patients of whom 30 percent were African American (National Institute of Neurological Disorders and Stroke rt-PA Stroke Study Group, 1995). In a post hoc analysis, a beneficial effect was also seen in the African American subgroup. A deliberate effort was made with this study to include adequate numbers of African Americans.

In 1998 enrollment in NIH-funded extramural research protocols included 32.2 percent men, 67 percent women, 54.8 percent White, 15.5 percent Black, 15.5 percent Asian, 7.8 percent Hispanic, and .9 percent American Indian (National Institutes of Health, NIH Tracking/Inclusion Committee, 2000).

Pharmaceutical Industry–Sponsored Research

The Food and Drug Administration (FDA) regulates drug research in the United States. The FDA encourages reporting of results by subgroups such as women and minorities. However, the FDA doses not require, as does the NIH, that women and minorities and their subpopulations be included in Phase III clinical trials in numbers adequate to allow for valid analyses of differences in intervention effect. In general, the percentage of African Americans in acute stroke studies sponsored by drug companies in the United States is close to the proportional representation in the overall population, but the numbers are usually too small to be able to draw a firm conclusion about efficacy.

In a safety study of a neuroprotective agent, tirilazad, there were 111 patients enrolled, of whom 84 percent were White (STIPAS Investigators, 1994). In the follow-up efficacy study with this drug 660 patients were enrolled, of whom 77 percent were White (RANTASS Investigators, 1996). In another study of a neuroprotective agent, lubeluzole, there were 1,786 patients enrolled, of whom 5 percent were Black (Diener et al., 2000). Because none of the many studies of neuroprotective agents had a positive result, there wasn't an issue of the effect in minorities. However, the trend for low numbers of minorities included in these pharmaceutical company–sponsored studies is disturbing.

Barriers to Participation in Clinical Trials by African Americans and Solutions

In a study of reasons for poor African American patient accrual in stroke research studies Harris et al. (1996) found the following barriers and suggested the following solutions:

- Lack of awareness about trials—speaker's bureau for churches and community organizations, community-based health fairs, church screenings, letters to private physicians, mass media, word of mouth
- Economic factors—travel reimbursement, accessible study site, extended office hours
- Communication issues—community-based information system, involvement of community members, information to community institutions and trusted individuals
- Mistrust—African American staff, involvement of African American representatives, show commitment, honesty, and patience

The NIH has listed five elements of outreach designed to increase retention and recruitment of minorities and women in clinical research (National Institutes of Health, NIH Outreach Notebook Committee, 1997).

- Understand the study population.
- Establish explicit goals for recruiting and retaining participants.
- Achieve agreement on research plans with investigators, medical and health-care staff, and community.
- Design and conduct evaluations to assess the efficacy of recruitment and retention strategies.

• Establish and maintain communications for keeping those involved in the study apprised of progress and study findings.

The NIH has shown progress in implementing policies to increase recruitment of minorities and women into clinical research that should lead to increases in representation of minorities and women in stroke research. The FDA has taken steps also but not to the extent of the NIH. Cultural sensitivity and participation of researchers within community groups and involvement of community groups in planning and implementation of research and having researchers from the community under investigation are important for enrolling adequate numbers of minorities in clinical stroke research.

GOVERNMENT POLICY

U.S. Goals for 2000 and 2010

Through an extensive consultative process in the late 1980s, the U.S. Department of Health and Human Services set a target goal for age-adjusted stroke mortality in Blacks for the year 2000 of 27 deaths per 100,000 (a nearly 50 percent decline from a 1987 baseline of 51.2). The 1996 rate for Blacks was 44.2, well short of the goal for 2000 (Figure 3.1). The two main goals for the year 2010 are eliminating (not merely reducing) health disparities among population groups together with increasing the years and quality of life (Gillum, 1999).

Stroke Act of 2002

The Stroke Treatment and Ongoing Prevention Act of 2002, passed by the Senate on February 6, 2002, provides programs for the prevention, treatment, and rehabilitation of stroke. This act recognizes African Americans as one of the high-risk groups for stroke and calls for research in disparities in the prevention, diagnosis, treatment, and rehabilitation of stroke among different populations.

SUMMARY

Stroke is the third leading cause of death in U.S. Black women and the sixth in Black men and an important cause of morbidity in Blacks. Mortality rates remain higher in Blacks than Whites in the United States. This situation will persist well into the twenty-first century. Strategies for primary and secondary prevention of stroke appropriate for particular segments of the Black population must be developed and vigorously implemented to reduce the burden of premature mortality and morbidity. Renewed efforts to prevent and control stroke risk factors, particularly elevated blood pressure, diabetes, and smoking, are urgently needed in the Black community. Increased research on stroke in Blacks is needed to develop more effective strategies for primary and secondary prevention of stroke to reduce the high burden of premature mortality and morbidity.

Access to medical care is a likely factor for excess stroke burden in African Americans. Therefore, access to medical care should be promoted at a national level because utilization of preventive services and treatments and maintenance of healthy lifestyles may lead to improvement in health outcomes.

In an editorial response to the paper on racial disparity in tPA treatment for stroke, it was recommended that "[w]hile further research may help us understand more specifically the racial disparity in stroke care, an education effort should take place immediately to identify and offer IV tPA treatment to appropriate Black stroke patients at all healthcare institutions. Perhaps a national initiative and registry specifically targeting the utilization of stroke care in minorities should be developed.

Policies, therefore, can be established to address the racial disparity in stroke care" (Wang, 2001, p. 1067). Also, as other new treatments for stroke are developed, we need to ensure that they are made available to African Americans and that we do not repeat the prior inequalities.

REFERENCES

Becker, C., et al. (1986). Community Hospital-Based Stroke Programs: North Carolina, Oregon, and New York, II: description of study population. *Stroke, 17*, 285–293.

Broderick, J., et al. (1998). The Greater Cincinnati/Northern Kentucky Stroke Study: Preliminary first-ever and total incidence rates of stroke among Blacks. *Stroke, 29*, 415–421.

Chiu, D., et al. (1998). Intravenous tissue plasminogen activator for acute ischemic stroke: Feasibility, safety, and efficacy in the first year of clinical practice. *Stroke, 29*, 18–22.

Cooper, R., Sempos, C., Hsieh, S.C., & Kovar, M.G. (1990). Slowdown of the decline of stroke mortality in the United States, 1978–1986. *Stroke, 21*, 1274–1279.

Diener, H.C., et al. (2000). Lubeluzole in Acute Ischemic Stroke Treatment: A double-blind study with an 8-hour inclusion window comparing a 10-mg daily dose of lubeluzole with placebo. *Stroke, 31*, 2543–2551.

Executive Committee for the Asymptomatic Carotid Atherosclerosis Study. (1995). Endarterectomy for asymptomatic carotid artery stenosis. *Journal of the American Medical Association, 273*, 1421–1428.

Feldman, D.J., Lee, P.R., Unterecker, J., Lloyd, K., Rusk, H.A., & Toole, A. (1962). A comparison of functionally oriented medical care and formal rehabilitation in the management of patients with hemiplegia due to cerebrovascular disease. *Journal of Chronic Disease, 15*, 297–310.

Friday, G., et al. (1989). Stroke in the Lehigh Valley: Racial/ethnic differences. *Neurology, 39*, 1165–1168.

Friday, G.H. (1994). *Cerebrovascular disease in Blacks.* In I. Livingston (Ed.), *Handbook of Black American health: The mosaic of conditions, issues, policies, and prospects* (pp. 33–45). Westport, CT: Greenwood Publishing.

Gaines, K., & Burke, G., for the SECORDS Investigators. (1995). Ethnic differences in stroke: Black–White differences in the United States population. *Neuroepidemiology, 14*, 209–239.

Gillum, R.F. (1997). Secular trends in stroke mortality in African Americans: The role of urbanization, diabetes and obesity. *Neuroepidemiology, 16*, 180–184.

Gillum, R.F. (1999). Stroke mortality in Blacks: Disturbing trends. *Stroke, 30*, 1711–1715.

Gillum, L.A., & Johnston, S.C. (2001). Characteristics of academic medical centers and ischemic stroke outcomes. *Stroke, 32*, 2137–2142.

Gillum, R.F., & Feinleib, M. (1993). Cardiovascular disease in the United States: Mortality, prevalence, and incidence. In A.S. Kapoor & B.N. Singh (Eds.), *Prognosis and risk assessment in cardiovascular disease* (pp. 49–59). New York: Churchill Livingston.

Gillum, R.F., & Sempos, C.T. (1997). The end of the long-term decline in stroke mortality in the United States? *Stroke, 28*, 1527–1529.

Goldstein, L.B., et al. (1994). Multicenter review of preoperative risk factors for carotid enardterectomy in patients with ipsilateral symptoms. *Stroke, 25*, 1116–1121.

Gordon, E.E., & Kohn, K.H. (1966). Evaluation of rehabilitation methods in the hemiplegic patient. *Journal of Chronic Disease, 19*, 3–16.

Gorelick, P.B. (1998). Cerebrovascular disease in African Americans. *Stroke, 29*, 2656–2664.

Harris, Y., Gorelick, P.B., Samuels, P., & Bempong, I. (1996). Why African Americans may not be participating in clinical trials. *Journal of the National Medical Association, 88*, 630–634.

Healy, B. (1992). Narrowing the gender gap in biomedical research. *Journal of Myocardial Ischemia, 4*, 14–37.

Heyman, A., Fields, W.S., & Keating, R.D. (1972). Joint study of extracranial arterial occlusion. *Journal of the American Medical Association, 222*, 285–289.

Horner, R.D., Matchar, D.B., Divine, G.W., & Feussner, J.R. (1991). Racial variations in ischemic stroke–related physical and functional impairments. *Stroke, 22*, 1497–1501.

Horner, R.D., Oddone, E.Z., & Matchar, D.B. (1995). Theories explaining racial differences in the utilization of diagnostic and therapeutic procedures for cerebrovascular disease. *Milbank Quarterly, 73*, 443–462.

Johnston, S.C., et al. (2001). Utilization of intravenous tissue-type plasminogen activator for ischemic stroke at academic medical centers: The influence of ethnicity. *Stroke, 32,* 1061–1068.

Karp, H.R., Flanders, W.D., Shipp, C.C., Taylor, B., & Martin, D. (1998). Carotid endarterectomy among Medicare beneficiaries: A statewide evaluation of appropriateness and outcome. *Stroke, 29,* 46–52.

Maxwell, G.J., et al. (1989). Infrequency of Blacks among patients having carotid endarterectomy. *Stroke, 20,* 22–26.

May, D.S., & Kittner, S.J. (1994). Use of Medicare claims data to estimate national trends in stroke incidence, 1985–1991. *Stroke, 25,* 2343–2347.

Mayberg, M.R., et al. for the Veterans Affairs Cooperative Studies Program 309 Trialist Group. (1991). Carotid endarterectomy and prevention of cerebral ischemia in symptomatic carotid stenosis. *Journal of the American Medical Association, 266,* 3289–3294.

McAnally, L.E., Corn, C.R., & Hamilton, S.F. (1992). Aspirin for the prevention of vascular death in women. *Public Health Nursing, 9,* 242–7.

Minino, A.M., Arias, E., Kochanek, R.D., Murphy, S.L., & Smith, B.L. (2002, September 16). Deaths: Final data for 2000. *National Vital Statistics Report, 50*(15).

Moore, W.S., et al. (1995). Guidelines for carotid endarterectomy: A multidisciplinary consensus statement from the Ad Hoc Committee, American Heart Association. *Circulation, 91,* 566–579.

National High Blood Pressure Education Program. The Sixth Report of the Joint National Committee on Prevention, Detection, Evaluation, and Treatment of High Blood Pressure. National Institutes of Health. NIH Pub. No. 98–4080, November 1997.

National Institute of Neurological Disorders (NINDS) and Stroke rt-PA Stroke Study Group. (1995). Tissue plasminogen activator for acute ischemic stroke. *New England Journal of Medicine, 333,* 1581–1587).

National Institutes of Health, NIH Outreach Notebook Committee. Outreach notebook for the NIH guidelines on inclusion of women and minorities as subjects in clinical research (NIH Pub.No. 97–4160). Bethesda, MD: National Institutes of Health 1997.

National Institutes of Health, NIH Tracking/Inclusion Committee. Monitoring adherence to the NIH policy on the inclusion of women and minorities as subjects in clinical research. Comprehensive report (Fiscal Years 1997–1998 Tracking Data). Bethesda, MD: National Institutes of Health. September 1, 2000.

NINDS t-PA Stroke Study Group. (1997). Generalized efficacy of t-PA for acute stroke: Subgroup analysis of the NINDS t-PA stroke trial. *Stroke, 28,* 2119–2125.

North American Symptomatic Carotid Endarterectomy Trial Collaborators. (1991). Beneficial effect of carotid endarterectomy in symptomatic patients with high-grade carotid stenosis. *New England Journal of Medicine, 325,* 445–453.

Oddone, E.Z., et al. (1998). Understanding racial variation in the use of carotid endarterectome: the role of aversion to surgery. *Journal of the National Mededical Association, 90,* 25–33.

Pinn, V.W. (1994). The role of the NIH's Office of Research on Women's Health. *Academic Medicine, 69,* 698–702.

RANTASS Investigators. (1996). A randomized trial of tirilazad mesylate in patients with acute stroke (RANTASS). *Stroke, 27,* 1453–1458.

Reed, S.D., Cramer, S.C., Blough D.K., Meyer, K., Jarvick J.G., & Wang D.Z. (2001). Treatment with tissue plasminogen activator and inpatient mortality rates for patients with ischemic stroke treated in community hospitals. *Stroke, 32,* 1832–1840.

Sacco, R.L., et al. (2001). Race-ethnic disparities in the impact of stroke risk factors: The Northern Manhattan Stroke Study. *Stroke, 32,* 1725–1731.

Sacco, R.L., et al. for the Northern Manhattan Stroke Study Collaborators. (1998). Stroke incidence among Whites, Black and Hispanic residents of an urban community: The Northern Manhattan Stroke Study. *American Journal of Epidemiology, 147,* 259–268.

Sacco, R.L., Kargman, D.E., Gu, Q., & Zamanillo, M.C. (1995). Race-ethnicity and determinants of intracranial atherosclerotic cerebral infarction: The Northern Manhattan Stroke Study. *Neurology, 26,* 14–20.

Saunders, E. (1995). Recruitment of African-American patients for clinical trials—the Allhat challenges. Antihypertensive and Lipid-lowering Trial to Prevent Heart Attack. *Journal of the National Medical Association, 87,* (8 Suppl): 627–629.

STIPAS Investigators. (1994). Safety study of tirilazad mesylate in patients with acute ischemic stroke (STI-PAS). *Stroke, 25*, 418–423.

Stroke Unit Trialists' Collaboration. (1997). Collaborative systemic review of the randomized trials of organised in-patient (stroke unit) care after stroke. *British Medical Journal, 314*, 1151–1159.

Wang, D.Z. (2001). It is time to implement stroke practice improvement programs and prevent the racial disparity in stroke care. *Stroke, 32*, 1061–1068.

Wityk, R.J., Lehman, D., Klag, M., Coresh, J., Ahn, H., & Litt, B. (1996). Race and sex differences in the distribution of cerebral atherosclerosis. *Stroke, 27*, 1974–1980.

CHAPTER 4

Hypertension: A Community Perspective

KEITH NORRIS AND DAVID MARTINS

INTRODUCTION

Hypertension or high blood pressure is a persistent and frequently progressive elevation in systolic and/or diastolic blood pressure. The level of blood pressure at which the diagnosis of hypertension is made is in evolution. The current classification of blood pressure as recommended in the sixth report of the Joint National Committee on Prevention, Detection, Evaluation, and Treatment of high blood pressure is shown in Table 4.1.

High blood pressure is a major risk factor for cardiovascular and vascular-related disease. The detection, treatment, and control of high blood pressure have been shown to reduce the risk of cardiovascular and vascular-related morbidity and mortality. Cardiovascular disease remains the leading cause of death in the nation, in part because most people with high blood pressure are still undetected, untreated, and/or uncontrolled (Burt et al., 1995). In spite of efforts at local and national levels to eliminate disparities in health and disease, there are significant racial and ethnic differences in the distribution of high blood pressure and its associated cardiovascular morbidity and mortality. In this chapter we examine the basis for some of these differences in racial and ethnic minorities with particular emphasis on the African American community. We also review strategies and programs, at both the individual and community levels, that are aimed at reducing the disproportionate burden of hypertension and its cardiovascular consequences in the community.

EPIDEMIOLOGY OF HYPERTENSION

Although the prevalence of hypertension varies with age and sex, it is estimated that 23 percent of adult Americans between the ages of 20 and 74 have hypertension. About 75 percent of women aged 75 and over have hypertension, and about 64 percent of men aged 75 and over have hypertension. At all ages and in both sexes African Americans have the highest prevalence of hypertension (NCHS, 2003). In African Americans hypertension tends to develop at an earlier age and tends to be more severe than in other racial/ethnic groups. In fact, a twofold to threefold increase in the prevalence of stage 3 hypertension has been reported among African Americans (Vaccaro et al., 1998). There is a direct relationship between the blood pressure level and the risk of stroke and

Table 4.1
The classification of blood pressure for adults

Blood Pressure Category	Blood Pressure Reading, mmHg	
Normal Range	Systolic	Diastolic
Optimal	< 120	< 80
Normal	120-129	80-84
High Normal	130-139	85-89
Hypertensive Range		
Stage 1	140-159	90-99
Stage 2	160-179	100-109
Stage 3	≥180	≥110

Source: Joint National Committee. *The Sixth Report on Prevention, Detection, Evaluation and Treatment of High Blood Pressure,* 1997.

coronary heart disease (MacMohon et al., 1990). Elevated blood pressure is also a major risk factor for heart failure and end-stage renal disease (World Health Organization-International Society of Hypertension, 1999; Martins et al., 2002). African Americans exhibit a greater increase in target organ damage than other ethnic minorities. The heart disease mortality rate is 50 percent higher, stroke mortality rate is 80 percent higher, and the incidence of hypertension-related end-stage renal disease is 320 percent higher in African Americans (Norris & Francis, 2000). In the African American community women have the highest mortality rates from stroke and coronary artery disease (American Heart Association, 2003).

It is apparent that hypertension, along with its cardiovascular morbidity and mortality, is an even greater challenge for the African American community than it is for the rest of the nation. Many of the factors responsible for the disparities in the incidence, prevalence, detection, treatment, and control of hypertension have been well described. These findings can be useful in the design and development of programs and policies targeted to the diagnosis and control of hypertension within the population. Public health strategies that incorporate these factors may alleviate some of the disproportionate burden of hypertension and its consequences within the African American community.

Review of Causative Factors

Blood pressure is a continuous variable determined by multiple factors and demonstrates a fairly normal distribution within the population. Family and twin studies suggest that only about 30–50 percent of the blood pressure variation in the general population can be explained by genetic factors (Lifton, 1996). It is our current understanding that elevated blood pressure reflects a complex interaction between genetic and environmental factors. The development of hypertension appears to require a genetic predisposition and/or an environmental precipitation. The search for specific genes responsible for hypertension has resulted in the discovery of some rare genetic causes of high and low blood pressure (Harrap, 1999), but the clear identification of a genetic basis of essential hypertension accounting for the disproportionately high prevalence in the African American community remains elusive.

Several lifestyle and environmental risk factors for hypertension have been identified with impor-

**Table 4.2
Lifestyle and
environmental risk factors
for hypertension**

| **Excess Body Fat** |
| High Sodium Intake |
| Low Potassium Intake |
| Physical Inactivity |
| Excess Alcohol Intake |
| Psychosocial Stress |

Source: Joint National Committee. *The Sixth Report on Prevention, Detection, Evaluation and Treatment of High Blood Pressure*, 1997.

tant differences among ethnic minorities within the population (see Table 4.2). Excess body fat, particularly in the upper body, is an important risk factor for hypertension. Excess body fat whether expressed as overweight or obesity is more common among African Americans (Flegal et al., 2002). Dietary salt intake in the form of sodium chloride has been associated with the level of blood pressure and the rise in blood pressure with age. As a group African Americans are more sensitive to changes in dietary salt intake (Elliott et al., 1996). Low potassium intake has been associated with hypertension, and there is evidence that high dietary potassium particularly in the form of fresh fruits and vegetables may protect from hypertension and perhaps reduce the need for antihypertensive drug therapy (Appel et al., 1997). Subgroup examination of the large meta-analysis of randomized controlled clinical trials on the effects of oral potassium on blood pressure suggests that the beneficial effects of high potassium intake may be enhanced in African Americans (Whelton et al., 1997).

Physical inactivity is a risk factor for hypertension and cardiovascular mortality. The American College of Sports Medicine recommends 20 to 60 minutes of rhythmical and aerobic large-muscle activity such as walking, running, and cycling three to five days a week for blood pressure control and cardiorespiratory fitness. More than 60 percent of U.S. adults do not engage in the recommended amount of activity, and about 25 percent are totally inactive. Physical inactivity is more common among older adults, women, less affluent people, Hispanic, and African American adults (CDC, 1999).

There are many reported psychosocial and health benefits of limited regular alcohol intake. However, the intake of three or more standard drinks of alcohol per day has been associated with serious adverse psychosocial and health consequences including hypertension. A standard drink of alcohol defined as about 14 grams of ethanol is contained in 1.5 ounces of distilled spirit, 5 ounce glass of table wine, and a 12-ounce glass of beer. Current estimates indicate that 62 percent of Americans ages 18 and over admitted to alcohol intake in the year 2000, and 32 percent had five or more drinks on the same occasion at least once in that year. Many of these Americans were African Americans (NCHS, 2003).

The low educational status and high unemployment rate prevalent among minority populations in the United States predispose African American communities to adverse political and socioeconomic conditions that contribute to environmental and psychosocial stress. Acute stress can transiently raise blood pressure, while chronic stress has been associated with sustained hypertension (Anderson, 1989). The contributory role of chronic stress to the development of hypertension is best illustrated by studies of job strain. The job-strain model of psychosocial conflict is specifically designed to assess occupational stress. The model employs work-related demands and the decision latitude of the workers to characterize jobs into high- and low-strain jobs. Workers with high decision latitudes are thought to have little or no distress because they have more flexibility in deciding how best to meet their work-related demands. The jobs most likely to cause distress are hypothesized to be those that combine high demands with low decision latitudes (Karasek et al., 1981).

National health surveys have shown that men in occupations high in demands and low in decision latitudes are more likely to have had a myocardial infarction (Karasek et al., 1988). Men employed in these typically blue-collar jobs have a threefold increase in hypertension, and those who remain in them for three or more years have a blood pressure that is 11/7mmHg higher than men in low-strain jobs. Hypertension has been suggested as the most likely mechanism by which job strain might cause coronary heart disease (Schnall et al., 1994).

Indigent lives and disfranchisement from the health-care system are notable contributors to psychosocial stress in African Americans. Some investigators have suggested that the increased incidence of hypertension in African Americans was due largely to internalized demands arising from socioeconomic stresses (Waitzman & Smith, 1994; Keil et al., 1977; Krieger & Sidney, 1996). This phenomenon is frequently termed "active coping" or "John Henryism." The Charleston Heart Study revealed an increased incidence of hypertension associated with darker skin color in African Americans (Keil et al., 1977). However, this association was abolished when adjusted for social class. Klag and associates reported an increased incidence of hypertension associated with darker skin color only in subjects in the lower levels of socioeconomic status, further supporting the overarching influence of environmental factors on blood pressure in African Americans (Klag et al., 1991).

Genetic and biologic differences may influence the distribution of the burden of hypertension within a population. The prevailing body of evidence seems to suggest that lifestyle and socioeconomic disparities have more influence on the prevalence of hypertension than genetic or biologic differences. Furthermore, the excess risk of hypertension in African Americans is more strongly linked to being born and living in the United States than with African ancestry. The greater burden of hypertension and its related cardiovascular morbidity and mortality within the African American population may in part be due to the greater probability of unemployment, low income, and high-strain occupational status within the community.

RECOMMENDATIONS

Primary Prevention

The rise in blood pressure with age and the higher prevalence of hypertension have been associated with weight gain, physical inactivity, excessive alcohol consumption, and high sodium and low potassium intake. Two complementary disease prevention models have been advocated for the primary prevention of hypertension (National High Blood Pressure Education Program Working Group Report on Primary Prevention of Hypertension, 1993). The first model directs the intervention at the population and aims to shift the blood pressure distribution curve downward. It has been estimated that a 2mmHg downward shift in the distribution of systolic blood pressure within the population could lower annual all-cause cardiovascular mortality by about 3 percent, with 4 percent and 6 percent reductions in annual mortality from stroke and coronary heart disease, respectively. The second model advocates targeting the intervention to groups most likely to develop hypertension within the population. Such targeted strategies should be aimed at "high-risk" populations such as African Americans and persons with additional cardiovascular risk factors and/or high normal blood pressure levels.

Strategies for Primary Prevention.   The strategies for the primary prevention of hypertension should focus on exercise and dietary changes and should be instituted in childhood and adolescence before the habitual dietary indiscretion and physical inactivity responsible for most of the obesity and overweight in adulthood are established.

Dietary Modification.   Dietary patterns high in fruits and vegetables and low in saturated fat and sweets have been shown to lower blood pressure and may reduce the rise in blood pressure with age. The beneficial effects of fruits and vegetables have been partly attributed to the high potassium and low sodium content of most fruits and vegetables. Although there is no evidence that excessive dietary fat directly raises blood pressure, increased serum levels of saturated fats such as low-density lipoproteins and cholesterol have been shown to add significantly to the risk of cardiovascular disease and death in patients with hypertension. The ingestion of high carbohydrate sweets and refined sugars may contribute to caloric excess and weight gain.

The high intake of salt and sugar in the developed countries is a direct consequence of the consumption of processed food. The successful implementation of dietary changes will require an active involvement of the food industry. It will be critical to reduce the salt and sugar content of processed foods. The food labels should provide an accurate and complete listing of content so that the consumers can make informed decisions on their consumption of processed food. Restaurants and meal service agencies should provide their customers with information on the salt, sugar, and saturated fat contents of their food selections. All food vendors should be encouraged and supported to promote food items lower in salt and sugar. The mass media can be used to educate and disseminate information on the role of dietary habits in the risk of developing hypertension.

Physical Activity.   Physical activity has been shown to lower blood pressure and to limit the rise in blood pressure with age. The benefits of physical activity require aerobic and rhythmic large muscle group activities such as walking, swimming, and cycling as recommended by the American College of Sports Medicine. Although the basis for the beneficial effects of physical activity is unknown, the decrease in cardiac output and peripheral resistance associated with regular physical activity may play a role.

The role of regular moderate physical activity in the maintenance of healthy weight and the prevention of hypertension need to be publicized in the community. Environmental inducement to physical activities, such as sidewalks with curb cuts and trails for cycling should be provided to high-risk communities. Physical activities should be encouraged within protected locations such as malls in bad weather. The use of schools is also effective in many instances, especially for adolescents. One semester of aerobic exercise reduced systolic blood pressure more than the standard physical education in high-risk (BP > 67th percentile), predominantly African American adolescent girls, reinforcing specialized physical education in the school setting as a feasible and effective health promotion strategy for high-risk adolescent girls (Ewart et al., 1998). The need for lifetime commitment to the adopted mode of exercise should be emphasized in the promotion of physical activity.

Secondary Prevention

The objectives of secondary prevention in persons with established diagnosis of hypertension are early detection and treatment. Early diagnosis and control of hypertension have been shown to reduce the cardiovascular mortality and morbidity associated with hypertension. Data from the third National Health and Nutrition Examination Survey (NHANES III) indicate that 32 percent of persons with hypertension are not aware of the disease, 15 percent are aware but are not receiving treatment, and only 45 percent that are aware and receiving treatment are controlled, leaving an estimated 76 percent of overall hypertensive persons in the United States with uncontrolled blood pressure levels (Burt et al., 1995). Subgroup analysis suggests that African American patients are less likely to be aware of the diagnosis of hypertension and more likely to be uncontrolled (Hyman & Pavlik, 2001). The

Table 4.3
Barriers to the diagnosis and control of hypertension

PATIENT-RELATED BARRIERS
Lack of awareness about consequences of hypertension
Lack of access to consumer medical information
Later diagnosis and greater burden of disease at diagnosis
Living in disadvantaged neighborhood
Inadequate resources to support healthy lifestyle choices
Inadequate recreational activity and facilities
Distrust of the medical establishment
Adverse medication reaction
PHYSICIAN-RELATED BARRIERS
Lower expectancy for favorable outcome for African American patients with hypertension
Limited evidence-based guidelines for treating hypertension in African Americans
Limited data to guide treatment decisions secondary to poor recruitment of African Americans into clinical trials
Failure to treat hypertension early and aggressively to target blood pressure goals
Low recognition of the greater prevalence of co-morbid disease(s) that require greater extent of medical intervention

Source: Adapted from J.G. Douglas, K.C. Ferdinand, G.L. Bakris, and J.R. Sowers, Barriers to blood pressure control in African-Americans, *Postgraduate Medicine* 112 (4) (2002): 51–70.

factors that perpetuate the unawareness and poor control of hypertension, particularly among African Americans, have been identified and characterized as shown in Table 4.3. Strategies for secondary prevention of hypertension must be aimed at overcoming the long and lengthening list of barriers to the diagnosis and control of hypertension.

Strategies for Secondary Prevention

The social context in which African Americans live and receive health care needs to be better understood in order to improve the cardiovascular outcome for African American patients with hypertension. Specific educational programs targeted to the community of patients and the providers responsible for their care can transcend most of the barriers to the diagnosis and control of hypertension. The education of the public and health providers on the disproportionate burden of hypertension and its associated cardiovascular risk in the African American community will raise awareness, mobilize the community of patients and providers, and foster patient–provider alliances needed for the elimination of the barriers to the diagnosis and control of hypertension. The Baltimore Alliance for the Prevention and Control of Hypertension and Diabetes, established to promote care and improve outcomes of hypertension and diabetes to the underserved community of West Baltimore and Maryland, is an example of this type of collaborate effort. This extensive collaboration of university, community health programs, church-based groups, managed care organizations, pharmaceutical companies, health policy and services research group is currently under evaluation and should better address cultural relevance and hopefully lead to improved outcomes in these communities (Gerber & Stewart, 1998).

Community Education

Community-based blood pressure screening programs should be staffed by individuals trained in accurate blood pressure measurement and experienced in the assessment and counseling of persons with high blood pressure. The use of registered nurses as church health educators led to a significant increase in knowledge scores and improved blood pressure levels from pre- to post-testing (Smith et al., 1997). The screening programs should be sponsored and supported by neighborhood health-care facilities that could serve as ready and accessible centers for referral and follow-up for persons with high blood pressure. The counseling for persons with high blood pressure and established diagnosis of hypertension should address the importance of dietary discretion, medication adherence, clinic attendance, smoking cessation and regular moderate physical activity in the control of blood pressure. Multiple counseling sessions may be required to emphasize and reaffirm the lifestyle changes required for blood pressure control.

A program of cardiovascular nutrition counseling every four months has been shown to reduce systolic blood pressure by about 7–11mmHg and diastolic blood pressure by about 4–7mmHg (Kumanyika et al., 1999). These educational programs can be conducted in town halls, city halls, senior citizen centers, barbershops, beauty salons, and local religious and educational institutions.

The church and local establishments such as barbershops have been particularly effective partners in the African American community for implementing health-care strategies. A church-based high blood pressure program for African American women led to improved blood pressure control in over 70 percent of participants and sustained weight loss in over 65 percent (Kumanyika & Charleston, 1992). A comprehensive work-site health promotion program among 4,000 city of Birmingham employees significantly reduced systolic blood pressure in African American participants. This study suggests that educational intervention tailored to the specific health perceptions and working conditions of a low literacy population is feasible and is an effective way to improve hypertension control (Fouad et al., 1997).

Community-wide intervention efforts and messages were shown to improve cardiovascular risk factor knowledge in a biracial South Carolina community with a low level of education. The greater changes observed among White adults in most of the behaviors and knowledge in this study support the need for different strategies to reach African Americans (Smith et al., 1996). Thus, community-based programs at various locations where people congregate such as churches, barbershops, beauty salons, firehouses, housing projects, and work sites can play a valuable role in improving cardiovascular health for African Americans (Kong, 1997). The involvement of the local media and local organizations should be sought and supported. Preprogram publicity ensures that the invitation to participate reaches the community at large. Live broadcast of counseling sessions ensures that the education reaches those who may not be able to attend. The incorporation of live question-and-answer sessions with panels of counselors invites and encourages the participation of the community. Actively engaging the community at multiple levels may be an effective strategy to promote and sustain responsible health decisions (Figure 4.1). The impact of programmatic activities in community education high blood pressure programs should be assessed using validated tools to ensure their effectiveness (Martins et al., 2001).

Provider Education

There is evidence that targeted clinic and office-based intervention programs can be incorporated into care plans for high-risk patients without disrupting the health care delivery. A community-oriented primary care approach for the detection, treatment, and control of hypertension was effective in every race-sex stratum of hypertensive patients utilizing a neighborhood health center; a particularly good response was noted for men and for African Americans (O'Connor et al., 1990).

Figure 4.1
Circle of influence model for health promotion

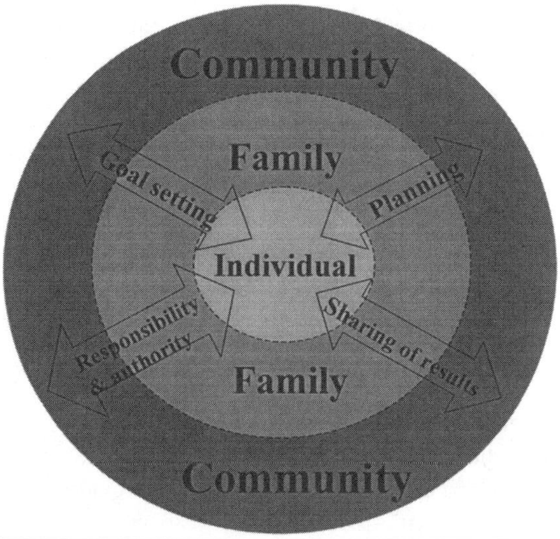

Source: This model was developed by L. Jones, D.S. Martins,
Y. Pardo, R. Baker, & K.C. Norris, © 2002.

Note: Community includes providers, health care agencies, and
so on.

Practice-based programs should seek active participation of both the patient and the provider. Lifestyle change goals and processes should be set and mutually agreed upon by both the patient and the provider. The recommendations for weight control, dietary salt reduction, moderation of alcohol intake, and regular physical activity should be provided in specific detail and design to suit the patient. The medication regimen should be simple and appropriate to provide for affordability, adherence, and efficacy. The patients should be forewarned about notable anticipated medication side effects. The provider should provide the patient with explanations and reasonable expectations for side effects that may interfere with quality of life as perceived by the patient. The use of home and herbal remedies should be explored because some of them may interfere with the control of blood pressure in patients with good medication adherence.

African American physician groups with expertise and experience in the treatment and control of hypertension in African American patients should make their knowledge and experience available in culturally and linguistically appropriate audiovisual formats. These materials could be distributed to providers responsible for the care of African American patients with hypertension, especially in local communities where midlevel providers provide most of the health-care services. Similar strategies are critical for other racial/ethnic groups within our nation. The participation of the providers in organizations dedicated to the issues of hypertension and its cardiovascular risk should be encouraged and supported. Scientific facts from annual meetings of these organizations should be made available in simple lay language to patients and providers in high-risk communities.

CONCLUSION

The education of the individual, family members, the health-care provider, and the community remains an essential component of both primary and secondary preventive strategies targeted at

African Americans. The incorporation of trusted and respected local establishments such as schools, barbershops, beauty salons, social clubs, and churches fosters and facilitates the awareness of hypertension and its cardiovascular risk in African American communities.

The use of local group settings and associated resources can often reinforce the health message with regard to appropriate diet, weight control, exercise, and high blood pressure control in a culturally sensitive manner that can seldom be duplicated in structured government-developed programs (Dressler et al., 1998; Shakoor-Abdullah et al., 1997). When feasible, the programs should be delivered in comprehensive cardiovascular risk reduction packages that include smoking cessation, moderation of alcohol intake, nutritional counseling, regular physical activities, and blood pressure screening. Such program packages, however, are unlikely to be sustained effectively without external resources in a predominantly minority setting (Shea et al., 1996).

Physicians, nurses, and other health-care professionals should be encouraged to lead and/or participate in these programs. They can often be invaluable resources for many medically related questions and concerns within the community. Secondary preventive measures can also be addressed through community programs, since most of these community-based risk reduction strategies will mirror those of primary prevention. Improving patients' knowledge of proven interventions to reduce blood pressure can stimulate them to enter into a more detailed dialogue with their primary care provider and hopefully improve their health. Since there is no evidence to support a different secondary prevention goal for African Americans in contrast to whites, it is important that health-care providers and health management systems make specific secondary prevention therapies widely available. Hopefully, by using innovative individual/family and community-based approaches for primary and secondary cardiovascular risk prevention with a focus on hypertension, we will soon see significant improvements in the health of the African American community.

NOTE

This research was supported by grants U54RR14616 and P20-RR11145 from the National Center for Research Resources, National Institutes of Health.

REFERENCES

American Heart Association (AHA). (2003). *Heart and Stroke Statistics—2004 Update*.

Anderson, N.B. Dallas Texas: American Heart Association. (1989). Racial differences in stress-induced cardiovascular reactivity and hypertension. Current status and substantive issues. *Psychological Bulletin, 105*, 89–105.

Appel, L.J., Moore, T.J., Obarzanek, E., Vollmer, W.M., Svetkey, L.P., Sacks, F.M., Bray, G.A., Vogt, T.M., Cutler, J.A., Windhauser, M.M., Lin, P.H., & Karanja, N. (1997). A clinical trial of the effects of dietary patterns on blood pressure. DASH Collaborative Research Group. *New England Journal of Medicine, 336*, 1117–1124.

Burt, V.L., Cutler, J.A., Higgins, M., Horan, M.J., Labarthe, D., Whelton, P., Brown, C., & Roccella, E.J. (1995). Trends in prevalence, awareness, treatment, and control of hypertension in the adult U.S. population: Data from the health examination surveys, 1960 to 1991. *Hypertension, 26*, 60–69.

Centers for Disease Control and Prevention (CDC). (1999). *National Physical Activity Initiative Fact Sheet*. Atlanta, GA: National Center for Chronic Disease Prevention.

Dressler, W.W., Bindon, J.R., & Neggers, Y.H. (1998). Culture, socioeconomic status, and coronary heart disease risk factors in an African American community. *Journal of Behavioral Medicine, 21(6)*, 527–544.

Elliott, P., et al., for the Intersalt Cooperative Reasearch Group. (1996). Intersalt revisited: further analyses of 24 hour sodium excretion and blood pressure within and across populations. *British Medical Journal, 312*, 1249–1253.

Ewart, C.K., Young, D.R., & Hagberg, J.M. (1998). Effects of school-based aerobic exercise on blood pressure in adolescent girls at risk for hypertension. *American Journal of Public Health, 88(6)*, 949–951.

Flegal, K.M., Carrol, M.D., Ogden, C.L., & Johnson, C.L. (2002). Prevalence and trends in obesity among U.S. adults. *Journal of American Medical Association, 288*, 1723–1727.

Fouad, M.N., Kiefe, C.I., Bartolucci, A.A., Burst M.N., Ulene, V., & Harvey, M.R. (1997). A hypertension control program tailored to unskilled and minority workers. *Ethnicity & Disease, 7(3)*, 191–199.

Gerber, J.C., & Stewart, D.L. (1998). Prevention and control of hypertension and diabetes in an underserved population through community outreach and disease management: A plan of action. *Journal of Association for Academic Minority Physicians, 9(3)*, 48–52.

Harrap, S.B. (1999). Known major genetic causes of high and low blood pressure. Genetics. In Oparil et al. (eds.), *Hypertension:companion to Brenner and Rector's The Kidney*. Philadelphia: W.B. Saunders.

Hyman, D.J., & Pavlik, V.N. (2001). Characteristics of patients with uncontrolled hypertension in the United States. *New England Journal of Medicine, 345(7)*, 479–486.

Intersalt Cooperative Research Group. (1996). Intersalt revisited; further analysis of 24 hour sodium excretion and blood pressure within and across population. *British Medical Journal, 312*, 1249–1253.

Joint National Committee (JNC). (1997). *Sixth Report on Prevention, Detection, Evaluation and Treatment of High Blood Pressure*. NIH Publication Number 98-4080.

Karasek, R.A., Theorell, T., Schwartz, J.E., Schnall, P.L., Pieper, C.F., & Michela, J.L. (1988). Job characteristics in relation to the prevalence of myocardial infarction. The U.S. Health Examination Survey (HES) and the Health and Nutrition Examination Survey (HANES). *American Journal of Public Health, 78*, 910–918.

Karasek, R.A., Baker, D., Marxer, F., Ahlbohm, A., & Theorell, T. (1981). Job decision latitude, job demands, and cardiovascular disease: A prospective study of Swedish men. *American Journal of Public Health, 75*, 694–705.

Keil, J.E., Tyroler, H.A., Sandifer, S.H., & Boyle, E., Jr. (1977). Hypertension: Effects of social class and racial admixture. *American Journal of Public Health, 64*, 634–639.

Klag, M.J., Whelton, P.K., Coresh, J., Grim, C.E., & Kuller, L.H. (1991). The association of skin color with blood pressure in U.S. Blacks with low socioeconomic status. *Journal of American Medical Association, 265*, 599–602.

Kong, B.W. (1997). Community-based hypertension control programs that work. *Journal of Health Care for the Poor and Underserved, 8(4)*, 409–415.

Krieger, N., & Sidney, S. (1996). Racial discrimination and blood pressure: The CARDIA Study of young Black and White adults. *American Journal of Public Health, 86(10)*, 1370–1378.

Kumanyika, S.K., Adams-Campbell, L., Van Horn, B., Ten Have, T.R., Treu, J.A., Askov, E., Williams, J., Achterberg, C., Zaghloul, S., Monsegu, D., Bright, M., Stoy, D.B., Malone-Jackson, M., Mooney, D., Deiling, S., & Caulfield, J. (1999). Outcomes of cardiovascular nutrition counseling program in African Americans with elevated blood pressure or cholesterol level. *Journal of American Dietetic Association, 99(11)*, 1380–1391.

Kumanyika, S.K., & Charleston, J.B. (1992). Lose weight and win: A church-based weight loss program for blood pressure control among Black women. *Patient Education and Counseling, 19(1)*, 19–32.

Lifton, R.P. Molecular genetics of human blood pressure variation. (1996). *Science, 272*, 676–80.

Livingston, I.L. (1993). Stress, hypertension and young Black Americans: The importance of counseling. *Journal of Multicultural Counseling, 4*, 132–142.

MacMohon, S., Peto, R., & Cutler, J. (1990). Blood pressure, stroke and coronary heart disease. Part 1. Prolonged differences in blood pressure; prospective observational studies corrected for regression dilutional bias. *Lancet, 335*, 765–774.

Martins, D., Gor, D., Teklehaimanot, S., & Norris, K.C. (2001). High blood pressure knowledge in an urban African-American community. *Ethnicity & Disease, 11*, 90–96.

Martins, D., Tareen, N., & Norris, K.C. (2002). The epidemiology of chronic renal disease in African Americans. *American Journal of Medical Sciences, 323(2)*, 65–71.

National Center for Health Statistics. (2000). *Health, United States* table 67. Hyattsville, MD: NCHS.

National Center for Health Statistics. (2000). *Health, United States* table 68. Hyattsville, MD: NCHS.

National Center for Health Statistics. (2003). *Health, United States, 2003 with chartbook on trends in the health of Americans*. Hyattsville, MD: NCHS.

National High Blood Pressure Education Program Working Group Report on Primary Prevention of Hypertension. (1993). *Archives of Internal Medicine, 153*, 186–208.

Norris, K.C., & Francis, C.K. (2000). Gender and ethnic differences and considerations in cardiovascular risk assessment and prevention in African Americans. In N. Wong, J.M. Gardin, and H.R. Black, *Practical Strategies in Preventing Heart Disease* (pp. 459–484). New York: McGraw-Hill.

O'Connor, P.J., Wagner, E.H., & Strogatz, D.S. (1990). Hypertension control in a rural community. An assessment of community-oriented primary care. *Journal of Family Practice, 30(4)*, 420–424.

Schnall, P.L., Landsbergis, P.A., & Baker, D. (1994). Job strain and cardiovascular disease. *Annual Review of Public Health, 15*, 381–411.

Shakoor-Abdullah, B., Kotchen, J.M., Walker, W.E., Chelius, T.H., & Hoffmann, R.G. (1997). Incorporating socio-economic and risk factor diversity into the development of an African-American community blood pressure control program. *Ethnicity & Disease, 7(3)*, 175–183.

Shea, S., Basch, C.E., Wechsler, H., & Lantigua, R. (1996). The Washington Heights-Inwood Healthy Heart Program: A 6-year report from a disadvantaged urban setting. *American Journal of Public Health, 86(2)*, 166–171.

Smith, E.D., Merritt, S.L., & Patel, M.K. (1997). Church-based education: An outreach program for African Americans with hypertension. *Ethnicity and Health, 2(3)*, 243–253.

Smith, N.L., Croft, J.B., Heath, G.W., & Cokkinides, V. (1996). Changes in cardiovascular disease knowledge and behavior in a low-education population of African-American and White adults. *Ethnicity & Disease, 6*, 244–254.

Vaccaro, O., Stamler, J., & Neaton, J.D. (1998). Sixteen-year coronary mortality in Black and White men with diabetes screened for the multiple risk factor intervention trial (MRFIT). *International Journal Epidemiology, 27(4)*, 636–641.

Waitzman, N.J., & Smith, K.R. (1994). The effect of occupational class transitions on hypertension: Racial disparities among working-age men. *American Journal of Public Health, 84*, 945–950.

Whelton, P.K., He, J., Cutler, J.A., Brancati, F.L., Appel, L.J., Follmann, D., & Klag, M.J. (1997). Effects of oral potassium on blood pressure; meta-analysis of randomized controlled clinical trials. *Journal of American Medical Association, 277*, 1624–1632.

World Health Organization-International Society of Hypertension Guidelines for the Management of Hypertension Guidelines Subcommittee. (1999). *Journal of Hypertension, 17*, 151–83.

CHAPTER 5

End-Stage Renal Disease

LAWRENCE Y.C. AGODOA

INTRODUCTION

The kidneys perform a multitude of functions, including removal of metabolic waste products, maintenance of acid-base homeostasis, control of fluid balance, immunological surveillance, and, very importantly, endocrine and hormonal regulation, including metabolism and regulation of insulin levels, erythropoietin synthesis, parathyroid hormone regulation, and gonadal function. When the kidneys fail, the functional alterations that pose immediate danger to life include accumulation of metabolic waste products and fluid and acid-base imbalance. These are functions that are regulated through urine output. With failure, metabolic waste products, such as urea, which are eliminated from the body through the urine, build up in the blood, hence, the term *uremia*, which refers to "urine in the blood." Because of the immediate threat to life, these functions were targeted early for remediation in renal replacement therapy (RRT) with hemodialysis and peritoneal dialysis. Terminal renal failure, also referred to as end-stage renal disease (ESRD), is defined as the stage at which RRT must be initiated to sustain life.

Unfortunately, however, RRT has not been able to restore life span to normal. Perhaps as a consequence of comorbid conditions accompanying ESRD, and/or as a complication of the RRT, patients on dialysis have a significantly diminished life span. Some of the comorbid conditions may appear early in the course of renal failure, and others may occur as renal disease progresses. Therefore, it is essential that patients with chronic renal insufficiency be identified early and that effective preventive management be initiated to slow down progression and abort the development of some of the comorbid conditions. The exact number of patients with chronic renal insufficiency is difficult to ascertain. However, analyzing data from the third National Health and Nutrition Examination Surveys (NHANES III), a cross-sectional nationally representative sample of the U.S. civilian noninstitutionalized population that uses a stratified, multistage probability cluster design with oversampling of Mexican Americans, African Americans, and elderly, Jones and colleagues reported that African Americans adults have a nearly three times higher prevalence of mild-moderate elevations of serum creatinine levels (≥ 2.0 mg/dl). They also estimated that there might be as many as 10–15 million persons in the United States with various levels of renal dysfunction (Jones et al., 1998).

In the 1960s the emerging new technology of dialysis gave the hope that ESRD need no longer be fatal. However, this new lifesaving technology was too expensive for those afflicted to afford. Therefore, in 1972, in the Social Security Amendments, PL 92-603, Section 299I, the Congress of the United States created an entitlement to Medicare for all persons with ESRD who were currently insured or eligible for benefits under Social Security, as well as for their spouses and/or dependent children. This entitlement for ESRD coverage was effective July 1, 1973. The law also mandated that providers must report some demographic and clinical information relevant to the ESRD treatment on the patients. This set the foundation for reporting and accurate accounting for ESRD care in the United States. In 1978, the Healthcare Financing Administration (HCFA) was established and given the responsibility for administering the Medicare ESRD program.

The National Institute of Diabetes and Digestive and Kidney Diseases (NIDDK) and the HCFA collaborated in 1988 to develop the U.S. Renal Data System (USRDS) database. The NIDDK, through a contract mechanism, established the USRDS database with the data reported to the HCFA (now the Centers for Medicare and Medicaid, CMS) on the Medicare ESRD patients. Additional data are added to the database through special studies carried out by the USRDS. The USRDS currently has information on over 96 percent of ESRD patients in the United States.

The six primary objectives under which the USRDS operates are (1) to characterize the total renal patient population and describe the distribution of patients by sociodemographic variables across treatment modalities, (2) to report on the incidence, prevalence, mortality rates, and trends over time of renal disease by primary diagnosis, treatment modality, and other variables, (3) to develop and analyze data on the effect of various modalities of treatment by disease and patient group categories, (4) to identify problems and opportunities for more focused special studies of renal research issues, (5) to conduct cost-effectiveness studies and other economic studies of ESRD, and (6) to make the data available to investigators and, by supporting investigator-initiated projects, to conduct biomedical and economic analyses of ESRD patients.

The Annual Data Report (ADR) of the USRDS presents nationally representative information on the incidence, prevalence, mortality, and survival for various subgroups of treated ESRD patients. The data are categorized by age, race, ethnicity, gender, and cause of ESRD. The ADR in its entirety is presented at the USRDS Web site at http://www.usrds.org. Abbreviated forms of the report are available on a CD ROM and in a hard copy. There is no comparable (i.e., complete) database in which patients with chronic renal failure are accurately accounted for. Most of the data presented in this chapter on ESRD are derived from the USRDS. Undoubtedly, some patients who develop ESRD never receive RRT prior to death. They are not accounted for in the USRDS; therefore, there is no appropriate way to accurately determine the total number of individuals who develop ESRD in the United States. Thus, the term "ESRD" in this chapter, for the most part, refers to individuals who receive RRT.

INCIDENCE AND PREVALENCE OF ESRD

It was estimated that the total number of beneficiaries in 1973 at the inception of the program was approximately 10,000. This number has dramatically increased to a period prevalence of 458,113 treated ESRD patients in 2000 (Figure 5.1). The incidence rate has also progressively increased, and 96,192 new cases were treated in 2000 (USRDS, 2002). Since its inception in 1988, the USRDS has reported data that racial and ethnic minorities in the United States, especially African Americans, are disproportionately afflicted with ESRD. Since the early days of the establishment of RRT in the United States and the Medicare program, racial and ethnic minorities, especially African Americans, have exhibited disproportionate affliction with renal disease. As shown in Figure 5.2, in 2000, the incidence rates, by race, were 269 per million population for Caucasians compared with 777 for

Figure 5.1
Time trends of prevalent count of patients treated for ESRD, 1991–2000

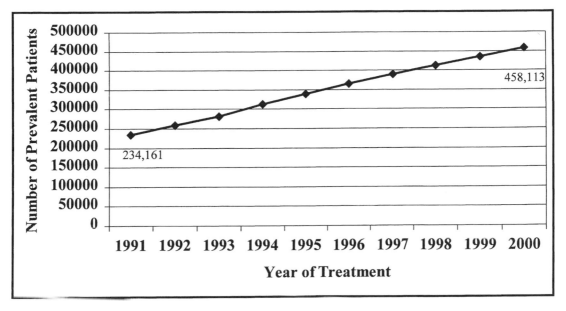

Source: USRDS 2002 Annual Data Report.

Figure 5.2
Incidence rate per million population of treated ESRD by race in the year 2000

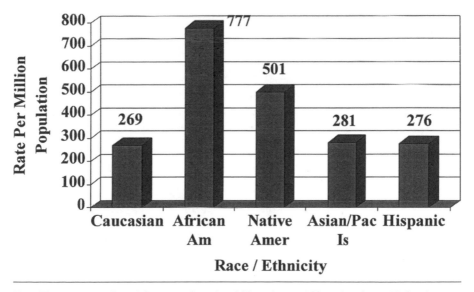

Note: The rates are adjusted for age and gender. African Am = African Americans, Native Amer = American Indians and Alaska Natives, Asian/Pac Is = Asian Americans and Pacific Islanders

Source: USRDS 2002 Annual Data Report.

Figure 5.3
Time trend of cause of ESRD, 1991–2000

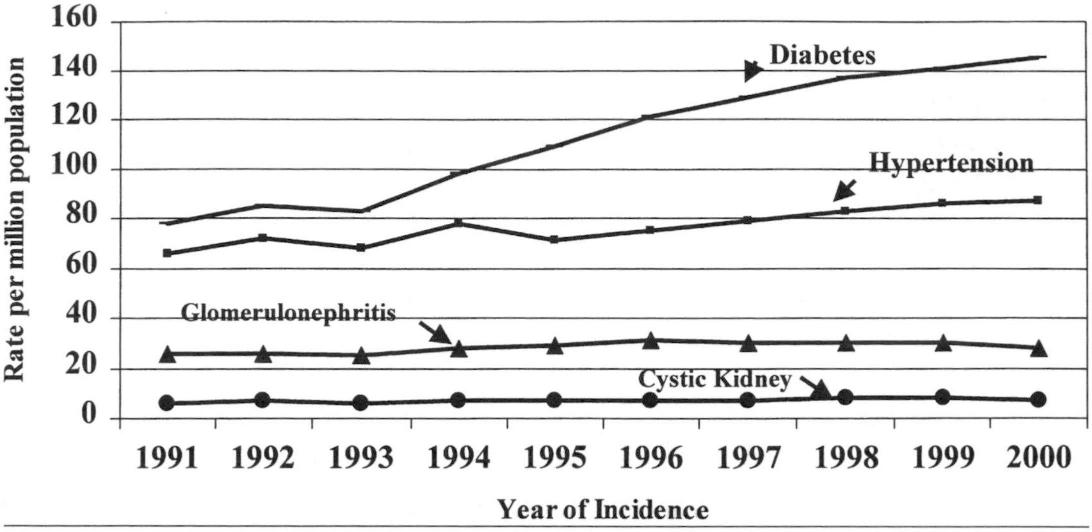

Note: Rates are per million population, adjusted for age, gender, and race.

Source: USRDS 2002 Annual Data Report

African Americans, 501 for American Indians and Alaska Natives, and 281 for Asian and Pacific Islanders (USRDS, 2002). The reported incidence rate of ESRD in Hispanic in 2000 was 276 per million population. Data reporting for Hispanics commenced in 1995, and there is reason to believe that this rate is lower than expected due to underreporting. The period and point prevalence rates, likewise, show higher rates of affliction of racial and ethnic minorities with ESRD.

CAUSES OF ESRD

Two diseases, namely diabetes mellitus and hypertension, cause approximately 70 percent of all new adult ESRD cases in the United States. Glomerulonephritis and cystic kidney diseases contribute about 10 percent (Figure 5.3). However, other "rarer" diseases causing ESRD, such as the human immunodeficiency virus (HIV), are also important contributors, especially in the African American community.

Diabetes Mellitus

Since the early 1970s diabetes mellitus has remained the leading cause of ESRD in the United States. Comparatively, it is a minor player in the causes of ESRD in Europe, Australia, and New Zealand. In the United States, the prevalence rate of diabetes in African American men is nearly 50 percent greater than that of White men; for African American women the rate is approximately 100 percent greater than in white women. Diabetes afflicts Hispanics (1.9 times that of non-Hispanic Whites) and Native American Indians (2.8 times that of non-Hispanic Whites) at an even higher rate (Harris et al., 1998; National Diabetes Fact Sheet, 1998).

Diabetes mellitus is the primary cause of ESRD in all racial and ethnic groups, but at a much higher rate in American Indians, Alaska Natives, and African Americans (USRDS, 2002), Figure

Figure 5.4
Incidence rate per million population of treated diabetic ESRD, 1997–2000

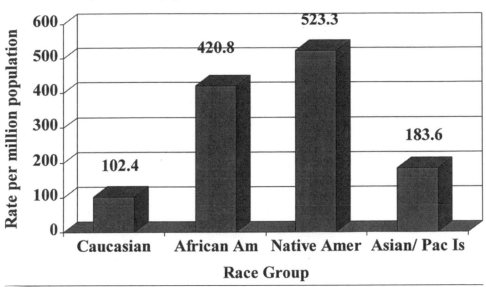

Note: Adjusted for age, gender and race. African Am = African American; Native Amer = American Indian and Alaska Native; Asian/ Pac Is = Asian and Pacific Islander.

Source: USRDS 2002 Annual Data Report.

5.4. In African Americans, especially, it was the second leading cause of ESRD prior to 1995. The age distribution is similar for all races in that the highest prevalence rates are in the 65–79 year age group, except for American Indians and Alaska Natives, where the highest incidence rate is in the 60–69 year age group. Curiously, however, even though this disease is practically unusual in children primarily because of the time it takes the established disease to cause sufficient injury to the kidneys to progress to end stage, there has been increasing frequency of the diagnosis of diabetic ESRD in African American girls and, to a minor extent, in Caucasian children. The gender difference is not the same in all the races. For Caucasians and Asians, men have a higher incidence rate of diabetic ESRD than women. In African Americans, American Indians, and Alaska Natives, women have a higher incidence rate than men.

It has been postulated that the continuing rise in the incidence of diabetic ESRD is due to a combination of increasing incidence rate of diabetes in the United States, as well as ineffective therapy to retard progression of diabetic renal disease in the early stages of development. The early effects of diabetes on the kidneys include microalbuminuria and hyperfiltration. Subsequently, the damage progresses to gross proteinuria and relentless decrease in glomerular filtration rate to end stage, as illustrated in Figure 5.5. Many investigators suggest that intervening early in the course of the disease would be more effective than after the disease has been established.

Unfortunately, primary care providers have typically waited until the later stages of the disease. Recently, three landmark studies in the nephropathy of Type 2 diabetes were completed and published. One of the studies conducted in the early phase of Type 2 diabetic nephropathy showed that treatment with angiotensin receptor blockers (ARBs) resulted in reduction of microalbuminuria and/or progression to gross proteinuria (Parving et al., 2001). The other two clinical trials were conducted in Type 2 diabetic patients with gross proteinuria and reduced glomerular filtration rate. Both studies

Figure 5.5
Schematic of the time course and progression of diabetic nephropathy

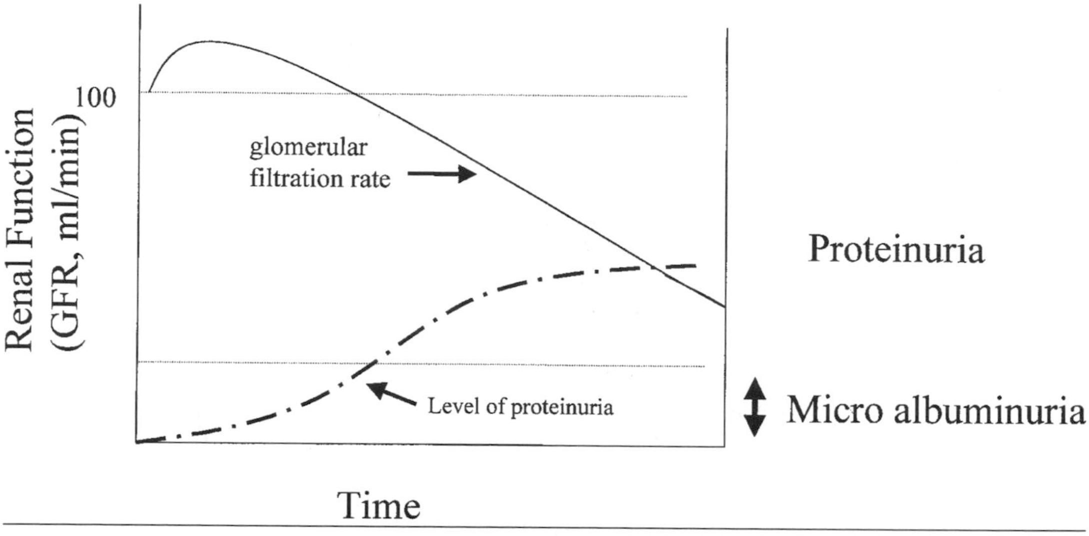

..... Level of microalbuminuria;—Time course for the glomerular filtration rate;—•—• Time course for the level of proteinuria.

showed that the use of ARBs in the late stages was effective in reducing, but not preventing, progression of the disease (Lewis et al., 2001; Brenner et al., 2001).

It can be concluded that diabetic ESRD can be delayed if patients in the advanced stages of the disease are treated with ARBs. There are also indications that treatment in the early stages of the disease with ARBs will probably reduce the incidence, and eventually the prevalence, of the disease.

Hypertension

Although the rate of rise in the incidence rate of hypertensive ESRD has diminished over the past decade, it remains a major cause of ESRD in the African American community. Among the racial and ethnic groups, only African Americans have shown a substantial increase in the prevalence of hypertension (Klag et al., 1977; Coresh et al., 2001). Mexican Americans, on the other hand, have shown poorer control of hypertension (65 percent that of African Americans or Whites, and this relatively poorer control may have implications for the future rates of ESRD development in this group (Burt et al., 1995).

The incidence of hypertensive end-stage renal disease is extremely high among younger African Americans, nearly 20 times the incidence for Caucasians in the 20–44 year old group (USRDS, 2001). As illustrated in Figure 5.3, the incidence rate of hypertensive ESRD has continued to increase, over the past two decades, but less dramatically in the last five. This rate of increase has been greatest in African Americans. It was the leading cause of ESRD prior to 1995 in African Americans, but currently the second leading cause of ESRD. In the year 2000, of the 96,192 new cases of ESRD, 24,566 (25.5 percent) were reported caused by hypertension. In the period 1997–2000, the incidence rates (per million population) of hypertensive ESRD by race were 554 for Caucasians, 778 for American Indians and Alaska Natives, 1,036 for Asians and Pacific Islanders, and 3,302 for African Americans, with a Black/White ratio of approximately 6:1, and the rate was higher in men than in women, for all races (Figure 5.6). Patients older than 80 years had the highest incidence rate of hypertensive ESRD (USRDS, 2002).

Figure 5.6
Incidence rate per million population of treated hypertensive ESRD, 1997–2000

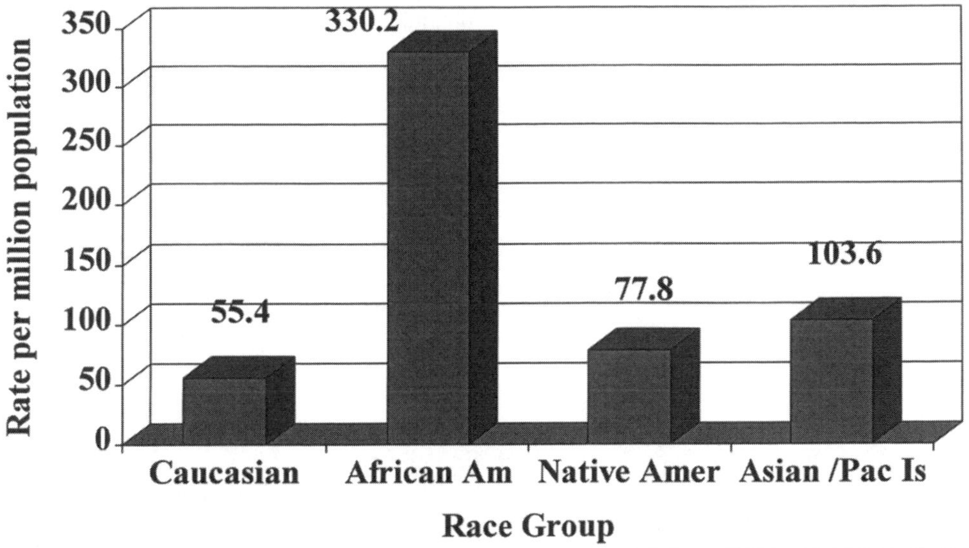

Note: Adjusted for age, gender and race. African Am = African American
Native Amer = American Indian and Alaska Native
Asian/ Pac Is = Asian and Pacific Islander.

Source: USRDS 2002 Annual Data Report.

At present, it is unclear whether the high incidence of hypertensive kidney disease, especially among African Americans, is a result of damage from severe essential hypertension potentiated by environmental nephrotoxins, use of illicit or prescribed drugs, or other factors (Perneger et al., 1994; Sandler et al., 1989; Norris, Thornhill-Joynes, & Robinson et al., 2001; Norris, Thornhill-Joynes & Tareen, 2001). Until recently, there was no effective way to halt progression to end stage once the disease developed. However, the results of the recently completed African American Study of Kidney Disease and Hypertension (AASK) clinical trial has shown that progression can be slowed even in the advanced stage of the disease by the use of angiotensin converting enzyme inhibitors (ACEI). In that study, patients without significant proteinuria showed no significant worsening of the disease with adequate control of the blood pressure. In the presence of proteinuria even at the level of 300 mg per 24 hours, however, the disease shows faster progression unless ACEI are used (Agodoa et al., 2001; Wright et al., 2002; Winston et al., 1998). There are no reported studies on the effect of intervention in the early phases of the disease. However, some investigators suggest that treatment of hypertension in the early phases of the disease will result in prevention of ESRD. The presence of proteinuria mandates the use of ACEI.

Glomerulonephritis

Primary and secondary glomerulonephritides constitute the third most frequently reported cause of ESRD in the United States. The incidence rate is higher in men than in women. Overall, African Americans have the highest rate of ESRD due to glomerulonephritis. However, the racial distribution varies by the type of glomerulonephritis. For example, IgA nephropathy and IgM nephropathy is less frequent in African American; on the other hand, focal and segmental glomerulosclerosis (FSGS) and nephropathy due to systemic lupus erythematosus (SLE) are more common in African Americans than Caucasians.

The current epidemic of infection with HIV has resulted in an important cause of ESRD. Although the total number of cases in the U.S. ESRD population is relatively few, it comprises the third leading cause of ESRD in African Americans and is as much as ten times the incidence rate in Caucasians (Monahan et al., 2001; Klotman, 1999; Maschio et al., 1996).

There are currently no consistent effective therapies for the glomerulonephritides. Immunosuppressive therapy was tried in patients with primary and some secondary (such as SLE) glomerulonephritides with inconsistent results. In general, however, these diseases are accompanied by proteinuria. Proteinuric kidney diseases have been shown to respond well to drugs that inhibit the rennin-angiotensin-aldosterone axis (GISEN Group, 1997; Ruggenenti et al., 1998; National Kidney Foundation K/DOQI Working Group, 2002). Therefore, therapeutic regimens for glomerular diseases usually contain ACEI.

Tubulo-Interstitial and Cystic Kidney Diseases

This is a group of diseases that are nonglomerular and nonvascular in origin, including autosomal dominant polycystic kidney disease (ADPKD), chronic pyelonephritis, hereditary nephritis, analgesics and other drugs, and heavy metals. Most of the individuals in this group have ADPKD. These diseases are usually insidious in onset. They constitute only about 4 percent of the total incident ESRD population. Even at this low incident rate, African Americans are afflicted at a higher rate than other racial and ethnic groups. There is approximately 25 percent higher incidence rate in men in all racial and ethnic groups. The peak incidence is in the 70–79 year age group (USRDS, 2002).

Treatment of this group of diseases is nonuniform. In instances where the causative agent is known, removal from exposure may diminish the rate of progression. ESRD is inevitable when patients are discovered at the stage 4 of the National Kidney Foundation's Kidney Disease Outcomes Quality Initiative (K/DOQI) (Boddanova et al., 2002). In the case of autosomal dominant polycystic kidney disease, treatment has been mostly symptomatic, primarily, treatment of hypertension that is frequently associated with this disease. However, because the pathogenic mechanisms include clonal expansion of partially differentiated epithelial cells that are dysregulated, undergo apoptosis, and have been shown to secret several growth factors, chemokines, proinflammatory cytokines, nucleotides, matrix metalloproteinases, lysosomal enzymes and vasoactive substances, there are many potential interventions. Many of these are in the initial stages of experimentation and will likely lead to the development of novel therapies that will prevent progression of the disease to end stage (Davis et al., 2001; Qian et al., 2001; Ifudu et al., 1999).

MODALITIES OF THERAPY FOR ESRD

The kidneys are primarily responsible for maintaining the body's homeostasis, including removal of metabolic waste products, conserving fluids when there is deficit, eliminating excess fluid, and maintaining acid base balance. They also produce growth factors, cytokines, proinflammatory mediators, and vasoactive substances. Therefore, a successful RRT should include all the functions lost when ESRD ensues. Early in the development of RRT, investigators focused primarily on correcting acid-base, fluid, and electrolyte disorders. Dialysis was the outcome of those early considerations. It is, therefore, not surprising that although dialysis has resulted in saving the patient with ESRD from immediate death, neither the quality of life nor the expected remaining life years are returned to the prerenal failure level. Successful renal transplant, on the other hand, returns the patient to near normal quality of life and life span. The remainder of this section focuses primarily on the racial differences in RRT.

Hemodialysis

Minorities, especially African Americans with the high incidence rate of ESRD, are also referred for specialist care later than Caucasians. Therefore, they are more likely to have more advanced disease and more complications from the renal failure. Compared with Caucasians, African Americans, by the time they see renal care specialists, are more likely to have hypoalbuminemia and severe anemia at the initiation of hemodialysis and are less likely to receive recombinant human erythropoietin therapy before dialysis (Schmidt et al., 1998). Some investigators also believe that this late referral results in more urgent and placement on hemodialysis (Stack, 2002; Winkelmayer et al., 2001; Astor et al., 2001). Furthermore, late referral is associated with an increased chance of dialysis catheter use (Stehman-Breen et al., 2000; Arora et al., 1999; NKF-DOQI, 1997).

The preferred vascular access for chronic hemodialysis is an autologous arteriovenous fistula rather than a synthetic arteriovenous graft or intravenous catheter due to the lower rates of thrombosis and infection (Hoen et al., 1998; Owen et al., 1998). Despite these recommendations and available outcome data, African Americans more commonly have synthetic grafts compared with White Americans. Late referral, which necessitates immediate access placement, may be one of the causes of this discrepancy (Arora et al., 1999; NKF-DOQI, 1997).

In 2000, of the 96,192 incident patients, 83,635 (87 percent) received hemodialysis as the initial modality of therapy. African Americans constituted 29 percent of the incident dialysis patient population and 38 percent of the prevalent dialysis population, compared with Caucasians, who constituted 63 percent of the incident dialysis population and only 54 percent of the prevalent dialysis population (USRDS, 2002). The decrease in the proportion of Caucasians in the prevalent population is mainly due to their referral for renal transplantation.

The prescribed dose, and hence the delivered dose, of dialysis is more likely to be suboptimal in African American hemodialysis patients despite clear guidelines for hemodialysis dose and frequent monitoring (Seghal, 1993; Frankenfield et al., 1999). A dialysis dose less than the recommended level is associated with higher mortality in patients with ESRD. Paradoxically, the survival of African Americans on hemodialysis is better than Whites (USRDS, 2002; Barker-Cummings et al., 1995). Interestingly, the relationship between dialysis dose and mortality risk appears to be weakest in Blacks (Seghal, 1993). However, there may be potential for improved survival with the combination of timely referral, optimal angio access, and appropriate dialysis delivery.

Peritoneal Dialysis

The two predominant modes of peritoneal dialysis in the United States are chronic ambulatory peritoneal dialysis (CAPD) and continuous cycling peritoneal dialysis (CCPD). In general, there has been a gradual decrease in the use of peritoneal dialysis in the United States. A decade ago, approximately 14 percent of the incidence of ESRD patients was treated with peritoneal dialysis; however, by the 2000, only 7.8 percent received this modality of treatment.

There are racial differences in peritoneal dialysis use; Whites and Asian Americans are more likely to choose peritoneal dialysis compared with African Americans and Native Americans (USRDS, 2002; Saade & Joglar, 1995; Nolph et al., 1987; Port et al., 1993). For example, in the Southeast, one study observed that African Americans were 50 percent less likely, compared with white Americans, to select peritoneal dialysis as an initial mode of ESRD treatment. The choice of peritoneal dialysis tends to be a function of education and socioeconomic status, cultural bias related to health behavior and body image, physician bias, and communication barriers (Saade & Joglar, 1995).

Renal Transplantation

Kidney transplantation is the treatment of choice for ESRD patients (Wolfe et al., 1999; Danielson et al., 1998). However, in the past two decades, the growing need for organs has outstripped the supply of kidneys. Therefore, the rate of transplantation has declined. In 1991, the rate of transplantation was approximately 8 per 100 patient years, and in the year 2000 the rate had declined to approximately 5 per 100 patient years (USRDS, 2002). The waiting time for African Americans to receive an organ is longer than that of Caucasians and is increasing at an even greater rate.

The shortage of organs is contributed to by the lower rate of organ donation among African American, Native American, and Hispanic American communities, compared with Caucasians (Epstein et al., 2000; Bleyer et al., 1996; Alexander & Sehgal, 1998), and six antigen matching is less frequent for African Americans than for Whites. With the faster rate of growth of ESRD incidence rate among African Americans, their chance of receiving a transplant is substantially lower than for Whites (Eggers, 1995; Gaylin et al., 1993; Soucie et al., 1992; Ayanian et al., 1999).

In the United States, the majority of renal transplants are cadaveric organs. The decline in the rate of cadaveric kidney transplants has been responsible for the overall decline in the transplantation rate. Living organ donor transplantation, on the other hand, has shown improvement, especially in living unrelated organs. In the period 1997–2000, the transplantation rate for first cadaveric transplant by race was 1.8 per 100 patient years for Caucasians, compared with 0.8 for African Americans, 0.9 for Native Americans, and 1.5 for Asians. The mean time to first cadaveric renal transplant for African Americans in the year 2000 was 1,360 days compared with 888 days for Caucasians, and 1,160 for Hispanic Americans. Overall, the first-year graft survival probabilities for cadaveric kidneys has substantially improved over the past decade from 77.1 percent in 1989 to 88.3 percent in 1998. However, the dramatic improvement seen in this short-term graft survival has not been maintained in the longer-term (i.e., 10-year), graft survival; 23.4 in 1980 to 34.5 in 1990.

The difference between African Americans and Caucasians is not significant in the short term; one-year graft survival probabilities in 1998 was 88.3 for Caucasians, and 87.0 for African Americans. On the other hand, the difference remains large in long-term graft survival; the ten-year graft survival in 1990 was 38.9 for Caucasians, compared with 21.6 in African Americans. The patient death rate for cadaveric donor renal transplants is higher for African Americans than for Caucasians (USRDS, 2002).

Living donor transplant rates in the period 1997–2000 were 1.7 per 100 patient years for Caucasians, 0.4 for African Americans, 0.6 for Native Americans, and 1.2 for Asians (USRDS, 2002). The mean time to first living donor transplant in the year 2000 was 583 days for African Americans, compared with 368 for Caucasians and 549 for Hispanic Americans. There has been notable improvement in both the short-term (one-year) and the long-term (ten-year) graft survival probabilities for living donor organs. However, as in the experience with cadaveric donor organs, the improvement in the ten-year graft survival is modest, compared with the one-year survival. African Americans have shorter graft survival in both the short term and long term compared with Caucasians. Patient death rate is also higher for African Americans (USRDS, 2002).

The major racial barriers that contribute to, and maintain, the large difference in the transplantation rates between African Americans and Caucasians include reluctance to accept transplants, comorbid conditions, limited access, lack of appropriate counseling by health-care providers, longer waiting times, sociodemographic characteristics, dialysis facility practice patterns, perceptions of care, and less trust in the health-care system (Ozminkowski et al., 1997; Sanfilippo et al., 1992; Hata et al., 1998; Ellison et al., 1993; Isaacs et al., 2000; Isaacs et al., 1999).

MORBIDITY AND MORTALITY IN ESRD

Morbidity

Morbidity in patients treated for ESRD is defined in terms of all causes and cause-specific hospitalization. Events such as acute myocardial infarction and problems with vascular access are frequent causes for hospitalization. In general, peritoneal dialysis patients spend more days, and transplant patients spend fewer days, in the hospital. Overall, there is not a significant difference between African Americans and Caucasians in the rate of first hospitalization for all ESRD patients. However, in dialysis patients, African Americans have a lower rate of first hospitalization but spend more time in the hospital when they receive renal transplants (USRDS, 2002).

Mortality

Despite advances in dialysis technology and transplantation, long-term survival in ESRD is dreadfully low. Almost half of all deaths are due to cardiovascular disease. The second most common cause of death is sepsis. Hypoalbuminemia at initiation of dialysis is an indicator for poor survival. Severe anemia and low dialysis dose are associated with poor prognosis in ESRD. Despite evidence that non-White patients are more likely to have these poor survival indicators as well as limited pre-ESRD care, the survival rates in dialysis are higher for racial and ethnic minorities compared with Caucasians. In the year 2000, the annual death rate for all ESRD patients (per 1,000 patient years) was 192.6 for Caucasians, compared with 157.3 for African Americans, 155.8 for Native Americans, and 130.4 for Asians. For hemodialysis patients, the annual death rate was 284.7 for Caucasians, 181.1 for African Americans, 192.8 for Native Americans, and 179.8 for Asians, as in Figure 5.7 (USRDS, 2002). Overall, the better survival of African Americans and other racial and ethnic minority groups is poorly understood and requires further exploration.

In general, kidney transplantation is associated with better survival and quality of life. Although African Americans have poorer survival than Caucasians, irrespective of graft function, there is a substantial survival benefit when compared with patients on the waiting list or on dialysis.

SUMMARY AND DISCUSSION

End-stage renal disease is a major public health problem in the United States. In spite of general improvement in health status of Americans and increased longevity, the incidence rate of ESRD continues to increase. The escalating incidence rate is seen in all racial and ethnic groups, but racial and ethnic minorities, especially African Americans, American Indians, and Alaska Natives, have the highest rate. They seem to develop ESRD at a younger age and suffer a higher burden of disease than Caucasians. Although the two most frequent causes of ESRD, namely Type 2 diabetes mellitus and hypertension, are also more common these minority groups, their higher prevalence does not entirely explain the disproportionate burden of renal disease. It is possible that other factors, including socioeconomic status, exposure to unidentified environmental agents, and genetic predisposition, play important roles in the development and progression of kidney disease in these groups.

It is quite intriguing that the racial and ethnic minorities that carry a disproportionate burden of ESRD have better survival than Caucasians. There is no ready explanation for this phenomenon, and requires further research. Finally, in addition to health education, such as the newly launched initiative, the National Kidney Disease Education Program, NKDEP, by the National Institute of Diabetes and Digestive and Kidney Diseases, there is need for increased funding for research into preventing the onset of kidney damage and for early detection and intervention.

Figure 5.7
Death rate per 1,000 patient years at risk of dialysis patients in the year 2000 by race

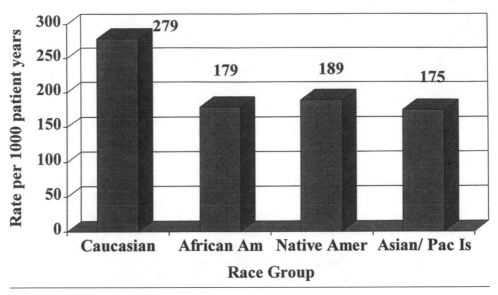

Note: Adjusted for age, gender and primary diagnosis. African Am = African American; Native Amer = American Indian and Alaska Native; Asian/ Pac Is = Asian and Pacific Islander.

Source: USRDS 2002 Annual Data Report.

REFERENCES

Agodoa, L.Y., et al., for the African American Study of Kidney Disease and Hypertension (AASK) Study Group. (2001). Effect of ramipril vs amlodipine on renal outcomes in hypertensive nephrosclerosis. A randomized controlled trial. *Journal of the American Medical Association, 285*, 2719–2728.

Alexander, G.C., & Sehgal, A.R. (1998). Barriers to cadaveric renal transplantation among Blacks, women, and the poor. *Journal of American Medical Association, 280*, 1148–1152.

Arora, P., et al. (1999). Prevalence, predictors, and consequences of late nephrology referral at a tertiary care center. *Journal of American Society of Nephrology, 10*, 1281–1286.

Astor, B.C., et al. (2001). Timing of nephrologist referral and arteriovenous access use: The CHOICE Study. *American Journal of Kidney Disease, 38*, 494–501.

Ayanian, J.Z., Cleary, P.D., Weissman, J.S., & Epstein, A.M. (1999). The effect of patients' preferences on racial differences in access to renal transplantation. *New England Journal of Medicine, 341*, 1661–1669.

Barker-Cummings, C., McClellan, W., Soucie, J.M., & Krisher, J. (1995). Ethnic differences in the use of peritoneal dialysis as initial treatment for end-stage renal disease. *Journal of American Medical Association, 274*, 1858–1862.

Bleyer, A.J., Tell, G.S., Evans, G.W., Ettinger, W.H., Jr., & Burkart, J.M. (1996). Survival of patients undergoing renal replacement therapy in one center with special emphasis on racial differences. *American Journal of Kidney Disease, 28*, 72–81.

Bogdanova, N., Markoff, A., & Horst, J. (2002). Autosomal dominant polycystic kidney disease—clinical and genetic aspects. Autosomal dominant polycystic kidney disease—clinical and genetic aspects. *Kidney and Blood Pressure Research, 25(5)*, 265–283.

Brenner, B.M., et al. (2001). Effects of losartan on renal and cardiovascular outcomes in patients with type 2 diabetes and nephropathy. *New England Journal of Medicine, 345*, 861–869.

Burt, V.L., et al. (1995). Prevalence of hypertension in the U.S. adult population. Results from the Third National Health and Nutrition Examination Survey, 1988–1991. *Hypertension, 3*, 305–313.

Coresh, J., et al. (2001). Prevalence of high blood pressure and elevated serum creatinine level in the United States: Findings from the Third National Health and Nutrition Examination Survey (1988–1994). *Archives of Internal Medicine, 161*, 1207–1216.

Danielson, B.L., LaPree, A.J., Odland, M.D., & Steffens, E.K. (1998). Attitudes and beliefs concerning organ donation among Native Americans in the upper Midwest. *Journal of Transplantation Coordination, 8*, 153–156.

Davis, I.D., MacRae, Dell, K., Sweeney, W.E., & Avner, E.D. (2001). Can progression of autosomal dominant or autosomal recessive polycystic kidney disease be prevented? *Seminars in Nephrology, 21(5)*, 430–40.

Eggers, P.W. (1995). Racial differences in access to kidney transplantation. *Health Care Financing Review, 17*, 89–103.

Ellison, M.D., Breen, T., Cunningham, P., & Daily, O. (1993). Blacks and whites on the UNOS renal waiting list: Waiting times and patients demographics compared. *Transplantation Proceedings, 25*, 2462–2466.

Epstein, A.M., et al. (2000). Racial disparities in access to renal transplantation—clinically appropriate or due to underuse or overuse? *New England Journal of Medicine, 343*, 1537–1544.

Frankenfield, D.L., Rocco, M.V., Frederick, P.R., Pugh, J., McClellan, W.M., & Owen, W.F., Jr. (1999). Racial/ethnic analysis of selected intermediate outcomes for hemodialysis patients: Results from the 1997 ESRD Core Indicators Project. *American Journal of Kidney Disease, 34*, 721–730.

Gaylin, D.S., et al. (1993). The impact of comorbid and sociodemographic factors on access to renal transplantation. *Journal of American Medical Association, 269*, 603–608.

GISEN Group. (1997). Randomized placebo-controlled trial of effect of ramipril on decline in glomerular filtration rate and risk of terminal renal failure in proteinuric, non-diabetic nephropathy. The GISEN Group (Gruppo Italiano di Studi Epidemiologici in Nefrologia). *Lancet, 349*, 1857–1863.

Harris, M.I., et al. (1998). Prevalence of diabetes, impaired fasting glucose and impaired glucose tolerance in U.S. adults. The Third National Health and Nutrition Examination Survey, 1988–1994. *Diabetes Care, 21(4)*, 518–524.

Hata, Y., Cecka, J.M., Takemoto, S., Ozawa, M., Cho, Y.W., & Terasaki, P.I. (1998). Effects of changes in the criteria for nationally shared kidney transplants for HLA-matched patients. *Transplantation, 65*, 208–212.

Hoen, B., Paul-Dauphin, A., Hestin, D., & Kessler, M. (1998). EPIBACDIAL: A multicenter prospective study of risk factors for bacteremia in chronic hemodialysis patients. *Journal of American Society of Nephrology, 9*, 869–876.

Ifudu, O., Dawood, M., Iofel, Y., Valcourt, J.S., & Friedman, E.A. (1999). Delayed referral of black, Hispanic, and older patients with chronic renal failure. *American Journal of Kidney Disease, 33*, 728–733.

Isaacs, R.B., et al. (1999). Racial disparities in renal transplant outcomes. *American Journal of Kidney Disease, 34*, 706–712.

Isaacs, R.B., Lobo, P.I., Nock, S.L., Hanson, J.A., Ojo, A.O., & Pruett, T.L. (2000). Racial disparities in access to simultaneous pancreas-kidney transplantation in the United States. *American Journal of Kidney Disease, 36*, 526–533.

Jones, C.A., et al. (1998). Serum creatinine levels in the US population: Third National Health and Nutrition Examination Survey. *American Journal of Kidney Diseases, 32*, 992–999.

Klag, M.J., Stamler, J., Brancati, F.L., Neaton, J.D., Randall, B.L., & Whelton, P.K. (1977). End-stage renal disease in African American and white men: 16-year MRFIT findings. *Journal of the American Medical Association, 277(16)*, 1293–8.

Klotman, P.E. (1999). HIV-associated nephropathy. *Kidney International, 56*, 1161–1176.

Lewis, E.J., et al. (2001). Renoprotective effect of the angiotensin-receptor antagonist Irbesartan in patients with nephropathy due to type 2 diabetes. *New England Journal of Medicine, 345*, 851–860.

Maschio, G., et al. (1996). Effect of the angiotensin-converting-enzyme inhibitor benazepril on the progression of chronic renal insufficiency. The Angiotensin-Converting-Enzyme Inhibition in Progressive Renal Insufficiency Study Group. *New England Journal of Medicine, 334 (15)*, 939–945.

Monahan, M., Tanji, N., & Klotman, P.E. (2001). HIV-associated nephropathy: An urban epidemic. *Seminars in Nephrology, 21(4)*, 393–402.

National Diabetes Fact Sheet: Incidence of diabetes. Web document: http://www.cdc.gov/diabetes/pubs/facts98.htm#incidence.

National Kidney Foundation K/DOQI Working Group. (2002). Clinical practice guidelines for chronic renal disease evaluation, classification, and stratification. *American Journal of Kidney Disease, 39*, S46–S75.

NKF-DOQI clinical practice guidelines for vascular access. (1997). National Kidney Foundation-Dialysis Outcomes Quality Initiative. *American Journal of Kidney Disease, 30*, S150–S191.

Nolph, K.D., Cutler, S.J., Steinberg, S.M., Novak, J.W., & Hirschman, G.H. (1987). Factors associated with morbidity and mortality among patients on CAPD. *American Society of Artificial Internal Organs Transactions, 33*, 57–65.

Norris, K.C., Thornhill-Joynes, M., Robinson, C., & Strickland, T., et al. (2001). Cocaine use, hypertension and end-stage renal disease. *American Journal of Kidney Disease, 38(3)*, 523–528.

Norris, K.C., Thornhill-Joynes, M., & Tareen, N. (2001). Cocaine use and chronic renal failure. *Seminars in Nephrology, 21(4)*, 362–366.

Owen, W.F., Jr., Chertow, G.M., Lazarus, J.M., & Lowrie, E.G. (1998). Dose of hemodialysis and survival: Differences by race and sex. *Journal of the American Medical Association, 280*, 1764–1768.

Ozminkowski, R.J., White, A.J., & Hassol, A. (1997). Murphy M. Minimizing racial disparity regarding receipt of a cadaver kidney transplant. *American Journal of Kidney Disease, 30*, 749–759.

Parving, H.H., Lehnert, H., Brochner-Mortensen, J., Gomis, R., Andersen, S., & Arner, P., (2001). The effect of irbesartan on the development of diabetic nephropathy in patients with type 2 diabetes. *New England Journal of Medicine, 345*, 870–878.

Perneger, T.V., Whelton, P.K., & Klag, M.J., (1994). Risk of kidney failure associated with the use of acetaminophen, aspirin and nonsteroidal anti-inflammatory drugs. *New England Journal of Medicine, 331*, 1675–1679.

Port, F.K., Wolfe, R.A., Mauger, E.A., Berling, D.P., & Jiang, K. (1993). Comparison of survival probabilities for dialysis patients vs. cadaveric renal transplant recipients. *Journal of American Medical Association, 270*, 1339–1343.

Qian, Q., Harris, P.C., & Torres, V.E. (2001). Treatment prospects for autosomal-dominant polycystic kidney disease. *Kidney International, 59(6)*, 2005–2022.

Ruggenenti, P., Perna, A., Gherardi, G., Gaspari, F., Benini, R., & Remuzzi, G. (1998). Renal function and requirement for dialysis in chronic nephropathy patients on long-term ramipril: REIN follow-up trial. Gruppo Italiano di Studi Epidemiologici in Nefrologia (GISEN). Ramipril Efficac in Nephropathy. *Lancet, 352*, 1252–1256.

Saade, M., & Joglar, F. (1995). Chronic peritoneal dialysis: Seven-year experience in a large Hispanic program. *Peritoneal Dialysis International, 15*, 37–41.

Sandler, D.P., et al. (1989). Analgesic use and chronic renal disease. *New England Journal of Medicine, 320*, 1238–1243.

Sanfilippo, F.P., et al. (1992). Factors affecting the waiting time of cadaveric kidney transplant candidates in the United States. *Journal of American Medical Association, 267*, 247–252.

Schmidt, R.J., Domico, J.R., Sorkin, M.I., & Hobbs, G. (1998). Early referral and its impact on emergent first dialyses, health care costs, and outcome. *American Journal of Kidney Disease, 32*, 278–283.

Seghal, A.R. (1993). Outcomes of renal replacement therapy among blacks and women. *American Journal of Kidney Disease, 35*, S148.

Soucie, J.M., Neylan, J.F., & McClellan, W. (1992). Race and sex differences in the identification of candidates for renal transplantation. *American Journal of Kidney Disease, 19*, 414–419.

Stack, A.G. (2002). Determinants of modality selection among incident U.S. dialysis patients: results from a national study. *Journal of American Society of Nephrology, 13*, 1279–1287.

Stehman-Breen, C.O., Sherrard, D.J., Gillen, D., & Caps, M. (2000). Determinants of type and timing of initial permanent hemodialysis vascular access. *Kidney International, 57*, 639–645.

U.S. Renal Data System (USRDS). (2001). *USRDS 2001 Annual Data Report: Atlas of End-Stage Renal Disease in the United States*. Bethesda, MD: National Institutes of Health, National Institute of Diabetes and Digestive and Kidney Diseases.

U.S. Renal Data System (USRDS). (2002). *USRDS 20021 Annual Data Report: Atlas of End-Stage Renal*

Disease in the United States. Bethesda, MD: National Institutes of Health, National Institute of Diabetes and Digestive and Kidney Diseases.

Winkelmayer, W.C., Glynn, R.J., Levin, R., Owen, W, Jr., & Avorn, J. (2001). Late referral and modality choice in end-stage renal disease. *Kidney International, 60,* 1547–1554.

Winston, J.S., Burns, G.C., & Klotman, P.E. (1998). The human immunodeficiency virus (HIV) epidemic and HIV-associated nephropathy. *Seminars in Nephrology, 18(4),* 373–377.

Wolfe, R.A., et al. (1999). Comparison of mortality in all patients on dialysis, patients on dialysis awaiting transplantation, and recipients of a first cadaveric transplant. *New England Journal of Medicine, 341,* 1725–1730.

Wright, J.T., Jr., et al., for the African American Study of Kidney Disease and Hypertension Study Group (2002). Effect of blood pressure lowering and antihypertensive drug class on progression of hypertensive kidney disease: Results of the AASK Trial. *Journal of the American Medical Association, 288,* 2421–2431.

CHAPTER 6

Diabetes-Related Disparities in African Americans

EUGENE S. TULL AND EARLE C. CHAMBERS

INTRODUCTION

The Report of the Secretary's Task Force on Black and Minority Health (1985) drew attention to the excess risk for diabetes that exists in minority groups compared to the European American population. Since that time the disparity that exists for African Americans has remained. National data published in 1998 suggest that the frequency of diabetes mellitus in adults age 20 and older is approximately 1.6 times higher for African than European Americans (Harris, Klein et al., 1998). In addition to the disparity in adults, it appears that African American youth are also disproportionately affected by the increase in the rate of diabetes that has been occurring among persons age 19 and younger since the mid-1990s (Kaufman, 2002).

Renewed interest in narrowing the gap between minorities and the majority population in the frequency and impact of diabetes mellitus has led to efforts to identify the antecedent causes of behaviors associated with increased risk for the disease. This area of focus holds promise for the development of research initiatives and community-based activities that may lead to better understanding of how social, behavioral, and biological factors are linked in the etiology of the disease and the most effective strategies to reduce risk within the context of individual communities and cultures. Until effective strategies for prevention and control of the illness and for narrowing the ethnic disparities are in place in communities across the United States, diabetes mellitus will continue to be a major health problem for the African American population. In this chapter, we describe the epidemiology and impact of diabetes mellitus on African Americans and provide suggestions for strategies that may help to eliminate the disparity.

Classification and Diagnosis

Diabetes mellitus is a heterogeneous group of disorders that are characterized by an abnormal increase in the level of blood glucose. The vast majority of diabetes cases that occur in the United States are due to the two major forms of the illness including Type 2 diabetes, or non-insulin-dependent diabetes mellitus (NIDDM), and Type 1 diabetes, or insulin-dependent diabetes mellitus (IDDM). In addition to these two, other forms of glucose intolerance have also been described,

Table 6.1
Diagnostic criteria for various forms of glucose intolerance

Type of Diabetes	Diagnostic Criteria	Description
Type 2	FPG ≥ 126mg/dl 2-hour OGTT ≥ 200mg/dl	Usually develops after age 40; associated with obesity and insulin resistance
Type 1	FPG ≥ 126mg/dl 2-hour OGTT ≥ 200mg/dl	Develops with insulinopenia and ketosis; associated with HLA genes and autoimmunity
IFG	FPG 110mg/dl - 125mg/dl	Associated with increased risk of microvascular complications
IGT	FPG ≥ 140mg/dl 2-hour OGTT 140-149 mg/dl	Increased risk of developing Type 2; high frequency of cardiovascular risk factors
GDM	FPG ≥ 140mg/dl 2-hour OGTT ≥ 200mg/dl	Diabetes during pregnancy will return to normal glucose status after delivery; associated with increased risk of developing Type 2 Diabetes
PDPD	FPG ≥ 140mg/dl 2-hour OGTT ≥ 200mg/dl	Cases present very thin; resistant to ketosis; shows phasic insulin dependence
FCPD	FPG ≥ 140mg/dl	Characteristics similar to PDPD but with pancreatic calcification

FPG, fasting plasma glucose; OGTT, oral glucose tolerance test; GDM, gestational diabetes mellitus; IFG, impaired fasting glucose; IGT, impaired glucose tolerance; PDPD, protein-deficient pancreatic diabetes; FCPD, fibrocalculus pancreatic diabetes. Diagnostic criteria are those recommended by the World Health Organization.

including impaired fasting glucose, impaired glucose tolerance, maturity-onset diabetes of youth (a genetically inherited form of Type 2 diabetes with onset in childhood), gestational diabetes, and other atypical diabetes. Classification of these diabetes subtypes is based on criteria published by the American Diabetes Association (ADA) (1997) and the World Health Organization (WHO, 1980). A diagnosis of diabetes is established by a fasting plasma glucose value ≥126 mg/dl (Expert Committee, 1997) or a value of 200 mg/dl two hours after a 75 gram glucose challenge on the oral glucose tolerance test (OGTT) (Expert Committee, 1997; WHO, 1980). Characteristics and distinguishing features of the different categories of glucose intolerance are presented in Table 6.1.

PREVALENCE AND INCIDENCE OF DIABETES MELLITUS IN AFRICAN AMERICANS

Type 2 Diabetes

The most reliable data on the prevalence of Type 2 diabetes among adults in the United States are based on the results of the National Health Nutrition and Examination Survey III (NHANES III), 1988–1994 (Harris, Flegal et al., 1998). These data indicate that approximately 1.5 million African Americans adults have diabetes (Harris, Flegal et al., 1998). As shown in Table 6.2, the prevalence of physician-diagnosed and-undiagnosed diabetes among African Americans increases with age, with rates being higher in women than men. The overall prevalence of diabetes peaks in the age group

Table 6.2
Prevalence of diagnosed and undiagnosed diabetes among African Americans in the National Health and Nutrition Examination Survey III, 1988–1994

	Age (years)						
	20-39	40-49	50-59	60-74	≥75	≥20	≥20*
Diagnosed Diabetes							
Men	1.6	5.5	13.0	16.8	14.7	5.9	7.3
Women	1.6	6.7	14.5	23.9	19.0	7.8	9.1
Both	1.6	5.2	13.8	20.9	17.5	6.9	8.2
Undiagnosed Diabetes							
Men	1.1	4.3	3.0	6.6	0.0	2.6	2.7
Women	1.7	3.7	8.5	8.5	7.6	4.0	4.5
Both	1.4	3.9	6.1	7.7	4.9	3.4	3.6

*Data from Harris, Flegal et al. (1998); Values are age- and sex-standardized.

60 through 74, where a quarter of the African American population has the disease. African Americans age 20 and older are 1.6 times more likely to have diabetes than European Americans.

There are no available national data comparing the prevalence of Type 2 diabetes for African American and European American children. However there are indications that the increase in the prevalence of childhood diabetes that began in the United States in the mid-1990s has disproportionately affected African American and other minority children (Fagot-Campagna et al., 2002). In a sample of children and youth from the NHANES III, in each five-year age group, beginning at age 5 through age 20, African Americans had significantly higher Hemoglobin A1c levels (an indication of the body's inability to regulate blood glucose) than European American children (Saaddine et al., 2002). Because the complications of diabetes are closely linked to the length of time one has the illness, an excess in the number of African Americans developing Type 2 diabetes at younger ages will add to the disparity that already exists in the frequency and impact of diabetes complications.

Type 1 Diabetes

Prior to 1992, most reports of the frequency of Type 1 diabetes (which develops primarily in childhood) indicated that the rates in European American children were nearly twice those of African American children (Lorenzi et al., 1985; LaPorte et al., 1986; Wagenknecht et al., 1989; Lipman, 1991). More recent reports (Libman et al., 1998; Lipton et al., 2002) suggest that in some communities in the United States the incidence of Type 1 diabetes in African American children is now similar to that of European American children. Across the United States there appears to be more variability in the frequency of Type 1 diabetes in African American children compared to European American. A similar variation in rates of childhood Type 1 diabetes also exists across Black populations in the Caribbean region (Tull et al., 1997). It has been suggested that the variability in the incidence of Type 1 diabetes among African American children might result from variations in degree of White admixture in the various communities (Tull et al., 1991).

Atypical Diabetes

Diabetic syndromes that are ketosis-resistant and are characterized by intermittent periods of normoglycemic remission appear to occur more frequently in African Americans. Banerji et al. (1994) identified an insulin-resistant variant of Type 2 diabetes that led to suggestions that the disease might occur in African Americans in an insulin-sensitive and an insulin-resistant form that differ genetically. Among Caribbean Blacks, a similar ketosis-resistant form of diabetes with phasic insulin dependence has been reported on the island of Jamaica (Morrison & Ragoobirsingh, 1992). Often described by such terms as "type 1 ½ diabetes," very little data exist on the frequency of these atypical diabetes syndromes, although they appear to occur more frequently in Western Hemisphere Blacks compared to people of White European decent.

FACTORS INFLUENCING THE OCCURRENCE OF DIABETES

Factors influencing the occurrence of diabetes mellitus in African Americans include personal characteristics such as genetics, age, and sex. Physiological factors and prediabetic states such as insulin resistance, the metabolic syndrome, hormones of the hypothalamic pituitary adrenal axis (HPA-axis), markers of systematic inflammation, other categories of glucose intolerance and natal and prenatal factors have been identified as risk factors for the development of Type 2 diabetes. Lifestyle behaviors such as physical inactivity and excess caloric intake are linked to the development of obesity and consequently to glucose intolerance. In recent years additional focus has been placed on elucidating the role of socioeconomic and cultural factors as contributors to the disparity in the frequency and impact of diabetes between ethnic groups. While the exact etiological interactions between these factors remain debatable, it is certain that a differential effect of some or most of these factors is responsible for creating the disparity in the frequency of diabetes mellitus between African Americans and European Americans.

Personal Characteristics

Genetic Factors.   An individual's risk of developing diabetes mellitus is, to a great extent, influenced by his or her genetic background. The influence of genetics appears to be stronger for Type 2 diabetes than for Type 1 diabetes. Evidence from twin studies suggests that genetic factors play an important role in the etiology of > 90 percent of Type 2 diabetes and approximately 50 percent of Type 1 diabetes cases (Barnett et al., 1981). The search for the genetic reasons that rates of diabetes vary in different ethnic groups has led to development of hypotheses that seek to account for racial differences in the frequency of Type 1 and Type 2 diabetes mellitus.

Thrifty Gene Hypothesis.   It has been hypothesized (Neel, 1962) that genetic selection for survival during harsh conditions such as famine may be a reason for higher rates of Type 2 diabetes among certain populations, including African Americans. Neel (1962) suggested that populations exposed to periodic famines would through natural selection increase the frequency of certain genetic trait(s), "thrifty genes," that predispose to energy conservation. The bodies of these individuals would be adept at storing fat during times of abundance. These fat stores would then help them survive during times of famine. In circumstances of relative plenty, in the absence of feast and famine cycles, these genes would become disadvantageous, predisposing to the development of obesity and an increased frequency of Type 2 diabetes. While the search for thrifty-genotype genes is ongoing, there are suggestions that alternative hypotheses (discussed later in this chapter) related to fetal nutrition may better explain the apparent increased risk for the development of Type 2 diabetes seen in African Americans and other minorities compared to European Americans.

Racial Admixture Hypothesis.   In 1975 MacDonald hypothesized that the frequency of Type 1 diabetes might be higher in U.S. Black children compared to Black African children because Type 1 diabetes susceptibility genes more common in the U.S. White population had become admixed into to the African American population (MacDonald, 1975). Studies using genetic markers (Reitnauer et al., 1982) and grandparental race (Tull et al., 1991) have shown that African American Type 1 diabetes patients have more White Caucasian admixture than nondiabetic African American controls. Possible genetic factors that admixture may have increased are genes in the major histocompatibility (MHC) region (the HLA complex) of chromosome 6. Genes this complex are involved in immunological rejection of foreign cells (Friedman & Fialkow, 1982). In support of the admixture hypothesis, African Americans with IDDM have been observed to have similar HLA allelic associations to those found in U.S. Whites, particularly for HLA-DR3 and DR4 (Dunston et al., 1989).

Age.   In most populations the prevalence of diabetes increases with age. In general, the insulin-dependent form of the disease occurs more frequently at younger age, while Type 2 diabetes predominates in the older age groups. Type 2 diabetes occurs most frequently among African Americans age 65 and older where the prevalence is three times greater than in the White population (Harris, Klein et al., 1998). For African Americans, the peak age range for diagnosis of Type 1 diabetes is approximately 15–19 years of age (LaPorte et al., 1986; Wagenknecht et al., 1989).

Sex.   In the United States Type 2 diabetes occurs more frequently in African American women than men. African American women age 20 and older are 1.2 times more likely to have diagnosed diabetes Type 2 diabetes and 1.6 times more likely to have undiagnosed Type 2 diabetes compared to Black men (Harris, Klein et al., 1998). A female excess has also been reported for Type 1 diabetes in the U.S. Black population compared to a male excess among European Americans (LaPorte et al., 1986; Wagenknecht et al., 1989). The sex differential for Type 2 diabetes probably reflects gender differences in the levels of associated risk factors such as obesity and physical inactivity. It has been suggested that the gender differences in Type 1 diabetes may be due to differences in susceptibility or exposure to etiologic agents (Dahlquist et al., 1985).

Physiological Factors

Metabolic Syndrome.   The clustering of metabolic abnormalities, including hypertension, glucose intolerance, high triglycerides, and low HDL cholesterol (HDLc), together with abdominal obesity, has been referred to as the metabolic syndrome (Hansen, 1999). Individuals with the metabolic syndrome are at increased risk of developing Type 2 diabetes mellitus (Laaksonen et al., 2002). Data from the NHANES III (Park et al., 2003) indicate that the prevalence of the metabolic syndrome in African American men (13.9 percent) is significantly lower than the prevalence in European American men (20.8 percent) while the rates for African American women (20.9 percent) and European American women (22.9 percent) do not differ significantly.

Insulin Resistance.   Insulin resistance is a strong risk factor for the development of Type 2 diabetes. In many populations, insulin resistance characterized by hyperinsulinemia can predate the development of Type 2 diabetes for years (Sicree et al., 1987). It has recently been demonstrated that, in addition to diabetes, insulin resistance may underlie a number of interrelated disorders including hypertension, body fat mass and distribution, and serum lipid abnormalities (Ferrannini et al., 1991). This has prompted speculation that hyperinsulinemia and/or insulin resistance may be the phenotypic expression of the "thrifty genotype" (Zimmet, 1992). Epidemiological studies suggest that African Americans are more insulin-resistant than European Americans (Saad et al., 1991).

Hormones of the Hypothalamic-Pituitary-Adrenal (HPA) Axis.   There is a link between malfunction of the hypothalamic-pituitary-adrenal (HPA) axis, with elevation in the level of the hormone cortisol and reductions in levels of sex steroid hormones, and the accumulation of visceral fat (Haffner et al., 1991). The increased visceral fat contributes to higher circulating levels of free fatty acids (Rebuffe-Scrive et al., 1985), and elevated levels free fatty acids are associated with the development of insulin resistance (Ferranni et al., 1983). Per Björntorp hypothesized that a defeat type response to chronic environmental stressors was an important contributor to malfunction of the HPA axis (Björntorp, 1997). There is an emerging body of evidence supporting Björntorp's hypothesis. Individuals with high levels of abdominal fat assessed by waist circumference show elevated salivary cortisol secretion when challenged by laboratory stressors (Epel et al., 2000), and an abnormal secretory pattern characterized by reduced salivary cortisol level in the morning has been associated with increased abdominal fat and other metabolic abnormalities (Rosemond & Björntorp, 2000; Ljung et al., 2000). Given that greater levels of psychosocial stress exist in African American communities, it is possible that at the population level African Americans may be more likely to experience HPA-axis dysfunction compared to European Americans.

Inflammatory Markers.   Serum levels of biological markers of inflammation, including C-reactive protein and PAI-1, are elevated in obese individuals, those with higher waist circumference and persons with diabetes (Ford, 1999). Cytokines such as Interlukin-6 (Il6) and tissue necrosis factor alfa (TNFα) are also elevated among persons with diabetes and abdominal obesity (Hotamisligil et al., 1995; Kern et al., 1995). IL6 also stimulates the HPA-axis—chronic activation of which is associated with central obesity and insulin resistance (Path et al., 2000).

Prior History of Glucose Intolerance.   A level of glucose intolerance such as impaired fasting glucose (IFG) or impaired glucose tolerance (IGT), where the fasting glucose or two-hour glucose tolerance test values are between normal and diabetic, is an important risk factor for Type 2 diabetes. African Americans are more likely to have impaired fasting glucose or impaired glucose tolerance compared to European Americans (Harris, Flegal et al., 1998). The risk of developing overt diabetes among individuals with IGT is related to the severity of impaired tolerance and presence of other risk factors including a positive family history of diabetes and obesity (Harris, 1989). Gestational diabetes (GDM) which refers to the development of diabetes during pregnancy and a subsequent return to normal tolerance following parturition is also a strong risk factor for diabetes. A number of risk factors for GDM have been identified among African American women, including age, gravidity, hypertension, obesity, and family history of diabetes (Roseman et al., 1991).

Behavioral Factors

Obesity.   Cross-sectional and longitudinal studies have demonstrated that obesity is a major risk factor for Type 2 diabetes in various ethnic groups, including African Americans. Recent studies of Black populations (Okosun et al., 1998; Okosun et al., 1999) reported that among Blacks from Nigeria, Jamaica, and the United States, the waist circumference is more strongly associated with Type 2 diabetes risk than BMI. It has been shown that, for a given waist-to-hip ratio, African American women have less visceral fat than European American women (Conway et al., 1995). However, quite paradoxically, African American women are more insulin-resistant than European American women despite the lower level of visceral fat (Lovejoy et al., 1996). The significant association of subcutaneous abdominal fat with fasting insulin and insulin sensitivity in African Americans (Lovejoy et al., 1996) suggests that other factors related to total obesity may influence insulin resistance in the Black population.

An association of skeletal muscle fat with increased insulin resistance (Phillips et al., 1996; Pan et al., 1997; Goodpaster et al., 1997), has also been reported. In a cohort of sedentary healthy White men and women, Goodpaster et al. (1997) showed that subcutaneous abdominal fat and thigh muscle fat predicted insulin sensitivity independent of visceral fat. A study of elderly (70–80 year olds) in the Health ABC study (Goodpaster et al., 2001), showed that Black men and women had higher absolute areas of intramuscular and subcutaneous thigh adipose tissue than White men and women.

Caloric Intake

A recent report from the study of dietary patterns among the Pima Indians (Williams et al., 2001) showed that consumption of a typically high-fat American diet was associated with increased incidence of Type 2 diabetes (Williams et al., 2001) when compared to a traditional Indian diet. Recent population studies have shown that the frequency of eating at fast-food restaurants is associated with higher total energy intake and higher percentage of fat energy (French et al., 2000) and that dietary fat is associated with insulin resistance (Harding et al., 2001). Irrespective of the type of foods consumed, the excess intake of calories is associated with weight gain, and obesity is associated with diabetes risk. Therefore, efforts to reduce the disparity in diabetes risk for African Americans will need to focus on promoting dietary change at the population level.

Physical Inactivity

Physical inactivity is associated with an increased risk of Type 2 diabetes in African Americans (James et al., 1998). National data from the 1988–1994 National Health Nutrition and Examination Survey (NHANES) III among adults age 20 and older indicate that the frequency of inactivity among African Americans (35 percent) was significantly higher than for European Americans (18 percent) (Crespo et al., 2000). Data from the NHANES III also show a similar pattern among children age 8–16 where the frequency of inactivity was higher for African American children, particularly girls (Crespo et al., 2001). While it appears that differences in levels of physical inactivity may contribute to the disparity in diabetes risk experienced by African Americans, there are some concerns about how activity is measured in most studies. Kriska (2000) suggests that low-level activities may form the greatest component of energy expended through physical activity in minority groups and therefore measurement of activity in these groups may require more objective methods of assessment other than questionnaires that assess leisure activity. However, the Diabetes Prevention Program demonstrated that moderate activity (150 minutes/week) together with caloric restriction was equally effective in reducing the three-year incidence of Type 2 diabetes for Black and White Americans (Diabetes Prevention Program Research Group, 2002).

Natal and Prenatal Factors.   Two underlying hypotheses have driven much of the research relating the prenatal intrauterine environment to the risk of developing diabetes. Freinkel (1980) hypothesized that exposure of the fetus to hyperglycemia in utero induces a "fuel mediated teratogenesis" that increases susceptibility to obesity and Type 2 diabetes. Epidemiological studies (Pettit et al., 1993) have provided some support for this hypothesis. Another hypothesis proposed by Barker (1992) suggests that undernutrition in the intrauterine and early postnatal environment predisposes to the development of Type 2 diabetes in the presence of overnutrition in adulthood. In support of this "thrifty phenotype" hypothesis, studies have shown that individuals who were low birth-weight infants are at increased risk of developing Type 2 diabetes as adults (Curhan et al., 1996). While cause-and-effect relationships in these hypotheses are yet unproven in humans, the hypothesized relationships between the prenatal factors and Type 2 diabetes might provide an explanation for the increased susceptibility of African Americans to Type 2 diabetes.

Socioeconomic and Cultural Factors

Socioeconomic Status (SES).   Higher levels of socioeconomic status are usually associated with a reduced risk of diabetes in developed countries and an increased risk in developing countries

(Marmot, 1999). The strong association of SES with Type 2 diabetes risk has led to the generalization that most of the disparity in diabetes risk between African Americans and European Americans is due to socioeconomic differences. Results of analyses of data from the NHANES III support this assertion for women, but not for men. Using the poverty income ratio (PIR; the ratio of total family income to the poverty threshold for a reference year) to measure socioeconomic status, Robbins et al. (2000) showed that adjusting for PIR reduced the odds ratio for diabetes risk by 34 percent among African American women but had little effect among African American men. Thus, it appears that while socioeconomic status is an important contributor to the disparity in diabetes risk in African American women, other factors contribute more to the disparity among Black men.

Psychological and Social Stress

A higher level of stress among African Americans with diabetes compared to European Americans with the disease has been suggested as a possible reason for disparity in diabetes-related morbidity between the groups (Bell et al., 1995). The contribution of stress to differences in the frequency of diabetes has not, however, been adequately studied. Three reasons that stress might be an important contributor to the disparity in diabetes risk between African Americans and European Americans are as follows: (1) cross-sectional (Wing et al., 1991; Raikkonen et al., 1996) and prospective (Raikkonen et al., 1999) studies have shown that measures of psychological stress, including depression, anxiety, mental fatigue, anger, and hostility, are significantly and positively related to larger waist size, a major risk factor for Type 2 diabetes; (2) collective social stress, as in the stress experienced by peoples or cultures experiencing Westernization, is associated with abnormal glucose homeostasis as measured by the Hemoglobin A1c level (Daniel et al., 1999); and (3) the disadvantaged position of African Americans (including exposure to racism) make African Americans as a group more likely to experience a chronic a level of stress not experienced by European Americans.

Surwit et al. (2002) reported that a significant relationship of hostility to fasting insulin and insulin sensitivity was partially dependent on BMI among European Americans, while the significant relationship of hostility to fasting glucose in African Americans was independent of BMI. In a study of African Americans in the U.S. Virgin Islands (Tull & Chambers, 2001) internalized racism and hostility were significantly associated with an increased risk of having newly diagnosed Type 2 diabetes. In another study among Black women on the Caribbean island of Dominica (Butler et al., 2002), hostility was not associated with abnormal fasting glucose independent of internalized racism, while the relationship of internalized racism to abnormal fasting glucose was independent of BMI but not waist circumference. It has been suggested that in African Americans social factors such as internalized racism are markers for dysfunction of the HPA-axis, which leads to abdominal obesity and associated metabolic abnormalities like Type 2 diabetes (Tull & Chambers, 2001).

DIABETES MORTALITY

In addition to the excess risk related to the development of the disease, a disparity exists in rates of death from diabetes. In a 22-year follow-up study of subjects who participated in the National Health and Nutrition Survey I (NHANES I) in 1971–1975, the age-adjusted mortality rate for diabetic African Americans was 27 percent higher than for diabetic European Americans (Gu et al., 1998). The disparity in Type 2 diabetes mortality may reflect the overall shorter duration of life for Blacks as well as possible earlier age of diabetes onset and or more rapid onset of complications because of poorer control of blood sugar, a higher frequency of hypertension, poorer nutrition, lower socioeconomic statue, and less access to good care. In a 34-year follow-up of Type 1 diabetes patients in Allegheny County, Pennsylvania, the mortality rate for African Americans was 2.43 times that of European Americans (Nishimura et al., 2001). Another study from the same cohort showed that much of the disparity in Type 1 diabetes mortality for African Americans is due to acute complications that are preventable (Tull & Barinas, 1996).

DIABETIC COMPLICATIONS

Diabetes mellitus is associated with a number of devastating complications that diminish the quality of life and lead to premature mortality. Data from the NHANES III (Harris, Klein et al., 1998) showed that the prevalence of diabetic retinopathy (eye disease) in African Americans was 46 percent higher than compared to European Americans. In a study (Arfken et al., 1998) of the risk of developing proliferative diabetic retinopathy (PDR) among Type 1 diabetic subjects, African American ethnicity was associated with an unadjusted odds ratio of 1.86. However, after adjusting for glycemic control, duration of diabetes, retinopathy grade, and length of follow-up, there were no ethnic differences in the rate of PDR. The rate of end-stage renal disease (ESRD) is four times higher in African Americans than European Americans (Nzerue et al., 2002). Rates of lower-extremity amputations have also been reported to be higher in African Americans than European Americans (Young et al., 2003).

In addition to disparities in diabetes-related mortality and morbidity, ethnic differences exist in the prevalence of risk factors for diabetes complications and premature death. Factors associated with an increased risk of diabetic complications include delay in diagnosis and treatment, poor control of blood sugar, limited access to care, and poor quality of care. Using data from the NHANES III cohort, Harris et al. (1999) reported that compared to European Americans, African Americans with diabetes had similar rates of health insurance coverage through governmental programs (91 percent vs. 89 percent, respectively), but significantly lower coverage through private insurance (81 percent vs. 56 percent, respectively). Poor control of blood sugar was highest among African American women compared to African American men and other race/ethnic groups in the NHANES III (Harris et al., 1999). African Americans with ESRD are less likely to receive simultaneous pancreas and kidney transplant than European Americans (Isaacs et al., 2000). In a study of 300,574 individuals enrolled in Medicare, African Americans with diabetes were significantly less likely to receive eye examinations than European Americans.

ELIMINATING THE DISPARITY

A Paradigm Shift

To begin to effectively address the disparity in diabetes risk, a paradigm shift is needed in which funding agencies and researchers alike place added value on understanding how culture influences both the frequency and impact of diabetes in African Americans. Moreover, studies that are designed to recruit and study only African Americans are needed and should be encouraged. There are some important considerations in this regard. First, it is possible that the risk factor(s) responsible for perpetuating the diabetes-related disparities in African Americans are active exclusively among African Americans. If this is the case, then studies comparing Black with White Americans are unlikely to yield the necessary clues for addressing the disparities. Internalized racism, for example, may be a promoter of HPA-axis dysregulation and diabetes risk in African Americans but not in European Americans. In addition, cultural context might alter the way social or behavioral risk factors operate in African and European Americans, thereby resulting in confusing results when Blacks and Whites are compared. A potential example of this situation is the differential effect seen when adjusting Black/White gender specific comparisons of diabetes prevalence for socioeconomic status in the NHANES III study. While adjusting for SES and other known risk factors substantially reduced the excess risk in Black women compared to White women, similar adjustment actually increased the disparity in Black males compared to White males (Robbins et al., 2000). Socioeconomic status and other risk factors might influence Black and White men differently within their specific cultural context.

Expanding the Pool of Investigators

There remains a dearth of investigators from ethnic minority groups who are actively engaged in diabetes research. Expanding the pool of minorities involved in diabetes research should continue to be the goal of established investigators and funding agencies. This might be accomplished through development of programs designed to (1) encourage young students at the college and graduate school level to pursue careers in various aspects of diabetes research, (2) encourage minority investigators in other fields to consider diabetes as an area of interest, and (3) encourage the development of interdisciplinary research teams that include social scientists, epidemiologists, and biomedical researchers to examine critical gaps in knowledge relative to the etiology of diabetes in African Americans.

Empowering the Next Generation of Potential Diabetics

For the African American population, "Generation Next" is facing the staggering possibility of a significantly lower average age at onset of Type 2 diabetes. The evidence suggests that risk factors such as obesity and physical activity are increasing in the population. There is a need for programs designed to increase the level of health consciousness in African American youth. Such programs should begin at the level of the primary school, where the youth are taught to care for their bodies and should show the long-term effects of sedentary lifestyle and poor diet. As one ancient Jewish writer wrote, "Where there is no vision, the people perish." African American youth and their parents must see the vision of a future without health disparities.

REFERENCES

American Diabetes Association (ADA). (1997). Report of the Expert Committee on the Diagnosis and Classification of Diabetes Mellitus. *Diabetes Care, 20,* 1183–1197.

Arfken C.L., et al. Santiago J.V., & Klein R. (1998). Development of proliferative diabetic retinopathy in African Americans and Whites with Type 1 diabetes. *Diabetes Care,* 792–795.

Banerji, M.A., & Lebovitz, H.E. (1990). Remission in non-insulin-dependent diabetes mellitus: Clinical characteristics of remission and relapse in Black patients. *Medicine, 69,* 176–185.

Banerji, M.A. et al. (1994). GAD antibody negative NIDDM in adult black subjects with diabetic ketoacidosis and increased frequency of human leukocyte antigen DR3 and DR4. Flatbush diabetes. *Diabetes, 43,* 741–745.

Barker, D.J.P. (Ed.). (1992). Fetal and infant origins of adult disease. London: *British Medical Journal* Books.

Barnett, A.H., et al. & Pyke, D.A. (1981). Diabetes in identical twins, a study of 200 pairs. *Diabetologia, 20,* 87–93.

Bell, R.A., et al. J.H., & Konen, J.C. (1995). Racial differences in psychosocial variables among adults with non-insulin-dependent diabetes mellitus. *Behavioral Medicine, 21,* 69–73.

Björntorp, P. (1997). Body fat distribution, insulin resistance, and metabolic diseases. (1997). *Nutrition, 13,* 795–803.

Björntorp P., & Rosemond, R. (2000). The metabolic syndrome—a neuroendocrine disorder? *British Journal of Nutrition, 83,* S49–S57.

Butler, C., Tull, E.S., Chambers, E.C., & Taylor, J. (2002). Internalized racism, body fat distribution, and abnormal fasting glucose among African-Caribbean women in Dominica, West Indies. *Journal National Medical Association, 94,* 143–148.

Conway, J.M., et al. (1995). Visceral adipose tissue differences in Black and White women. *American Journal of Clinical Nutrition, 61*, 765–71.

Crespo, C.J., et al. (2000). Race/ethnicity, social class and their relation to physical inactivity during leisure time: results from the Third National Health and Nutrition Examination Survey, 1988–1994. *American Journal of Preventive Medicine, 18*, 46–53.

Crespo, C.J., et al. (2001). Television watching, energy intake and obesity in U.S. children: Results from the Third National Health and Nutrition Examination Survey, 1988–1994. *Archives of Pediatrics and Adolescent Medicine, 155*, 360–365.

Curhan, G.C., et al. (1996). Birth weight and adult hypertension, diabetes mellitus, and obesity in U.S. men. *Circulation, 15*, 3246–3250.

Dahlquist, G., Blom, L., Holgren, G., Hogglof, B., Larsson, Y., Sterky, G., & Wall, S. (1985). The epidemiology of diabetes in Sweedish children 0–14 years: A six year prospective study. *Diabetologia, 28*, 802–808.

Daniel, M., O'Dea, K., Rowley, K.G., McDermott, R., & Kelly, S. (1999). Glycated hemoglobin as an indicator of social environmental stress among indigenous versus Westernized populations. *Preventive Medicine, 29*, 405–413.

Diabetes Prevention Program (DPP) Research Group (2002). The Diabetes Prevention Program (DPP): Description of lifestyle intervention. *Diabetes Care, 25*, 2165–2171.

Dunston, G.M., Henry, L.W., Christian, J., Ofosu, M.D., & Callender, C.O. (1989). HLA-DR3, DQ heterogeneity in American blacks is associated with susceptibility and resistance to insulin-dependent diabetes mellitus. *Transplantation Proceedings, 21*, 653–655.

Epel, E.S., Mc Ewen, B., Seeman, T., Matthews, K., Castellazzo, G., Brownell, K.D., Bell, J., & Ickovics, J.R. (2000). Stress and body shape: Stress-induced cortisol secretion is consistently greater among women with central fat. *Psychosomatic Medicine, 62*, 623–632.

Fagot-Campagna, A., Pettitt, D.J., Engelgau, M.M., Burrows, N.R., Geiss, L.S., & Valdez, R. (2002). Type 2 diabetes in North American children and adolescents: An epidemiologic review and a public health perspective. *Journal of Pediatrics, 136*, 664–672.

Ferland, M., Despres, J.P., Tremblay, A., Pinault, S., Nadeau, A., Moorjani, S., Lupien, P., Thériault, G., & Bouchard, C. (1989). Assessment of adipose tissue distribution by computed axial tomography in obese women: Association with body density and anthropometric measurements. *British Journal of Nutrition, 61*, 139–148.

Ferrannini, E., Barett, E.J., Bevilaqua, M.P., & DeFronzo, R.A. (1983) Effects of fatty acids on glucose production and utilization in man. *Journal of Clinical Investigation, 72*, 1737.

Ford, E.S. (1999). Body mass index, diabetes, and C-reactive protein among U.S. adults. *Diabetes Care, 22*, 1971–1977.

Freinkel, N. (1980). Of pregnancy and progeny. *Diabetes, 29*, 1023–1035.

French, S.A., et al. (2000). Fast food restaurant use among women in the Pound of Prevention study: Dietary, behavioral and demographic correlates. *International Journal of Obesity and Related Metabolic Disorders, 24*, 1353–1359.

Friedman, J.M., & Fialkow, J. (1982). Genetics. In B.N. Broduff & S.J. Bleicher (Eds.), *Diabetes Mellitus and Obesity* (pp. 364–373). Baltimore, MD: Williams/Wilkins.

Goodpaster, B.H., et al. (2001). Attenuation of skeletal muscle and strength in the elderly: The Health ABC Study. *Journal of Applied Physiology, 90*, 2157–2165.

Goodpaster, B.H., et al. (1997). Subcutaneous abdominal fat and thigh muscle composition predict insulin sensitivity independent of visceral fat. *Diabetes, 46*, 1579–1585.

Gu, K., et al. (1998). Mortality in adults with and without diabetes in a national cohort of the U.S. population, 1971–1993. *Diabetes Care, 21*, 1138–1145.

Haffner, S.M., Katz, M.S., & Dunn, J.F. (1991). Increased upper body obesity and overall adiposity is associated with decreased sex hormone binding globulin in postmenopausal women. *Int J Obes, 15*, 471–478.

Hansen, B.C. (1999). The metabolic syndrome X. *Annals of the New York Academy of Sciences, 892*: 1–24.

Harding, A.H., et al. (2001). Is the association between dietary fat intake and insulin resistance modified by physical activity? *Metabolism, 50*, 1186–1192.

Harris, M.I. (1989). Impaired glucose tolerance in the U.S. population. *Diabetes Care, 12*, 464–474.

Harris, M.I. (1999). Racial and ethnic differences in health insurance coverage for adults with diabetes. *Diabetes Care, 22,* 1679–1682.

Harris, M.I., Eastman, R.C., Cowie, C.C., Flegal, K.M., & Eberhardt, M.S. (1999). Racial and ethnic differences in glycemic control of adults with Type 2 diabetes. *Diabetes Care, 22,* 403–408.

Harris, M.I., Flegal, K.M., Cowie, L.L., et al. (1998). Prevalence of diabetes, impaired fasting glucose, and impaired glucose tolerance in U.S. adults. The Third National Health and Nutrition Examination Survey, 1988–1994. *Diabetes Care, 21,* 518–524.

Harris, M.I., Klein R., Cowie C.C., Rowland M., & Byrd-Holt, D.D. (1998). Is the risk of diabetic retinopathy greater in non-Hispanic blacks and Mexican Americans than in non-Hispanic whites with Type 2 diabetes. *Diabetes Care, 21,* 1230–1234.

Hotamisligil, G.S., Arner, P., Caro, J.F., Atkinson, R.L., & Spiegelman, B.M. (1995). Increased adipose tissue expression of tumor necrosis factor alpha in human obesity and insulin resistance. *Journal of Clinical Investigation, 95,* 2409–2415.

Isaacs, R.B., Lobo, P.I., Nock, S.I., Hanson, J.A., Ojo, A.O., & Pruett, T.L. (2000). Racial disparities in access to simultaneous pancreas-kidney transplation in the United States. *American Journal of Kidney Disease, 36,* 526–633.

James, S.A., et al. (1998). Physical activity and NIDDM in African Americans. The Pitt County Study. *Diabetes Care, 21,* 555–562.

Kaufman, F.R. (2002). Type 2 diabetes mellitus in children and youth: A new epidemic. *Journal of Pediatric Endocrinology Metabolism, 15,* 737–744.

Kendall J., Hatton, D. (2002). Racism as a source of health disparity in families with children with attention deficit hyperactivity disorder. *Advances in Nursing Science, 25,* 22–39.

Kern, P.A., Saghizadeh, M., Ong, J.M., Bosch, R.J., Deem, R., & Simsolo, R.B. (1995). The expression of tumor necrosis factor in human adipose tissue: Regulation by obesity, weight loss and relationship to lipoprotein lipase. *Journal of Clinical Investigation, 95,* 2111–2119.

Kriska, A.K. (2000). Ethnic and cultural issues in assessing physical activity. *Research Quarterly for Exercise and Sport, 71,* 47–53.

Laaksonen, D.E., Lakka, H.M., Niskanan, L.K., Kaplan, G.A., Salonen, J.T., & Lakka, T.A. (2002). Metabolic syndrome and development of diabetes mellitus: Application and validation of recently suggested definitions of the metabolic syndrome in a prospective cohort study. *American Journal of Epidemiology, 156,* 1070 1077.

LaPorte, R.E., et al. (1986). Differences between Blacks and Whites in the epidemiology of insulin-dependent diabetes mellitus in Allegheny County, Pennsylvania. *American Journal of Epidemiology, 123,* 592–603.

Libman, I.M., Pietropaolo, M., Trucco, M., Dorman, J.S., LaPorte, R.E., Becker, D. (1998) Islet cell autoimmunity in white and black children and adolescents with IDDM. *Diabetes Care, 21(11),* 1824–1827.

Lipman, T.H. (1991). The epidemiology of Type 1 diabetes in children 0–14 years of age in Philadelphia. Doctoral dissertation, University of Pennsylvania.

Lipton, R., Keenan, H., Onyemere, K.U., & Freels, S. (2002). Incidence and onset features of diabetes in African-American and Latino children in Chicago, 1985–1994. *Diabetes Metabolism Research & Review, 18,* 135–142.

Ljung, T., et al. (2000). The activity of the hypothalmic-pituitary-adrenal axis and the sympathetic nervous system in relation to waist/hip circumference ratio in men. *Obesity Research, 8,* 487–495.

Lorenzi, M., Cogliero, E., & Schmidt, N.J. (1985). Racial differences in the incidence of juvenile-onset Type 1 diabetes: Epidemiological studies in southern California. *Diabetologia, 28,* 734–738.

Lovejoy, J.C., de la Bretonne, J.A., Klemperer, M., & Tulley, R. (1996). Abdominal fat distribution and metabolic risk factors: Effects of race. *Metabolism, 45,* 1119–1124.

MacDonald, M.J. (1975). Lower frequency of diabetes among hospitalized Negro than white children. Theoretical implications. *Acta Geneticae Medicae et Gemellologiae 24,* 119–126.

Marmot, M. (1999). Epidemiology of socioeconomic status and health: Are determinants within countries the same as between countries? *Annals of the New York Academy of Science, 896,* 16–29.

Morrison, E.Y., & Ragoobirsingh, D.J. (1992). Type diabetes revisited. *Journal of the National Medical Association, 84,* 603–608.

Neel, J.V. (1962). Diabetes mellitus—A "thrifty genotype" rendered detrimental by "progress"? *American Journal of Human Genetics, 14*, 353–362.

Nishimura, R., LaPorte, R.E., Dorman, J.S., Tajima, N., Becker, D., & Orchard, T. (2001). Mortality trends in Type 1 diabetes: The Allegheny County (Pennsylvania) Registry 1965–1999. *Diabetes Care, 24*, 823–827.

Nzerue, C.M., Demissochew, H., & Tucker, J.K. (2002). Race and kidney disease: Role of social and environmental factors. *Journal National Medical Association, 94(8 Suppl)*: 28S–38S.

Okosun, I.S., Cooper, R.S., Prewitt, T.E., & Rotimi, C.N. (1999). The relation of central adiposity to components of the insulin resistance syndrome in a biracial U.S. population sample. *Ethnicity and Disease, 9*, 218–29.

Okosun, I.S., Cooper, R.S., Rotimi, C.N., Osotimehin, B., & Forrester, T. (1998). Association of waist circumference with risk of hypertension and Type 2 diabetes in Nigerians, Jamaicans, and African-Americans. *Diabetes Care, 21*, 1836–1842.

Pan, D.A., Lillioja, S., Kriketos, A.D., Milner, M.R., Baur, L.A., Bogardus, C., Jenkins, A.B., & Storlien, L.H. (1997). Skeletal muscle triglyceride levels are inversely related to insulin action. *Diabetes, 46*, 983–988.

Park, Y.W., Zhu, S., Palanippan, L., Heshka, S., Carnethon, M.R., & Heymsfield, S.B. (2003). The metabolic syndrome: Prevalence and associated risk factor findings in the U.S. population from the Third National Health and Nutrition Examination Survey, 1988–1994. *Archives of Internal Medicine, 163*, 427–436.

Path, G., Scherbaum, W.A., & Bornstein, S.R. (2000). The role of interleukin-6 in the human adrenal gland. *European Journal of Clinical Investigation, 30*, Suppl 3, 91–95.

Pettit, D.J., Nelson, R.G., Saad, M.F., Bennett, P.H. & Knowler, W.C. (1993). Diabetes and obesity in the offspring of Pima Indian Women with diabetes during pregnancy. *Diabetes Care, 16*, 310–314.

Phillips, D.I.W., Caddy, S., Ilic, V., Fielding, B.A., Frayn, K.N., Borthwick, A.C., & Taylor, R. (1996). Intramuscular triglyceride and muscle insulin sensitivity: Evidence for a relationship in nondiabetic subjects. *Metabolism, 45*, 947–950.

Pomerleau, J., McKeigue, P.M., Chaturvedi, N. (1999). Relationships of fasting and postload glucose levels to sex and alcohol consumption: Are American Diabetes Association criteria biased against detection of diabetes in women? *Diabetes Care, 22*, 430–433.

Raikkonen, K., Hautenen, A., & Keltikangas-Jarvinen, L. (1994). Association of stress and depression with regional fat distribution in healthy middle-age men. *Journal of Behavioral Medicine, 17*, 605–616.

Raikkonen, K., Mathews, K.A., Kuller, L.H., Reiber, C., & Bunker, C.H. (1999). Anger, hostility and visceral adipose tissue in healthy postmenopausal women. *Metabolism* 48, 146–1151.

Rebuffe-Scrive, M., Lundholm K., & Bjorntorp, P. (1985). Glucocoid hormone binding in human adipose tissue. *European Journal of Clinical Investigation, 15*, 267–271.

Reitnauer, P.J., Go, R.C.P., Acton, R.T., Murphy, C.C., Budowle, B., Barger, B.O. & Roseman, J.M. (1982). Evidence of genetic admixture as a determinant in the occurrence of insulin-dependent diabetes mellitus. *Diabetes, 31*, 532–537.

Report of the Expert Committee on the Diagnosis and Classification of Diabetes Mellitus. (1997). *Diabetes Care*, 20(7), 1183–1197.

Report of the Secretary's Task Force on Black and Minority Health. (1985). Volume 1: Executive Summary. DHHS Publication No. 017-090-00078. Washington, DC: U.S. Government Printing Office.

Robbins, J.M., et al., (2000). Excess type 2 diabetes in African-American women and men aged 40–74 and socioeconomic status: Evidence from the Third National Health and Nutrition Examination Survey. *Journal of Epidemiology and Community Health, 54*, 39–45.

Rose, K.M., Newman, B., Mayer-Davis, E.J., Selby, J.V. (1998). Genetic and behavioral determinants of waist-hip ration and waist circumferentc in women twins. *Obesity Research, 6*, 383–392.

Roseman, J.M., Go, R.C.P., Perkins, L.L., Barger, B.D., Beel, D.A., Goldenberg, R.L., DuBard, M.B., Huddlestone, J.F., Sedacek, C.M., & Acton, R.T. (1991). Gestational diabetes among African American women. *Diabetes and Metabolism Review, 7*, 93–104.

Rosemond, R., & Bjorntorp, P. (2000). Occupational status, cortisol secretory pattern and visceral obesity in middle-age men. *Obes Res*, 8, 445–450.

Ross, R., Dagnone, D., Jones, P.J., Smith, H., Paddags, A., Hudson, R., & Janssen, I. (2000). Reduction in obesity and related comorbid conditions after diet-induced weight loss or exercise-induced weight loss in men. A randomized, controlled trial. *Annals of Internal Medicine, 18*, 133, 92–103.

Saad, M.F., Lillioja, S., Nyomba, B.L., Castillo, C., Ferraro, R., & De Gregorio, M. (1991). Racial differences in the relation between blood pressure and insulin resistance. *New England Journal of Medicine, 324,(11)*, 733–739.

Saaddine J.B., Fagot-Campagna, A., Rolka, D., Narayan K.M.V., Geiss, L., Eberhardt, M., & Flegal, K.M. (2002). Distribution of HbA1c levels for children and young adults in the U.S.: Third National Health and Nutrition Examination Survey. *Diabetes Care, 25*, 1326–1330.

Sicree, R.A., Zimmet, P., King O.M., & Coventry, J.S. (1987). Plasma insulin response among auruans: Prediction of deterioration in glucose tolerance over 6 years. *Diabetes, 36*, 179–186.

Surwitt, R.S., Williams, R.B., Siegler I.C., Lane, J.D., Helms, M., Applegate K.I., Zucker, N., Feinglos, M.N., McCaskill C.M., & Barefoot, J.C. (2002). Hostility, race and glucose metabolism in nondiabetic individuals. *Diabetes Care, 25*, 835–839.

Tull, E.S., & Barinas E. (1996). A twofold excess mortality among black compared with white IDDM patients in Allegheny County, Pennsylvania. *Diabetes Care, 19*, 1344–1347.

Tull, E.S., & Chambers, E.C. (2001). Internalized racism is associated with glucose intolerance among Black Americans in the U.S. Virgin Islands. *Diabetes Care, 24*, 1498.

Tull, E.S., Jordan, O.W., Simon, L., Laws, M., Smith, D.O., Vanterpool, H., & Butler C. (1997). Incidence of childhood-onsed IDDM in Black African-heritage populations in the Caribbean. The Caribbean African Heritage IDDM Study (CAHIS) Group. *Diabetes Care, 20*, 309–310.

Tull, E.S., Roseman, J.M., & Christian C.L.E. (1991). Epidemiology of childhood IDDM in the U.S. Virgin Islands from 1979–1988: Evidence of an epidemic in the early 1980's and variation by degree of racial admixture. *Diabetes Care, 14*, 558–564.

Wagenknecht, L.E., Roseman J.M., & Alexander W.J. (1989). Epidemiology of IDDM in Black and White children in Jefferson County, Alabama, 1979–1985. *Diabetes, 38*, 29–633.

Williams, D.E., Knowler, W.C., Smith, C.J., Hanson, R.L., Roumain, J., Saremi, A., Kriska, A.M., Bennett, P.H., & Nelson, R.G. (2001). The effect of Indian or Anglo dietary preference on the incidence of diabetes in Pima Indians. *Diabetes Care, 24*, 811–816.

Wing, R.R., Matthews, K.A., Kuller, L.H., Meilahn, E.N., & Plantinga, P. (1991). Waist to hip ratio in middle-aged women. Associations with behavioral and psychosocial factors and with changes in cardiovascular risk factors. *Arteriosclerosis and Thrombosis, 11*, 1250–1257.

World Health Organization (WHO). (1980). Report of expert committee on diabetes mellitus. Technical Report Series, Series no. 646. Geneva: World Health Organization.

Yamanouchi, K., (1995). Daily walking combined with diet therapy is a useful means for obese NIDDM patients not only to reduce body weight but also to improve insulin sensitivity. *Diabetes Care, 18(6)*, 775–778.

Young, B.A., Maynard, C. Reiber, G., & Boyko E.J. (2003). Effects of ethnicity and nephropathy on lower-extremity amputation risk among diabetic veterans. *Diabetes Care, 26*, 495–501.

Zaldivar, A., & Smolowitz, J. (1994). Perceptions of the importance placed on religion and folk medicine by non-Mexican-American Hispanic adults with diabetes. *Diabetes Education, 20*, 303–306.

Zimmit, P. (1992). Kelly West Lecture 1991. Challenges in diabetes epidemiology—From West to the rest. *Diabetes Care, 15*, 232–251.

PART II

General Chronic Conditions

CHAPTER 7

Cancer Status in Black Americans

KI MOON BANG

INTRODUCTION

Cancer accounts for one out of every four deaths in the United States. During the period 1992–1999, trends of cancer incidence and mortality rates have decreased for both Blacks and Whites. The age-adjusted cancer incidence rate was 526.6 per 100,000 population for Blacks and 480.4 for Whites (NCI, 2002). The mortality rate was 267.3 per 100,000 population for Blacks compared with 205.1 for Whites (NCI, 2002). The five-year survival rate for cancer in Blacks diagnosed from 1992 through 1998 was about 53 percent compared with 64 percent for Whites (ACS, 2003). A considerable part of this difference in survival can be attributed to late diagnoses.

Strategies for reducing cancer incidence and mortality in Blacks have been developed and intervention and prevention programs targeted for high-risk populations, including Black Americans. The Department of Health and Human Services has established an objective of reducing cancer mortality to less than 202.4 per 100,000 population as the baseline in 1998 for Healthy People 2010 (USDHHS, 2000). Achieving this goal depends on the development and implementation of cancer prevention and control strategies directed at specific populations.

Cancer rates where Blacks have significantly higher incidence and mortality rates than Whites include lung, esophagus, stomach, colon, liver, prostate, larynx, cervix uteri, pancreas, and multiple myeloma. In contrast, cancer sites that Blacks have significantly lower incidence than Whites include breast and corpus uteri. The excessive incidence of these sites in Blacks might be explained by smoking, alcohol consumption, diet, physical activity, socioeconomic status, and lack of medical care. These factors are associated with an increased risk of cancer, but the precise cause–effect relationship has not been well addressed. This chapter reviews the epidemiology of cancer for Black Americans (i.e., current status and risk factors) and also proposes recommendations to reduce the incidence of cancer and related mortality rates.

Data Sources

The data in this chapter were derived from the latest available sources. Incidence and survival data were obtained from the Surveillance, Epidemiology and End Results (SEER) program of the

Table 7.1
Age-adjusted cancer incidence rates (per 100,000 population) by race and sex, 1992–1999

	Incidence rate			Trend (Annual % Change)		
	All races	Blacks	Whites	All races	Blacks	Whites
Total	475.8	526.6	480.4	-0.9	-1.3	-0.9
Males	570.5	703.6	568.2	-2.3	-2.7	-2.4
Females	413.6	404.8	424.4	+0.3	+0.1	+0.4

*Rates are adjusted to the 2000 U.S. standard population.

Source: National Cancer Institute, Cancer Control & Population Sciences, 2002.

National Cancer Institute (NCI, 2002). The National Cancer Institute collects data from 12 population-based tumor registries on all newly diagnosed patients and follow-up information on persons previously diagnosed. The geographic areas that make up the SEER program's database represent approximately 26 percent of the U.S. population (NCI, 2002). The estimated cancer incidence and five-year survival rates were obtained from the American Cancer Society (ACS, 2003). The mortality data were obtained from the National Center for Health Statistics vital statistics system (NCHS, 2002). Information on each death occurring in the United States includes cause of death, age at death, gender, and geographic area of residence at time of death.

CANCER STATUS

Incidence

The American Cancer Society (ACS) estimated that 1,334,100 Americans would be diagnosed with cancer in 2003 (ACS, 2003). About 185,000 of these new cases would be Black Americans. The age-adjusted incidence rate of cancer was 475.8 per 100,000 population for the period 1992–1999 based on the SEER program. The incidence rate decreased 0.9 percent per year for this period. The overall incidence in Blacks was 526.6 per 100,000 population compared with 480.4 for Whites (NCI, 2002) (Table 7.1). However, the magnitude of the overall cancer incidence rate among Blacks is about 9 percent higher than among Whites for the period 1992–1999. During this period, the age-adjusted incidence rate for Black males was 703.6 per 100,000 population compared with 568.2 for White males. In the case of females, the rate for Black females was 404.8 per 100,000 population compared with 424.4 for White females (Table 7.1). For the five years 1995–1999, the age-adjusted rate for Blacks declined 5.6 percent compared with 3.8 percent for Whites (Table 7.2).

The top five rank-ordered sites for cancer incidence among Blacks include the lung, prostate, breast, colon, and pancreas. The age-specific incidence rate increased with increasing age: for Black

Table 7.2
Age-adjusted cancer incidence rates (per 100,000 population) by race and sex, 1995–1999

	Blacks			Whites		
Year	Both	Males	Females	Both	Males	Females
1995	269.6	372.8	206.0	207.8	261.8	173.7
1996	264.9	365.3	202.3	205.3	256.8	172.1
1997	262.1	354.7	204.4	202.2	251.9	170.0
1998	256.8	345.4	201.4	200.7	248.6	168.8
1999	254.4	340.5	200.2	199.8	246.5	168.6

*Rate are per 100,000 population and are age-adjusted to the 2000 U.S. standard population.

Source: National Cancer Institute, 2002.

males, 160.4 per 100,000 population, for age group 40–44 compared with 2,509.9 per 100,000 population for age group 65–69. The overall age-adjusted incidence rate of lung cancer is 82.6 per 100,000 population during the period 1992–1999. The percent change of lung cancer incidence over this time interval is 1.4 percent decrease. The age-adjusted incidence rate of lung cancer for Black males is 124.1 per 100,000 population compared with 53.2 for Black females. Black men have a lung cancer rate 2 times higher than that of women and 1.3 times higher that of White men (Table 7.3). Prostate cancer incidence is the highest in Blacks. The incidence rate of prostate cancer is 275.3 per 100,000 population for Blacks compared with 172.9 for Whites. Black American men have a higher risk for developing prostate cancer than Whites.

During the period 1992–1999, the frequently diagnosed cancer sites in males are prostate, followed by lung and colon. Cancer incidence at these sites is higher for Black males than for males of other racial groups (NCHS, 2002). Female breast cancer incidence rate in Blacks was 120.7 per 100,000 population compared with 137.0 in White females. Black women over 65 years have much higher incidence of breast cancer than Black women less than 65 years. Colon cancer incidence rate in Blacks is 47.8 per 100,000 population compared with 39.1 for Whites during the period 1992–1999. Black men experience higher incidence of colon cancer than that of Black women. The annual percent change in colon cancer during the period 1992–1999 is 0.6 percent decrease, 1.6 percent decrease for men and 0.3 percent decrease for women. Pancreas cancer incidence is 16.2 per 100,000 population compared with 10.7 for Whites. The pancreas incidence rate for Blacks is higher for men (17.6 per 100,000) than for women (15.0 per 100,000) (NCI, 2002) (Table 7.3).

Mortality

The total number of cancer death was 549,838 in 1999 compared with 416,509 in 1980 (NCHS, 2002). The age-adjusted cancer mortality rate for Blacks is 267.3 per 100,000 population compared

Table 7.3
**Age-adjusted incidence rates (per 100,000 population) by
primary cancer site, 1992–1999**

	Blacks			Whites		
Site	Both	Males	Females	Both	Males	Females
All sites	526.6	703.6	404.8	480.4	568.2	424.4
Lung	82.6	124.1	53.2	64.3	82.9	51.1
Prostate	-	275.3	-	-	172.9	-
Breast	-	-	120.7	-	-	137.0
Colon/ Rectum	61.9	70.7	55.8	53.9	64.4	46.1
Colon	47.8	52.9	44.3	39.1	45.3	34.5
Pancreas	16.2	17.6	15.0	10.7	12.2	9.5
Corpus uteri	-	-	17.7	-	-	26.0
Cervix uteri	-	-	13.2	-	-	9.6
Stomach	13.9	19.6	9.9	7.9	11.7	5.2
Esophagus	8.0	12.9	4.4	4.2	7.1	1.9
Larynx	7.0	12.9	2.8	4.1	7.3	1.6
Leukemia	9.9	12.6	7.9	12.8	16.9	9.8
Liver	6.2	9.6	3.5	4.2	6.4	2.5
Multiple myeloma	11.4	13.1	10.3	5.2	6.5	4.2

Incidence rates per 100,000 population are adjusted to the 2000 U.S. standard population.

Source: National Cancer Institute, 2002.

with 205.1 for Whites for the period 1992–1999 (Table 7.4). The overall age-adjusted mortality rate decreased 5.6 percent, from 269.6 per 100,000 population in 1995 to 254.4 in 1999 (NCHS, 2002) (Table 7.5). The decrease is higher for males (8.7%) than for females (2.9%) during this period.

For major cancer sites, age-adjusted mortality rates per 100,000 population are 68.9 for lung cancer, 29.1 for colon and rectum, 37.3 for breast, 75.1 for prostate, 10.1 for stomach, and 14.7 for pancreas during the period 1992–1999 (NCI, 2002). Trends in cancer mortality rates during the period 1995–1999 are summarized in Table 7.5. During this period, age-adjusted cancer mortality for Blacks decreased 5.6 percent compared with 3.8 percent for Whites.

Differences between Blacks and Whites

The overall difference in cancer incidence, mortality, and survival rates between Blacks and Whites are summarized in Tables 7.1, 7.4, and 7.6. For all sites combined, Blacks experience 23 percent

Table 7.4

Age-adjusted cancer mortality rates (per 100,000 population) by race and sex, 1992–1999

	Mortality rate			Trend (Annual % Change)		
	All races	Blacks	Whites	All races	Blacks	Whites
Total	208.7	267.3	205.1	-0.9	-1.8	-0.9
Males	264.7	369.0	258.1	-1.5	-1.9	-1.4
Females	172.7	204.5	171.2	-0.6	-0.4	-0.6

Rates are adjusted to the 2000 U.S. standard population.

Source: National Cancer Institute, Cancer Control & Population Sciences, 2002.

Table 7.5

Age-adjusted cancer mortality rates (per 100,000 population) by race and sex, 1995–1999

	Blacks			Whites		
Year	Both	Males	Females	Both	Males	Females
1995	269.6	372.8	206.0	207.8	261.8	173.7
1996	264.9	365.3	202.3	205.3	256.8	172.1
1997	262.1	354.7	204.4	202.2	251.9	170.0
1998	256.8	345.4	201.4	200.0	248.6	168.8
1999	254.4	340.5	200.2	199.8	246.5	168.6

Rates are per 100,000 population and are age-adjusted to the 2000 U.S. population.

Source: National Center for Health Statistics, Health United States, 2002.

Table 7.6
Five-year cancer survival rates (percent) by race, 1992–1998

Site	Blacks	Whites
Brain	40	32
Breast	73	88
Cervix uterine	60	72
Colon	53	63
Esophagus	8	15
Leukemia	38	47
Liver	4	7
Lung	12	15
Multiple myeloma	33	30
Pancreas	4	4
Prostate	93	98
Stomach	20	21
Testis	85	96
Urinary bladder	65	82

Source: American Cancer Society, Cancer Facts and Figures, 2003.

higher mortality than Whites. Individual cancer sites for which there are particularly notable excesses in incidence and mortality in Blacks are esophagus, cervix uteri, larynx, prostate, stomach, lung (males), multiple myeloma, oral cavity, and liver. The cancer sites for which Blacks have less incidence and mortality than Whites are breast, leukemia, testis, brain, and melanoma of skin (NCI, 2002; NCHS, 2002; ACS, 2003) (Table 7.3).

Cancer survival rates are different between Blacks and Whites based on the data from SEER areas (Table 7.6). The overall five-year survival rate during the period 1992–1998 was 53 percent for Blacks compared with 64 percent for Whites (ACS, 2003). Blacks have more favorable survival than Whites for cancers of the brain and multiple myeloma. Cancer rates for which Whites have more than a 10 percent greater survival rate than Blacks include: colon/rectum, oval cavity, larynx, melanoma, female breast, cervix uteri, corpus uteri, prostate, and urinary bladder.

In examining survival trend, it is desirable to observe changes in survival rates as related to the stage of disease at diagnosis. The stage can be classified as localized or regional cancer. Survival rate is much better in cases of localized cancer than regional cancer. For example, a vast difference is the five-year survival rate of stomach cancer, which was observed according to stage (i.e., 59 percent for localized versus 22 percent for regional) (ACS, 2002). One of the reasons for poor survival in Blacks may be that the disease is diagnosed and treated at a late stage (White et al., 1981).

Low socioeconomic status can be a strong determinant of poor survival rates in Blacks (Bang, Perlin, & Sampson, 1987). Also, the observed difference in survival rates between Blacks and Whites may be attributed to a number of factors, including, but not limited to, inadequate medical care, cancer treatment, and cancer screening programs for Blacks than Whites (Bang, White, Gause, & Leffall, 1988). A recent study showed that Black cancer patients tend to have higher relative risk of cancer death than the other racial groups (Clegg et al., 2002). Relative survival rates for Whites exceed those for Blacks by 15 percent for most stages.

Risk Factors

Multiple risk factors contribute to cancer in Black Americans. The major risk factors include (1) lifestyle factors, (2) occupational/environmental exposure, (3) familial predisposition and genetic factors, and (4) socioeconomic status. A discussion of these factors follows.

Lifestyle Factors.   Lifestyle factors include cigarette smoking, alcohol consumption, and eating habits. The higher cancer incidence for Blacks might be the result of lifestyle (ACS, 2003; Baquet et al., 1991; McWhorter et al., 1989; Hargreaves et al., 1989; Bang et al., 1988; Gullatte, 1989). Higher cancer rates in the lung, head and neck, stomach, liver, and esophagus in Blacks can be attributed exclusively to smoking and drinking. Other risk factors include inadequate diet and being obese.

Smoking.   Smoking accounts for at least 30 percent of all cancer deaths. Smoking is a risk factor for the lung, lip, tongue, mouth, larynx, esophagus, bladder, pancreas, and cervix uteri. Smoking is the most preventable cause of cancer death in our society. It is estimated that cigarette smoking is responsible for 87 percent of lung cancer (ACS, 2003). Between 1997 and 2000, current smoking prevalence declined for Blacks (26.7 percent to 23.2 percent and Whites (25.3 percent to 24.1 percent) (CDC, 2003). Between 1983 and 1999, smoking among college graduates decreased almost 50 percent from 21 percent to 11 percent, but among adults without a high school education the percentage decreased only 22 percent from 41 percent to 32 percent (ACS, 2002). Currently, it is estimated that there are approximately 47 million smokers in the United States. Men were more likely to smoke (26 percent) than women (21 percent).

Smoking prevalence is different between Blacks and Whites. In 2001, the Centers for Disease Control reported that 28.7 percent of Black males in the United States smoked compared with 25.4 percent of White males (USDHHS, 2001). For those between the ages of 35 and 44 years, 35.0 percent of Black men smoked compared with 29.5 percent of White men. When Black and White women were compared, 29.0 percent of Blacks compared with 27.0 percent of White women smoked. At ages 45 to 64, however, the percentage of Black women who smoked was 22.6 percent compared with 21.3 percent for White women. For ages 65 and over, the smoking prevalence was 13.6 percent for Blacks compared with 10.4 percent of White women. Smoking rates are higher among Blacks, blue-collar workers, and people with few years of education. The higher prevalence of smoking in Blacks is associated with an increased risk of lung cancer and other cancer sites. A recent issue concerns the health effects of passive smoking. The U.S. Environmental Protection Agency report on the respiratory health effects of passive smoking indicates that secondhand smoke is responsible for approximately 3,000 lung cancer deaths per year in nonsmoking adults (EPA, 1992).

Drinking.   Alcohol drinking has been reported to be associated with colon, breast, prostate, and esophageal cancers. People who drink alcohol should limit themselves to no more than two drinks per day for men and one drink a day for women (ACS, 2003). The National Health and Nutrition Examination Survey (NHANES), conducted by the National Center for Health Statistics, showed that Black men report heavier drinking than do White men of comparable age (Mettlin, 1980). The incidence rate of esophageal cancer in Blacks is almost four times higher than in Whites. One of the reasons for this might be a higher alcohol consumption rate among Blacks than Whites. A recent case-control study by the National Cancer Institute showed that the major factors responsible for the excess of esophageal cancer in the District of Columbia was alcoholic consumption, and the risk increased with the amount of ethanol consumed and was highest among drinkers of hard liquor (Potter et al., 1981). Besides esophageal cancer, alcohol consumption is associated with cancer of the larynx, stomach, colon/rectum, pancreas, and breast.

Diet.   Cancer deaths in the United States that are associated with diet range from 10 to 70 percent (DHHS, 1988). The most consistent evidence is that higher intake of fruits and vegetables reduces the risk of specific cancers. Many reported evidences show that meat or animal fat intake is associated with risks of colon and prostate cancers (Willett, 1996). Prior research has examined the role diet and nutrition may play in the development of cancer. Poor eating habits and the nutritional status of Black Americans are a national problem that could contribute to higher incidence and mortality rates from cancer. Blacks have different eating patterns from those of Whites. The NHANES data showed that Blacks consume higher levels of fats and lower levels of vegetables than Whites. Among men aged 18 to 44 years, 37 percent of Blacks report that they usually eat fruits and vegetables two or more times a day compared with 53 percent of Whites (Mettlin, 1980).

Numerous studies have shown that daily consumption of vegetables and fruits is associated with a decreased risk of lung, prostate, bladder, esophagus, and stomach cancers. For the majority of Blacks who do not smoke, dietary choices and physical activity are the most important modifiable determinants of cancer risk. The American Cancer Society recommended dietary guidelines to reduce cancer risk (ACS, 2003). The guidelines include (1) eat five or more servings of vegetables and fruit each day, (2) choose whole grains in preference to processed grains and sugars, and (3) limit consumption of red meats, especially high-fat and processed meats.

Obesity.   Dietary consumption is directly related to excessive body weight and cancer. Diets high in fat and low in fiber and obesity are associated with various cancers, particularly colon, breast, and prostate cancers. Survey data suggest that Blacks consume diets high in fat (Hargreaves et al., 1989). High-fiber diets may reduce risk of colon cancer. A diet high in fat may be a risk factor for colon, breast, and prostate cancers (ACS, 2002). Both obesity and the various nutritional deficiency states are potentially favorable for cancer growth. Obesity is associated with cancers of the endometrium, breast, colon, and ovary (Hargreaves et al., 1989). Cellular immune deficiency, a possible outcome of protein-calories malnutrition and zinc deficiency, may facilitate the development of head, neck, and gastric cancers (Hargreaves et al., 1989).

Occupational/Environmental Risk Factors.   The contribution of occupational exposure to the cause of cancer in Blacks may be even greater than 4 percent of all cancer deaths that have been estimated (Doll & Peto, 1981; DHHS, 1985). For many historical reasons, Blacks are believed to have higher occupational exposures compared with Whites because of placement in less skilled and more hazardous jobs. Various occupational hazards, especially ionizing radiation and chemicals like asbestos, benzene, chromium, lead, nickel, beta-naphthylamine, bischloromethyl ether, and vinyl chloride are known to cause cancer (Frumkin & Levy, 1983).

Asbestos, another known carcinogen, is known to cause lung cancer and mesothelioma (Lee, et al., 2002). Previous epidemiologic studies have documented the carcinogenic effects of exposure to asbestos in the workplace. These data provide the basis for assessing the potential impact of general environmental asbestos exposures in the form of insulation for new buildings and asbestos-contained water (Decoufle', 1982). Ambient air pollution has been identified as carcinogenic for humans. Among the many organic particulates in polluted air, polycyclic aromatic hydrocarbons have been most intensively studied for potential carcinogenicity. Among carcinogenic polycyclic organic compounds identified in the air, benzo(a)pyrene is known to be the most potent carcinogen in humans. The sources of benzo(a)pyrene are inefficient, smoldering combustors of carbonaceous solid fuels, such as home boilers, cokes ovens, and smoky coal refuse and forest fires (Shy & Struba, 1982). The International Agency for Research on Cancer (IARC) has established human carcinogens for which exposure is mainly occupational including 26 exposures (i.e., asbestos, crystalline silica, 4-aminibiphenyl) (Vainia et al., 2002).

Familial Predisposition and Genetic Factors.   The aggregation of cancer in families is a long-observed and well-documented phenomenon, but it is still subject to debate. The large bowel is the site of more familial and heritable cancers than perhaps any other site. This is evidenced by the threefold to fourfold rates of the disease in relatives of patients than in some control groups. Specifically, what is seen are the numerous inherited polyposis syndromes that have long been associated with the familial occurrence of large bowel cancer (Anderson, 1982). Other genetic evidence comes from the occurrence of gastric carcinoma as an associated neoplasm in several inherited disorders, including diffuse gastrointestinal polyposis, juvenile polyposis, hereditary adenocarcinomatosis, and Torre's syndrome (Anderson, 1978). This list also includes ataxia telangiectasis (Frais, 1979). Gastric cancer may also aggregate in families as the sole neoplasm. An example is Napoleon Bonaparte's family, where his father, his sister and himself were documented as having stomach cancer, and his paternal grandfather was suspected of having the neoplasm as well (Sokoloff, 1938).

The role for genetic predisposition in cancer is most evident by familial transmission of retinoblastoma, dysplastic nervus syndrome, multiple endocrine neoplasia, and polyposis coli, where there is essentially a 100 percent chance of developing cancer in one's lifetime for persons who have inherited the trait (Shields, 1993). The Li-Fraumeni cancer family syndrome is among the most dramatic because family members are at risk for multiorgan cancers including breast, bone sarcomas, brain, leukemia, and adrenocortical neoplasm (Li, 1990; Garber et al., 1991) which suggests a germ line mutation accounting for the multiorgan involvement. These inheritable syndromes involve genetic sequences for proto-oncogenics and tumor suppressor genes, metabolic capacity to activate or detoxify carcinogens, and the repair of DNA damage.

Socioeconomic Status.   Socioeconomic status is an important factor in cancer incidence, survival, and mortality. The poor have less ability to practice good health habits and less access to good health care. Because of poor health habits, the incidence of cancer is high (Bang et al., 1988). Low socioeconomic status correlates with poor survival rates from cancer (Smith et al., 1990; Lipworth et al., 1970). A study in the District of Columbia showed that cancer mortality in the southwestern area of the city was greater than in the northwestern area (White & Parker, 1981). People of higher socioeconomic status live in the northwestern section than in the southeastern section. Another epidemiologic study showed that the incidence of lung cancer was found in Blacks with lower income and less education (Devesa & Diamond, 1982).

It appears that Blacks tend to be less knowledgeable about cancer than Whites. In 1980, an American Cancer Society's study of Black Americans' attitude toward cancer was conducted by EVAXX, Inc., a Black-owned evaluation organization (EVAXX, 1981). The study indicated that Blacks believe cancer is the main concern of Whites, while hypertension and sickle-cell disease are the primary health concerns of Blacks. In particular, the study revealed that lower-income Blacks are less likely to have specific cancer tests and are less familiar with them. The study also showed that 69 percent of Blacks, as compared with 55 percent of Whites, think that they are not likely to get cancer, and only 25 percent of Blacks, as compared with 54 percent of Whites, could name five to seven of cancer's seven warning signs.

Other Risk Factors.   Other risk factors not mentioned previously include hormones and immunologic factors. Hormones (i.e., estrogen, progestogen) are associated with increased risk of cancers of the breast, endometrium, prostate, ovary, and testis (Bernstein & Henderson, 1996). Epidemiological hypothesis is that neoplasia is the consequence of excessive hormonal stimulation of the particular target or organ. These hormone-related cancers account for more than 20 percent of all newly diagnosed male cancers and more than 40 percent of all newly diagnosed female cancers in the United States. Cervical cancer incidence rate for Black females is higher than that for White females. However, it has not been well addressed if higher cervical incidence rate for Black females is associated with the heavy use of hormones.

Immunologic factors is concerned with cancer etiology recently. More recently, the acquired immunodeficiency syndrome (AIDS) has underlined the relevance of the immune function to malignancy (Kinlen, 1996). Kaposi's sarcoma has been frequently found among AIDS patients (Beral et al., 1990). Epidemiologic evidence suggests that the immune system does not play a major role in all cancers, but it is important in certain malignancies. Non-Hodgkin's lymphoma shows increases in a variety of different immunological disturbances (Kinlen, 1996). The evidence on cancer and immune impairment suggests that immunosurveillance in humans is important if malignancies are related with either viral in origin or possibly antigenic in nature.

RECOMMENDATIONS

Epidemiologic Studies

Numerous descriptive studies have adequately documented differences in incidence and mortality between Blacks and Whites. However, more comprehensive epidemiologic studies should be conducted to identify etiologic factors associated with higher rates of cancer of the prostate, esophagus, pancreas, multiple myeloma, and lung. A large population-based case-control study of pancreas, esophageal, prostate cancers, and multiple myeloma is in progress to evaluate the excess risk of these cancers among Blacks (Baquet & Gibbs, 1992). A comparison of Blacks and Whites should take into account socioeconomic or occupational difference. Additionally, biochemical and genetic epidemiologic studies should be conducted using case-control designs.

Basic Research and Clinical Trials

Basic laboratory research projects are needed to determine the risk factors of cancer sites that disproportionately affect Blacks. Cancer sites that should be examined for this research include prostate and multiple myeloma. These sites have a high incidence of cancer for Blacks. An internal NCI breast cancer work group was formed to study breast cancer in Black women, and one of its objectives is to analyze potential molecular markers (Baquet & Gibbs, 1992).

More research on cellular oncogenes is needed. Oncogenes are genes that are specifically turned on for only a brief moment during the cell cycle, and they become altered by mutations. Also, oncogenes may operate continuously, thereby resulting in unregulated cell growth.

Lifestyle Change and Risk Reduction

Lifestyle and risk factors can increase an individual's risk of developing cancer. Therefore, lifestyle factors that are related to cancer incidence and mortality should be changed, and risk reduction activities should be performed. The Department of Health and Human Services established the Healthy People 2010 objectives for cancer reduction as follows: (1) reduce cigarette smoking to a prevalence of no more than 18 percent among Blacks aged 20 years and older, (2) reduce dietary fat intake to an average of 30 percent of calories or less and average saturated fat intake to less than 10 percent of calories among people aged 2 and older, (3) increase complex carbohydrate and fiber-containing foods in the diets of adults to five or more daily servings for vegetables and fruits and to six or more daily servings for grain products, and (4) increase 60 percent for breast examination and mammogram for Black females 50 years and over (DHHS, 2001).

Socioeconomic status is related to cancer incidence and mortality. However, the exact interaction between socioeconomic status and cancer is not known. Further research is required to specify and define the relationship of socioeconomic status to cancer incidence and survival. Since lower socioeconomic factors have been known to be associated with the risk of various cancers, cancer education is essential to reduce the risk of cancer in Blacks. NCI developed education materials and services for special populations as well as for the general population. The Cancer Prevention Awareness Program for Black Americans was developed to provide cancer information through the mass media and intermediary organizations. The Cancer Information Service is a nationwide program that offers current information about cancer prevention and treatment. By using the toll-free telephone number (1-800-4-CANCER or 1-800-ACS-2345), a variety of cancer information can be obtained (ACS, 2003; Baquet & Gibbs, 1992) and, hopefully, utilized.

Cancer prevention studies should be conducted to identify the factors related to reducing cancer incidence and mortality. One of the largest cancer prevention studies ever carried out in the United States is the American Cancer Society's Cancer Prevention Study II (ACS, 1992). This prospective study has been conducted since 1982 to examine the habits and exposures of more than one million Americans. The goal of this study was to identify those factors that affect a person's chance of developing cancer by comparing mortality rates in various exposed groups. Results from this study showed that exercise was associated with reduced cancer mortality, that, among women, smokers die of lung cancer at a rate 12 times that of nonsmokers, and that men who smoke have an increased risk of myeloid leukemia (ACS, 1992).

Psychosocial and Behavioral Research

Research on behavioral modifications is having a significant impact on symptoms of cancer and its treatment. Research with humans on the role of stress has centered on either the ability of stress to cause cancer or the role of stress during the disease to encourage a preexisting cancer to spread more rapidly. Although there are many studies about bereaved people who developed cancer following the death of their spouse, there is no scientific report to support this evidence. Experimental stress can alter immunity and cancer growth in animals, with stress generally favoring increased tumor growth in most experimental studies (Allen & Brickman, 1983). Whether or not these observed changes in laboratory measures of immunity have clinical relevance to resistance to human cancer growth remains to be proved. Stress is an important risk factor to be scientifically investigated for the potential association with cancer.

Occupational Cancer Surveillance

Occupational surveillance of exposed workers is useful for identifying hazards and to protect workers at increased risk. Screening for occupational cancer in exposed populations for purpose of early diagnosis is rarely applied but has been tested in some situations. Cancer surveillance at the workplace has been explored for bladder cancer among people exposed to 2-napthylamine and to benzidine and for lung cancer among workers exposed to asbestos. Lung cancer remains still the leading cause of death from cancer in Blacks. For lung cancer screening, the use of spiral computed tomography (CT) has been developed. The use of biomarkers to identify the early clinical phase of progression of lung cancer in high-risk populations has been also proposed to detect earlier than possible with spiral CT (Vainio et al., 2002). A hybrid CT-biomarker approach may improve the detection of any types of lung cancer early (Mulshine & Henschke, 2000).

CONCLUSION

It is clear that the overall trend in cancer incidence and mortality among Blacks have been decreasing for recent years. The overall cancer mortality for Blacks is approximately 30 percent higher than those for Whites (ACS, 2003). The reasons for these disparities are complex and involve issues related to differential exposures and risk factors. However, risk factors that may explain the large difference in cancer rates between Blacks and Whites include (1) smoking habits, (2) alcohol consumption, (3) dietary habits, (4) exposure to occupational/environmental carcinogens, (5) physical activity, and (6) low socioeconomic status.

The burden of cancer is disproportionately distributed among Blacks compared with Whites in the United States. One of the major goals of the year 2010 objectives for the nation is to reduce health disparities among Americans. To reduce cancer incidence and mortality in Blacks, national cooperative efforts including research collaboration, intervention studies, epidemiologic and clinical trials, basic research, training, education, and information distribution must be continue. NCI should take a national leadership role to implement cancer prevention and control activities in the Black population. Furthermore, there should be cooperative agreements between various sectors, for example, the federal government, Black medical schools, professional organizations, cancer research institutes, and pharmaceutical companies regarding research and education. Also, culturally appropriate cancer control, prevention strategies, and guidelines for the Black community should be developed. Medical and related personnel must, while emphasizing the importance of primary and secondary prevention, at the same time, use innovative and effective approaches to focus their efforts toward educating the poor on the signs, symptoms, and dangers of cancer. The important future challenging direction in cancer prevention and control will be the improved technology application for identifying genotypic and phenotypic markers of cancer susceptibility and risk factors for specific types of cancer in Black Americans.

REFERENCES

Allen, W., & Brickman, M. (1983). Stress, personality, and cancer. In E.H. Rosenbaum (Ed.), *Can you prevent cancer?* (pp. 213–222). St. Louis: C.V. Mosby Company.

American Cancer Society (ACS). (1992). Cancer Facts and Figure 1992. New York, American Cancer Society.

American Cancer Society (ACS). (2002). Cancer Facts and Figure 2002. Atlanta, American Cancer Society.

American Cancer Society (ACS). (2003). Cancer Facts and Figure 2003. Atlanta, American Cancer Society.

Anderson, D.E. (1978). Familial cancer and cancer families. *Seminars in Oncology, 5,* 11–16.

Anderson, D.E. (1982). Familial predisposition. In Schottenfeld, D., & Fraumeni, J., Jr. (Eds.), *Cancer epidemiology and Prevention* (pp. 318–335). Philadelphia: W.B. Saunders Company.

Bang, K.M., Perlin, E., & Sampson, C.C. (1987). Increased cancer risks in Blacks: A look at the factors. *Journal of National Medical Association, 79,* 383–388.

Bang, K.M., White, J.E., Gause, B.L., & Leffall, L.D., Jr. (1988). Evaluation of recent trends in cancer mortality and incidence among Blacks. *Cancer, 61,* 1255–1261.

Baquet, C.R. & Gibbs, T. (1992). Cancers and Black Americans. In R.L. Braithwaite and S.E. Taylor (Eds.), *Health Issues in the Black community.* San Francisco: Jossey-Bass.

Baquet, C.R., Horm, J.W., Gibbs, T., & Greenwald, P. (1991). Socioeconomic factors and cancer incidence among Blacks and Whites. *Journal of National Cancer Institute, 83,* 551–557.

Beral, V., Peterman, T.A., Berkelman, R.L., & Jaffee, H.W. (1990). Kaposi's sarcoma among persons with AIDS: A sexually transmitted infections? *Lancet, 335,* 123–128.

Bernstein, L., & Henderson, B.E. (1996). Exogenous hormones. In D. Schottenfeld & J.F. Fraumeni, Jr. (Eds.), *Cancer epidemiology and prevention* (pp. 462–488). New York: Oxford University Press.

Centers for Disease Control (CDC). (2003). Smoking prevalence among U.S. adults. (http://www.cdc.gov/tobacco/research_data/adults_pre/prevali.htm.)

Clegg, L.X., Li, F.P., Hankey, B.F., Chu, K., & Edwards, B.K. (2002). Cancer survival among U.S. *whites* and minorities. *Archives of Internal Medicine, 162,* 1985–1993.

Decoufle', P. (1982). Occupation. In D.A. Schottenfeld & J. Fraumeni, Jr. (Eds.), *Cancer Epidemiology and Prevention* (pp. 318–335). Philadelphia, W.B. Saunders Company.

Department of Health and Human Services (DHHS). (1988). Surgeon General's report on nutrition and health. DHHS Publication No. (PHS) 88-50210, Washington, DC, U.S. Government Printing Office.

Department of Health and Human Services (DHHS). (2001). Healthy People 2000. Final Review, DHHS Publication No. 01-0256.

Devesa, S.S., & Diamond, F.L. (1982). Socioeconomic and racial difference in lung cancer incidence. *American Journal of Epidemiology, 118,* 818–831.

Doll, R., & Peto, R. (1981). The causes of cancer: Quantitative estimates of available risk of cancer in the United States today. *Journal of National Cancer Institute, 66,* 1192–1308.

Environmental Protection Agency (EPA). (1992). Respiratory health effects of passive smoking: Lung cancer and other disorders. Washington, DC: U.S. Environmental Protection Agency, Office of Health and Environmental Assessment, Office of Atmospheric and Indoor Air Programs, Publication No. EPA/600/8-90/006F.

EVAXX, Inc. (1981). Black Americans' attitudes toward cancer and cancer tests: Highlights of a study. *CA, 31(4),* 212–218.

Frais, M.A. (1979). Gastric adenocarcinoma due to ataxia-telangiectasis (Louis-Bar Syndrome). *Journal of Medical Genetics, 4,* 160–161.

Frumkin, H., & Levy, B.S. (1983). Carcinogens. In B.S. Levy and D.H. Wegman (Eds.), *Occupational Health* (pp. 145–175). Boston: Little, Brown.

Garber, J.E., Goldstein, A.M., Kantor, A.F., Dreyfus, M.G., Fraumeni, J.F., Jr., & Li, F.P. (1991). Follow-up study of twenty-four families with Li-Fraumeni syndrome. *Cancer Research, 51,* 6094–6097.

Gullatte, M.M. (1989). Cancer prevention and early detection in Black Americans: Colon and rectum. *Journal of National Black Nurses Association, 3,* 49–56.

Hargreaves, M.K., Baquet, C., & Gamshadzahi, A. (1989). Diet, nutritional status, and cancer risk in American Blacks. *Nutrition and Cancer, 12,* 1–28.

Kinlen, L.J. (1996). Immunologic factors, including AIDS. In D. Schottenfeld & J.F. Fraumeni, Jr. (Eds.), *Cancer epidemiology and prevention* (pp. 532–545). New York: Oxford University Press.

Lee, Y.C.G., Klerk, N.H., Henderson, D.W. & Musk, A.W. (2002). Malignant mesothelioma. In D.J. Hendrick, P.S. Burge, W.S. Beckett, & A. Churg (Eds.), *Occupational disorders of the lung* (pp. 359–379). New York: W.B. Saunders.

Li, F.P. (1990). Familial cancer syndrome and clusters. *Current Problems in Cancer, 14,* 73–114.

Lipworth, L., Abelin, T., & Connelly, R.R. (1970). Socio-economic factors in the prognosis of cancer patients. *Journal of Chronic Disease, 23,* 105–116.

McWhorter, W.P., Schatzkin, A.G., Horm, J.W., & Brown, C.C. (1989). Contribution of socioeconomic status to Black/White differences in cancer incidence. *Cancer, 63,* 982–987.

Mettlin, C. (1980). Nutritional habits of Blacks and Whites. *Preventive Medicine, 9,* 601–606.

Mulshine, J.L. & Henschke, C.L. (2000). Prospects for lung cancer screening. *Lancet, 355,* 592–593.

National Cancer Institute (NCI). (2002). Cancer control & population sciences: SEER Cancer Statistics Review, 1973–1999.

National Center for Health Statistics (NCHS). (2002). Health United States, 2002. U.S. Department of Health and Human Services, DHHS Publication No. 1232.

Potter, L.M., Morris, L.E., & Blot, W.J. (1981). Esophageal cancer among Black men in Washington, DC: Alcohol, tobacco, and other risk factors. *Journal of National Cancer Institute, 67,* 777–783.

Shields, P.G. (1993). Inherited factors and environmental exposures in cancer risk. *Journal of Occupational Medicine, 35,* 34–41.

Shy, C.M., & Struba, R.J. (1982). Air and water pollution. In D. Schottenfelf and J. Fraumeni, Jr. (Eds.), *Cancer epidemiology and prevention* (pp. 336–363). Philadelphia: W.B. Saunders Company.

Smith, C.D., Shipley, M.J., & Rose, G. (1990). Magnitude and causes of socioeconomic differentials in mortality: Future evidence from the Whitehall study. *Journal of Epidemiology and Community Health, 44*, 265–270.

Sokoloff, B. (1938). Predisposition to cancer in the Bonaparte family. *American Journal of Surgery, 11*, 673–678.

U.S. Department of Health and Human Services (USDHHS). (2000). Healthy People 2010: Tracking Healthy People 2010. U.S. Government Printing Office.

U.S. Department of Health and Human Services (USDHHS). (2001). Health United States, 2001. DHHS Publication No. (PHS) 01-1232.

Vainio, H., Fletcher, T. & Boffetta, P. (2002). Occupational causes of cancer. In A. Malcolm (Ed.), *The cancer handbook* (pp. 413–419). New York: Nature Publishing Group.

White, J.E., Enterline, J.P., Alam, Z., & Moore, F.M. (1981). Cancer among Blacks in the United States: Recognizing the problem. In A.I. Helleb (Ed.), *Cancer among Black populations* (pp. 35–53). New York: Alan R Liss.

White, J.E., & Parker, D. (1981). The distribution of cancer mortality in Washington, DC, 1971–76. Cancer Coordinating Council for Metropolitan Washington, Washington, DC.

Willett, W.C. (1996). Diet and nutrition. In D. Schottenfeld & J.F. Fraumeni, Jr. (Eds.), *Cancer epidemiology and prevention* (pp. 438–461). New York: Oxford University Press.

CHAPTER 8

The Epidemiology of Chronic Obstructive Pulmonary Disease and Asthma in African Americans

KI MOON BANG

INTRODUCTION

Chronic obstructive pulmonary disease (COPD) and asthma are the fourth and fifth leading causes of death in the United States (USDHHS, 2001). There were 124,153 deaths in 1999, as shown in Table 8.1. The age-adjusted mortality rate for COPD and asthma increased by 13.1 percent from 1995 to 1999. A recent study reported that the cost due to job-related COPD and asthma is estimated to be $6.6 billion in 1996 (Leigh et al., 2002). COPD is projected to rank fifth in 2020 as a worldwide burden of disease (Murray & Lopez, 1996). COPD and asthma are important causes of morbidity and mortality in African Americans in the United States. This chapter reviews the epidemiology of COPD and asthma in African Americans and examines the risk factors for COPD and asthma in African Americans that may explain racial differences in COPD and asthma.

CHRONIC OBSTRUCTIVE PULMONARY DISEASE

COPD is a major cause of chronic morbidity and disability in the United states (USDHHS, 2001; Feinleib et al., 1989). It is a significant cause of morbidity and mortality in African Americans (Mays, 1975; USDHHS, 2000). Over 120,000 people die each year because of this condition (USDHHS, 2001), as shown in Table 8.1, and cigarette smoking accounts for 82 percent of these deaths (Office on Smoking, 1989). Mortality rates from COPD have paralleled those for lung cancer and have increased progressively over the last 25 years.

The Department of Health and Human Services has established an objective of reducing COPD deaths to less than 25 per 100,000 population by the year 2000 (USDHHS, 2000). Additionally, the Healthy People 2010 objective is to reduce deaths from COPD among adults aged 45 years and older (USDHHS, 2000). In 1999, the COPD death rate per 100,000 population in African Americans was 50.2 for males and 23.9 for females, as shown in Table 8.2 (USDHHS, 2001). Although published studies indicate racial differences in COPD, there remains a need for more research in this area.

Table 8.1
Deaths of chronic obstructive pulmonary disease by race and gender in 1999

Race	Total	(%)	Male	(%)	Female	(%)
African Americans	7,909	(6.4)	4.502	(7.2)	3,407	(5.5)
Whites	114,717	(92.4)	56,982	(91.3)	57,735	(93.5)
Other	1,527	(1.2)	912	(1.5)	615	(1.0)
All races	124,153	(100.0)	62,396	(100.0)	61,757	(100.0)

Source: National Center for Health Statistics, Health United States, 2001.

Table 8.2
Age-adjusted mortality rates (per 100,000 population) of chronic obstructive pulmonary disease by race and gender, 1995–1999

	African Americans				Whites		
Year	Total	Male	Female		Total	Male	Female
1995	30.0	47.0	20.5		41.8	56.1	33.6
1996	30.8	46.1	21.8		42.4	55.5	34.9
1997	30.3	45.8	21.1		43.0	55.9	35.5
1998	30.8	45.2	22.3		43.6	55.4	36.5
1999	33.7	50.2	23.9		47.5	59.6	40.2

Source: National Center for Health Statistics, Health United States, 2001.

EPIDEMIOLOGY OF CHRONIC OBSTRUCTIVE PULMONARY DISEASE

Definition

In this chapter, the term chronic obstructive pulmonary disease, or COPD, includes rubrics 490 to 496 of the ninth revision of the International Classification of Diseases (ICD-9). COPD consists of bronchitis (ICD-9 490-491), emphysema (ICD-9 492), asthma (ICD-9 493), and other conditions (ICD-9 494-496). COPD is clinically defined as obstructive airways disease manifested by a forced expiratory volume in one second (FEV_1) that is less than 65 percent of the predicted value (Higgins et al., 1984). A recent workshop report on Global Strategy for the Diagnosis, Management, and Prevention of Chronic Obstructive Pulmonary Disease recommends to define COPD as FEV_1/FVC<70 percent and FEV_1>=80 percent predicted (Pauwels et al., 2001).

Prevalence

The prevalence of COPD in the United States has been increasing in recent decades. Estimates are about 14 million people with COPD, and the COPD cases have increased by 41 percent since 1982 (ATS, 1995). Approximately 12.5 million people have chronic bronchitis, and 1.7 million people have emphysema. Prevalence estimates of COPD are available from the data obtained through national surveys of the National Center for Health Statistics (NCHS). These surveys include the annual National Health Interview Survey (NHIS) and the periodic National Health and Nutrition Examination Survey (NHANES). NHIS presents one-year-period prevalence, which is equivalent to point prevalence for chronic diseases (NCHS, 1986). NHANES may provide cumulative or lifetime prevalence because of the several-year survey period (NCHS, 1981). A recent report on data based from NHANES III shows that the prevalence of COPD is 4 percent among nonsmokers and 11 percent among smokers in the United States (USDHHS, 1999). The prevalence of COPD among African Americans in age groups 45 years and over was lower than Whites based on data from the 1990 NHIS (Gillum, 1990).

A study on the spirometry data obtained from NHANES I reported that prevalence of COPD in African Americans was 5.4 percent—3.7 percent for males and 6.7 percent for females. The prevalence was significantly higher with age for both males and females (Bang, 1993). NHANES I spirometry was performed using an electronic spirometer on all examinees aged 25 to 74 years in the detailed sample (NCHS, 1978). In NHANES I, sex ratios (male/female) for history of chronic bronchitis or emphysema were 0.5 for African Americans and 0.9 for Whites, ages 35 to 74 (Gillum, 1990). The reason for the higher ratio in African Americans may be related to African American women's immune defenses and familial or genetic factors or other related risk factors.

Mortality

Table 8.1 shows deaths from COPD by race and gender in 1999. Table 8.2 shows age-adjusted mortality rates of COPD in African Americans and Whites from 1995 to 1999. In 1999, there were 124,153 deaths due to COPD, as shown in Table 8.1. The total number of deaths from COPD in African Americans was 7,909 compared to 114,717 in whites. The age-adjusted COPD mortality rate for African Americans increased 12.3 percent from 1995 to 1999. The mortality rate for COPD was higher in males than in females. The mortality rate for COPD in Whites was higher than that in African Americans.

COPD mortality is disproportionately distributed at older ages. Approximately 87 percent of the deaths from COPD in 1999 occurred in people over the age of 65. Although men and women have

Table 8.3

Mortality rates (per 100,000 population) of chronic obstructive pulmonary disease among African Americans by age group and gender, 1995–1999

Age group and Gender	1995	1996	1997	1998	1999	1995-1999 % Change
All ages						
Male	47.0	46.1	45.8	45.2	50.2	+ 6.8 %
Female	20.5	21.8	21.1	22.3	23.9	+16.6 %
35-44 years						
Male	4.3	5.2	4.8	5.0	4.8	+11.6 %
Female	5.4	5.0	5.0	5.3	4.6	-14.8 %
45-54 years						
Male	17.3	15.4	14.9	15.1	16.1	-6.9 %
Female	12.9	13.2	12.2	14.2	12.8	-0.8 %
55-64 years						
Male	62.0	63.2	56.6	56.6	62.1	+0.2 %
Female	34.7	34.8	35.8	33.8	34.8	+0.3 %
65-74 years						
Male	175.1	161.6	170.7	164.2	177.7	+1.5 %
Female	78.3	84.3	81.4	84.8	88.3	+12.8 %
75-84 years						
Male	366.5	380.7	374.9	372.1	423.5	+15.6 %
Female	136.6	137.6	136.9	148.9	173.9	+27.3 %

Source: National Center for Health Statistics, Health United States, 2001.

similar rates of COPD prior to 55 years of age, men have twice higher rates than women after age 55, as shown in Table 8.3.

Different mortality trends for COPD existed between African Americans and Whites during the period 1995–1999, as shown in Table 8.2. The age-adjusted mortality rate in African Americans rose 12.3 percent compared with 13.6 percent in Whites during this period. The increase for COPD death rates was 16.6 percent for African American females compared with 6.8 percent for African American males. A recent study reported racial difference of COPD mortality from 1979 to 1998 (Levine et al., 2001). African Americans to Whites mortality ratio for COPD, 1979–1998, was 0.06 in males and 0.02 in females, suggesting that COPD mortality in African Americans increased slightly compared to those in Whites.

When all races are looked at by age group during the period 1995–1999, the mortality rate increased by 2.1 percent for those 55 to 64 years of age, by 11.6 percent for those 65 to 74 years of age, by 13.8 percent for those 75 to 84 years of age, and by 21.8 percent for those more than 85 years of age. As seen in Table 8.3, the age-specific mortality rates for African American females increased more than 13 percent compared with those in African American males in ages 65 years and older during the period 1995–1999.

RISK FACTORS FOR CHRONIC OBSTRUCTIVE PULMONARY DISEASE

Age and Sex

COPD mortality rate increases with age. In 1999, COPD mortality rate for ages 75 to 84 years was 400.4 per 100,000 population compared with 179.2 for ages 65 to 74, 48.3 for ages 55 to 64, 8.7 for ages 45 to 54, and 2.0 for ages 35 to 44. Sex ratios (male/female) of age-adjusted mortality rates for COPD were 2.1 in African Americans and 1.5 in Whites (USDHHS, 2001). Many studies have shown that ventilatory lung function increases with age to about ages 25 to 30 years and then declines progressively in relationship with COPD. The decline is usually considered to be linear, though some studies have suggested that there may be interactions with age and height (Higgins, 1980).

Cigarette Smoking

Cigarette smoking is a major risk factor for COPD. Cigarette smoking accounts for 80 percent to 90 percent of the risk of developing COPD in the United States (U.S. Surgeon General, 1984). Numerous papers show that cigarette smokers have higher death rates from chronic bronchitis, emphysema, and asthma than nonsmokers. Differences between cigarette smokers and nonsmokers in crease as cigarette consumption increases. Pipe and cigar smokers have higher morbidity and mortality rates for COPD than nonsmokers (Higgins, 1984). There is a significant relationship between the number of cigarettes smoked per day and decrement of pulmonary function (Benowitz et al., 1983).

Trends in cigarette-smoking prevalence have been published for African Americans and Whites (CDC, 1987; NCHS, 1989; Fiore et al., 1989; Novotny et al., 1988). In 1987, 43 percent of African American men aged 45 and older smoked cigarettes compared with 30 percent of White men (NCHS, 1989). The prevalence of cigarette smoking has been declined since 1987. In 2001, the prevalence of cigarette smoking in African Americans was 22.2 percent, compared with 16 percent in Hispanics and 24.5 percent in Whites (NCHS, 2002). African American women aged 20 to 24 smoked more than African American men the same age (Fiore et al., 1989).

Although the importance of cigarette smoking as a cause of COPD is clearly known, some facets of the health effects are not fully understood. The health effects of cigarette smoking are not of equal frequency and severity in all smokers. The cigarette smoke–COPD relationship may be influenced by personal factors as well as by other environmental hazards.

The effect of involuntary exposure to cigarette smoke also has attracted recent attention. Passive smoking was reported to be significantly related to lower FEV_1 and forced vital capacity (FVC) values among Frenchwomen (Kauffmann et al., 1989). Mean levels of ventilatory lung function were significantly lower, and prevalence rates of respiratory symptoms and disease were higher in nonsmoking wives of smoking husbands and in nonsmoking children of smoking parents than in non-smoking households (USDHHS, 1979; Lefioe et al., 1984). Although the effect of passive smoking appears to be small, it is important to investigate the effect of involuntary exposure of smoking in relation to COPD.

Although smoking prevalence is higher in African Americans than in Whites, lower COPD mortality and morbidity are reported in African Americans compared with Whites. These differences in race-related prevalence and health outcomes may enhance understanding of the pathophysiology and etiology of COPD and the effects of smoking (Gillum, 1990; Novotny et al., 1988).

Environmental/Occupational Exposures

Many studies have shown the adverse effects of pollution on the respiratory tract. Occupational exposure is a known risk factor for COPD. Occupational exposure to inorganic and organic dusts and chemical agents can increase the risk of developing COPD (Becklake, 1989; Oxman et al., 1993). Some specific occupations have high risk of COPD. For example, farmworkers increase the risk of developing chronic bronchitis due to dust and chemical exposures, and in combination with smoking the risk increase to sixfold (Frost et al., 1994; Melbostad et al., 1997).

Temporal and spatial variations in mortality, morbidity, the prevalence of respiratory symptoms, lung functions values, and sickness absence from work have been shown to correlate with various indices of pollution in different populations. Past studies have examined the acute effects of daily air pollution concentrations on daily morbidity and mortality. Some of the earlier studies were initiated in London in 1958. In these studies moderately high correlations (r = 0.6) were seen between daily concentration of smoke and sulfur dioxide and daily morbidity and mortality (Higgins, 1980). Presently, African Americans have more exposure experience to air pollution than Whites. In 1980, African Americans (59.7 percent) were more likely than Whites (27 percent) to live in central cities, where air pollution exposure is usually greater than in rural areas. Relatedly, indoor air pollution and passive smoking effects may be associated with the increased risk of COPD, especially asthma, in African Americans.

Death rates for chronic respiratory diseases are higher than expected among men in certain occupations and industries. Epidemiologic surveys have shown that exposures at work to cotton, hemp, or grain dust; firefighting; and work involving exposure to asbestos are associated with respiratory symptoms and reduced lung function. Comparison of prevalence rates of respiratory symptoms and mean levels of FEV_1 in miners and nonminers in West Virginia showed that respiratory function was poorest in miners who smoked and best in nonsmoking nonminers (Higgins, 1970). Interaction between certain occupational hazards and cigarette smoking results in increased rates of COPD. African Americans may have been employed more frequently than Whites in occupations with the above-mentioned and other health hazards.

Genetic Factors

Several reports show the familial occurrence of COPD (Higgins & Keller, 1975; Hubert et al., 1982; Cohen et al., 1975). It has been reported that COPD patients have a higher frequency of Pi variant phenotypes than those without lung disease (Cohen et al., 1975). Also, alpha-antitrypsin deficiency (PiZ homozygote) was reported to be less frequent in African Americans than Whites (Lieberman et al., 1976; Young et al., 1978). No study has reported on familial aggregation of COPD or pulmonary function in African Americans, although familial aggregation was reported on for Whites (Redline et al., 1987). Bronchial asthma probably results from the interaction of multiple gene loci with one or more factors in the environment (NIH, 1981).

Infection

Patients with COPD are more susceptible to respiratory infections. For example, persons with chronic bronchitis usually have a history of frequent attacks of pneumonia and pleurisy. However, the role of infectious agents in recurrent exacerbations of chronic bronchitis is uncertain. There is a significant increase in bacterial, viral, and mycoplasmal pathogens during exacerbations. The extent to which respiratory infections contribute to the initiation of COPD is less certain (Speizer & Tager, 1979), but several studies report that childhood respiratory illness may be associated with reduced lung function at older ages (USDHHS, 1979). Incidence rates of obstructive airways disease and chronic bronchitis were higher in those with a history of respiratory tract infections in Tecumseh (Higgins, 1984).

Influenza and pneumonia mortality rates are reported to be higher in African Americans than in Whites (Gillum & Liu, 1984). NHANES I showed that African American children aged 1 to 5 years had more episodes of pneumonia than White children. At ages 6 to 11, 12.9 percent of African American girls compared with 9.5 percent of White girls had a history of treatment for pneumonia (Gillum, 1991).

Allergies

A recent study based on the data from NHANES III-Phase I survey, 1988–1991, reported that African Americans have higher allergen reactivity than Whites and Mexican Americans (Bang et al., 1993). The prevalence of asthma in children and young adults was higher in African Americans than in Whites. In NHANES I, a history of treatment for allergens other than asthma was more prevalent in White children ages 1 to 11 than in African American children of similar ages. These findings may be explained by a different presentation of atopy in African Americans compared to Whites or differential access to medical care resulting in diagnosis of more severe forms of atopy in African Americans compared to Whites (Witting et al., 1978).

The relationship between allergies and COPD has not been clearly determined. There are a number of questions to be resolved. For example, is the reported association between higher blood eosinophil count and both lower lever and faster decline of pulmonary function among nonsmokers a reflection of an adverse effect of environmental antigens on allergies? Do allergies have a significant impact on lung growth and development during childhood? If so, does this influence the risk of COPD in later life? Research in these areas will hopefully provide important insights into the pathogenesis of COPD.

Other Risk Factors

Other potential risk factors include socioeconomic status, nutrition, alcohol consumption, and climate. However, these factors are less important than the risk factors discussed before.

Chronic bronchitis, emphysema, and asthma were reported to be more frequent in persons with low socioeconomic status (Evans et al., 1987). Several surveys have noted a higher prevalence of respiratory symptoms, chronic bronchitis, and lower ventilatory lung function in less-educated persons (Higgins, 1980).

Periodontal disease has been shown to be inversely related to FEV in men and women. Upper abdominal surgery, especially when performed in an emergency, is also associated with an increased risk of chronic respiratory disease (Higgins, 1980).

Table 8.4
Prevalence of asthma by race in 2000

Race	Prevalence (%)
African Americans	12.1
Whites	10.4
Hispanics	9.8
Other	10.2
All races	10.5

Source: CDC, Behavioral Risk Factor Surveillance System, 2000.

ASTHMA

Asthma is a respiratory disease characterized by variable airflow obstruction with airway hyper-responsiveness including cough, wheezing, and shortness of breath (CDC, 1995). Asthma is a mutifactorial disease that has been associated with respiratory infection, genetics, socioeconomic, nutritional, air pollution, and occupational risk factors. Asthma affects approximately over 17 million Americans (CDC, 1998). Based on the finding from recent CDC's Behavioral Risk Factor Survey, African Americans had higher prevalence of asthma than that in Whites (CDC, 2002) as shown in Table 8.4.

EPIDEMIOLOGY OF ASTHMA

Prevalence and Mortality

A recent report based on data from the National Health Interview Survey (NHIS) shows that asthma prevalence for all ages is 4.1 percent, with the rate for children under 18 years being 5.7 percent. These prevalence rates are based on responses to a question as to whether the individual had seen a physician for asthma within the past year (Weiss, 1998). The CDC's Behavioral Risk Factor Survey shows that asthma prevalence was 10.5 percent. By race, the prevalence for African Americans was 12.1 percent compared with 10.4 percent for Whites, as shown in Table 8.4 (CDC, 2002). In the 1970 NHIS, asthma rates per 1,000 population were 36.4 for African Americans compared with 27.9 for Whites among persons less than 6 years old. For ages 6 to 16 years, the rates were 25.2 for African Americans compared with 26.3 for Whites; and for ages 4 to 64 years, the rates were 44.5 for African Americans compared with 31.9 for Whites. Between 1979 and 1981, asthma ranked fourth among African Americans and eighth among Whites in prevalence of 19 conditions on the NHIS checklist (NCHS, 1986). Asthma prevalence rates per 1,000 population were 31 for Whites and 32 for non-Whites.

Although no incidence studies have been performed in the United States for the last 10 years, old investigations suggest that roughly half of all asthma causes are diagnosed before the age of 10 years

(Broder et al., 1974). African Americans have almost three times more hospitalization rate of asthma for treatment than that in Whites (Essien et al., 2001). The male African Americans to Whites mortality rate ratio for asthma increased from 2.38 in 1979 to 3.78 in 1998. For females, the ratio also increased from 2.50 in 1979 to 3.17 in 1998. The net change in African Americans to Whites mortality ratio for COPD was 1.40 in males and 0.67 in females, suggesting that asthma mortality rate in female African Americans increased more than those in males (Levine et al., 2001).

RISK FACTORS FOR ASTHMA

Age and Sex

Asthma rates have been increasing in very young and very old individuals. Individuals at old age have lower levels of lung function, such that milder degrees of airway inflamation and smaller changes in lung function may precipitate symptoms and the diagnosing of asthma. Asthma in children is predominantly a male disease. The gender ratio for a doctor's diagnosis of asthma is approximately 2 to 1, male to female in younger ages. Following puberty, asthma incidence is greater in females. Mostly diagnosed cases of asthma in subjects after age 40 years are females, and there is now evidence that estrogen use is a risk factors for asthma in adults (Weiss, 1998).

Race

Asthma prevalence is higher in African Americans than in Whites. Hospitalization and mortality rates are consistently higher in African Americans than in Whites. Whether these racial difference are due to inadequate treatment and access to medical care remains unclear.

Socioeconomic Status

Lower socioeconomic status is associated with an increase in asthma prevalence. A recent report showed that people in households with the lowest income (less than $9,000 per year) had a highest prevalence of asthma (16 percent) than those in the highest income households (12 percent) (Northridge et al., 2002). Low socioeconomic status may be important in explaining the higher asthma mortality in African Americans (Evans et al., 1987). However, studies show that asthma morbidity and mortality are not significantly different between African Americans and Whites soldiers (Ward, 1992), suggesting that ethnic differences may disappear by adjusting for similar living conditions.

Young Maternal Age and Prematurity

Infants born to mothers who are less than 20 years have an increased incidence of asthma (Martinez et al., 1992). It is known that prematurity and low birth weight are more common in these young mothers. Infants born prematurely carry a fourfold increased risk of the development of asthma (Von Mutius 2000). Prematurity is associated with bronchopulmonary dysplasia, a disease characterized by increased airway responsiveness and asthma symptoms. African Americans have lower birth weights and higher rates of prematurity than Whites; therefore, prematurity may contribute to racial differences in asthma prevalence and morbidity.

Cigarette Smoking

A number of cross-sectional, population-based epidemiologic studies have examined the relationship between cigarette smoking and asthma. Population-based studies in England and Australia found an increased occurrence of asthma among current smokers compared to former or never smokers (Burney, 1987; Woolcock, 1986). A population-based study reported that cigarette smoking increased serum IgE concentration and also increased risk of occupational asthma in workers who smoked (Zetterstrom et al., 1981). Maternal cigarette smoking is a risk factor for the development of asthma in the first year of life (Weiss, 1994). The risk is about twofold in infants born to smoking mothers without an allergic history but increase to almost fourfold in infants of allergic parents with mothers who smoke. The predominant effect of maternal cigarette smoking is due to in utero exposure with decreased lung function at birth. Maternal cigarette smoking has been associated with an increase in peripheral blood eosinophilia, serum immunoglobulin E (IgE) levels, and skin test reactivity. It is clear that maternal cigarette smoke exposure is associated with a greater occurrence of lower respiratory tract infections. In adults, active cigarette smoking is associated with increased airway responsiveness, elevations in total serum IgE level, and peripheral blood eosinophilia. However, there is no clear evidence suggesting that active cigarette smoking does lead to the development of asthma in adults. Smoking might be a risk factor in sensitization of high-molecular-weight agents to induce asthma (Banks & Wang, 2000).

Respiratory Infection

The relationship between asthma and respiratory illness has been investigated in a number of studies. These studies have demonstrated a prominent association between lower respiratory tract viral infections in early life and wheezing illness (Busse et al., 1995). Respiratory syncytial virus (RSV) has been the major cause of bronchitis in children, and RSV infection is associated with IgE production, airway inflammation, and increased airway responsiveness. These studies showed that RSV bronchitis in children is associated with the development of chronic wheezing in later life (Sigurs et al., 1995). Asthma was founded in 23 percent of parents who had experienced infantile RSV bronchitis as versus 1 percent of controls when evaluated at age three years. Although the association between viral respiratory tract infection and asthma is well documented, it is not still clear that this relationship is based on cause and effect. The alternative possibility is that patients with abnormal lung function or an underlying asthmatic condition may be predisposed to viral respiratory tract infection in childhood.

Another important relationship between respiratory illness and asthma relates to the ability of respiratory illnesses to trigger asthmatic exacerbations. A number of studies have demonstrated a close temporal relationship between viral infection and asthma exacerbation (Bjornsdottir & Busse, 1992; Pattemore et al., 1992; Stark & Grazinano, 1995). It is clear that viral respiratory infections are important triggers of acute asthmatic symptomatology.

Genetic Factors

Asthma is a complex genetic disorder. Several studies showed increased prevalence of asthma among first-degree relatives of asthmatic subjects (20 percent to 25 percent), compared with a general population prevalence (4 percent) (Sanford et al., 1996; Sibbald & Turner-Warwick, 1979; Hopp et al., 1988) and greater concordance rates among monozygotic than dizygotic twins (Hopp et al., 1984; Duffy et al., 1990). It is well demonstrated that people with a family history of asthma are more likely to develop asthma (Horwood et al., 1985) and that parental asthma is a stronger predictor of asthma in the offspring than parental atopy (Von Mutius & Nicolai, 1996). The increasing prevalence of asthma indicates that genetic factors alone are unlikely to account for a substantial proportion of asthma causes.

Air Pollution

Many studies reported the association between air pollutants and asthma. Studies of major air pollution episodes have reported increased symptoms and an increase in hospital admission for asthma (Wardlaw, 1993). Air pollution includes SO_2, NO_2, and airborne particulates with a size of 10 Φm or less that can be inhaled into the lung (Dockery & Pope, 1997). Especially, NO_2 related to increasing motor vehicle use. An association between traffic density on residential streets and asthma symptoms has been found in studies in several countries (Duhme et al., 1996; Pershagen et al., 1995; Livingstone et al., 1996). The reported evidence does not support a major role for outdoor air pollution as a determinant of asthma prevalence, although the possibility of interaction between pollutants and the possibility of a very different alveoli response to ultrafine particles suggests that further studies are required.

Indoor Allergens

Indoor allergens includes house dust mite, cat and dog allergens, cockroach, and fungi. These allergens are associated with elevated risk of asthma. A recent study in Los Alamos, New Mexico, shows the importance of exposure and sensitization to cat and dog allergens (Sporik et al., 1995). This study demonstrated that the strongest associated risk for asthma was cat sensitization. The prevalence of mite and cockroach sensitization reflected low levels of exposure. A recent study suggested that in the inner-city areas with a high proportion of cockroach-infected houses, sensitization to cockroach allergens was common, highlighting the importance of these allergens as a risk factor for asthma (Call et al., 1992). High prevalence of cockroach sensitization (up to 70 percent) was found among asthmatic patients in several U.S. cities (Kang et al., 1979; Mendoza & Snyder, 1970; Menon et al., 1991). It is unknown whether African Americans have higher or lower prevalence of cockroach sensitization than that in Whites.

Diet

Several studies reported the relationship between asthma and diet including coffee, vitamins, and other factors. A study showed that subjects who drank coffee on a regular basis had a 29 percent reduction in the odds of having current asthma symptoms, compared with non-coffee drinkers (Schwartz & Weiss, 1992). There appears to be some evidence that coffee drinking does have beneficial effects on asthma and asthma symptoms. Several studies have assessed the relationship of vitamin C intake to asthma or wheeze. A study based on NHANES II data found an inverse association between serum vitamin C and the prevalence of wheeze (Schwartz & Weiss, 1992). Another study examined the effect of vitamin C intake on the subsequent development of asthma among women in the Nurses Health Study, but no significant relationship between vitamin C intake and asthma was found in the study (Troisi et al., 1995).

The study of diet as a risk factor and a potential modifier of the effect on asthma is in its infancy. A study reported on the protective effects of breast feeding on recurrent wheezing at age 6 years in the Tuscon Birth cohort (Wright et al., 1995). A total of 988 children were followed for six years, and breast feeding was unrelated to serum IgE levels or to skin test reactivity and was protective against wheezing. To date, the number of large-scale epidemiologic investigations is small, most are cross-sectional, and most are focused on adults. It is estimated that over one-half of all asthma cases are diagnosed by age 6. Therefore, truly identifying the role of dietary factors in the development of asthma requires studies that focus on young subjects.

Occupational Factors

Asthma is associated with occupational exposures. There are more than 200 known occupational causes of asthma, and asthma is the most common occupational respiratory disease in developed countries (Chan-Yeung & Malo, 1994; Chan-Yeung, 1995). Estimates of the proportion of adult asthma that is thought to be of occupational origin range from 2 percent to 15 percent in the United States (Chan-Yeung & Malo, 1995). Recent studies show that potentially work-related asthma is estimated to be 13 to 26 percent (Blanc et al., 1996; Milton et al., 1998). A recent study on data from the NHANES III reported that the prevalence of work-related asthma in African Americans was 4 percent compared to 3.7 percent in Whites (Arif et al., 2002). These data suggest that African American workers might be potentially exposed more to hazardous asthmagens in the workplace. It is important to distinguish between occupational asthma that is triggered by nonspecific irritants in patients with preexisting or concurrent asthma and asthma that arises as a consequence of exposure to a specific etiologic agent. A number of natural and synthetic chemicals are known to cause asthma by IgE-mediated mechanisms, as well as by nonallergic mechanisms of unknown origin.

Occupational asthma, with a latency period, involves the variable of time, depending on the agent involved (Malo et al., 1991). Typically, the onset of occupational asthma may occur one to three years after initial exposure, although some exposures may induce occupational asthma in some workers in less than one month (Anto et al., 1996). Some workplace agents can directly induce asthma by effects similar to those of pharmacologic agonists (Chan-Yeung & Lam, 1986). However, most occupational exposures probably cause asthma through sensitization and IgE mediated mechanisms (Burney, 1987). Tobacco smokers may be particularly sensitive to some occupational allergens (Zetterstrom et al., 1981).

The diagnosis of occupational asthma normally relies on combined sources of information. The presence of work-related respiratory symptoms is suggestive of occupational asthma. There are symptoms that are reported to be worse at work and better on rest days and holidays. Epidemiologic studies are usually based on respiratory symptoms questionnaires, particularly with regard to work-related chest tightness, wheeze, and shortness of breath. Only half of workers considered to have occupational asthma from questionnaire responses will have this diagnosis confirmed by other means (Malo et al., 1991). Thus, epidemiological studies are important to investigate some workers further with serial measures of lung function across the working day and throughout the working week. The most common method of recording serial measures of lung function is for the worker to record peak expiratory flow. There are many strategies used to diagnose occupational asthma using this techniques (Moscato et al., 1995). A critical factor in determining how asthma is associated with occupational exposures depends on the definition of occupational or work-related asthma. The National Institute for Occupational Safety and Health recently has published a case definition of work-related asthma (Jajosky et al., 1999). This definition includes two types of asthma: (1) work-aggravated asthma, which occurs in subjects who have a history of symptomatic asthma or who have been treated for asthma within two years of entering the workplace; and (2) new-onset asthma, which occurs in people with either no history of asthma or a history of preexisting asthma that was either untreated or asymptomatic for at least two years before entering the workplace.

CONCLUSION AND RECOMMENDATIONS

The apparent continuing rise in COPD mortality among African Americans requires more attention and further investigation to determine to what extent the rise is real and to what extent it is an artifact of changing fashion and practices in diagnosis and exposures to environmental/occupational risk factors. Population-based studies have shown that age and cigarette smoking are risk factors for

COPD in African Americans. Other potential risk factors for COPD, previously discussed, should be investigated using comprehensive epidemiologic approaches. Since NHANES was a cross-sectional study, longitudinal studies of changes in lung function and the development of respiratory symptoms with increasing age in African American smokers and nonsmokers are needed. These studies must utilize state-of-the-art statistical, epidemiological, and other methodologies. Repeated measurements of the prevalence of COPD are required in order to monitor secular changes on morbidity. The data from continuous NHANES and NHIS will be important sources for COPD studies regarding racial disparities in the future.

Prevention and treatment of COPD in African Americans are important areas of scientific pursuit. Especially occupational COPD should be a preventable disease in African Americans if exposures to causal agents are carefully controlled. When the risks of occupational COPD in the workplace are not quantified, proper surveillance approach need to be considered. For example, periodic spirometry measurements at two- to five-year intervals are necessary (Stenton, 2002). Workers with a rapid decline of FEV_1 can be removed from further exposure or provided with appropriate respiratory protection in the workplace.

The higher prevalence of cigarette smoking in African Americans (vs. Whites) is associated with a higher prevalence of, and mortality from, COPD. The control of cigarette smoking is a key to prevent and manage COPD. The prevalence of cigarette smoking among adult African Americans is 23.2 percent (CDC, 2002). Smoking cession for smokers and education for nonsmokers are necessary to reduce the prevalence of COPD in African Americans. Therefore, smoking prevention and cessation programs for African Americans should be expanded at the national, state, and local levels. With cessation of smoking, the rate of pulmonary functional loss declines, but lost function cannot be regained. However, timely smoking cessation (e.g., through effective health promotional/education campaigns, especially in the African American community) can prevent the development of symptomatic disease.

Reduction of air pollution is clearly desirable. Strict enforcement of the National Ambient Air Quality standards in the United States should contribute to the elimination of general air pollution as a factor in the development and progression of respiratory disease.

Greater regulatory and enforcement policies are needed for federal, state, and local governments. For example, more stringent control of occupational exposures should be mandated by the Occupational Safety and Health and Mining Safety and Health Acts. Also, legislative requirements to restrict the use of potentially hazardous materials used in occupations should help to ultimately eliminate occupational irritants as risk factors for COPD.

Aggressive specific and supportive management can improve survival from COPD. Recently, a workshop report on Global Strategy for the Diagnosis, Management, and Prevention of COPD (Pauwels et al., 2001) recommends the four components of COPD management: (1) assess and monitor disease; (2) reduce risk factors; (3) manage stable COPD; and (4) manage exacerbations. Additionally, effective education for patients with COPD needs to be determined. Future research should be focused on a better understanding of molecular and cellular pathogenic mechanism of COPD and also improved methods for early detection.

The mortality and morbidity due to asthma are associated with multifactors, but in many instances they can be related to the lack of control of chronic asthma activity and the delayed or ineffective treatment of the acute exacerbation. In this sense, a preventive approach is important to avoid asthma causing agents and conditions. When workers cannot avoid airborne sensitizers in the workplace, the risks could be limited by monitoring the exposure and antibody levels. Increasing levels of IgE antibodies in workers indicate a potential exposure risk and new occupational asthma might be developed (Hendrick & Burge, 2002). The control of exposure is essential to reduce the prevalence of asthma in the workplace. The prevention of asthmatic exacerbations is the primary goal of a therapeutic program. There is a multifactorial process to reduce morbidity and potential mortality of asthma. This multifactorial process includes environmental control and avoidance of causative agents, appropriate medications, education of patient and family in the asthmatic process and its treatment, and early identification of exacerbations. Further study is needed to identify the true causal factors of asthma, although many risk factors have been reported.

For prevention of COPD and asthma, there are three preventive methods; (1) primary prevention; (2) secondary prevention; (3) tertiary prevention (Chan-Yeung & Malo, 1997). Primary prevention is to eliminate the sensitizing agents, such as isocyanates, through reducing exposure and other control methods. Secondary prevention is the early detection of disease. For example, questionnaire and assessment of bronchial hyperresponsiveness are better methods for workers exposed to low-molecular-weight agents and skin-prick testing for workers exposed to high-molecular weight agents. Tertiary prevention is prevention of permanent damage. Once the diagnosis of asthma or COPD is made, the patient needs to be removed from the environment (e.g., the workplace) in order to prevent further exposure and the risk of permanent damage. These preventive approaches should be implemented early, especially for African American workers who are potentially exposed to hazardous chemicals and who are also currently smoking. These prevention efforts could help reduce African Americans' risks for asthma and COPD.

Lastly, prompt and adequate treatment of acute respiratory infection and of exacerbations of chronic bronchitis and asthma will reduce mortality and morbidity and also reduce the economic costs associated with loss from work. Again, these and other important prevention activities, as well as those mentioned before, will have the potential of contributing to a reduction in the overall incidence and prevalence of COPD and asthma in the African American population.

REFERENCES

American Thoracic Society (ATS) (1995). Standards for the diagnosis and care of patients with chronic obstructive pulmonary disease. *American Journal of Respiratory and Critical Care Medicine, 152*, S77–S121.

Anto, J.M., Sunyer, J., & Newman-Taylor, J.A. (1996). Comparison of soybean epidemic asthma and occupational asthma. *Thorax, 51*, 743–749.

Arif, A.A., Whitehead, L.W., Delclos, G.L., Tortolero, S.R., & Lee, E.S. (2002). Prevalence and risk factors of work related asthma by industry among United States workers: Data from the third national health and nutrition examination survey (1988–1994). *Occupational and Environmental Medicine, 59*, 505–511.

Bang, K.M. (1993). Prevalence of chronic obstructive pulmonary disease in blacks. *Journal of the National Medical Association, 85*, 51–55.

Bang, K.M., Gergen, P., & Turkeltaub, P. (1993). Allergen skin test reactivity in a United States national sample: Results from phase I of the third National Health and Nutrition Examination Survey (NHANES III), 1988–1991. *Proceedings of the 1993 annual meeting of American Academy of Allergy & Immunology*, Chicago.

Banks, D.E., & Wang M.L. (2000). Occupational asthma: The big picture. In D.E., Banks, E. & M.L. Wang (Eds.), *Occupational Medicine: State of the Art Reviews, 15*, 335–357.

Becklake, M. (1989). Occupational exposures: Evidence for a causal association with chronic obstructive pulmonary disease. *American Review of Respiratory Disease, 140*, S85–S91.

Benowitz, N.K., Hall, S.M., & Herning, R.I. (1983). Smokers of low-yield cigarettes do not consume less nicotine. *New England Journal of Medicine, 309*, 139–142.

Bjornsdottir, U.S., & Busse, W.W. (1992). Respiratory infections and asthma. *Clinical Allergy, 76*, 895–915.

Blanc, P.D., Cisternas, M., Smith, S., & Yelin, E. (1996). Occupational asthma in a community-based survey of adult asthma. *Chest, 109*, 56S–57S.

Broder, I., Higgins, N.W., & Matthews, K.P. (1974). Epidemiology of asthma and allergic rhinitis in a total community: Tecumseh, Michigan. III. Second survey of the community. *Journal of Allergy and Clinical Immunology, 53*, 127.

Burney, P.G.J. (1987). Descriptive epidemiology of bronchial reactivity in an adult population: Results from a community study. *Thorax, 42,* 38.

Busse, W.M., Banks-Schlegel, S.P., & Larsen, G.L. (1995). NHLBI workshop summary, childhood-versus adult-onset asthma. *American Journal of Respiratory and Critical Care Medicine, 151,* 1635–1639.

Call, R.S., Smith, T.F., Morris, E., Chapman, M.D., & Platts-Mills T.A.E. (1992). Risk factors for asthma in inner city children. *Journal of Pediatrics, 121,* 862–866.

Centers for Disease Control and Prevention (CDC). (1987). Cigarette smoking among Blacks and other minority population. *Mortality and Morbidity Weekly Report, 36,* 404–407.

Centers for Disease Control and Prevention (CDC). (1995). Current trends asthma—United States, 1982–1992. *Morbidity and Mortality Weekly Report, 43,* 952–955.

Centers for Disease Control and Prevention (CDC). (1998). Forecasted state-specific estimates of self-reported asthma prevalence-United States. *Mortality and Morbidity Weekly Report, 47,* 1022–1025.

Centers for Disease Control and Prevention (CDC). (2002). Behavioral Risk Factor Surveillance System, prevalence data-Nationwide 2000 asthma. http://apps.nccd.cdc.gov/brfss.

Chan-Yeung, M. (1995). Assessment of asthma in the workplace. *Chest, 108,* 1084–1117.

Chan-Yeung, M., & Lam, S. (1986). Occupational asthma. *American Review of Respiratory Disease, 133,* 686–703.

Chan-Yeung, M., & Malo, J.L. (1994). Aetiological agents in occupational asthma. *European Respiratory Journal, 7,* 346–371.

Chan-Yeung, M., & Malo, J.L. (1995). Epidemiology of occupational asthma. In W. Busse & S. Holgate (Eds.), *Asthma and rhinitis* (pp. 44–57). Oxford: Blackwell Scientific.

Chan-Yeung, M., & Malo, J.L. (1997). Occupational asthma. In P.J. Barnes et al. (Eds.), *Asthma* (pp. 2143–2155). Philadelphia: Lippincott-Raven.

Cohen, B.H., et al. (1975). Genetic-epidemiologic study of chronic obstructive pulmonary disease. *Johns Hopkins Medical Journal, 137,* 95–104.

Dockery, D.W., & Pope, C.A. (1997). Outdoor air: Particulates. In K. Steenland & D.A. Savits (Eds.), *Topics in environmental epidemiology* (pp. 119–166). New York: Oxford University.

Duffy, D.L., Martin, N.G., & Battistutta, D. (1990). Genetics of asthma and hay fever in Australian twins. *American Review of Respiratory Disease, 142,* 1351–1358.

Duhme, H., Weiland, S.K., & Keil, U. (1996). The association between self-reported symptoms of asthma and allergic rhinitis and self-reported traffic density on street of residence in adolescents. *Epidemiology, 7,* 578–582.

Essien, J., Mobley, C.N., Griffith, M., Creer, T.L., & Celler, R.L. (2001) Pediatrics asthma in African American Children. In R.L. Braithwaite & S.E. Taylor (Eds.), *Health issues in the Black community* (pp. 282–305). San Francisco: Jossey-Bass.

Evans, R., III, et al. (1987). National trends in mortality of asthma in the U.S.A.: Prevalence, hospitalization, and death from asthma over two decades, 1965–1984. *Chest, 91 (supp.),* 65s–74s.

Feinleib, M., Rosenber, H., Collins, J.G., Delozier, J.E., Pokras, R., & Chervarley, F.M. (1989). Trends in COPD morbidity and mortality in the United States. *American Review of Respiratory Disease, 140,* s9–s18.

Fiore, M.C., Novotny, T.E., Pierce, J.P., Hatziandreu, E.J., Patal, K.M., & Davis, R.M. (1989). Trends in cigarette smoking in the United States: The changing influence of gender and race. *Journal of the American Medical Association, 261,* 49–55.

Frost, F., Tollestrup, K., & Starzyk, P. (1994). History of smoking from the Washington State death certificate. *American Journal of Preventive Medicine, 10,* 335–339.

Gillum, G.F. (1990). Chronic obstructive pulmonary disease in Blacks and Whites: Mortality and morbidity. *Journal of the National Medical Association, 82,* 417–428.

Gillum, G.F. (1991). Chronic obstructive pulmonary disease in Blacks and Whites: Pulmonary function norms and risk factors. *Journal of the National Medical Association, 83,* 393–401.

Gillum, G.F., & Liu, K.C. (1984). Coronary heart disease mortality in United States Blacks, 1940–1978: Trends and unanswered questions. *American Heart Journal, 108,* 728–732.

Hendrick, D.J., & Burge, P.S. (2002). Asthma. In D.J. Hendrick, P.S. Burge, W.S. Beckett, & A. Churg (Eds.), *Occupational disorders of the lung: Recognition, management, and prevention* (pp. 33–76). New York: W.B. Saunders.

Higgins, I. (1970). Occupational factor in chronic bronchitis and emphysema. In N.G.M. Orie & R. Van Der Lende (Eds.), *Bronchitis III: Proceedings of the third international symposium on bronchitis*. Springfield, IL: Charles C. Thomas.

Higgins, I. (1980). Respiratory disease. In J.M. Last (Ed.), *Public health and preventive medicine*, 11th ed. New York: Appleton-Century-Crofts.

Higgins, M. (1984). Epidemiology of COPD: State of the art. *Chest, 85*, 35–85.

Higgins, M.W., & Keller, J.B. (1975). Familial occurrence of chronic respiratory disease and familial resemblance in ventilatory capacity. *Journal of Chronic Disease, 28*, 239–251.

Higgins, M.W., et al. (1984). Risk of chronic obstructive pulmonary disease. *American Review of Respiratory Disease, 130*, 380–385.

Hopp, R.J., Bewtra, A.K., & Riven, R. (1988). Bronchial reactivity pattern in nonasthmatic parents of asthmatics. *Annals of Allergy, 61*, 184–186.

Hopp, R.J., Bewtra, A.K., & Watt, C.D. (1984). Genetic analysis of allergic disease in twins. *Journal of Allergy and Clinical Immunology, 73*, 265–270.

Horwood, L.J., Fergusson, D.M., & Shannon, F.T. (1985). Social and familial factors in the development of early childhood asthma. *Pediatrics, 75*, 859–868.

Hubert, H.B., Fabsitz., R.R., & Feinleib, M. (1982). Genetic and environmental influences on pulmonary function in adult twins. *American Review of Respiratory Disease, 125*, 404–415.

Jajosky, R., Harrison, R., Reinisch, F., & Flattery, J. (1999). Surveillance of work-related asthma in selected U.S. states using surveillance guidelines for state health departments—California, Massachusetts, Michigan, and New Jersey, 1993–1995. *Morbidity and Mortality Weekly Report, 48*, 1–20.

Kang, B., Vellody, D., Homburger, H., & Yunginger, J.W. (1979). Cockroach cause of allergic asthma. Its specificity and immunologic profile. *Journal of Allergy and Clinical Immunology, 63*, 80–86.

Kauffmann, F., Dockery, D.W., Speizer, F.E., & Ferris, B.G. (1989). Respiratory symptoms and lung function in relation to passive smoking: A comparative study of American and French women. *International Journal of Epidemiology, 18*, 334–344.

Lefioe, N.M., Ashley, M.J., Pederson, L.I., & Keays, J.J. (1984). The health risks of passive smoking. *Chest, 1*, 90–95.

Leigh, J.P., Romano, P.S., Schenker, M.B., & Kreiss, K. (2002). Costs of occupational COPD and asthma. *Chest, 121*, 264–272.

Levine, R.S., Foster, J.E., Fullilove, R.E., Fullilove, M.T., Briggs, N.C., Hull, P.C., Husaini, B.A., & Hennekens, C.H. (2001). Black–White inequalities in mortality and life expectancy, 1933–1999: Implications for healthy people 2010. *Public Health Reports, 116*, 474–494.

Lieberman, J., Gaidulis, L., & Roberts, L. (1976). Racial distribution of alpha 1-anti-trypsin variants among junior high school students. *American Review of Respiratory Disease, 114*, 1194–1198.

Livingstone, A.E., Shaddick, G., Grundy, C., & Elliott, P. (1996). Do people living near inner city main roads have more asthma needing treatment? *British Medical Journal, 312*, 676–677.

Malo, J.L., Ghezzo, H., & L-Archeveque, J. (1991). Is the clinical history a satisfactory means of diagnosing occupational asthma? *American Review of Respiratory Disease, 143*, 528–532.

Martinez, F.D., Wright, A.L., & Holberg, C.J. (1992). Maternal age as a risk factor for wheezing lower respiratory illness in the first year of life. *American Journal of Epidemiology, 136*, 1258.

Mays, E.E. (1975). Pulmonary diseases. In R.A. Williams (Ed.), *Textbook of black-related diseases* (pp. 429–436). New York: McGraw-Hill Book Company.

Melbostad, E., Eduard, W., & Magnus, P. (1997). Chronic bronchitis in farmers. *Scandinavian Journal of Work Environmental Health, 23*, 271–280.

Mendoza, J., & Snyder, F.D. (1970). Cockroach sensitivity in children with bronchial asthma. *Annals of Allergy, 28*, 159–163.

Menon, P., Menon, V., Hilman, B., Stankus, R., & Lehrer, S.B. (1991). Skin test reactivity to whole body and fecal extracts of American and German cockroaches in atopic asthmatics. *Annals of Allergy, 67*, 573–577.

Milton, D.K., Solomon, G.M., Rosiello, R.A., & Herrick, R.F. (1998). Risk and incidence of asthma attributable to occupational exposure among HMO members. *American Journal of Industrial Medicine, 33*, 1–10.

Moscato, G., Godnic-Cvar, J., & Maestrelli, P. (1995). For the Subcommittee on Occupational Allergy of

European Academy of Allergy and Clinical Immunology: Statement of self-monitoring of peak expiratory flows in the investigation of occupational asthma. *Journal of Allergy and Clinical Immunology, 96,* 295–301.

Murray, C.J.L. & Lopez, A.D. (1996). Evidence-based health policy—lessons from the global burden of disease study. *Science, 274,* 740–743.

National Center for Health Statistics (NCHS). (1978). Plan and operation of the NHANES I. Augmentation survey of adults 25–74 years, United States, 1974–75. *Vital and Health Statistics, USHHS, DHEW Publication No. (PHS) 78-1314; Series 1, No. 14.* Washington, DC: U.S. Government Printing Office.

National Center for Health Statistics (NCHS). (1981). Plan and operation of the second National Health and Nutrition Examination Survey, 1976–80. *Vital and Health Statistics, DHHS Publication No. (PHS) 81-1317, Series 1, No. 15.* Washington, DC: U.S. Government Printing Office.

National Center for Health Statistics (NCHS). (1986). Prevalence of selected chronic conditions, United States, 1979–81. *Vital and Health Statistics, DHHS Publication No. (PHS) 86-1583, Series 10, No. 155.* Washington, DC: U.S. Government Printing Office.

National Center for Health Statistics (NCHS). (1989). Health United States, 1988. *DHHS Publication No. (PHS) 89-1232.* Washington, DC: U.S. Government Printing Office.

National Center for Health Statistics (NCHS). (2002). Smoking prevalence: Early release of selected estimates based on data from the 2001 NHIS. http://www.cdc.gov/nchs/about/major/nhis/released200207/table08_1.htm.

National Institutes of Health (NIH). (1981). Epidemiology of Respiratory Disease Task Force Report. *NIH Publication 82-2019.* Bethesda, MD: U.S. Government Printing Office.

Northridge, M.E., Myer, I.H., & Dunn, L. (2002). Overlooked and underserved in Harlem: A population-based survey of adults with asthma. *Environmental Health Perspectives, 110,* 217–220.

Novotny, T.E., Walker, K.E., Kendrick, J.S., & Remington, P.L. (1988). Smoking by Blacks and Whites: Socioeconomic and demographic differences. *American Journal of Public Health, 78,* 1187–1189.

Office on Smoking and Health. (1989). Reducing the health consequences of smoking: 25 years of progress. A report of the surgeon general. *DHHS Publication No. (CDC) 89-8411.* Washington, DC: U.S. Government Printing Office.

Oxman, A.D., Muir D.C.F., Shannon, H.S., Stock, S.R., Hnizdo, E., & Lange, H.J. (1993). Occupational dust exposure and chronic obstructive pulmonary disease. A systematic overview of the evidence. *American Review of Respiratory Disease, 148,* 38–48.

Pattemore, P.K., Johnston, S.L., & Bardin, P.G. (1992). Viruses as precipitants of asthma symptoms: 1. Epidemiology. *Clinical and Experimental Allergy, 22,* 325–336.

Pauwels, R.A., Buist, A.S., Calverley, P.M.A., Jenkins, C.R., & Hurd, S.S. (2001). Global strategy for the diagnosis, management, and prevention of chronic obstructive pulmonary disease: NHLBI/WHO Global Initiative for Chronic Obstructive Lung Disease (GOLD) Workshop Summary. *American Journal of Respiratory and Critical Care Medicine, 163,* 1256–1276.

Pershagen, G., Rylander, E., & Norberg, S. (1995). Air pollution involving nitrogen dioxin exposure and wheezing bronchitis in children. *International Journal of Epidemiology, 24,* 1147–1153.

Redline, S., Tishler, P.V., Lewitter, F.I., Tager, I.B., Munoz, A., & Speizer, F.E. (1987). Assessment of genetic and nongenetic influences on pulmonary function: A twin study. *American Review of Respiratory Disease, 135,* 217–222.

Sanford, A., Weir, T., & Pare, P. (1996). State of the art: The genetics of asthma. *American Journal of Respiratory and Critical Care Medicine, 153,* 1749–1765.

Schwartz, J., & Weiss, S.T. (1992). Caffeine intake and asthma symptoms. *Annals of Epidemiology, 2,* 627–635.

Sibbald, B., & Turner-Warwick, M. (1979). Factors influencing the prevalence of asthma among first degree relatives of extrinsic and intrinsic asthmatics. *Thorax, 34,* 332–337.

Sigurs, N., Bjarnason, R., & Sigurbergsson, F. (1995). Asthma and immunoglobulin E antibodies after respiratory syncytial virus bronchiolitis: A prospective cohort study with matched controls. *Pediatrics, 95,* 500–505.

Speizer, F.E., & Tager, I.B. (1979). Epidemiology of chronic mucus hypersecretion and obstructive airways disease. *Epidemiologic Review, 1,* 124–142.

Sporik, R., Ingram, M.J., & Price, W. (1995). Association of asthma with serum IgE and skin test reactivity to allergens among children living at high altitude: Tickling the dragon's breath. *American Journal of Respiratory and Critical Care Medicine, 151*, 1388–1392.

Stark, J.M., & Grazinano, F.M. (1995). Lower airway response to viruses. In W.W. Busse & S.T. Holgate (Eds.), *Asthma and rhinitis* (pp. 1229–1243). Oxford: Blackwell Scientific.

Stenton, C. (2002). Chronic obstructive pulmonary disease (COPD). In D.J. Hendrick, P.S. Burge, W.S. Beckett, & A. Churg (Eds.), *Occupational disorders of the lung: Recognition, management, and prevention* (pp. 77–91). New York: W.B. Saunders.

Troisi, R.J., Willet, W.C., Weiss, S.T., Trichopoulos, D., Rosner, B., & Speizer, F.E. (1995). A prospective study of diet and adult onset asthma. *American Review of Respiratory and Critical Care Medicine, 151*, 1401–1408.

U.S. Department of Health and Human Services (USDHHS). (1979). *Smoking and health. A report of the surgeon general. DHHS Publication No. (PHS) 79-50066*. Washington, DC: U.S. Government Printing Office.

U.S. Department of Health and Human Services (USDHHS). (1999). National Institute for Occupational Safety and Health. *Work-related Lung Disease Surveillance Report, 1999. DHHS (NIOSH) No. 2000-05*.

U.S. Department of Health and Human Services (USDHHS). (2000). *Healthy People 2010: Tracking Healthy People 2010*. Washington, DC: U.S. Government Printing Office.

U.S. Department of Health and Human Services (USDHHS). (2001). Centers for Disease Control and Prevention. *Health, United States, 2001 with Urban and Rural Health Chartbook, Publication No. (PHS) 01-1232*. Washington, DC: U.S. Government Printing Office.

U.S. Surgeon General. (1984). *The health consequences of smoking; Chronic obstructive lung disease*. U.S. Department of Health and Human Services, Publication No. 84-50205.

Von Mutius, E. (2000). The burden of childhood asthma. *Archives of Disease in Childhood, 82(Suppl II)*, ii2–ii5.

Von Mutius, E., & Nicolai, T. (1996). Familial aggregation of asthma in a South Bavarian population. *American Journal of Respiratory and Critical Care Medicine, 153*, 1266–1272.

Ward, D.L. (1992). An international comparison of asthma morbidity and mortality in U.S. soldiers, 1984 to 1988. *Chest, 101*, 613–620.

Wardlaw, A. (1993). The role of air pollution in asthma. *Clinical Experiment of Allergy, 23*, 81–96.

Weiss, S.T. (1994). Smoking and asthma. *Comparative Therapy, 20*, 606–610.

Weiss, S.T. (1998). Asthma: Epidemiology. In A.P. Fishman (Ed.). *Fishman's pulmonary disease and disorders*, 3rd ed. (pp. 735–743). New York: McGraw-Hill.

Witting, H.J., McLaughlen, E.T., Leifer, K.L., & Belloit, J.D. (1978). Risk factors for the development of allergic disease: Analysis of 2190 patient records. *Annals of Allergy, 41*, 84–88.

Woolcock, A.J. (1986). Prevalence of bronchial hyperresponsiveness and asthma in a rural adult population. *Thorax 41*: 283.

Wright, A.L., Holberg, C.J., Taussig, L.M., & Martinez, F.D. (1995). Relationship of infant feeding to recurrent wheezing at age 6 years. *Archives of Pediatric and Adolescent Medicine, 149*, 758–763.

Young, R.C., Headings, V.E., Henderson, A.L., Bose, S., & Hackney, R.L., Jr. (1978). Protease inhibitor profile of Black Americans with and without chronic cardiopulmonary disease. *Journal of National Medical Association, 70*, 849–856.

Zetterstrom, O., Osterman, K., Machado, L., & Johansson, S.G.O. (1981). Another smoking hazard: Raised serum IgE concentration and increased risk of occupational allergy. *British Medical Journal, 283*, 1215–1217.

CHAPTER 9

Sickle-Cell Disease: Biosocial Aspects

JOSEPH TELFAIR

INTRODUCTION

Sickle-cell disease (SCD) refers to a group of genetic disorders in which sickling of red blood cells due to loss of oxygen gives the cell a sicklelike shape and results in a chronic anemia and obstruction of the body's smaller circulatory system (NHLBI, 2002). In the United States, the disease occurs mostly (but not exclusively) in African Americans (see Table 1). It is the most common genetic disorder within a specific population, having an incidence of 1 in every 500 live Black births (Davis et al., 1997; Castro, 1999). To date there are about 75,000 individuals with the disorder (NHLBI, 2002). Unexpected, intermittent, and at times life-threatening complications characterize the course of the disease (Wagner & Vichinsky, 1989). Like individuals with similar chronic conditions, these variations are reported to have a profound impact on the biological, psychological, and social development of these individuals, as well as implications for their overall management (Telfair, 1994; Hague & Telfair, 2000). The disease's inheritance type is autosomal recessive.

As Figure 9.1 illustrates, individuals must inherit a sickle-cell gene from both parents in order to have sickle-cell disease (symptomatic), but if they inherit both a normal and a sickle-cell gene, they have only sickle-cell trait and are asymptomatic. Prognostic expectations for morbidity, mortality, and life expectancy of patients with the disease have improved significantly over the past 20 years with improvements and wider availability of medical care to infants and young children with the condition (Platt et al., 1994; NHLBI, 2002). However, significant disparities in the attention to social and psychological issues (e.g., relationships with families, employment, school, research in trying to understand those who live comparatively well with the condition as compared to those who do not, etc.) and overall improvements in the sociocultural aspects of access to, and utilization of, supportive care (as compared to clinical care) continue to greatly compromise the quality of life of persons with SCD.

Understanding the impact that sickle-cell disease has on the lives of those with the condition and the areas where disparities exists must begin with a basic understanding of the condition itself. This chapter provides an overview of the geographic, historical, and bioclinical aspects of the condition. Please note that since SCD predominantly affects African Americans, all references to treatments, clinical care, biosocial issues, and concerns refer to this population. Understanding of these aspects

Figure 9.1
Inheritance patterns of sickle-cell trait and anemia

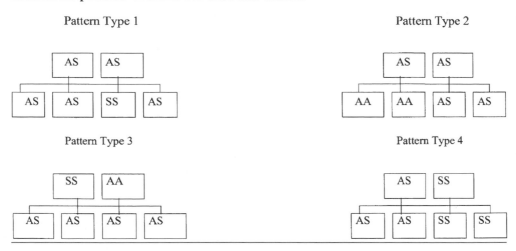

Source: Nash & Telfair (1994), Sickle cell disease (126–127).

Note: If both parents have sickle-cell anemia (SS) or any combination of sickle-cell disease (i.e., SC, Sβ^+ thalassemia, etc.) the child will inherit sickle-cell disease. Likewise if both parents have normal hemoglobin (AA), the chance of the child inheriting sickle-cell disease is zero.

of SCD provides insights into the experiences of African Americans with chronic conditions, especially those with genetic disorders.

THE BIOSOCIAL PERSPECTIVE

A biosocial model for understanding and working with a chronic genetic condition such as sickle-cell anemia is imperative for a holistic approach toward services. As individuals move through the life cycle, they encounter frequently increasing physical, psychological, and social problems that can affect their quality of life. A biosocial model, as seen in Figure 9.2, visualizes the individual in continuous interaction with internal (physical and psychological) and external (social) influences (Schwartz, 1982). The impact of any one influence can support the overall response of the individual to the chronic condition either positively or negatively. Outside influences, such as the provision of services, can help offset the deleterious impact. The negative interaction of these systems can depress, demoralize, and offset the individual's and his or her family's sense of purpose and direction.

The transaction among the elements that affect the functional status of individuals with sickle-cell disease is viewed as a spinning top (Figure 9.2). The elements are the physical (molecular, genetic, cellular, and organ systems) and psychological (cognitive, affective, and behavioral). The conceptual framework offers a broader perspective than the physical and psychological by incorporating an ecological perspective. Ecology's concern is with the relationship between organisms and their environment (Germain, 1979; Bronfenbrenner, 1979). Attention is focused on the influence of social and physical environments on adaptation and coping behaviors of people (Garbarino, 1985). Lack of fit between individual and environment can negatively affect a person's physical and mental health (Werthiem, 1975). Likewise, ill health can negatively affect the degree of congruence between the individual and the environment. Therefore, understanding a condition such as sickle-cell disease from a biosocial perspective allows one to formulate a holistic approach vital to competent comprehensive care (Schwartz, 1982). African Americans experience complex health disadvantages that are com-

Figure 9.2
Biosocial model of health and illness

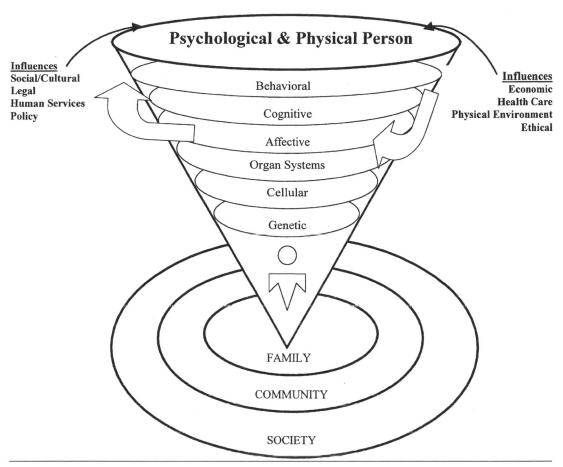

Source: Dillworth-Anderson, P., Harris, L.H., Holbrook, C.T., Konrad, R., Kramer, K.D., Nash, K.B., Phillips, G. (1993), Graphical Representation of Biopsychosocial Model of Health and Illness, *Journal of Health and Social Policy* (1994) (re-drawn).

pounded by a combination of poverty, racial bias, ignorance, and lack of access to quality health care. Having sickle-cell disease only exacerbates these conditions. This chapter focuses on the utilization of the biosocial model, not only in understanding sickle-cell disease and its various current and future treatments but also in the delivery of services to those with the condition.

OVERVIEW OF SICKLE-CELL ANEMIA

Geographic Distribution

It is unclear whether or not the sickle-cell gene (Hgb S) arose as a single mutation that spread through migration or from identical mutations in different areas throughout the world (Serjeant, 1992). It is recognized that the gene is widespread and not racially linked. The common factor in its spread is falciparurn malaria; the sickle gene existed in high concentrations in the equatorial regions of Africa and several Mediterranean regions, areas where malaria is endemic (Serjeant, 1992). In these areas the heterozygote (the individual with a single Hgb S gene or sickle-cell trait) has a natural resistance to malaria. Consequently, these individuals had a greater chance to transmit the gene. Serjeant (1992) suggests that migration from, and exploration of, equatorial and West Africa were key in spreading the gene to India, Saudi Arabia, Spain, southern Italy, and other Mediterranean regions (p. 380). Gaston (1987) notes that the slave trade was a primary catalyst in bringing the gene to the New World. This explains the high incidence of the various sickle hemoglobinopathies among African Americans and peoples of the Caribbean.

Historical Aspects

In the 1910 edition of the *Archives of Internal Medicine*, Dr. James Herrick of Chicago presented the first accepted report of the blood disorder "sickle-cell disease" in North America (Serjeant, 2001). It was suspected that the disease was present in North America before Dr. Herrick's report but had gone unrecognized (Scott, 1983; Gaston, 1987). This was due to misdiagnosis resulting from the disease's clinical manifestations being similar to those of other tropical diseases and "the infrequency of microscopic examination of peripheral blood smears" (Serjeant, 1992). Other case reports followed Dr. Herrick's, and in 1922 Dr. V.R. Mason summarized these reports and entitled this new disease entity "sickle-cell anemia" (Serjeant, 1992). Major milestones in understanding the pathology and pathophysiology of the disease occurred during the five decades following Dr. Herrick's first report (Scott, 1983). Gaston (1987) states that during the 1920s, investigations led to the recognition that sickle-cell anemia were an inherited clinical entity "with a characteristic blood picture" (p. 150).

Serjeant points to Diggs' (1935) recognition in 1935 of the processes that lead to the "splenic sequestration crises" as one of the first arguments for the differentiating between symptomatic gene carriers (sickle-cell disease) and asymptomatic cases (sickle-cell trait). This led to the conclusion that "the sickle-cell phenomenon was inherited as a Mendelian autosomal dominant characteristic" (Serjeant, 1992). Other hemolytic aspects of the disease, such as jaundice, gallstones associated with increased bilirubin secretions, and bony changes, were also first recognized during the 1920s and 1930s (Serjeant, 1992). The research of Ham and Castle in the 1940s brought recognition of the cyclical aspects of the sickling process (Gaston, 1987). Understanding this concept of the "vicious cycle of erythrostasis" led to early and later research and treatment of the most common clinical symptom, the vaso-occlusive (pain) episode. The work of Pauling et al. (1949) and others (Ingram, 1956), demonstrating the difference in electrophoretic separation between normal and sickle hemoglobins, led to the understanding that an abnormal hemoglobin was responsible for the sickling phenomenon. Ingram (1956) noted that the changes in this abnormal hemoglobin were due to an unusual substitution in the amino acid sequence of polypeptide chains that make up the hemoglobin molecule (giving the cell its "sickled shape") (Gaston, 1987).

Serjeant (2001) notes that J.F. Neel and E.A. Beet, working independently of each other, clarified the disease's heterozygous-homozygous pattern of inheritance (p. 346). The elucidation of the genetic difference between these gene-present states led to the development of laboratory tests that allowed for prenatal and infant screening and some understanding of the clinical variability of the various hemoglobin S genotypes (Whitten & Nisihura, 1985; Edelstein, 1986; Davis et al., 1997). Other early discoveries of disease characteristics noted by Serjeant (1992) included (a) the relationship between sickle-cell disease and leg ulcers and the adverse effect of the disease on pregnancy in the late 1930s; (b) the retardation of physical and sexual development in children and adults; and (c) recognition, much later, of priapism, retinal, and cerebral vascular complications (strokes).

BIOCLINICAL AND TREATMENT ASPECTS OF THE DISEASE

Bioclinical Aspects

The most common types of sickle-cell disease are Hemoglobin SS (homozygous sickle-cell disease), SC, Sβ^0, and Sβ^+ Thalassemia (heterozygous types) (Sickle-Cell Disease Guideline Panel, 1993; AAP Committee on Genetics, 2002) (see Table 9.1). The inheritance pattern for all forms of sickle-cell disease is autosomal recessive. The disease results from an abnormality in the structure of the main oxygen-carrying compound in the red blood cell (hemoglobin). Under low oxygen conditions, sickle hemoglobin polymerizes, changing the red cell from the usual flexible disc shape to a hard, jagged, irregular shape. This increased rigidity, due to polymerization, results in early cell breakdown (Castro, 1999). These cells pass through the individual's blood system with much difficulty, often collecting at the junctures in the smaller veins and capillaries, causing blockage, resulting in the disease's most common symptom, the sickle-cell "pain episode" (Ballas, 1994). These pain episodes are often severe and unpredictable, lasting from several hours to several days (Wagner & Vichinsky, 1989; Ballas, 1994).

Developmentally, the ever-present sickling condition with underlying hemolysis and secondary vaso-occlusion in early life may lead to dactylitis (hand-foot syndrome), stroke, osteomyelitis, anernia, priapism, aseptic necrosis, and in older patients the potential for blindness, cardiopulmonary problems, renal failure, and other major organ damage (e.g., spleen, liver) (Wagner & Vichinsky, 1989). Complications associated with the disease vary in severity and frequency across all individuals and disease types (Hemoglobin SS being the most common and most severe) (NHLBI, 2002). With the advances in the early detection and treatment of these complications over the past 25 years, the severity of most has been reduced (Davis et al., 1997; AAP Committee on Genetics, 2002).

Treatments

Current and experimental techniques of the management of sickle-cell disease are directed at early prevention, early detection, and prevention before major irreparable damage is done and supportive management once damage has occurred (Steinberg, 1999). Most are discussed later.

Oral Penicillin.   Before newborn screening for sickle-cell disease and the initiation of prophylaxis with oral penicillin, hundreds of children died each year due to severe bacterial infections (Wagner & Vichinsky, 1989). Currently, children with sickle-cell disease begin to receive prophylactic oral penicillin by four months of age to decrease the risk of mortality associated with infections (Falletta et al., 1995).

Exchange Transfusion.   Exchange transfusion therapy, in many cases, is the treatment of choice for reducing the concentration of sickle hemoglobin and thereby the rate of progressive organ damage or conditions such as stroke, aseptic necrosis, and chronic pain (Steinberg, 1999). It is an immediate management tool of priapism, acute chest syndrome, splenic sequestration, and other conditions that require emergent intervention but not long-term management (Vichinsky et al., 1995). Exchange transfusion therapy has also proven to be a veritable tool in the prevention of recurrent vaso-occlusive events, which happens to be the most serious complications of sickle-cell disease. The aim of transfusion is to reduce the hemoglobin S concentration to less than 30 percent and maintain it at this level for three to five years (Steinberg, 1999). The rationale for this approach is based on the following facts: (a) in sickle-cell patients, exchange transfusion improves exercise capacity without a substantial rise in their hematocrit (Miller et al., 1980), suggesting improved tissue oxygenation; (b) complications such as chest syndrome, priapism, and pain crises are rare in those patients who are on transfusion program for stroke; and (c) incidence of vaso-occlusive complications is reduced in pregnant sickle-cell patients who are on prophylactic transfusions (Koshy et al., 1988).

Table 9.1

Prevalence of sickle-cell disease (Hb SS, sickle cell-hemoglobin C disease and sickle beta-thalassemia syndromes) by racial or ethnic group, per 100,000 live births, United States, 1990 and unspecified years

Racial or ethnic group	Mean prevalence	95 percent confidence interval
White	1.72	1.06 - 2.66
Black	289	277 - 300
Hispanic, total	5.28	2.60 - 9.61
Hispanic, Eastern States	89.8	27.0 – 190.0
Hispanic, Western States	3.14	1.19 - 6.86
Asian	7.61	1.85 - 57.20
Native American	36.20	0.04 - 182

Source: Abbreviated and modified from results of Bayesian meta-analysis published by Sickle Cell Disease Guideline Panel, 1993.

Because of the risk of iron overload (Embury et al., 1994), concurrent chelation therapy with deferoxamine (Desferal) is used to rid the body of excess iron that could cause severe damage to vital blood-profuse organs (Lubin & Vichinsky, 1991; Vichinsky et al., 1995; Styles & Vichinsky, 1997). Relatedly, the improved preparation of blood products has reduced the incidence of secondary viral infection and alloimmunization (NHLBI, 2002).

New Drug Therapies.   The vaso-occlusive episode and its complications are the most common symptom associated with sickle-cell disease (Schecther et al., 1987; Serjeant, 1992; Ballas, 1994).

For a number of years, clinical researchers have been investigating methods that can possibly decrease the frequency of these events, such as the use of new drug therapies aimed at decreasing the amount of hemoglobin S cells in the individual's circulatory system. Two of these experimental drugs are Erythropoietin (EPO) and hydroxyurea (HU).

Erythropoietin (EPO) is a hormone that is produced by the kidney and stimulates the bone marrow to increase the production of red blood cells (Noguchi, 1988; Brunara et al., 1990). Recent experiments have shown that EPO, when given in sufficient doses, will enhance the synthesis of fetal hemoglobin (Hgb F) (Noguchi et al., 1988). Fetal hemoglobin is a normal hemoglobin present at birth and is gradually replaced by adult hemoglobins between 6 and 18 months of age (Noguchi et al., 1988). The fetal hemoglobin genes are normal in individuals with sickle-cell disease. It is argued that by using agents that stimulate Hgb F synthesis, this "hemoglobin switch" can be reversed, therefore increasing the percentage of cells in the individual's circulatory system containing normal fetal hemoglobin and decreasing the percentage of hemoglobin S (sickle hemoglobin) (Brunara et al., 1990; Rodgers, 1990).

Hydroxyurea (HU) is a medication that has been used for several years in the treatment of Polycythemi avera and other myeloproliferative disorders (Charache et al., 1987). Recent experiments have shown that EPO or HU, when given in sufficient doses, will enhance the synthesis of fetal hemoglobin (Hgb F) (Noguchi et al., 1988). The hypothesized end result is the improvement in general health by reduction of the rate of organ damage from vaso-occlusion and other complications related to hemolysis (Dover et al., 1986). The response of patients to hydroxyurea depends on the capacity of the bone marrow to withstand moderate doses of the drug (Steinberg, et al., 1997). Based on these results, the U.S. Food and Drug Administration (FDA) approved its use as an effective palliative treatment for adults with sickle-cell anemia. However, there remain uncertainties regarding potentials of teratogenicity, mutagenicity, and leukaemogenicity. A key factor in HU therapy resides not only in taking the medication but also in complying with the necessary laboratory follow-up to ensure safe use of the medication and to avoid toxicity (Charache et al., 1995a; Charache et al., 1995b).

Cost is a factor that must be weighed against the cost of frequent painful crises. Hydroxyurea, therefore, should be reserved for those patients whose complications are sufficiently severe to justify the burdens of treatment and who can comply with the regimen. Also research is under way to evaluate the combined use of HU and EPO to increase and maintain the level of Hgb F (Brunara et al., 1990; Chrache et al., 1995b).

Concern regarding the potential risk of carcinogenesis and other chronic long-term complications is raised by clinical Investigators and social scientists alike (Vichinsky, 1992). Because of these concerns, the drug is currently recommended only for individuals who have had a severe disease course (Charache et al., 1987; Vichinsky, 1992). Also, studies have shown the potential for EPO to augment the increase in Hgb F obtained by HU alone, and research is under way to evaluate the combined use of HU and EPO to increase and maintain the level of Heb F (Noguchi, 1988; Brunara et al., 1990). This combined therapy could be extremely beneficial (Lubin & Vichinsky, 1991).

Lastly, HU has been studied in both adults and children, and the results were remarkably similar (Ferster et al., 1996). HU's use over long years, however, has not been studied in children. Clinical trails of HU in children, such as the HUG-KIDS study, are under way (Wang et al., 2002). While promising, these studies are not without controversy, particularly in regard to the unknown effects of HU on child growth and development (Ohene-Frempong & Smith-Whitney, 1997).

Bone Marrow Transplantation.   Another alternative therapy, bone marrow transplantation, has recently been reported as the "cure" for sickle-cell disease (Vermylen et al., 1988; Walters et al., 2000). Young children who have experienced few complications secondary to their condition are considered ideal candidates for the procedure (Kodish et al., 1990; Billings, 1989; Walters et al., 2000). Johnson et al. (1984) reported on the first such transplant, successfully performed on an 8-

year-old child with sickle-cell anemia and acute myeloblastic leukemia. Relatively few bone marrow transplants have been used for persons with sickle-cell disease (Hoppe & Walters, 2001).

A recent report by the Multicenter Investigation of Bone Marrow Transplantation for Sickle Cell Disease (Walters et al., 2000) and research in Eurpoe (Lucarelli et al., 1990) suggest that children suffering from a major complication, such as stroke, who demonstrate full recovery would be suitable candidates for an attempt at cure with bone marrow transplantation because of the inevitable risk of another stroke with debilitating results.

Bone marrow transplant has great promise and can cure children with sickle-cell disease, but at what cost? Bone marrow transplantation has an inherent risk of death from complications associated with the procedure and immediate side effects such as infection and graft-versus-host disease (Kodish et al., 1991; Hoppe & Walters, 2001).

Cost-benefit decisions also must consider the psychological, legal, ethical, and nonmedical cost (i.e., out-of-pocket cost borne by parents) and quality-of-life issues (Williams, 1984; Vaughan et al., 1986; Durbin, 1988; Billings, 1989; Stevens & Pletsch, 2002; Walters et al., 2002). Knowing that many children with sickle-cell anemia survive into adulthood with limited problems and become productive citizens and parents makes this a difficult choice for parents and professionals alike (Billings, 1989; Kodish et al., 1990).

Future Treatments and Promising Research.   Future research includes the development of genetic therapy that can be effectively administered without complication. The purpose of the therapy will be act as "switch" to regulate or turn off the sickle gene (Van Raamsdonk, 2002). Gene therapy involves the transfer of normal genes into certain marrow cells. Unlike bone marrow transplantation, gene therapy does not require chemotherapy to destroy marrow. It only adds the normal gene in place of the defective gene. The question is, Can the gene be altered to maintain the production of fetal hemoglobin instead of increasing synthesis of sickle hemoglobin and reduce the overall clinical severity based on persistence of fetal hemoglobin? If effective, this therapy would prove less complicated and cheaper than bone marrow transplantation (Bertrand, 2002). The use of genetic therapy in young children before the onset of organ failure is also conceptually possible (Ryan et al., 1990). Although the technology for gene therapy is not yet available, much progress is being made in the area, and such therapy could possibly be available within the next decade (Bertrand, 2002). Despite its potential, genetic therapy implies the treatment of a fetus in utero as one means of altering the genetic outcome. Use of this therapy raises ethical issues that must be addressed before the therapy can be sanctioned as an option for expectant parents.

PSYCHOLOGICAL AND SOCIAL SICKLE-CELL DISEASE LITERATURE

Sociopsychological issues can significantly affect the overall well-being of the person with SCD (Telfair, 1994; Telfair & Nash, 1996; Vavasseur, 1987; Whitten & Nishiura, 1985; Lemanek et al., 1986; Hurtig & White, 1986; Barrettt et al., 1988). Compared to the biomedical and bioclinical areas, few empirical studies exist that address the question of how these issues may contribute to the life course of these individuals (Hurtig & White, 1986; Moise, 1986; LePontis, 1986; Nash & Telfair, 1994; Thompson, 1995). It is well known that as the physical aspects of SCD become progressively more manageable, the sociopsychological problems associated with this chronic illness assume greater importance (Abrams et al., 1994; Burlew et al., 2000).

Unfortunately, research on this aspect of SCD has been "scarce and fragmented" (Telfair, 1994). In addition, individuals with SCD have to deal with provider and public lack of knowledge and understanding of their condition, the stereotype of being socially dysfunctional, and the stigmatization of their condition as the "Black disease" (Vavasseur, 1987; Telfair & Nash, 1996). Having a chronic condition such as SCD, while struggling with issues of being an African American or a person of color in this society, compounds the already complex task of day-to-day functioning (Kellerman, 1980; Gibbs, 1990; Nash & Telfair, 1994).

The outcome of this lack of attention has been significant gaps in research and policies designed to understand and improve access and utilization of clinical and supportive services for this population, especially adults and those living in rural areas (Abrams et al., 1994; Hague & Telfair, 2000).

Critical and Emerging Psychological and Social Research Issues

Family Research.   A small but recent body of literature has examined the relationship between children's conditions and their families. The primary focus of these studies has been on the effects of the disease on overall family dynamics that include family social support, coping style, parental self-esteem, kinship network, parental relations, and parent–child relations. Dilworth-Anderson and Slaughter (1986) in their study of the impact of the child with sickle-cell disease on extended family functioning, examined variables of family social support and coping style. Family is the most frequently studied social-ecological variable (Thompson et al., 1999).

Recently Evans et al. (1988), explored how the presence of a child with sickle-cell disease affects parental relations, parent–child relations, and parent's perceptions of the child's behavior. Evans et al. (1988) concluded that the child's illness may cause interpersonal difficulties for the parent, particularly single female-headed households, which the researchers postulate are at risk for family dysfunction. Evans et al. (1988) advocate an aggressive outreach program that includes a parent education support group that emphasizes understanding the cognitive and psychological development of the child, parenting a child with sickle-cell disease, and effective family communication (p. 130). Findings from previous research suggest that family factors such as cohesion (Kliewer & Lewis, 1995), organization and control (Burlew et al., 1989), family support (Wallander et al., 1989), and parent–child relationships may be important social ecological factors for understanding adaptation.

Child and Adolescent Research.   The increased life expectancy due to recent medical advances has heightened the need to understand more fully the psychosocial aspects of living with sickle-cell (Fischoff & Jenkins, 1987; Telfair et al., 1994; Wojciechowski et al., 2002) and the threat to adaptation during childhood and adolescence (Armstrong et al., 1993; LePontois, 1986). Previous researchers have demonstrated that chronic illness in general (Lavigne & Faier-Routman, 1992) and sickle-cell disease in particular (Bennett, 1994; Brown, Doepke, et al., 1993; Brown, Kaslow et al., 1993; Gil et al., 1997; Kliewer & Lewis, 1995; Thompson, 1995; Thompson et al., 1999; Thompson et al., 1993) are risk factors for child and adolescent adaptation. Adaptation is used here in a broad sense to refer to both psychological functioning (e.g., anxiety, depression) and personal adjustment (e.g., behavior problems) (Brown, Doepke, et al., 1993).

Previous findings have been inconsistent regarding whether SCD adolescents differ from peers on these adaptation constructs (Brown, Kaslow, et al., 1993; Iloeje, 1991; Morgan & Jackson, 1986; Siegel et al., 1990; Schoenherr et al., 1992; Treiber et al., 1987; Morgan & Jackson, 1986; Noll et al., 1992). One explanation put forth by Burlew and her colleagues (Burlew et al., 2000) is that children and adolescents with SCD or other chronic illnesses may indeed vary in their psychosocial adaptation to the unpredictability and seriousness of the complications (e.g., intermittent pain crises) and the various treatment issues associated with the condition. In fact, in recent studies using within group designs, researchers have documented this variability in adaptation to sickle-cell (Thompson et al., 1993; Thompson, Gil, Keith et al., 1994). However, studies that include both biomedical and psychosocial factors in the same regression models provide convincing evidence that biomedical factors account for very little of the variability, while psychosocial factors account for considerably more of the variability in adaptation to sickle-cell (Thompson et al., 1993; Thompson et al., 1999) and other chronic illnesses (Bennett, 1994; Lavigne & Faier-Routman, 1992).

Two theoretical models from the stress and coping literature provide a useful framework for conceptualizing the interrelationships of biomedical factors, psychosocial factors, and adaptation. The transactional stress and coping model by Thompson is grounded in ecological-systems theory (Thompson & Gustafson, 1996, p. 143). Variables consistent with this model have been demonstrated to account for 30 to 68 percent of the variance in psychosocial adaptation among children with sickle-cell disease (Thompson et al., 1993). The Disability-Stress-Coping model also includes biomedical factors along with psychosocial resistance factors (Wallander & Varni, 1992; Wallander et al., 1989). Prior literature has applied this model to adaptation among children with sickle-cell disease (Brown, Doepke, et al., 1993) and other chronic illnesses such as diabetes, JRA, and spina bifida (Wallander & Varni, 1992; Wallander et al., 1989). Both theoretical models imply that psychosocial factors might serve as potential protective mechanisms by buffering the impact of the stressor (e.g., medical severity) on adaptation. However, the issue of whether psychosocial resistance factors buffer the relationship between biomedical risk factors and adaptation is largely unexplored among children and adolescents with sickle cell (Thompson, 1995; Telfair & Gardner, 1999).

Transition to Adult Care.   Transition encompasses both medical and life transition. It is defined as the process involved in the movement of adolescents from a focus on pediatric life skills issues to adult life skills issues, for example, from pediatric or child-centered care to adult health-care services. Transition readiness is defined as the specific decisions made, and actions taken, in building capacity by preparing the adolescent and his or her primary medical care provider, parental caretakers/ family, and other social and education services providers to begin, continue, and finish the process of transition. Given the fact that much of the adolescent's life is spent outside of the medical system and the reality of existing adult medical care systems (that of few providers and related services), an expected outcome of a well-planned and implemented transition program is that adolescents/young adults will have the ability and skills to practice effective social and self-care skills and negotiate their care within any medical care system that they enter (Telfair et al., 1994; NHLBI, 2002; Wojciechowski et al., 2002).

Newborn Screening and the Community.   Genetic services related to SCD have been offered to individuals and the communities at risk for several decades. The screening of newborn babies for SCD followed by parental health education, enrollment in comprehensive care programs, penicillin prophylaxis, and antipneumococcal vaccination has been the most significant public health activity conducted in SCD. The main purpose of testing newborns for SCD is to detect those with the disease early so that prophylactic antibiotic treatment and parental education can be started within the first two months of life, early enough to prevent death from severe infections. (Consensus Development Conference, 1987) The success of this program, developed largely through Maternal and Child Health Bureau support, in saving lives has been well established (Shafer et al., 1996).

In addition to detecting those with the disease, the newborn screening program detects thousands of babies with sickle-cell trait and carriers of other hemoglobin variants. An infant with trait provides a genetic window into a family that may be at risk for having a child with SCD. However, in the United States, follow-up of babies with SCD and those with sickle-cell trait or another abnormal hemoglobin trait is an uneven public health service with a wide variation in standards and practices in different states. While most state newborn screening programs have plans for follow-up of babies with disease, almost all of them fall short of the guidelines recommended by the Council of Regional Networks for Genetic Services for the follow-up of babies with sickle-cell trait and other hemoglobin variants (Pass et al., 2000).

Many babies with SCD are never entered into appropriate programs of comprehensive care and do not receive even the minimum standards of care established for infants with SCD. In most of the trait follow-up programs, parents are notified of the results of the carrier baby's abnormal test, but they are left on their own to seek education, testing, and genetic counseling. Most of the parents are never tested or counseled. There is no coordinated program at the national level to encourage and ensure uniformity of standards and services in the newborn trait follow-up programs. Despite guidelines set forth by the Council of Regional Networks for Genetic Services (CORN) (Pass et al., 2000), there are no organized preconception screening and counseling programs for SCD in the country. It is therefore not unusual to find that many mothers of newborns with SCD were unaware of the fact that they could have a child with the disease, even if they had had a previous child with sickle-cell trait. Unfortunately, some state SCD newborn screening programs fall short of these guidelines.

CHALLENGES AND PROMISE OF BIOSOCIAL RESEARCH AND SERVICES

Sickle-cell anemia is a lifelong stressor that influences an individual and his or her family's medical and psychological and social functioning. Currently, management of SCD is directed at prevention, early detection before major irreparable damage is done, and supportive management once damage has occurred. According to the CORN, the urgency of identifying genetic conditions as early as possible is of utmost importance, and a protocol for the newborn screening system must be followed to maximize the quality of life potential for children with special health care needs (Pass et al., 2000).

Biosocial services are divided into four categories: medical, educational, counseling (psychotherapy), and support services. Such services enable the individual (and family) to better manage the physical condition and mediate stressful situations that promote a higher level of coping. It is anticipated that this will facilitate the better adaptation of the individual to his or her chronic condition. Such adaptation allows individuals to define their limitations and to achieve goals they set for themselves. The range and number of services that are required to help the individual and family cope may be multiply dimensional and offered by several different providers (Nash & Telfair, 1994). An overarching problem that needs to be addressed by those serving persons with SCD is the lack of a coordinated, uniformed effort, as well as a lack of data that allows for the documentation and evaluation of the effectiveness of these efforts.

Health-Care Access and Disparities

Compared to all areas of SCD research and practice, issues addressing health and human services outcomes research (e.g., access, utilization and cost-of-care, etc.) have received almost no attention in the published literature (Sprinkle et al., 1994; Hague & Telfair, 2000). In the current atmosphere of medical and health-care reform, this dearth of research has presented a very serious problem for those in the SCD community (clients, families, providers, and researchers). Comprehensive care centers serving persons with SCD (like those with other chronic conditions) are finding themselves ill prepared to address many of the new demands of the rapidly changing system (Blumenthal & Meyer, 1996; Zelman, 1996). A major reason for this is the lack of existing information on (a) nonmedical characteristics of person's with SCD; (b) their knowledge of existing services available through their local and state health care systems; and (c) their care utilization patterns (Hughes & Konrad, 1994; Midence & Elander, 1994). The health reform literature is clear—information on client characteristics and patterns of care utilization is the key to planning, developing, and implementing health-care financing, quality guidelines, and access (how and for whom) decisions (Zelman, 1996).

The reality is that there are too many unknowns specific to health system changes and no mechanisms in place within the sickle-cell community to address or study problems specific to these changes. The latter is especially relevant since persons with SCD are differentially dependent upon publicly supported programs. Lack of attention to these issues has led to differential access and utilization of services, particularly in regard to age and geographic location (Blendon et al., 1989;

Hague & Telfair, 2000; Telfair et al., in press). Thus, for persons with SCD there are many very practical difficulties of implementing a number of the recommended regimens of care that make the promotion of ideal health very problematic in many communities (e.g., in rural or medically under-served communities).

CONSIDERATIONS AND RECOMMENDATIONS FOR ADDRESSING BARRIERS TO BIOSOCIAL CARE FOR PERSONS WITH SICKLE-CELL DISEASE

Barriers to biosocial care of African Americans with chronic conditions have been systematically scrutinized in the past. These barriers can be examined through the dimensions of the individual, institution, and society. Many believe that it is easier to change the personal barrier (meaning client barriers) and institutional barriers (meaning staff and agency policy) than societal barriers.

Minimizing these disparities and the delivery of services require multiple strategies that affect the individual and family, the institution that provides the services, and the societal context in which the population lives. Considerations necessary to deliver services to this population include:

1. Regarding the day-to-day lives of persons with SCD, greater recognition of cultural factors, economic factors, problems of access to services, a generalized suspicion and fear of government controls, and language differences.
2. Regarding newborn screening, there are infants with SCD who do not enter into appropriate programs of comprehensive care and do not receive the requisite interventions (Sprinkle et al., 1994). Further, follow-up of infants who are carriers is suboptimal (Sprinkle et al., 1994). It is thus imperative that carrier notification and counseling be undertaken with sensitivity and accuracy (Newborn Screening Committee, 1994).
3. Regarding provider and patient differences, the provider should make an effort to minimize these differences through:
   a. reexamination of the nature of the relationship between practitioner and patient;
   b. exploration of mutual role expectations;
   c. exploration of the nature of the power in the relationship in terms of gender, class, and racial differences;
   d. development of a capacity to cope with cultural value differences;
   e. development of a capacity to work with patients' perception of services; and
   f. response to the patients' needs, both physical, psychological and social.

CONCLUSION

Sickle-cell anemia is a varied and complicated disorder. Insights into its history, biology, patho-physiology, and treatment serve to emphasize this complexity. Although its origins remain a point of much debate, advances in the detection and treatment of many of its symptoms (NHLBI, 2002) have highlighted the variability of the disease across individuals and groups. Until a cure is found, further research on biomedical and bioclinical aspects of sickle-cell disease and the promotion of effective treatment must be done.

Because of the unique ethnic, religious, and racial makeup of persons with sickle-cell disease it is critical that the influence of cultural issues on health service delivery be a part of any treatment plan and a culturally competent system of care. Individuals with sickle-cell disease as part of a diverse group share a myriad of historical experiences, which commonly bind them together as a unique group within our society. However, many experience varying degrees of complex health disadvantages, which are exacerbated by a combination of poverty, racial bias, ignorance, and a history of barriers to the attainment (access) of adequate, quality medical and health services. It is notable that individuals experience these problems from different economic, class, and interpersonal perspectives. These factors affect the individual's (or their family's) relationship with providers and their adherence to treatment regimens. Therefore, it is important to separate the effects of general societal experiences (e.g., discrimination, classism) and the effects of cultural experiences on the lives of individuals (and families) with sickle-cell disease from diverse backgrounds (Telfair & Nash, 1996).

NOTE

The author would like to express his gratitude to those persons with sickle-cell disease who have unselfishly shared insights into their lives and allowed for work such as this chapter to be written. Thanks are given to professional colleagues who give of themselves to make successful work with this population a reality. Thanks to my wife, Adrena, for her clinical insights, patience, and support. This chapter is dedicated posthumously to Dr. Kermit Nash, who was in the forefront of keeping the biosocial model of sickle-cell disease alive.

REFERENCES

Abrams, M.R., Phillips, G., & Whitworth, E. (1994). Adaptation and Coping: A look at a sickle cell patient population over age 30—An integral phase of the life-long developmental process. In K. Nash, (Ed.). *Psychosocial aspects of sickle cell disease: Past, present and future directions of research* (pp. 141–160). Binghamton, NY: Haworth Press.

American Academy of Pediatrics (AAP) Committee on Genetics, Section on Hematology/Oncology (2002). Health supervision for children with sickle cell disease. *Pediatrics, 109*, 526–535.

Armstrong, F.D., Lemanek, K.L., Pegelow, C.H., Gonzalez, J.C., & Martinez, A. (1993). Impact of lifestyle disruption on parent and child coping, knowledge, and parental discipline in children with sickle cell anemia. *Children's Health Care, 22*, 189–203.

Ballas, S.K. (1994). Neurobiology and treatment of pain. In S.H. Embury, R.P. Hebbel, N. Mohandas, & M.H. Steinberg, eds. *Sickle cell disease: Basic principles and clinical practice* (pp. 745–772). New York: Raven Press.

Barrett, D.H., Wisotzek, I.E. Abel, G.G., Rouleau, J.L. Plait, A.F. Plooand, W.E., & Eckman, J.R. (1988). Assessment of psychosocial functioning of patients with sickle cell disease. *Southern Medical Journal, 81*, 745–750.

Bennett, D.S. (1994). Depression among children with chronic medical problems: A meta-analysis. *Journal of Pediatric Psychology, 19*, 149–169.

Bertrand, D. (2002). Gene therapy may lead to cure for sickle cell patients. *Journal of the National Medical Association, 94*, A9–10.

Billings, F.T. (1989). Treatment of sickle cell anemia with bone marrow transplantation-Pros and cons. *Transactions of the American Clinical and Climatological Association, 10*, 8–20.

Blendon, R.J., Aiken L.H., Freeman H.E., & Corey C.R. (1989). Access to medical care for Black and White Americans: A matter of continuing concern. *Journal of the American Medical Association, 26*, 278–281.

Blumethal, D., & Meyer, G.S. (1996). Academic health centers in a changing environment. *Health Affairs, 15(2)*, 200–215.

Bronfenbrenner, U. (1979). *The ecology of human development: Experiments by nature and design.* Cambridge: Harvard University Press.

Brown, R.T., Doepke, K.J., & Kaslow, N.J. (1993). Risk-Resistance-Adaptation model for pediatric chronic illness: Sickle cell syndrome as an example. *Clinical Psychology Review, 13*, 119–132.

Brown, R., Kaslow, N., Doepke, K., Buchanan, I., Eckman, J., & Baldwin, K. (1993). Psychological and family function in children with sickle cell and their mothers. *Journal of American Academy of Child and Adolescent Psychiatry, 32*, 545–552.

Brunara, C., Goldberg, M.A., Dover, G.J., & Bunn, H.F. (1990). Evaluation of hydroxyurea and erythropoietin therapy in sickle cell disease. Paper presented at the 15th Annual Meeting of the National Sickle Cell Disease Centers, Berkeley, CA.

Burlew, A.K., Evans, R., & Oler, C. (1989). The impact of a child with sickle cell disease on family dynamics. *Annals of New York Academy of Sciences, 565*, 161–171.

Burlew, A.K., Telfair, J., Colangelo, L., & Wright, L. (2000). Factors that influence psychosocial functioning in adolescents with sickle cell disease. *J of Pediatric Psychology, 25*, 287–99.

Castro, O. (1999). Management of sickle cell disease: Recent advances and controversies. *British Journal of Heamatology, 107*, 2–11.

Charache, S., Dover, G.J., Moyer, M.A., & Moore, J.W. (1987). Hydroxyurea-induced augmentation of fetal hemoglobin production in patients with sickle cell anemia. *Blood, 30*, 109–116.

Charache, S. et al. (1995a). Effect of hydroxyurea on the frequency of painful crises in sickle cell disease. *New England Journal of Medicine, 332*, 1317–1322.

Charache, S. et al. (1995b). Design of the multicenter study of hydroxyurea in sickle cell anemia. Investigators of the Multicenter Study of Hydroxyurea. *Control Clinical Trials, 16*, 432–446.

Consensus Development Conference. (1987). Newborn screening for sickle cell disease and other hemoglobinopathies. *Journal of the American Medical Association, 258*, 205–1209.

Davis, H., Schoendorf, K.C., Gergen, P.J., & Moore, R.M., Jr. (1997). National trends in the mortality of children with sickle cell disease, 1968 through 1992. *American Journal of Public Health, 87*, 1317–1322.

Diggs, L.W. (1935). Atrophy of spleen is a late complication. *Journal of the American Medical Association, 104*, 538.

Dillworth-Anderson, P., & Slaughter, D.T. (1986). Sickle cell anemic children and the Black extended family. In A.L. Hurtig & C.T. Viera (Eds.), Sickle cell disease: Psychological and psychosocial issues (pp. 114–130). Urbana and Chicago: University of Illinois Press.

Dover, G.J., Humphries, R.K., Moore, J.G., Young, N.S., Charache, S., & Nienhaus, A.W. (1986). Hydroxyurea induction of hemoglobin F production in sickle cell disease: Relationship between cytoxicity and F cell production. *Blood, 67*, 735.

Durbin, M. (1988). Bone marrow transplantation: Economic, ethical and social issues. *Pediatrics, 82*, 774–783.

Edelstein, S.J. (1986). *The sickled cell: From myth to molecules*. Cambridge: Harvard University Press.

Embury, S.H., Hebbel, R.P., Mohandas, N., & Steinberg, M.H. (Eds.). (1994). *Sickle cell disease: Basic principles and clinical practice*. New York: Raven Press.

Evans, R.C., Burlew, A.K., & Oler, C.H. (1988). Children with sickle cell anemia: Parental relations, parent–child relations and child behavior. *Social Work, 33*, 127–130.

Falletta, J.M., et al. (1995). Discontinuing penicillin prophylaxis in children with sickle cell anemia. Prophylactic Penicillin Study II. *Journal of Pediatrics, 127*, 685–690.

Ferster, A., Vermylen, C., Cornu, G., Buyse, M., Corazza, F., Devalck, C., Fondu, P., Toppet, M., & Sariban, E. (1996). Hydroxyurea for treatment of severe sickle cell anemia: A pediatric clinical trial. *Blood, 88*, 1960–1964.

Fischoff, J., & Jenkins, D.S. (1987). Sickle cell anemia. In E. Noshipts (Ed.), *Basic handbook of child psychiatry* (pp. 97–102). New York: Basic Books.

Garbarino, J. (1985). Human ecology and competence in adolescence. In J. Garbarino (Ed.), *Adolescent development: An ecological perspective* (Chapter 2). Columbus: Charles E. Merrill.

Gaston, M.H. (1987). Sickle cell disease: An overview. *Seminars in Roentgenology, 22*, 150–159.

Germain, C. (1979). *Social work practice: People and environment*. New York: Columbia University Press.

Gibbs, J.T. (1990). Developing intervention models for Black families: Linking theory and research. In H.E. Cheatham and J.B. Stewart (Eds.), *Black families: Interdisciplinary perspectives* (pp. 325–351). New Brunswick, NJ: Transaction.

Gil, K.M., Wilson, J.J., & Edens, J.L. (1997). The stability of pain coping strategies in young children, adolescents, and adults with sickle cell disease over an 18-month period. *The Clinical Journal of Pain, 13*, 110–115.

Hague, A., & Telfair, J. (2000). Socioeconomic distress and health status: The Urban-Rural dichotomy of services utilization for people with sickle cell disorders in North Carolina. *Journal of Rural Health, 16*, 43–55.

Hoppe, C.C., & Walters, M.C. (2001). Bone marrow transplantation in sickle cell anemia. *Current Opinion in Oncology, 13*, 85–90.

Hughes, M., & Konrad T.R. (1994). Epilogue. In K.B. Nash (Ed.), *Psychosocial aspects of sickle cell disease: Past, present and future directions of research*. New York: Haworth Press.

Hurtig, A.L. (1986). The invisible chronic illness in adolescence. In A.L. Hurtig & C.T. Viera (Eds.), *Sickle cell disease: Psychological and psychosocial issues* (pp. 42–61). Urbana and Chicago: University of Illinois Press.

Hurtig, A.L., & White, L.S. (1986). Psychological adjustment in children and adolescents with sickle cell disease. *Journal of Pediatric Psychology, 11*, 411–427.

Iloeje, S.O. (1991). Psychiatric morbidity among children with sickle cell disease. *Developmental Medicine and Child Neurology, 11*, 1087–1094.

Ingram, V.M. (1956). A special chemical difference between globin of normal human and sickle cell anemia hemoglobin. *Nature, 178*, 792–794.

Johnson, F.L., Look, A.T., Gockerman, J. Ruggiero, M.R., Dalla-Pozza, L., & Billings, F.T. (1984). Bone-marrow transplantation in a patient with sickle cell anemia. *New England Journal of Medicine, 311*, 780–783.

Kellerman, J. (1980). Psychological effects of illness in adolescence. I. Anxiety, self-esteem, and perception of control. *Journal of Pediatrics, 97*, 126–131.

Kliewer, W., & Lewis, H. (1995). Family influences on coping processes in children and adolescents with sickle cell disease. *Journal of Pediatric Psychology, 20*, 511–525.

Kodish, E., Lantos, J., Siegler, M., Kohrman, A., & Johnson, F.L. (1990). Bone marrow transplantation in sickle cell disease: The trade-off between early mortality and quality of life. *Clinical Research, 38*, 694–700.

Kodish, E., Lantos, J., Stocking, C., Singer, P.A., Siegler, M., & Johnson, F.L. (1991). Bone marrow transplantation for sickle cell disease: A study of parents' decisions. *New England Journal of Medicine, 325*, 1349–1353.

Koshy, M., Burd, L., Wallace, Moawad, & Baron, J. (1988). Prophylactic red cell transfusions in pregnant patients with sickle cell disease: A randomized cooperative study. *New England Journal of Medicine, 319*, 1447–1152.

Lavigne, J.V., & Faier-Routman, J. (1992). Psychological adjustment to pediatric physical disorders: A meta-analytic review. *J. of Pediatric Psychology, 17*, 133–157.

Leavell, S.R., & Ford, C.V. (1983). Psychopathology in patients with sickle cell disease. *Psychosomatics, 24*, 23–25, 28–29, 32, 37.

Lemanek, K.L., Moore, S., Gresham, F., Williamson, D., & Kelly, H. (1986). Psychological adjustment of children with sickle cell anemia. *Journal of Pediatric Psychology, 11*, 397–410.

LePontois, J. (1986). Adolescents with Sickle cell anemia: Developmental issues. A.L. in Hurtig and C.T. Viera (Eds.), *Sickle cell disease: Psychological and psychosocial issues*, (pp. 75–83). Urbana and Chicago: University of Illinois Press.

Lubin, B., & Vichinsky, E. (1991). Sickle cell disease. In R. Hoffman, E.J. Benz, S.J. Shattil, B. Furie, & H.J. Cohen (Eds.), *Hematology: Basic Principles and Practice* (pp. 450–471). New York: Churchill Living stone.

Lucarelli, G., Galimberti, M., Polchi, P., Angelucci, E., Baronciani, D., Giardini, C., Politi, P., Durazzi, S.M., Muretto, P., & Albertini, F. (1990). Bone marrow transplantation in patients with thalassemia. *New England Journal of Medicine, 322*, 417–421.

Midence, K., & Elander, J. (1994). *Sickle cell disease: A psychosocial approach.* New York: Radcliffe Medical Press.

Miller, D.M., Winslow, R.M., Klein, H.G., Wilson, K.C., Brown, F.L., & Statham, N.J. (1980). Improved exercise performance after exchange transfusion in subjects with sickle cell anemia. *Blood, 56*, 1127–1131.

Moise, J.R. (1986). Toward a model of competence and coping. In A.L. Hurtig & C.T. Viera (Eds.), *Sickle cell disease: Psychological and psychosocial issues* (pp. 7–23). Urbana and Chicago: University of Illinois Press.

Morgan, S.R., & Jackson, J. (1986). Psychological and social concomitants of sickle cell anemia in adolescents. *Journal of Pediatric Psychology, 11*, 429–440.

Nash, K.B. (1986). Ethnicity, race and the health care delivery system. In A.L. Hurtig & C.T. Viera (Eds.), *Sickle cell disease: Psychological and psychosocial issues* (pp. 131–146). Urbana and Chicago: University of Illinois Press.

Nash, K.B. (1992). Diagnosis and management of psychosocial problems in the sickle cell patient and family. In V.N. Mankad & R.B. More (Eds.), *Sickle cell disease* (pp. 389–402). Westport, CT: Praeger.

Nash, K.B., & Telfair, J. (1994). Sickle cell disease: A biopsychosocial model. In I. Livingston (Ed.), *Handbook of Black American health: The mosaic of conditions, issues, policies, and prospects* (pp. 123–139). Westport, CT: Greenwood Publishing Group.

Newborn Screening for Sickle Cell Disease and Other Hemoglobinopathies. National Institutes of Health Consensus Development Conference Statement. *Journal of the American Medical Association, 258*, 1205–1209.

Newborn Screening Committee. (July 1994). *The Council of Regional Networks for Genetic Services (CORN), National Newborn Screening Report—1991*. New York: CORN.

NHLBI. (2002). *The management of sickle cell disease*. Division of Blood Disease and Resources, National Heart, Lung and Blood Institute, National Institutes of Health. NIH Publication, No. 02-2117.

Noguchi, C.T. (1988). Levels of fetal hemoglobin necessary for effective therapy of sickle cell disease. *New England Journal of Medicine, 318*, 96–99.

Noll, R., Bukowski, W., Davies, W.H., Koontz, K., & Ris, D. (1992). Social interactions between children with cancer or sickle cell disease and their peers: Teacher rating. *Developmental and Behavioral Pediatrics, 13*, 187–193.

Ohene-Frempong, K., & Smith-Whitney, K. (1997). Use of hydroxyurea in children with sickle cell disease: what comes next? *Seminars in Hematology, 34(Suppl 3)*, 30–41.

Pass, K.A., et al. (2000). U.S. newborn screening system guidelines II: Follow-up of children, diagnosis, management, and evaluation. Statement of the Council of Regional Networks for Genetic Services (CORN). *J. of Pediatric, 137*, S1–S345.

Pauling, L., Itano, H., Singer, S.J., & Wells, I. (1949). Sickle cell anemia, A molecular disease. *Science, 110*, 543–548.

Perrine, S.P., Miller, B.A., Cohen, L., Vichinsky, E.P., Hurst, D., & Lubin, B. (1989). Sodium butyrate enhances fetal hemoglobin gene expression in erythroid progenitors of patients with HbSS and beta thalassemia. *Blood, 74*, 454.

Platt, O.S., Brambilla, D.J., Rosse, W.F., Milner, P.F., Castro, O., Steinburg, M.H., Klug, P.P. (1994). Mortality in sickle cell disease: Life expectancy and risk factors for early death. *New England Journal of Medicine, 330*, 1639–1644.

Rodgers, G.P. (1990). Hydroxyurea therapy in sickle cell disease: An update on the NIH experience. Paper presented at the 15th Annual Meeting of National Sickle Cell Disease Centers, Berkeley, CA.

Ryan, T.M., Townes, T.M., Reilly, M.P., Asakurat, T., Palmiter, R.D. Bfinsted, R.L., & Behringer, R.R. (1990). Human sickle hemoglobin in transgenic mice. *Science, 247*, 566.

Schecther, A.N., Noguchi, C.T., & Rodgers, G.P. (1987). Sickle cell anemia. In G. Stamatoyannopoulos, A.W. Nienhaus, P. Leder, & P.W. Majerus (Eds.), *Molecular basis of blood diseases* (pp. 179–218). Philadelphia: W.B. Saunders Co.

Schoenherr, S., Brown, R., Baldwin, K., & Kaslow, N. (1992). Attributional styles and psychopathology in pediatric chronic illness groups. *Journal of Clinical Child Psychology, 21*, 380–387.

Schwartz, G.E. (1982). Testing the biosocial model: The ultimate challenge facing behavioral medicine. *Journal of Consulting and Clinical Psychology, 50*, 1040–1053.

Scott, R.B. (1983). Sickle cell anemia: Problems in education and mass screening. In H. Abramson et al., (Eds.), *Sickle cell disease: Diagnosis, management, education and research* (pp. 285–292). St. Louis: C.V. Mosby Company.

Serjeant, G.R. (1992). *Sickle cell disease*, 2nd ed. Oxford: Oxford University Press.

Serjeant, G.R. (2001). Historical Review: The emerging understanding of sickle cell disease. *British Journal of Heamatology, 112*, 3–18.

Shafer, F.E., Lorey, F., Cunningham, G.C., Klumpp, C., Vichinsky, E., & Lubin, B. (1996). Newborn screening for sickle cell disease: 4 years of experience from California's newborn screening program. *Journal of Pediatric Hematology/Oncology 8*, 36–41.

Sickle Cell Disease Guideline Panel. (1993). *Sickle cell disease screening: Management and counseling in newborns and infants. Clinical practice guideline No. 6*. AHCRP Pub. No. 93-0562. Rockville, MD:

Agency for Health Care Policy and Research, Public Health Service, U.S. Department of Health and Human Services.

Siegel, W., Golden, N., Gough, J., Lashley, M., & Secker, I. (1990). Depression, self-esteem, and life events in adolescents with chronic diseases. *Journal of Adolescent Health Care, 11*, 501–504.

Sprinkle, R.H., Hynes, D.M., & Konrad, T.R. (1994). Is universal neonatal Hemoglobinopathy screening cost-effective? *Archives of Pediatric and Adolescent Medicine, 148*: 461–469.

Steinberg, M.H. (1999). Management of sickle cell disease. *New England Journal of Medicine, 340(13)*, 1021–1030.

Steinberg M.H., Lu, Z.H., Barton, F.B., Terrin, M.L., Charache S., & Dover G.J. (1997). Fetal hemoglobin in sickle cell anemia: Determinants of response to hydroxyurea. *Blood, 89*, 1078–1088.

Stevens, P.E., & Pletsch, P.K. (2002). Ethical issues of informed consent: Mothers' experiences enrolling their children in bone marrow transplantation research. *Cancer Nursing, 25*, 81–87.

Styles, L.A., & Vichinsky, E.P. (1997). New therapies and approaches to transfusion in sickle cell disease in children. *Current Opinion in Pediatrics, 9*, 41–46.

Telfair, J. (1994). Factors in the long-term adjustment of children and adolescents with sickle cell disease. *Journal of Health and Social Policy, 5*, 69–96.

Telfair, J., & Gardner, M. (1999). African American adolescents with sickle cell disease: Support groups and psychological well-being. *J of Black Psychology, 25*, 378–390.

Telfair, J., Hague, A., Etienne, M., Tang, S., & Strasser, S. (in press). Urban and rural differences of access to and utilization of services among persons with sickle cell disease in Alabama. *Public Health Reports, 118*.

Telfair, J., Myers, J., & Drezner, S. (1994). Transfer as a component of the transition of adolescents with sickle cell disease to adult care: Adolescent, adult and parent perspectives. *Journal of Adolescent Health, 15(11)*, 558–565.

Telfair, J., & Nash, K.B. (1996). African American culture. In N.L. Fisher (Ed.), *Cultural and ethnic diversity: A guide for genetic professionals* (pp. 36–59). Baltimore, MD: Johns Hopkins University Press.

Thompson, R.J. Jr. (1995). Commentary: Sickle cell disease. *Journal of Pediatric Psychology, 20*, 403–406.

Thompson, R.J. Jr., Armstrong, F.D., Kronenberger, W.G., Scott, D., McCabe, M.A., Smith, B., Radcliffe, J., Colangelo, L., Gallagher, D., Islam, S., & Wright, E. (1999). Family functioning, neurocognitive functioning, and behavior problems in children with sickle cell disease. *Journal of Pediatric Psychology, 4*, 491–498.

Thompson, R.J., Jr., Gil, K.M., Burbach, D.J., Keith, B.R., & Kinney, T.R. (1993). Role of child and maternal processes in the psychological adjustment of children with sickle cell disease. *Journal of Consulting and Clinical Psychology, 61*, 468–474.

Thompson, R.J., Jr., Gil, K.M., Keith, B.R., Gustafson, K.E., George, L.K., & Kinney, T.R. (1994). Psychological adjustment of children with sickle cell disease: Stability and change over a 10-month period. *Journal of Consulting and Clinical Psychology, 62*, 856–860.

Thompson, R.J., Jr., & Gustafson, K.E. (1996). *Adaptation to chronic childhood illness*. Washington, DC: American Psychological Association.

Treiber, F., Mabe, A., & Wilson, G. (1987). Psychological adjustment of sickle cell children and their siblings. *Children's Health Care, 16*, 82–88.

Van Raamsdonk, J. (2002). Treatment of sickle cell disease with anti-sickling gene therapy. *Clinical Genetics, 61*, 258–259.

Vaughan, W.P., Purtilo, R.B., Butler, B.B.A., & Armitage, J.O. (1986). Ethical and financial issues in autologous marrow transplantation: A symposium sponsored by the University of Nebraska Medical Center. *Annals of Internal Medicine, 105*, 134–135.

Vavasseur, J.W. (1987). Psychosocial aspects of chronic disease: Cultural and ethnic implications. *Birth Defects, 23*, 144–153.

Vermylen, C., Ninane, J., Robles, E.F., & Cornu, G. (1988). Bone marrow transplantation in five children with sickle cell anemia. *Lancet, 1(8600)*, 1427–1428.

Vichinsky, E.P. (1992). Personal communication, June.

Vichinsky E.P., Haberkern C.M., Neumayr L., Earles A.N., Black D., Koshy M., Pegelow, C., Abboud, M., Ohene-Frempong, K., & Iyer, R.V. (1995). A comparison of conservative and aggressive transfusion regimens the preoperative management of sickle cell disease. *New England Journal of Medicine, 333*, 206–213.

Wagner, G.M., & Vichinsky, E.P. (1989). Sickling syndromes and unstable hemoglobin diseases. In W.C. Mentzer & G.M. Wagner (Eds.), *The hereditary hemolytic anemias* (Chapter 4). New York: Churchill Livingstone.

Wallander, J.L., & Varni, J.W. (1992). Adjustment in children with chronic physical disorders, programmatic research on a disability-stress-coping model. In A.M. LaGreca, L. Siegel, J. Wallander, & C. Walker (Eds.), *Stress and coping with pediatric conditions* (pp. 279–298). New York: Guilford Press.

Wallander, J.L., Varni, J., Babani, L. Banis, H.T., Varni, J.W., & Wilcox, K.T. (1989). Family resources as resistance factors for psychological maladjustment in chronically ill and handicapped children. *Journal of Pediatric Psychology, 14*, 157–173.

Walters, M.C., et al. (2000). Impact of bone marrow transplantation for symptomatic sickle cell disease: An interim report. Multicenter investigation of bone marrow transplantation for sickle cell disease. *Blood, 95*, 1918–1924.

Wang, W.C., et al. (2002). Effect of hydroxyurea on growth in children with sickle cell anemia: Results of the HUG-KIDS Study. *Journal of Pediatrics, 140*, 225–229.

Werthiem, E.S. (1975). Person-environment interaction: The epigenesis of autonomy and competence. 1. Theoretical considerations (normal development). *British Journal of Medical Psychology, 48*, 1–8.

Whitten, C.F., & Nisihura, E.N. (1985). Sickle cell anemia. In N. Hobbs & J.M. Perrin (Eds.), *Issues in the care of children with chronic illnesses* (pp. 236–260). London: Jossey-Bass.

Williams, T.E. (1984). Legal issues and ethical dilemmas surrounding bone marrow transplantation in children. *American Journal of Pediatric Hematology/Oncology, 6*, 83–88.

Wojciechowski, E.A., Hurtig, A., & Dorn, L. (2002). A natural history study of adolescents and young adults with sickle cell disease as they transfer to adult care: A need for case management services. *Journal of Pediatric Nursing, 17*, 18–27.

Zelman, W.A. (1996). *The changing health care marketplace*. San Francisco: Jossey-Bass.

CHAPTER 10

Ophthalmic Disease in Blacks: Prospects for Eliminating Racial and Ethnic Disparities in Health in the Public Health Context

SHAFFDEEN A. AMUWO, MAURICE F. RABB, AND
ROBERT G. FABIAN

INTRODUCTION

In this chapter we discuss some of the major causes of visual impairment and blindness in Blacks from a public health perspective. These are sickle-cell disease, HIV/AIDS, diabetes, glaucoma, and cataract. As pointed out by McLeod and Rabb (1994), the leading causes of blindness among Blacks are treatable, whereas with Whites, untreatable age-related macular degeneration is the principal cause. Thus, in the case of Blacks, it is especially important that timely treatment be available. Only access to quality vision health services and correct diagnosis can make this possible, however, which generally means consultation with a primary-care physician followed by referral to an ophthalmologist. Equally important is the availability of services that could prevent or ameliorate the impact of blindness and visual impairment. Recent work by Bazargan et al. on "the recency of eye examination suggests that the amount of preventive care in place may not be adequate" (1998, p. 91).

Blacks live primarily in medically underserved areas. Additionally, it is often the case that cultural and social differences create barriers between medical professionals and the minority populations they serve (Freid, Praeger, & Xia, 2003; Smedley, Stith, & Nelson, 2002). These differences add a public health dimension to the problem of caring for the eye health of Blacks and other minorities, as it does for minority health concerns in general. The key to breaking down barriers between health-care providers and the Black community resides in developing community structures that they trust as serving these interests and that foster knowledge of health problems that will permit care providers to serve them effectively.

The Healthy People 2010, a prevention agenda for the United States, following its predecessors such as Healthy People in 1979 and Healthy People 2000 in 1980, provides a framework of support for access to quality vision services. It recognizes vision as one of the 28 focus areas with a specific target to be achieved nationally by 2010 (USDHHS, 2000a). Starting in 1979 from national goals for reducing premature deaths and preserving independence for older Americans and prescribing 226 targeted health objectives for the nation to achieve within ten years, and culminating in 2000 with over-arching goals of increasing quality and years of healthy life and eliminating health disparities, these documents are a framework for the pursuit of quality of life for all Americans. They further emphasize that the quality of eye vision for Blacks would definitely contribute to the elimination of health disparities.

Vision impairment is defined as "having 20/40 or worse vision in the better eye even with eye glasses" (USDHHS, 2002, p. 3). Blindness, on the other hand, is "typically defined as visual acuity with best corrections in the better eye worse than or equal to 20/200 or a visual field extent of less than 20 degrees in diameter" (USDHHS, 2002, p. 3). Both vision impairment and blindness represent a significant morbidity and economic burden in the United States affecting approximately 3.4 million of the U.S. population age 40 and over, a significant proportion of whom are Blacks, who are more affected than Whites (USDHHS, 2002).

Focus of the Chapter

This chapter is written from a public health perspective, which we intend to be complementary to the ophthalmology chapter by McLeod and Rabb in the 1994 edition of this text. Thus, we stress "issues and policies" more than "conditions" referred to in the subtitle of the 1994 edition. We have followed a different organization from the previous chapter in order to highlight the behavioral and other public health issues involved in eye health among African Americans.

SICKLE-CELL DISEASE

The Epidemiology of Sickle-Cell Disease and Related Outcomes

Approximately one of ten African Americans is a carrier of sickle-cell trait; about one in 400 is affected. Global mortality for sickle-cell disease is estimated to be 800,000 annually. This is generally caused by infections and secondary complications (Amuwo, 2002). In this country, sickle-cell disease affects about 72,000 persons, mostly of African descent. About two million Americans, or one in 12 African Americans, carry sickle-cell trait (USDHHS, 1996). Only those who inherit the trait from both parents have the likelihood of becoming ill and experience some other problems (as described in Chapter 9 of this book); others, however, can pass the trait on to their offspring. Sickle-cell disease is, symptomatically, very complex. These symptoms, in addition to visual impairment and possible eventual blindness, "include chronic anemia [and accompanying fatigue], acute chest syndrome, stroke, splenic and renal dysfunction, pain crises and susceptibility to bacterial infections, particularly in children" (Ashley-Koch et al., 1998, p. 2). Delayed growth and puberty in children and slight build in adults also occurs (USDHHS, 1996).

Living with Sickle-Cell Disease

"There appears to be age variations due to genders in sickle cell disease. For instance, males between the ages of 15 and 24 years and females between the ages of 20 and 39 years are mostly affected. However, regardless of age, the greatest risk is between 25 and 39 years for both sexes" (Fox et al., 1990). As for central visual loss, it occurs in approximately 12 percent of eyes with PSR (Condon & Serjeant, 1980). Several studies have shown that in a non-U.S. population, 50 percent of patients with sickle-cell disease had PSR, 18 percent had vitreous hemmorhage, and 8 percent had gone on to retinal detachment. Four percent of the total population had a blind eye, which included 6 percent of the sickle-cell population (Van Meurs, 1991; McLeod & Raab, 1994, pp. 149–150).

The disease is difficult to live with; it is painful, "characterized by chronic anemia and periodic episodes of pain" (USDHHS, 1996), and it is deadly. With good health habits and good health care, "in the past 30 years, the life expectancy of people with sickle cell anemia has increased. Many patients with sickle cell anemia now live into their mid- forties and beyond" (USDHHS, 1996). For many people, it requires major life adjustments simply to face the possibility of these realities, a necessary prelude to doing the screening, which is only the first step. Fully responsible life choices, such as the marriage decision, can be influenced by the knowledge gained by the first step that one must take to combat sickle-cell disease.

Prevention Efforts Associated with Sickle-Cell Disease

Early-life recognition is particularly important. It requires that parents respond to early-life complications caused by sickle-cell disease, and this is often difficult in medically underserved areas, where many of the most susceptible live.

Because of the complexity of the sickle-cell symptoms, prevention and treatment of eye symptoms cannot be considered in isolation; carriers of sickle-cell trait must be prepared to deal with a multifaceted problem. Indeed, from a public health perspective, encouraging members of susceptible communities to test for presence of sickle-cell trait is itself a major task. Many people are likely to have conflicting feelings about acquiring knowledge that they carry the trait or must face the prospect of becoming sick from the disease. Special efforts must be made to reach them. Testing infants for sickle-cell disease is particularly important. Most states are now doing this in response to a law passed by congress in 1972 (Ashley-Koch et al., 1998) and subsequent laws that provide for states to now conduct neonatal testing for the presence of sickle-cell hemoglobinopathy. Survival rates among one- to three-year olds have improved in recent years, in large part because of screening programs and attention to other psychological issues brought upon by the sickle-cell disease.

That eye health among the African American population is significantly affected by sickle-cell disease underscores the fact that the eye health problem is a very complicated one. The solution to this eye-health problem is found in a community that has the institutions and well-trained and culturally sensitive personnel who enjoy the confidence of the people living in the community. Such a community can accomplish essential eye-care needs: (a) the development of a screening infrastructure technically capable of flagging the almost certain need for eye care among every at-risk member of the population; (b) the development of ophthalmic interventions, which, if applied within minutes to hours after the onset of symptoms, would prevent blindness from occurring (c) the provision of special care within 2 to 48 hours of symptoms that can prevent loss of vision from hemorrhage and /or retinal attachment (Harlan & Goldberg, 1996); (d) the ongoing development of medicines and medical and surgical techniques; (e) possibly even the discovery of a cure for the disease in this age of molecular and genetic medicine. All of these advances are moving forward day by day as a result of scientific and technological progress. But blindness from central retinal artery occlusion is taking place today in neighborhoods almost in the shadow of the buildings—for example, research institutions and hospitals—that house the knowledge and tools to defeat the malady.

The health economist Victor Fuchs (1998) said that differences in health levels among populations are not importantly related to differences in medical care. Rather, "other socioeconomic and cultural variables are now much more important than differences in the quantity and quality of medical care" (Fuchs, 1998, p. 16). The other socioeconomic and cultural variables pertain to the networks of community groups and organizations that can reach people with eye illness, who can place the problem in its larger medial context, and motivate them to make the life-altering choices necessary to make the best of their life situation. This requires professional people who can instill a great deal of confidence and trust. As Fuchs observed in his 1998 book, the extension of responsibility for achieving health care to a broader group of health care professionals, including those in public health, is perhaps the most important change that he has observed since his book was first published in

1974. Scientific progress in medicine is a seamless worldwide accomplishment. Delivery of medical services is a problem that is essentially local in nature and most challenging when professional personnel must reach people with cultural backgrounds not well represented in the professional community.

Workable Community Education Programs

A community education project supported by the National Heart, Lung and Blood Institute devoted to sickle-cell anemia in Chicago illustrates the kind of community-oriented program that can make the care of eye and other sickle-cell disorders more effective. It was a 16-month-long education program involving of 4,232 individuals from 253 culturally and socially heterogeneous community groups throughout Chicago. The program contributed basic medical knowledge of the blood disorder and symptoms caused by the illness, and it contributed knowledge of popular misconceptions about the disease that can contribute to stigmatization of persons who carry the trait or suffer from the disease. The program assisted people in adjusting their lives to their conditions and in making decisions about dealing with their conditions in a positive manner (Amuwo & Jenkins, 2001).

Treatment of eye disease fits in this overall community framework. There is no escaping the necessity of viewing sickle-cell-related eye health and care from a community perspective. This is especially true when the community is medically underserved and, consequently, lacking the basic knowledge and resources to make fundamental life decisions and to respond to crises that may require care within hours to ward off grave consequences.

HIV/AIDS

The Epidemiology of HIV/AIDS

The global estimates of HIV/AIDS, especially among predominantly Black African countries and sub-Saharan Africa, are alarming. The World Health Organization (2002) estimated that over 40 million people worldwide are living with HIV/AIDS in 2001; over 38.1 million are from sub-Saharan Africa, and close to one million in North America, a substantial number of whom are Black (WHO Reports, 2002).

In the United States, about 690,000 cases of AIDS had been reported to CDC by the end of 1998, although substantial declines in U.S. AIDS incidence and deaths have been reported in recent years (HIV/AIDS Statistics, 1999a). While incidence numbers have been declining overall, nevertheless the Black experience has been worsening. Between 1993 and 1998, the percentage of AIDS in Whites was down from 60 percent to 33 percent, while in Blacks the percentage was up from 25 percent to 45 percent. Hispanic incidence has stayed about the same at 20 percent (McLeod & Rabb, 1994). According to a recent conference at the Harvard AIDS Institute, more than 50 percent of AIDS cases will be among Blacks by the turn of the century (HIV/AIDS Continues to Decimate African-Americans, 1998), even though Blacks constitute about 13 percent of the population. People with AIDS per 100,000 population break down as follows: Whites 18, Blacks 125, Hispanics 58; among women the numbers are Whites 2, Blacks 50, Hispanics 17. AIDS is the fifth leading cause of death in the United States among people aged 25 to 44; among women in this age group, AIDS is the third leading cause of death, and among Black women it is the leading cause of death (Women's Interagency HIV Study, n.d.). Thus, while AIDS is coming under greater control overall in the United States, it is becoming an increasingly serious problem among Blacks, particularly women. To this extent, HIV/AIDS is one of the six focus areas of the U.S. Department of Health and Human Services' initiative to eliminate racial and ethnic disparities in health (USDHHS, 2000b).

HIV/AIDS and Related Eye Disease

Sight-threatening disease cytomegalovirus (CMV) retinitis is associated with late-stage AIDS (Lee, 2001). Yet AIDS-related eye illness has not always been given due attention. "For most public health authorities, particularly in developing countries, the fact that the . . . HIV affects the eye is simply a curiosity" (Courtright, 1996, p. 496). The epidemiology of the ocular manifestations of AIDS is not well understood. Furthermore, it differs between developed and underdeveloped countries (Courtright, 1996).

CMV retinitis, if left untreated, can cause retinal detachment and blindness within two to six months. CMV retinitis has occurred in about one-fourth of active-AIDS patients (Lee, 2001). All patients with HIV should be screened for CMV retinitis (Gallemore & Boyer, 2001). "A person newly diagnosed with CMV retinitis can expect to visit the specialist every two to four weeks" (Lee, 2001, p. 2). The patient should do a vision check each day (Lee, 2001).

Treatments of the various eye illnesses related to AIDS are available. For example, impaired vision can be remedied, and blindness can be avoided. However, careful monitoring of the patient's health status, by both patient and doctor, is essential.

There are four essential elements to maintaining eye health among AIDS patients: (1) availability of adequate personnel and facilities; (2) knowledge about the disease that is required of patient and provider; (3) confidence on the part of patients that providers have their best interest at heart. The first three elements are often lacking, as we observed in our discussion of sickle-cell disease. The fourth element, also essential in the battery of weapons against sickle-cell disease, is equally important in combating AIDS-related eye illness: (4) the need on the part of the patient, or potential patient, to have a strong altruistic regard for the well-being of persons, and potential persons, close to the patient. This element also can be lacking in some patients, though certainly not all.

We note initially that adequate care for eye health among Blacks is often coextensive with prevention and care for diseases that have serious consequences other than eye disease. Thus, when we speak about combating eye diseases originating in sickle-cell disease, HIV/AIDS, and diabetes, we unavoidably must talk about prevention of the underlying disease itself as much as specific measures required for caring for eye health. A discussion follows briefly about each of these elements.

Availability of Adequate Resources.   Concerning the first element needed for eye care—availability of adequate resources—once again, we face the fact that many African Americans live in underserved areas. There is a shortage of resources where demand for those resources is growing the most rapidly. Nationally, Blacks are underrepresented in all health professions. The situation is especially worse when it comes to specialized areas of medicine such as ophthalmology. Even among nurses and other ancillary health services professions, shortages are becoming endemic. While there is dearth of literature, a recent Harvard School of Public Health and Vanderbilt School of Nursing analysis of discharged records of more than six million patients at 799 hospitals in 11 states in 1997 documents a correlation between nursing shortage and patient illness (Grady, 2002). Certainly, morbidity due to eye problems, even if it is secondary to the underlying illness, such as HIV/AIDS, makes the elimination of health disparity an additional challenge if access is very limited. Adequate community resources mean more than well-equipped clinics and highly skilled nurses and ophthalmologists, however. It also means a community infrastructure of people who can convey knowledge and a concomitant sense of optimism that applying that knowledge can work. This is often called empowerment. Various public health professionals with skills and connections at the community and individual levels can contribute to this vital link.

Knowledge about the Disease.   Knowledge about the disease, the second element, is essential because the patient must be competent to recognize symptoms and the necessity of timely response. Floaters, flashing lights, or blurred vision, for example, could signal onset of CMV retinitis and requires immediate medical attention. A solid knowledge about eye disease could mean the difference between successful medical intervention and rationalized fearful procrastination with disastrous consequences.

Eye illness, we have noted, is only one of a number of manifestations of the chronic diseases being considering in this chapter. While it might seem artificial to single out eye illness in considering these diseases, nevertheless, it is quite possible that eye illness could be focal among some people who are making behavioral decisions about health that are likely to affect others. Each of these diseases has numerous dreaded consequences. Different consequences are likely to have different cognitive effects among people. Blindness might well capture the imagination of some people more than other disease consequences, even to the point of being approximately on par with death. Therefore, it is important that people know that serious eye illness is one of the consequences of many diseases that have many dreaded consequences. Some people are likely to respond with positive behavior to mental promptings about blindness that other dreaded consequences don't elicit.

Needed Confidence.   Confidence in health-care providers is the third element. What has already been said about community and interpersonal skills describes part of what goes into confidence building. Adequate levels of confidence, however, will not be established in a Black community without the adequate presence of Black health-care professionals.

Patrick Allen, a microbiologist at the University of Colorado, says that "fear and suspicion in the Black community of the biomedical establishment is a major health problem that reaches beyond these diseases, such as hypertension, sickle-cell anemia, certain types of cancer and AIDS. What we really need is a massive cultural shift to take place for such changes to occur [raised health consciousness in the Black community]" (Scott, n.d., p. 3). Allen is often asked by young Black people if the AIDS virus was developed to rid the world of African Americans. He says he used to dismiss the idea out of hand, but this response turned his audience against him. Now he hedges his answer, saying he doubts it and believes the epidemic could hardly have happened that way.

The need for confidence among community members in the professions that serve them has long been recognized, and medical schools and schools of public health have programs to attract Blacks and other minorities into the health professions. Those students tend to return to underserved areas populated by their own ethnic groups (Cantor et al., 1996).

Altruistic Concerns.   We identified altruistic concern for others as a fourth element essential to combating eye illness caused by diseases that are transmitted from one person to another. Among the diseases considered in this chapter, altruistic concern is most important in combating sickle-cell disease and HIV/AIDS. Because there is, as yet, no vaccine for HIV/AIDS, preventing the spread of the disease is a behavioral matter. Different lifestyles generate different degrees of likelihood that a person is infected or not or is likely to become infected. These different degrees of disease risk, in turn, generate different kinds of behavior; some persons are more likely to avoid risky behavior than others. Some feel they have nothing to lose; others have serious concerns about protecting themselves and/or others (Philipson & Posner, 1993). Health professionals can help individuals protect themselves against self-centered, high-risk sex or drug-use partners. They can help altruistic persons, whether at high or low risk of infection, adapt behavior that can protect others for whom they care against risk of infection. Eye disease is an important consequence of infection. Greater awareness that prompts attention to symptoms is beneficial and can therefore protect the eye health of persons in a community and also help protect the community from the much more wide-ranging consequences of HIV infection.

DIABETES

The Epidemiology of Diabetes

The worldwide distribution of diabetes is extensive and affects, among others, populations in Africa and Latin America. In the Unites States, diabetes is the seventh leading cause of death. It is a very serious public health problem affecting approximately 16 million adults and children. According to the Centers for Disease Control and Prevention (CDC) estimates, 10.3 million Americans have diagnosed diabetes, while an additional 5.4 million have undiagnosed diabetes (USDHHS, 2002). The U.S. Department of Health and Human Services (2000b) has estimated its economic burden in the United States to be over $100 billion. Among Blacks, the prevalence of diabetes is approximately 70 percent higher than Whites, while among Hispanics, it is nearly double that of Whites (USDHHS, 2000b).

"Diabetes Mellitus is a chronic, sometimes severe disease of sugar metabolism. A major long-term complication is damage to small and large blood vessels throughout the body, leading to premature atherosclerosis, heart attack, stroke, and kidney failure and eye disease" (Diseases of the Eye, n.d., p. 38). Insulin deficiency, or resistance to insulin action, causes elevated blood sugar and without preventive treatment can cause eye disease and blindness, as well as other complications.

Diabetic Retinopathy

According to the U.S. Department of Health and Human Services (2002), there are gaps among racial and ethnic groups, not only in the rate of diabetes but also in the rates of associated complications, one of which is diabetic retinopathy. Blacks are disproportionately affected by diabetes, and diabetic retinopathy is the leading cause of new cases of blindness among Blacks 20 to 44 years of age (Eliminate disparities in diabetes, n.d.). The report further states that clinical trials have demonstrated that approximately 60 percent of diabetes-related blindness can be prevented through the control of blood glucose and through early detection and laser photocoagulation treatment. However, not only are people unaware as to how to control diabetes, but the widely available photocoagulation treatment is largely underused.

Eye illness does not develop in all diabetics; diabetic retinopathy usually doesn't develop until a person is diabetic for at least ten years. Diabetic eye disease is similar to the other sources of eye illness discussed so far in that it is one of numerous complications caused by the underlying condition. Careful attention to eye symptoms can, therefore, protect the patient not only from eye problems but also from numerous other serious threats to health and life as well.

In addition to being the leading cause of blindness, diabetes is the leading cause of end-stage renal disease (ESRD) and nontraumatic amputations (USDHHS, 2002). In 1999, the diabetes-related death rate among African Americans was 139 per 100,000. Blacks are two times more likely to die from diabetes than Whites (USDHHS, 2000b). Blacks also suffer higher rates of diabetes complications for eye disease, as well as kidney failure and amputations (New Awareness Campaign Targets the African American Diabetes Epidemic, 1998).

Lack of adequate diagnosis contributes to making diabetes one of the most serious health problems in the United States. About one-third of diabetes cases are undiagnosed among Blacks, similar to other groups in the United States. Lack of adequate diagnosis is part of a larger problem of poor resources used in the treatment of diabetes: "[D]iabetes is not being managed aggressively: physician practices do not meet recommended standards of care; patients do not know how to manage their diabetes; and the health care system is poorly equipped to manage diabetes. The diabetes problem lacks efficacious and efficient prevention strategies. . . . Strategies that would lessen the burden of diabetes are not being used widely or regularly utilized in daily care" (Vinicor, 1999, p. 3).

The primary epidemiologic and public health considerations of diabetic retinopathy include the identification of patients at risk and patients with disease, the minimization of risk factors for the development and progression of disease, and treatment when necessary. All patients with diabetes are patients at risk. Therefore, all diabetic patients must be referred for examination by an ophthalmologist regularly. A study of Black and Hispanic diabetic patients referred for initial ophthalmologic evaluation found that 37.3 percent of Black patients had severe retinopathy (either pre-proliferative or proliferative disease) at the time of initial evaluation. Indeed, many of these patients had not been referred in a timely fashion by their internist, but had sought care because of decreased visual acuity. (McLeod & Raab, 1994, pp. 147–149)

Community Involvement in Diabetes Care

The links between eye health and diabetes in the African American population are similar to the linkages in the other diseases discussed so far. Eye illness is one of numerous complications likely to arise and not necessarily the most important, as in sickle-cell disease and HIV/AIDS. Because these diseases have many manifestations, knowledge is vital, and this is most important at the local level, as Fuchs has emphasized (Fuchs, 1998). The role of the public health professional should, therefore, be emphasized, probably more than it has been in the past. Underutilization of public health professionals is perhaps principally a result of widespread ignorance of their roles and functions (Taylor, 1997). Those areas of public health that stress the many aspects and dimensions of community involvement should be in strong demand. Schools of public health, in turn, have recognized the importance of minority representation among health professionals in making health care a vital concern in underserved minority communities (Bureau of Health Professions, 1998).

Efforts are being made to improve the effectiveness of diabetes care in underserved communities. The National Institutes of Health have been investigating comprehensive community efforts to reduce diabetes among high-risk minority populations. NIH is conducting diabetes research that focuses on the norms and lifestyles of minority communities and has the objective of involving minority staff and research investigations. The goal of the research is to improve interventions to the cultural norms of minority communities. CDC is developing surveillance systems to investigate the diabetes burden on Blacks and other minorities for use at state, regional, and local levels.

The Agency for Healthcare Research and Quality has supported research into the functioning of community health centers in diabetes control (Ocampo & Foster, 2001). These health centers mainly serve poor patients and have limited resources. Chin et al. (2000) found that only 26 percent of patients at 55 midwestern community health centers received dilated eye exams, making eye care the lowest-priority monitoring objective among the major services offered. A Harvard School of Public Health study found that diabetic eye care was lowest in managed care plans among the major forms of care reported on, with the exception of follow-up mental health care (Study Finds Significant Racial Disparities in Quality of Care for Participants in Medicare Managed Care Plans, 2002). The Chi et al. (1989) study found that the community health centers had difficulty meeting American Diabetes Association standards. The study found that deficient diabetes care is not limited to community health centers. The study's authors suggested that improving quality of care is largely a local problem, with needed strategies varying from setting to setting.

Health Career Opportunity Programs and other health diversity-related programs sponsored by the health resources and service administration of the U.S. Department of Health and Human Services, with their emphasis on drawing disadvantaged minorities into medical and public health schools, is a long-term strategy that should be pursued to improve care in underserved communities. A principal reason for pursuing this strategy is that minority graduates return to underserved communities in disproportionate numbers. While it is documented that minority health professionals return disproportionately to their ethnic communities (Komaromy et al., 1996), nevertheless there is an urgent need to increase the supply of Black health professionals to Black communities.

GLAUCOMA

The Epidemiology of Glaucoma

Glaucoma is a group of eye diseases in which, for unknown reasons, normal fluid pressure inside the eye slowly rises, causing damage to the optic nerve. Open-angle, or chronic glaucoma, is the most common form of the disease. It appears that the elevated fluid pressure within the eye (intraocular pressure) is common to all cases (USDHHS, n.d.). Acute, closed-angle glaucoma is a medical emergency, requiring attention within hours to avoid permanent vision damage. Glaucoma is an end-stage condition, where narrowed field of vision is a serious symptom that eventually emerges. Other symptoms include headaches, blurred vision, difficulty adapting to darkness, and halos around lights. Because of the lack of early symptoms, about half of Americans affected by glaucoma are unaware that they have the disease. Risk factors include high intraocular pressure (not a sure sign of glaucoma), family history, severe myopia, diabetes, hypertension, and African ancestry. Blacks over age 40 are at elevated risk.

According to the U.S. Department of Health and Human Services (USDHHS, n.d.), glaucoma is the second leading cause of irreversible blindness in the U.S., and the leading cause of blindness among African Americans (USDHHS, 1996b). Evidence is presented that Blacks are 5 times more likely to have glaucoma than Whites and 4 times more likely to suffer blindness from glaucoma than Whites. Among people aged 45–64, blindness is 15 times more likely among Blacks than among Whites (USDHHS, n.d.). Furthermore, the disparity in the rates of glaucoma and glaucoma blindness among White and Black Americans may also reflect greater access to effective treatment among Whites, although the higher prevalence of glaucoma among Blacks may have a biologic basis as well (USDHHS, 1996, p. 3).

Detection and Control of Glaucoma

Although glaucoma can be controlled and vision loss slowed or halted, preventive measures to avoid glaucoma have not been devised. However, age, race, diabetes, eye trauma, and long-term use of steroid medications increase its risk. Therefore, from a public health perspective, when factors that can be controlled are controlled, morbidities associated with glaucoma are substantially reduced. Routine screening for glaucoma in a primary-care setting has not been proved efficacious. Screening is most likely to be effective among groups at elevated risk of glaucoma. Blacks, hypertensives, diabetics, and relatives of glaucoma patients are among those who should receive primary-care screening for glaucoma. Younger Black men and women (age 20–39) should receive an eye examination every three to five years by an ophthalmologist because of their higher risk of glaucoma (USDHHS, 1996b).

Specific features [of care] include the general population's access to screening, the competence of screeners (especially in the evaluation of the optic disc), and follow-up and treatment of glaucoma suspects and patients. Though mass screenings staffed by volunteers can reach a great many people, the staff are usually inexperienced observers, detection rates are low, and follow-up is often poor. . . . [P]ublic health departments can play a useful role in well-organized detection programs, though follow-up remains a problem.

The environment best suited for the detection and referral for treatment of glaucoma is probably the primary physician's office. Internists and family practitioners should be educated in the risk factors for glaucoma, trained in the recognition of suspicious optic discs, and encouraged to routinely check intraocular pressure (Levi & Schwartz, 1983). As they follow the general condition of the patient, they can ensure that patients with suspicious features or a diagnosis of glaucoma are indeed under the care of an ophthalmologist. (McLeod & Rabb, 1994, p. 144)

Barriers to Detection and Treatment

"Even when glaucoma has been identified, it is suggested that Blacks might not receive adequate therapy. A study of Medicare clinics demonstrated that the rate of glaucoma surgery in Blacks was 45 percent lower than the expected rate and that Whites were receiving proportionally higher rates of treatment (Javitt et al., 1991). It is not at all clear why a disparity in the delivery of care to identified Black and White glaucoma patients should exist, but a great deal of interest has arisen in the possible social and economic contributors to this phenomenon. It is important that ophthalmologists recognize the aggressive nature of the disease in Blacks and that primary physicians concern themselves with timely referrals and follow-up" (McLeod & Rabb, 1994, p. 144).

"The psychology of the disease is in some respects comparable to that of systemic hypertension: both diseases tend to be asymptomatic for much of their course, therapy is inconvenient to irritating, if not frankly noxious, and successful treatment as perceived by the patient is undramatic. It is therefore tremendously important that patients understand the nature of the disease, its natural history and its potentially devastating consequences. Therefore, patient and physician education is paramount" (McLeod & Rabb, 1994, p. 144).

Glaucoma is a major eye health problem among African Americans because it is the leading cause of blindness and has prevalence rates that are much higher than in the general population. Recognition and diagnosis of the disease, which is really a group of diseases, are difficult and complex. Dealing with glaucoma as a chronic problem requires knowledge that racial background and age are significant factors. This knowledge, when presented in a clear and trustworthy way, leads generally to nonemergency care that can detect developing problems. But in the Black community, there is often a sense of being separated from the sources of care, even when they are geographically close by. Sources of care must also be psychologically close by. Once again, in the case of glaucoma, overcoming psychological barriers is a major step in achieving improved eye health in African American communities.

Specific knowledge about symptoms is also important, even though symptom presentation can be subtle and complex. Nausea and vomiting, for example, are symptoms of acute glaucoma, along with eye pain, headaches, vision loss, and others. Thus, it could be easy to misinterpret, and perhaps rationalize, serious symptoms. A high price can be paid: "These signs may last for a few hours, and then return again for another round. Each attack takes with it part of your field of vision" (Lee & Bailey, n.d.). Armed with this knowledge, perhaps acquired in a supportive community setting, should prompt at-risk individuals (e.g., African Americans) to seek immediate help from an ophthalmologist or hospital emergency room.

Chronic glaucoma and acute glaucoma require recognition of different and appropriate responses. Congenital glaucoma is yet another manifestation of the disease in the glaucoma group. Its special complicating factor is that it involves children who are too young to understand the problem. Recognition of symptoms by parents can lead to timely consultation with a pediatrician or eye care specialist (Lee & Bailey, n.d.).

In summary, glaucoma can, like other eye diseases considered in this chapter, be regarded in large part as a public health problem, where effective contact with health professionals in a community setting can be invaluable.

CATARACT

The Epidemiology of Cataract

Cataract is a clouding of the eye's naturally clear lens. Early effects are slight blurring or clouding of vision, which grows worse over time. Cataract heightens the glare from sunlight or auto headlights at night. Colors may not appear as bright as they once did.

"The most common type and, therefore, the most important to examine in terms of public health issues is senile cataract. This can be defined as the presence of lens opacity in a person over 45 years of age in the absence of other causes for cataract" (McLeod & Rabb, p. 145). "1.2% of the entire population of Africa is blind, with cataract causing 36% of this blindness" (Ocampo, and Foster, 2002).

The tragedy of this experience is heightened by the fact that cataract is a reversible condition. "Cataract surgery is very successful in restoring vision. In fact, it is the most frequently performed surgery in the United States. . . . Nine out of 10 people who have cataract surgery regain very good vision, somewhere between 20/20 and 20/40" (Lee & Bailey, n.d., p. 3).

Several epidemiologic studies have "attempted to define demographic, environmental, and other risk factors for senile cataracts. Under demographic factors, age is the most obvious. Both the Framingham and the HANES studies have demonstrated an increasing prevalence of senile cataracts with advancing age. Numerous studies have also suggested that women over 60 years of age are at a slightly higher risk of cataracts than are men. . . ."

Geographic variations in the age-adjusted prevalence of cataracts have suggested that environmental factors might contribute to cataract formation. The HANES data showed cataracts to be more common in rural than in urban dwellers, though it should be noted that this assessment was based on current residence rather than history. Ultraviolet light has been shown to be a risk factor for cataract formation in numerous studies in different parts of the world (Hollows & Moran, 1981). Current research addresses the contribution of poor nutrition to cataract formation and the role of supplements in retarding cataract formation.

There is general consensus in the current literature that Blacks are at an increased risk of cataract formation and subsequent visual debilitation. The HANES study found that Blacks had an age-adjusted relative risk of 1.50 compared to Whites. The Baltimore Eye Survey found unoperated cataract to be the leading cause of blindness in Blacks (nearly one-third of the total) as opposed to age-related macular degeneration, which is the leading cause in Whites. The age-adjusted risk of cataract blindness in Blacks was 5.25 times that of Whites. The study also noted that the White subjects rendered blind by cataract were all at least 80 years old, while the Black subjects included much younger people (Sommer et al., 1991).

"The relative prevalence of cataract and consequent blindness is a particularly interesting public health concern because it depends not only upon the relative risk of cataract development but also upon the risk of curative cataract extraction" (McLeod & Rabb, 1994, p. 146).

Detection and Treatment of Cataracts

Analysis of the Baltimore Eye Survey data with regard to socioeconomic status indicated that in this population, where approximately 40 percent of blindness was potentially correctable, visual impairment was associated with lower socioeconomic status (Tielsch et al., 1991). More specifically, both the HANES and the Framingham studies found poor education to be a risk factor for cataract. It is not clear what environmental or personal features marked by education and socioeconomic factors contribute to risk of cataract formation, but one might postulate that poorer or less-educated people might be less informed about health care issues in general, including cataract and available treatment centers.

The identification, diagnosis, and treatment of visual impairment due to cataract are comparatively straightforward in individual cases. The pressing issue is that of providing service to communities as a whole. A person who sits at home blinded by potentially curable cataracts either does not know about the cure, does not want it, or cannot get it. . . . The question of why people with reversible disease go untreated, even in urban areas where people are aware of the disease entity and treatment centers are available, is a difficult one. . . . [But this] sociologic and epidemiologic question demands further investigation. (McLeod & Rabb, 1998, pp. 145–147)

DISCUSSION AND FUTURE NEEDS

Americans understand better than ever the importance of their own behavior, their own life choices, to the maintenance of good health. They are accustomed to being reminded of the warning signs of a great variety of illnesses and the importance of early response to these signs. The need for regular examinations once they have reached certain ages or have family histories that make them vulnerable to certain illnesses has been impressed upon them. Americans taking increased responsibility for their own health has been a major factor in bringing about the health improvements that have occurred in recent years.

In discussing some of the major causes of eye illness affecting African Americans in this chapter, we have noted their typically subtle and insidious nature. Knowledge and awareness are particularly important in combating eye disease. We have repeatedly stressed that for people to acquire and apply this knowledge requires access, greater inclusion of African Americans in health professions training, cultural sensitivity and awareness, and trust and confidence in the health-care system. Yet for all of the progress that has been made in achieving better health among Americans, Blacks continue to lag seriously behind Whites. Why is this? Is it because of economic differences? Perhaps racism explains the health differences (and the economic inequality)? (Health News Feed #1779, n.d.).

The Harvard Study

Commenting on the Harvard study of over 300,000 Medicare recipients, Johns Hopkins researcher Leiyu Shi doubts that these explanations can bear the burden of explanation: "[T]he real culprit may be providers who don't realize that different ethnic groups have different medical vulnerabilities." (Health Newsfeed #1779, n.d., p. 1). These vulnerabilities manifest themselves in various ways. Eye health among African Americans is, to a significant degree, a group of distinct medical problems requiring distinct modes of care and a distinct research agenda. Blacks sometimes have excessive eye-health problems compared to Whites because of genetic predisposition. There is also the problem of access to medical care, which we have argued is essentially a problem of effectively linking patients to the community.

The Harvard Medicare study shows that much remains to be accomplished even after solving the access problems; "both races received similar insurance" among the subjects of their study (Health News Feed # 1779, p. 1). The Harvard study found that Blacks tended to belong to poorer-quality health plans than Whites. It also found that Blacks tended to receive poorer care within a given health-care program. The study observed a deficit in eye examinations among Black diabetics, compared with Whites. Socioeconomic reasons could account for only part of these disparities. Differences in race-related preferences for medical care were observed. While the study controlled for various demographic characteristics, it did not consider provider demographics. Caregiver characteristics are not an explanatory variable in accounting for differences in quality of care (Schneider et al., 2002).

Dr. Eric Schneider, coauthor of the *JAMA* report on the Harvard study, says that "the possible explanations include racial bias among doctors and cultural differences, including a tendency among some blacks to shun some preventive health care measures" (Blacks Get Poorer Care Than Whites Even In Similar Health Plans, n.d.). Dr. Karen Scott Collins, lead author of a recent Commonwealth Fund study, reports "that minorities are more likely to report having trouble communicating with doctors, feeling disrespected in a doctor's visit, and not understanding or not following a doctor's instructions" (Barnard, 2002, p. 2).

The Need For More Black Health Professionals

A major lesson to be drawn from the considerations discussed in this chapter is that there is a major need for a greater presence of Black health-care professionals in Black underserved communities. It has been noted that Black doctors, as well as other minority doctors, are highly likely to serve in their own ethnic communities (Komaromy et al., 1996). Recruitment of Black students into medical school through such means as the Health Career Opportunity Programs and the Medical Minority Education Programs are also widely recognized. This kind of recruitment of health professionals through schools of public health is much less extensive, however, and should be greatly extended as a means of deepening and broadening Black participation in health care at the community level. Victor Fuchs' (1998) observation that the broadening of the professional health-care base is one of the most important developments in recent years needs to be incorporated with greater emphasis in Black communities. The study of provision of equal-quality eye care to African Americans serves to underscore these needs.

Lastly, a word about medical research. Medical research lays the foundation for benefits to all, and although racial differences have not been totally ignored, they have not played center stage. But lack of Black involvement in medical research, nevertheless, has health consequences in the Black community. Patrick Allen, a biomedical researcher at the University of Colorado, observes that "less than one percent of U.S. biomedical researchers are black—'a disenfranchisement that directly affects health' " (Scott, n.d., p. 2). The reason is that an influx of African Americans into biomedical research would significantly raise health consciousness in the Black community, he believes. There is also a potential for altering the balance of research affecting Black health. Allen, a leader in the recently formed Black Biomedical Research Movement, says that "[t]he fear and suspicion in the black community of the biomedical establishment is a major public health problem that reaches beyond these diseases" (Scott, n.d., p. 3). Community involvement of African Americans in the promotion of their own good health must be a complex, many-layered experience, nowhere better exemplified than in the promotion of eye health.

REFERENCES

Amuwo, S.A. (2004). *The effectiveness of an experimental learning strategy: An approach to culturally specific health education.* Manuscript under review.

Amuwo, S.A. & Flay B. (2001, November). Community empowerment: The Aban Aya Experience. Paper presented at the meeting of the American Public Health Association, New York.

Amuwo, S.A. & Jenkins, E. (2001). True partnership evolves over time. In M. Sullivan & J. Kelly (Eds.), *Collaborative Research: University and Community Partnership* (pp. 25–43). Washington, DC: American Public Health Association.

Ashley-Koch, A., Yang, Z., & Olney R.S. (1998). Sickle hemoglobin (Hb S) allele and sickle cell disease. *HuGE Review.* Retrieved June 6, 2002, from http://www.cdc.gov/genomics/hugenet/reviews.sickle.htm

Barnard, Anne. (2002, March). Study says Blacks get poorer medical care. The ad hoc committee to defend health care. (2002, March 13). Retrieved from http://216.36.252.42/news_study_poorercare.htm

Bazargan, M., Baker, R., & Bazargan, S. (1998). Correlates of recency of eye examination among elderly African-Americans. *Ophthalmic Epidemiology, 5,* 91–100.

Blacks get poorer care than Whites even in similar health plans: Study. (n.d.). Associated Press. Retrieved from http://www.msnbc.com/news/722946.asp

Bureau of Health Professions Division of Disadvantaged Assistance. (1998, February). *HCOP digest: Fiscal year 1997.*

Cantor, J.C., Miles E.L., Baker L.C., & Barker D.C. (1996). *Physician service to the underserved: Implications for Affirmative Action in Medical Education.* Blue Cross and Blue Shield of the Rochester Area.

Chi, T., Ritch, R., Stickler, D., Pitman, B., Tsai, C., & Hsish, F.Y. (1989). Racial differences in optic nerve head parameters. *Archives of Ophthalmology, 107,* 836–839.

Chin, M.H., et al. (2000). Quality of diabetes care in community health centers. *American Journal of Public Health, 90*, 431–434.

Condon, P.I., & Serjeant, G.R. (1980). Behavior of untreated proliferative sickle retinopathy. *British Journal of Ophthalmology, 64*, 404–411.

Courtright, Paul. (1996, June). The challenge of HIV/AIDS related eye disease. *British Journal of Ophthalmology, 80*, 496–498.

Diseases of the Eye. (n.d.). Iowa Department for the Blind. Retrieved on June 18, 2002, from http:www.blind.state.ia.us/eye_disease.htm

Don't lose sight of glaucoma. (n.d.) USDHHS (M.D.) NIH Publication No. 91-3251. Retrieved from http://www.openseason.com/annex/library/cic/X))77_sight.txt.html

Eliminate disparities in diabetes. (n.d) Retrieved from http://www.rstl.com/goal4.htm.

Forum. *Environmental Health Perspectives*, 106. (1998, December). Retrieved on June 4, 2002, from http://ehpnet1.niehs.nih.gov/docs/1998/106-12/forum.html

Fox, P.D., Dunn, D.T., Morris, J.S., & Serjeant, G.R. (1990). Risk factors for proliferative sickle retinopathy. *British Journal of Ophthalmology, 74*, 172–176.

Freid, Praeger, MacKay, & Xia (2003). Health, United States, 2003. *Chartbook on Trends in the health of Americans*. Hyattsville: Maryland, NCHS. Also can be accessed at (1/25/04) http://www.cdc.gov/nchs/data/hus/hus03.pdf

Fuchs, V.R. (1998). *Who shall live?: Health, economics and social choice* (expanded ed.). London World Scientific.

Gallemore, R.P., & Boyer D.S. (2001, December). Save your sight: Eye disease and HIV. *Positive Living*. Retrieved July 2, 2002, from http://www.thebody.com/apla/dec01/sight.html

Grady, D (2002, May 30). Study first to document correlation between nursing shortage and patient death/illness. *New York Times*, p. A14.

Harlan, J.B., Jr., & Goldberg, M.F. (1996). Management and therapy of eye disorders in sickle cell disease. Retrieved June 25, 2002, from http://sickle.bwh.harvard.edu/eye.html

Health News Feed # 1779. (N.d.). A study finds that elderly Blacks receive worse health care than similarly insured Whites. Retrieved on June 6, 2002, from http://www.hopkinsmedicine.org/healthnewsfeed/hnf_1779.htm

Helsing, Karen. (2001) *2000 annual data report: Applications, new enrollments and students fall 2000 graduates, 1999–00 with trends, 1989–2000*. Associations of Schools of Public Health.

HIV/AIDS continues to decimate African-Americans; church leaders and gospel radio respond to challenge. (1998, February). *Business Wire*. Retrieved June 13, 2002, from http://www.aegis.com/news/bw/1998/BW980205.html

HIV/AIDS Statistics. (1999a). *Black Health Care.Com*. Retrieved June 6, 2002, from http://www.blackhealthcare.com/BHC/AIDS/Emidemiology.asp

HIV/AIDS Statistics. (1999b). *McLeod health*. Retrieved July 2, 2002, from http://www.mcleodhealth.org/library/hivi/4623

Hollows, F., & Moran, D. (1981). Cataract: The ultraviolet risk factor. *Lancet, 2*, 1249–1250.

Javitt, J.C., McBean, A.M., Nicholson, G.A., Babish, J.D., Warren, J.L., & Krakauer, H. (1991). Undertreatment of glaucoma among black Americans. *New England Journal of Medicine, 325*, 1418–1422.

Komaromy, M., et al. (1996, May 16). The role of Black and Hispanic physicians in providing health care for underserved populations. *The New England Journal of Medicine, 334*, 1305–1310.

Lee, Judith. (2001, June). CMV Retinitis and AIDS. *All about vision.com*. Retrieved July 2, 2002, from http://www.allaboutvision.com./conditions/cmv_retinits_aids.htm

Lee, Judith, & Bailey, Gretchyn. (n.d.a). Cataracts. *All about vision.com*. Retrieved on June 18, 2002, from http://allaboutvision.com/conditions/cataracts.htm

Lee, Judith & Bailey, Gretchyn. (n.d.b). Glaucoma. *All about vison.com*. Retrieved on June 18, 2002, from http://www.allaboutvision.com/conditions/glaucoma.htm

Levi, L., & Schwartz, B. (1983). Glaucoma screening in the health care setting. *Survey of Ophthalmology, 28*, 64.

McLeod, S.D., & Rabb, M.F. (1994). Ophthalmology in blacks: A survey of major entities. In I.V. Livingston (Ed.), *Handbook of Black American health: The mosaic of conditions, issues, policies, and prospects* (pp. 140–154). Westport, CT: Greenwood Press.

New awareness campaign targets the African American diabetes epidemic. (1998, September). Retrieved on June 13, 2002, from http:www.niddk.nih.gov.welcome/releases/9_19_98.htm

Nickerson, R.J., Pool, J., Colton, T.L., Ganley, J.P., Lowenstein, J.I., & Darber, J.R. (1980). The Framingham eye study monograph. *Survey of Ophthalmology, 24,* (supp.), 355–707.

Ocampo, Vicente V., & Foster, C.S. (2002, July). Cataract, Senile. *eMedicine Journal.* Retrieved on June 4, 2002, from http://www.emedicine.com/oph/topic49.htm

Philipson, T.J., & Posner R.A. (1993). *Private choices and public health: The AIDS epidemic in an economic perspective.* Cambridge: Harvard University Press.

Procaare: HIV vs. AIDS incidence, USA. (1998). Retrieved June 6, 2002, from http://www.essentialdrugs.org/programs/procaarehma/procaare.199804.msg0023.html

Schneider, Eric, Zaslavsky, Alan & Epstein, Arnold. (2002, March). Racial disparities in quality of care for enrollees in Medicare managed care. *Journal of the American Medical Association, 287,* 1288–1294.

Scott, Jim. (N.d.). Pat Allen targets AIDS research, raising health consciousness in the Black community. (N.d.). *Black biomedical research movement.* Retrieved on June 13, 2002, from http://www.bbrm.org/articles/coloradan_article.html

Smedley, B.D., Stitch, A.Y., & Nelson, A.R. (2002). *Unequal treatment: Confronting racial and ethnic disparities in health care.* Institute of Medicine. Washington, DC: National Academies Press.

Sommer, A., et al. (1991). Radical differences in the cause-specific prevalence of blindness in East Baltimore. *New England Journal of Medicine, 325,* 1412–1417.

Study finds significant racial disparities in quality of care for participants in Medicare managed care plans. (2002, March). Harvard School of Public Health Press Releases. Retrieved on June 6, 2002, from http://www.hsph.harvard.edu/press/release/press031222002.html

Study finds that elderly Blacks receive worse health care than similarly insured Whites. (N.d.) Health Newsfeed #1779 Retrieved on June 6, 2002, from http://216.239.33.100/search?q=cachse:n5imMrDiTcED:www.hopkinsmedicine.org/healthnews

Taylor, Humphrey. (1997, January). *"Public Health": Two words few people understand Even though almost everyone thinks public health functions are very important.* New York: Louis Harris and Associates.

Tielsch, J.M., Sommer, A., Katz, J., Quigley, H., & Ezrine, S. (1991). Socioeconomic status and visual impairment among urban Americans. *Archives of Ophthalmology, 109,* 637–641.

U.S. Department of Health and Human Services (USDHHS). (1996). *Sickle cell anemia* (NIH Publication No. 96-4057).

U.S. Department of Health and Human Services (USDHHS). (2000a, November). *Healthy people 2010: Objectives for improving health.* Volume II, Part A Focus Areas 1–14. Washington, DC: U.S. Government Printing Office.

U.S. Department of Health and Human Services (USDHHS). (2000b, November). *Healthy people 2010: Objectives for improving health.* Volume II, Part B Focus Areas 15–28. Washington, DC: U.S. Government Printing Office.

U.S. Department of Health and Human Services (USDHHS). (2001). *Healthy people 2000: Final review.* National Center for Health Statistics. Publication no. 01-0256. Hyattsville, MD: Public Health Service.

U.S. Department of Health and Human Services (USDHHS). National Eye Institute. National Institutes of Health. (2002). *Vision problems in the U.S.: Prevalence of adult vision impairment and age-related eye disease in America.* Bethesda, MD.

U.S. Department of Health and Human Services (USDHHS). (n.d.). *Don't lose sight of glaucoma.* National Institutes of Health. Public Health Service. NIH Publication no. 91-3251.

Van Meurs, J.C. (1991). Relationship between peripheral vascular closure and proliferative retinopathy in sickle cell disease. *Archives of Clinical Experimental Ophthalmology, 229(6),* 543–8.

Vinicor, Frank. (1999, September). Diabetes. Assistant Secretary for Legislation Department of Health and Human Services. Retrieved June 13, 2002, from http://www.hhs.gov/asl/testify/t990908a.html

WHO Reports. Joint United Nations Programme on HIV/AIDS (UNAIDS) and World Health Organization (WHO) (2002).

Women's Interagency HIV Study. (n.d.). What in the WIHS? Retrieved June 6, 2002, from https:statepiaps.Jhsph.edu/wihs/wihs/

CHAPTER 11

Immunological Disorders

MARGUERITE E. NEITA AND LATEEF A. OLOPOENIA

INTRODUCTION

The concept of immunity and resistance to disease has engaged humankind for centuries. Modern science has elucidated many of the mechanisms of disease resistance and immune responsiveness; however, the basic premise remains that the immune response, which consists of specialized cells, tissues, and effector molecules (cell chemicals), exists to "keep us safe" from substances that the body docs not recognize as "self." These substances include mutant cells, foreign microscopic antigens (bacteria, viruses, and parasites), and self-proteins altered by drugs and infections, all of which have the potential for causing life-threatening malignancies, infections, and autoimmune disorders (Sigal & Ron, 1994; Sigal, 1994).

When the immune response goes awry, disease and tissue damage occur. Disorders of the immune system may be either diminished (immunodeficiency) or exaggerated (hypersensitivity). Immunodeficiency reactions may be congenital or acquired because of damage to the immune system by chemicals, drugs, radiation, infection, or inadequate nutrition (Rosen, 2001; Weller, 2001). The acquired immunodeficiency syndrome (AIDS) is the best-known immunodeficiency disorder today. AIDS is caused by infection with the human immunodeficiency virus (HIV), which severely destroys the immune system, leaving an infected person with no resistance to infection or malignant disease.

In hypersensitivity reactions, the immune system overreacts and loses its ability to distinguish "self" from "nonself." Because of the overwhelming, adverse immunological reaction, tissues of the body are damaged with devastating consequences for the host if treatment is unavailable or delayed (Janeway & Travers, 1997; Platts-Mills, 2001). Systemic diseases, with underlying immunological mechanisms, can be classified as hypersensitivity type reactions (Greenwood & Whittle, 1981; Hay & Westwood, 2001; Roitt et al., 1985).

Studies indicate a familial and racial susceptibility to the immune hypersensitivity disorders. The data implicate the immune response genes of the major histocompatibility complex (MHC) as well as some genes outside the MHC, with an increased predisposition to developing immune system disorders (Brodsky, 2001; Cooke, 2001; Janeway & Travers, 1997). The environment and interrelated socioeconomic factors may also play a role in the development and incidence of the immunological disorders discussed here.

Table 11.1
Hypersensitivity classification, mechanisms, and associated immune disorders

Hypersensitivity Classification	Immune Mechanism	Immune System Mediator	Immune Disorders
Type 1	Atopy	IgE antibody	Allergy, Asthma
Type II	Cytotoxic	IgM and IgG antibodies	Grave's disease Hashimoto's Thyroiditis
Type III	Immune Complex Deposition	IgM and IgG antibodies	Systemic Lupus Erythematosus (SLE)
Type IV	Cell Mediated Immunity (CMI)	T- lymphocytes and Macrophages	Sarcoidosis, Tuberculosis, Leprosy
Unclassified Disorders	CMI & Auto antibody Antibody overproduction	T-cells Plasma cells (B-lymphocytes)	Progressive Systemic Sclerosis (PSS) Multiple Myeloma

This chapter describes the hypersensitivity disorders that predominantly affect Black Americans and reviews the genetic, environmental, and socioeconomic factors that result in the disproportionate incidence and unfavorable outcomes in the Black population.

HYPERSENSITIVITY REACTIONS

Classification

In 1963, British immunologists P.G.H. Gell and R.R. Coombs classified hypersensitivity reactions into four types (I, II, III, and IV) based on the various immunologic mechanisms involved. Hypersensitivity reactions types I, II and III are mediated by specific, circulating serum proteins (antibodies/immunoglobulins) and are considered immediate-type hypersensitivity reactions because of the rapidity of the immune response, which occurs within minutes. In contrast, Type IV is a cell-mediated delayed type reaction that takes more than 12 hours to develop. While the Gell and Coombs classifications are convenient, in some disease states, a clearly defined separation of hypersensitivity reactions is not always possible (Goldsby et al., 2000; Greenwood & Whittle, 1981; Roitt et al., 1985). Disorders such as progressive systemic sclerosis (PSS) and multiple myeloma (MM) do not fit precisely into the Gell and Coombs classification (Table 11.1).

FACTORS THAT PREDISPOSE TO IMMUNE DISORDERS

Genes of the Major Histocompatibility Complex (MHC)

The genes that regulate and control immune responsiveness are located on human chromosome 6; this region of the genome is referred to as the major histocompatibility complex (MHC). The highly polymorphic gene products of the MHC are cell membrane proteins, also known as human leukocyte antigens (HLA). They are classified as Class I (HLA-A, -B and -C), Class II (HLA-DP,-DQ,-DR, -DM), and Class III (C2, C4, Bf) proteins.

The MHC/HLA genes are inherited as a pair of codominant alleles from both parents. Family and twin studies of this gene complex have helped to link the presence of certain MHC alleles and HLA proteins, especially the Class II proteins, with disorders of the immune system (Brodsky, 2001; Cooke, 2001; Goldsby et al., 2000; Janeway & Travers, 1997). By comparing the frequency of an allele in the general population with its frequency in individuals with a specific disease, the relative risk (RR) or probability of developing that disease can be determined. Relative risk values greater than 1 indicate that an individual, with that allele, is at increased risk for developing a particular disease (Goldsby et al., 2000; Cooke, 2001).

Three important concerns with regard to the association between HLA antigens and immune disorders must be noted. First, the mere presence of a particular HLA allele does not imply that an individual will develop the associated disease; second, other non-MHC genes may also be involved in disease susceptibility. Third, relative risk values are reported from studies mainly of the Caucasian population and vary based on different populations and geographic locations (Brodsky, 2001; Cooke, 2001; Janeway & Travers, 1997).

The issue of genetic susceptibility to immune disorders is complex. Cooke (2001) suggests that for each population, a collection of various MHC gene products in combination with different environmental factors contribute to the development of disease. The combination of MHC-regulated genetic predisposition, non-MHC genetic susceptibility, and environmental impact may provide an explanation for the prevalence of these immune disorders in the Black population.

Environmental and Socioeconomic Factors

The evidence from several studies has shown that the interaction between genetic susceptibility and environmental factors plays a significant role in the development of hypersensitivity reactions.

Although Black people in the diaspora share a common genetic ancestry, the immunological disorders prevalent in Black Americans are reportedly rare on the African continent (Adebajo & Davis, 1992, 1994; Greenwood & Whittle, 1981; Newsome & Choudhuri, 1984). The high prevalence of some disorders among Black Americans is also seen in the Black Caribbean population living in Great Britain (Hosoda et al., 1997; Petri, 1998). This suggests that other factors may interact with the underlying genetic susceptibility to promote disease development.

While Adebajo and Davis (1992, 1994), report that the immune hypersensitivity disorders are more common in the larger African cities than in rural villages, they also hypothesize that the decreased prevalence observed in Africa may result from inadequate testing, underdiagnosis, and increased mortality due to greater severity of symptoms. They also suggest that chronic infections with malaria and other parasites appear to protect the immune system and prevent hypersensitivity-associated immune disorders (Adebajo & Davis, 1992, 1994; Greenwood & Whittle, 1981).

Epidemiological data indicate an increasing incidence of the hypersensitivity immune disorders in the industrialized nations when compared with the less developed countries of the world. In an attempt to explain the increasing incidence of asthma and other immunological disorders in the industrialized world, researchers are currently directing their attention to the hygiene hypothesis initially proposed in 1989. The hypothesis suggests that early stimuli to the immune system, from viral infections, bacterial toxins, and parasitic infestations, direct the immune system to produce fewer of the effector chemicals or cytokines involved in allergic and autoimmune diseases.

As a direct result of modernization, improved sanitation, and higher socioeconomic status in modern industrialized countries, children are less exposed to bacterial infections and parasitic infestations. This underexposure results in an inappropriately elevated immune response to environmental stimuli, with a concomitant increase in hypersensitivity reactions and the associated disorders (Bach, 2002; Braun-Fahrländer et al., 2002; Janeway & Travers, 1997; Pongracic & Evans, 2001; Weiss, 2002).

Since it is often difficult to separate environmental and socioeconomic issues, they are discussed together in this chapter.

IMMUNE HYPERSENSITIVITY REACTIONS

Type I Hypersensitivity Reactions

In Type I, or immediate type hypersensitivity reactions, the immune system overreacts to seemingly innocuous environmental stimuli by producing large amounts of specific immunoglobulin E (IgE) antibodies and other immunological mediators. Type I hypersensitivity reactions are associated with allergic (atopic) and asthmatic responses to common substances. Atopy is defined as the genetically predetermined hypersensitivity response to these environmental agents (Janeway & Travers, 2001; Platts-Mills, 2001; Terr, 2001).

Allergies   Allergic or atopic reactions occur after exposure to common substances usually regarded as harmless. These substances called (allergens), which may be inhaled or ingested, include foods (shellfish, eggs, milk, chicken, and peanuts), pollens (hay fever), dust mite feces, insect venom (bites) and some drugs (Janeway & Travers, 2001; Platts-Mills, 2001; Terr, 2001).

DeLeo et al. (2002) and Dickel et al. (2001) report that any racial differences seen in the response to specific allergens occur as a result of increased occupationally or culturally based exposure to the specific allergen. However, no overall difference in the prevalence of allergic contact dermatitis and irritant contact dermatitis between Black and White Americans is found.

Asthma   Asthma, the most common, chronic childhood disease today, is rapidly increasing in incidence, morbidity, and mortality in the inner cities of the industrialized world. Epidemiological data also indicate that asthma occurs more often and with greater severity in the Black American community (Crater et al., 2001; Joseph et al., 2000; Halterman et al., 2001; Pongracic & Evans, 2001).

Black American children with asthma tend to have higher levels of IgE antibody, greater airway hyperresponsiveness (Joseph et al., 2000; Pongracic & Evans, 2001), more severe symptoms, more absences from school (Rand et al., 2000; Lieu et al., 2002; Joseph et al., 2000), higher mortality rates, and more emergency room visits and hospitalizations (Eggleston, 1998; Joseph et al., 1998; Joseph et al., 2000; Lieu et al., 2002; Mannino et al., 2002; Thomas & Whitman, 1999). They are also less likely to receive and/or use long-term, preventive medication (Cooper & Hickson, 2001; Diaz et al., 2000; Eggleston, 1998; Halterman et al., 2002; Lieu et al., 2002; Sarpong et al., 1996).

Genetics of Asthma.   The genetics of asthma is complicated by the number of associated genes and environmental factors involved (Platts-Mills, 2001). While the gene–environment interaction is a significant contributor to the prevalence of asthma, researchers believe that the continued steady increase in asthma incidence in the industrialized nations cannot be attributed to genetic change only;

this emphasizes the importance of environmental and other factors in the development of asthma (Crater et al., 2001; Platts-Mills, 2001).

Socioeconomic and Environmental Factors Associated with Asthma.   Data collected in nation-wide studies indicate that urban living played a greater role than race in the incidence of asthma in at-risk children (Aligne et al., 2000; Pongracic & Evans, 2001). This is supported by other studies, which find that urban dwelling and Black American children are sensitized to a greater degree by exposure to mold, decaying cockroach skeletons, mice, and dust mite allergens present in older, substandard, urban housing units (Call et al., 1992; Eggleston & Arruda, 2001; Kuster, 1996; Ortega & Calderon, 2000; Platt-Mills et al., 1991; Pongracic & Evans, 2001; Rauh et al., 2002; Sarpong et al., 1996; Stevenson et al., 2001).

Other aspects of urban living that exacerbate asthma morbidity include outdoor pollution (sulfur dioxide, smog, particulate matter) and indoor pollution (secondhand cigarette smoke and nitrogen dioxide from space heaters and gas stoves). Studies show that at least 50 percent of inner-city children are exposed to indoor secondhand smoke (Eggleston, 1998; Pongracic & Evans, 2001). Other studies show that when systemic levels of cotinine (a nicotine metabolite) are used as a measure, Black children are more susceptible to the effects of secondary tobacco smoke than White children (Knight et al., 1996).

The psychosocial stresses of inner-city living, such as low-income, single-parent homes, depression, anxiety, crime, alcoholism, and drug abuse, have been implicated in reduced compliance with medication use, poor asthma control, and increased morbidity and mortality (Eggleston, 1998; Pongracic & Evans, 2001). It seems, therefore, that while there may be an underlying genetic predisposition, environmental and social factors play a definitive role in the development, prevalence, and severity of asthma among urban-dwelling Black Americans.

Type II Hypersensitivity Reactions

Type II hypersensitivity reactions involve antibodies directed against specific cells and tissues and are most often the cause of hemolytic transfusion reactions as well as some autoimmune or connective tissue disorders (Roitt et al., 1985). Two such disorders, Grave's disease and Hashimoto's thyroiditis, involve the thyroid gland (Janeway & Travers, 2001; Roitt et al., 1985). While these occur more commonly in women than in men, there is no significant difference in racial distribution either in the United States or worldwide (Floyd, 2002; Lahita, 2000; Odeke & Nagelberg, 2002).

Type III Hypersensitivity Reactions

A typical Type III hypersensitivity mechanism is involved in other autoimmune disorders such as systemic lupus erythematosus (SLE). This Type III hypersensitivity mechanism is characterized by formation of immune complexes of antibodies (IgM and IgG) with antigens such as foreign-proteins, self-proteins, and the products of infectious agents. Normally, specialized cells and proteins of the immune system remove or clear the complexes. When clearance is defective, the complexes persist, deposit in the tissues, and cause an unabated inflammatory response that results in severe tissue damage (Hay & Westwood, 2001; Janeway & Travers, 2001).

Systemic Lupus Erythematosus.   Systemic lupus erythematosus (SLE) or "lupus" is a systemic autoimmune disorder of unknown etiology, characterized by the production of autoantibodies, primarily to the deoxyribonucleic acid (DNA) in the cell nucleus. Immune complex deposition often occurs in the glomerular capillaries of the kidneys causing lupus glomerulonephritis (Hahn, 2001; Roitt et al., 1985; Roitt, 2001).

The prevalence of SLE is higher in the Black population than in the White population, and higher in females than in males. Black women are therefore at the highest risk for developing the disorder. This is supported by data such as the results from the 1995 study by McCarty et al. of racial differences and prevalence of SLE in a Pennsylvania patient cohort. Rough frequencies, for the annual incidence of SLE in that study, were as follows: Black females, 9.2; White females, 3.5; Black males, 0.7; White males, 0.4.

The female-to-male incidence, reportedly as high as 11:1 during the childbearing years (ages 20–50), declines during the postmenopausal years to approximately 2:1 (Manzi, 2001; Sanchez-Guerrero et al., 1995). The sex hormones (estrogen, androgens, and progesterone) are linked to the genetic control and immunomodulation of the immune system and to the development of SLE and other autoimmune diseases (Cutolo & Wilder, 2000; Lahita, 2000, Petri, 1998).

Cutolo and Wilder (2000) indicate that immune responsiveness is usually intensified by estrogens (female hormones) and inhibited by the androgens (male hormones) and progesterone. Symptoms of SLE worsen when normal estrogen levels increase during the second half of the menstrual cycle and during or after pregnancy (Bruce & Laskin, 1997; Julkunen, 1991). Sensitivity to estrogen may therefore explain the predominance of SLE in women, especially during the childbearing years. This clearly has implications for the use of oral contraceptives (OC) and postmenopausal hormone replacement estrogen therapy (HRT) in Black women. Both of these reportedly worsen the symptoms of, or precipitate, SLE in women (Bruce & Laskin, 1997; Julkunen, 1991; Sanchez-Guerrero et al., 1995).

Initial symptoms of SLE are vague and may include fatigue, weight loss, joint pains, and an erythematous rash on exposure to sunlight. Eventually, all organ systems are involved. Renal involvement (glomerulonephritis) affects a majority of patients with SLE; other sequelae include pleurisy, vasculitis, arthritis, hypertension and nervous system damage (Hahn, 2001; Molina et al., 1997; Sack & Fye, 2001; Sacks et al., 2002). Black Americans with lupus tend to have more severe symptomatology; greater organ system damage; a higher incidence of central nervous system and cardiac involvement; more severe renal disease, musculoskeletal damage, and bone necrosis. In Black American patients, the age of onset and initial diagnosis is often lower, and the death rate higher than in other groups (Adebajo & Davis, 1994; Cooper et al., 2002; Gedalia et al., 1999; Petri, 1998; Walsh et al., 1995; Walsh et al., 1996).

Data from the Centers for Disease Control (CDC) on morbidity and mortality for 1979–1998 show that while the overall death rate from SLE increased from 39 to 52 per ten million, the highest increase was among Black women aged 45–64 years. Mortality among the racial and gender groups shows that the death rate was threefold higher among Blacks than Whites, and fivefold higher in women than in men (Sacks et al., 2002). Walsh et al. (1996) report that for Black patients, especially Black women, renal involvement was the major cause of death. Increased renal involvement was also found among African patients with SLE (Adebajo & Davis, 1994).

Walsh et al. (1995) report that White women receive better medical care and live longer after the initial diagnosis of SLE. In contrast, for Black women the combination of higher prevalence, barriers to effective health care, unvarying risk in young Black women (<45 years old), and an increasing risk in older Black women (>55 years old) contribute to the increasing mortality seen in Black Americans.

Genetics of SLE.   The MHC/HLA genes appear to be among the major risk factors in the genetic predisposition to SLE. Associations have been made with several gene alleles including HLA-DR2, -DR3, and the Class III allele C4AQO (Hahn, 2001; Roitt, 2001). Several studies currently link the presence of specific HLA alleles such as HLA-DR7 and -DQ_β with the production of specific autoantibodies, which are implicated in increased severity of the disease (Hahn, 2001; Wilson et al., 1984). While HLA-B8 and -DR3 are consistently associated with SLE in White populations, the same is not true in other ethnic groups (Sullivan, 2000).

Other studies show a strong association with defects in other alleles (FcγRIIA and DRB*1501/ 15.3 and DBQ1*0602) and the predisposition of Black Americans to SLE when compared with White Americans (Hahn, 2001; Petri, 1998; Sullivan, 2000).

Molina et al. (1997) report that Black Afro-Caribbean and South African patients had similar distributions of autoantibodies associated with SLE. In a recent report, Smikle et al. (2002) report that different MHC alleles were associated with SLE in the Black Jamaican population when compared with other Black populations.

These variations in genetic association suggest that while genetic predisposition, race, and gender are linked to the development of SLE, other factors are required to promote development of the disease. Hahn (2001) suggests that individual variations in the interaction between an assortment of genes and different environmental factors may activate a Type III immune response, which results in the kind of disorder classified as SLE.

Socioeconomic and Environmental Factors Associated with SLE.   Environmental agents, such as sunlight, are known to exacerbate the symptoms of SLE (Hahn, 2001); attempts have been made to implicate other environmental substances as causative agents. Petri (1998) reports no relationship between hair dyes and hair relaxers and the development of SLE in Black Americans. However, there is positive association between cigarette smoke, the prevalence of the discoid form of "lupus," and the increased musculoskeletal damage seen in the Black American patient with SLE.

The modifiable social factors that contribute to the morbidity and mortality of SLE in the Black American population are lack of access to appropriate health care, delayed diagnosis, and inappropriate management of the organ damage and associated disability (Petri, 1998; Sacks et al., 2002; Walsh et al., 1995).

The disparity seen between the Black and White population in the prevalence of SLE and the prognosis for those affected are complicated by the interplay between the variations in genetic predisposition, environmental factors, and hormonal interactions.

Type IV Hypersensitivity Reactions

Type IV reactions are cell-mediated, and the response is delayed; the reaction becomes apparent after 12 or more hours. Diseases associated with the Type IV hypersensitivity mechanism include sarcoidosis, tuberculosis, and leprosy, as well as skin reactions to poison ivy, latex, hair dyes, and nickel.

The mechanism involved is mediated by the T-cells of the immune response unlike the B-cell-mediated, antibody dependent reactions described above. Diseases caused by Type IV mechanisms include conditions in which the pathogen, usually an infectious agent, persists in the body, causing constant activation of the monocyte/macrophage cells and the concomitant production of activation products that damage the tissues. This unremitting activation of the cellular components of the immune system results in the formation of characteristic granulomatous or nodular inflammatory lesions (Britton, 2001; Maliarik et al., 2000; Roitt et al., 1985).

The antigens or infectious agents that cause tuberculosis, *Mycobacterium tuberculosis*, and leprosy, *Mycobacterium leprae*, are well known. These diseases are also classified as infectious diseases and will not be discussed in this chapter.

Sarcoidosis.   Sarcoidosis is an immunological disorder of unknown etiology. The disease is characterized by mild chest discomfort, dry cough, fatigue, weight loss and shortness of breath (Crystal, 2001; English et al., 2001; Torrington et al., 1997). The lungs are primarily affected, but no association with smoking has been found; in fact sarcoidosis, may be more common in non-smokers (Crystal, 2001; English et al., 2001). Other tissues affected include the skin, liver, spleen, lymph nodes, heart, nerves, muscle, joints and bone marrow (Crystal, 2001; Gould & Callen, 2001; Hosoda et al., 1997; Kerdel & Moschella, 1984; Scofield & Sadanandan, 2001).

Kerdel and Moschella (1984) report an increased prevalence in developed countries. Studies of various population groups in the United States, including U.S. Army and Navy personnel, indicate that the prevalence of the disease is highest in the Black population, with the number of Blacks (35.5 per 100,000) disproportionately affected when compared to Whites (10.9 per 100,000). The reported ratio of Black:White individuals affected in the United States ranges from 4:1 to 17:1 (Baughman et al., 2001; Crystal, 2001; Gould & Callen, 2001; Hosoda et al., 1997; Kerdel & Moschella, 1984; Rybicki et al., 1999; Scofield & Sadanandan, 2001).

The highest incidence is in Black women aged 30 to 39 years and 45 to 65 years, and the lowest is in White males (English et al., 2001; Rybicki, 1997; Torrington et al., 1997). In the Northern European White population, the prevalence is high (Crystal, 2001; Gould & Callen, 2001). Newsome and Choudhuri (1984) and Crystal (2001) state that the disease is reported rarely in Africa. However, an early study of sarcoidosis indicates that the prevalence in the Black and Colored South African population was similar to that in Black Americans when compared to the White population (Benatar, 1977).

Although the death rate from sarcoidosis is low (~ 10%), Black Americans, especially inner-city Black patients, exhibit more severe symptoms, including skin and hematological involvement, increased airway obstruction, and shortness of breath than White patients (Baughman ct al., 2001, Kerdel & Moschella, 1984; Torrington et al., 1997). The ACCESS (A Case Control Etiologic Study of Sarcoidosis) research group, which examined 736 sarcoidosis patients from clinical centers in the United States, reports that the degree and type of organ involvement is predicated mainly by race (Baughman et al., 2001).

Morbidity and mortality data are worse for females when compared with males and for Black patients when compared with White patients (English et al., 2001, Israel et al., 1997; Kerdel & Moschella, 1984).

Genetics of Sarcoidosis.   The incidence of the disease in related family members, monozygotic and dizygotic twins, siblings, mother and child pairs, and same-sex relatives supports the suggestion of a genetic predisposition to sarcoidosis (Crystal, 2001; Elford et al., 2000; Maliarik ct al., 2000; Rybicki et al., 1999; Rybicki et al., 2001). The presence of certain MHC/HLA alleles has been associated with the predisposition to sarcoidosis and with the patients' prognosis. Elford and colleagues (2000) report the presence of HLA-A2 in three of five family members affected with sarcoidosis.

Associations have also been made between HLA-DRB1 and HLA-DR5 with increased susceptibility; HLA-A1, HLA-B8 and acute sarcoidosis and spontaneous remission from the disease; HLA-DR-3 and better patient outcomes; HLA-B13 and early onset and chronicity; HLA-1, -B8, DR-3, and HLA-B27 and the development of lung disease (Elford et al., 2000; English et al., 2001; Kerdel & Moschella, 1984).

While much of the genetic evidence is based on studies in Northern European and Japanese populations, recent studies have examined the link between various MHC/HLA alleles and non-MHC genes and the development of sarcoidosis in the Black population. Maliarik et al. (1998) report that substitutions of amino acid sequences in the HLA-DPB1 protein showed weak associations with increased risk of developing sarcoidosis. Rybicki et al. (1999) and Maliarik et al. (2000), report associations between non-MHC genes that code for immune system regulatory proteins and the susceptibility to sarcoidosis in Black Americans.

More research is necessary to identify the genes associated with the predisposition of Black Americans to sarcoidosis. In addition, the role of environmental and socioeconomic factors that contribute to the prevalence of the disease in Black Americans needs to be clarified.

Socioeconomic and Environmental Factors.   Reports of clustering of the disease in unrelated individuals in the same geographic area and in married couples strongly suggest an environmental component to this disease. Epidemiological data support the link between several environmental agents and the development of the disease, and attempts have been made to implicate infectious agents (mycobacteria, fungi, bacteria, and viruses), mycobacterial deoxyribonucleic acid (DNA), chemicals (zirconium and beryllium), dust from antiskid materials on aircraft carriers, clay, soil, talc, and pine pollens without definitive confirmation (English et al., 2001; Gould & Callen, 2001; Hosoda et al., 1997; Kerdel & Moschella, 1984).

The disease has also been associated with medications; malignancies; and other immunological disorders such as SLE, RA, autoimmune thyroiditis and PSS (English et al., 2001; Scofield & Sadanandan, 2001).

Other reports suggest a seasonal relationship, like the observation that the disease appears to occur more frequently during the early spring, when the temperature begins to rise after the colder winter months (English et al., 2001; Hosoda et al., 1997).

There are no reports to indicate a direct causative relationship between socioeconomic status and sarcoidosis. Kajdasz et al. (1999) report that while the incidence of sarcoidosis among South Carolinians showed regional variations, no significant link was found between SES and the development of sarcoidosis. However, indicators of poor SES such as low income, lack of health insurance, or inadequate health insurance are associated with more debilitating disease and greater physical and emotional impairment (Rabin et al., 2001).

More intensive research is required to elucidate the relationship between the MHC and non-MHC genes, the environment, and the role of any associated socioeconomic issues in the high prevalence of sarcoidosis in the Black American population.

Unclassified Disorders.   Progressive systemic sclerosis (PSS) and multiple myeloma (MM) are two disorders that do not readily fit the Gell and Coombs classification for diseases associated with hypersensitivity mechanisms. In particular, individuals with PSS may sometimes present with characteristics of other autoimmune diseases such as lupus erythematosus. This is referred to as the *overlap syndrome* (Gilliland, 2001; LeRoy et al., 1988). PSS and MM are discussed here because they primarily affect Black Americans.

Progressive Systemic Sclerosis (PSS).   PSS or scleroderma is another systemic autoimmune disorder. This disease is characterized by accretion of connective tissue in the skin and fibrosis or hardening of the internal organs.

There are two subsets of scleroderma. One is the milder, limited cutaneous scleroderma, or CREST syndrome, which primarily affects the skin and is characterized by *C*alcinosis, *R*aynaud's phenomenon, *E*sophageal dysmotility, *S*clerodactyly, and *T*elangiectasia (CREST). A more severe form of the disease, diffuse cutaneous scleroderma, causes thickening of the skin with internal organ involvement. PSS is more common in women, especially young Black women, with a female-to-male ratio of 3:1. The ratio of female-to-males affected increases during the childbearing years to approximately 8:1 (Gilliland, 2001; LeRoy et al., 1988; Mayes, 1996).

Studies indicate that the incidence of scleroderma was higher, the age of diagnosis lower, the severe diffuse cutaneous subset twice as frequent, and the age of onset earlier in young Black women when compared to White women (Laing et al., 1997; Mayes, 1996). These factors were associated with a significantly decreased survival rate seven years post diagnosis (Laing et al., 1997). Survival rates are dependent on the degree of internal organ involvement, especially the pulmonary involvement associated with the diffuse cutaneous subset. African Americans are at increased risk for pulmonary interstitial fibrosis, which is the primary cause of death in sarcoidosis (Gilliland, 2001; Greidinger et al., 1998; Kuwana et al., 1999).

Genetics of PSS.   The link between HLA antigens and the incidence of scleroderma is not strong; however, there has been some association made with the HLA-A1, -B8, -DR3, -DRB1, and HLA-DQ alleles. Some studies link disease susceptibility with C4AQ0 and HLA-DQA2 (Gilliland, 2001; Kuwana et al., 1999; LeRoy et al., 1988; Mayes, 1996). Okano (1996) reports the association of HLA-DR11 and -DQ7 with the milder CREST syndrome and the presence of HLA-DR-1, -4, and -8 with anticentromere autoantibodies seen in the CREST syndrome. Several types of autoantibodies are specifically associated with PSS, the anticentromere, anti-RNA polymerase, and anti-DNA to-poisomerase 1 (antitopo 1) or Scl-70 antibodies are designated as marker antibodies for PSS (Gil-liland, 2001; Okano, 1996). African Americans have a higher incidence of autoantibodies to DNA topoisomerase 1 (antitopo 1), which is associated with the more severe lung, skin, joint, vascular and pulmonary involvement (Greidinger et al., 1998; Mayes, 1996; Okano 1996).

Socioeconomic and Environmental Factors.   Geographic and occupation-related clustering of the disease suggests interplay between genetics and an environmental component. While no definitive agent has been identified, studies implicate exposure to silica dust (coal mines), aromatic hydrocar-bons (benzene and toluene), chemotherapeutic drugs, and residence in an industrial district (Gilliland, 2001; Mayes, 1996).

As with the other immune disorders discussed here, the development of PSS in Black Americans shows tenuous genetic associations, suggested links with environmental agents, and similar gender-related issues. The genetic predispositions seen in Black Americans with PSS are also adversely impacted by socioeconomic factors such as occupation, living conditions, and the lack of access to appropriate health care, which result in more severe morbidity and mortality.

Multiple Myeloma.   Multiple myeloma (MM) is a malignancy of the antibody-producing B-cells or plasma cells of the immune system. The disorder causes the plasma cells to manufacture large amounts of a single type of antibody, most commonly IgM or IgG. The perturbations caused by the plasma cell tumor include organ dysfunction, bone pain, fractures, anemia, increased susceptibility to infection, and renal failure (Longo, 2001).

After a steady climb during the preceding 30 years, the incidence and mortality rates for multiple myeloma in the United States peaked in the 1980s (Baris et al., 2000). The incidence is highest in men older than 40 years and is approximately twice as high in Black Americans compared to White Americans (Baris et al., 2000; Brown et al., 1997; Brown et al., 2001; Lewis et al., 1994; Longo, 2001).

While the etiology of multiple myeloma is unknown, it is suggested that there is a link to chronic antigenic stimulation (CAS), environmental factors, and socioeconomic status (SES) (Baris et al., 2000; Lewis et al., 1994; Longo, 2001). In a 1994 study Lewis and colleagues indicate no significant increase in MM among black subjects with CAS, defined as the sum of the number of childhood infections, vaccinations, allergic reactions, and autoimmune diseases. However, there was a strong correlation with allergic responses, especially to penicillin, and the development of multiple myeloma in Black men.

Genetics of Multiple Myeloma.   Results from a 1992 study by Pottern and colleagues indicate that the presence of HLA-Cw2 is positively associated with the development of multiple myeloma in both Black and White patients. HLA-Bw65, -Cw2, and -DRw-14 were present more frequently in Black MM patients when compared to Black controls. The presence of the HLA-Cw2 allele in healthy controls suggests that while people with HLA-Cw2 may have a genetic predisposition to MM, development of the disease requires the presence of unidentified environmental factors (Pottern et al., 1992).

Socioeconomic and Environmental Factors Associated with Myeloma.   Several studies indicate a correlation between development of MM and occupation-based SES. Longo (2001) reports an increased incidence in farmers, leather workers and woodworkers, and those exposed to radiation and petroleum products. Among female housekeepers who are exposed to cooking fumes and other household pollution factors, the risk of multiple myeloma was twice as high as for women with higher SES (Koessel et al., 1996).

For both Black and White subjects, education, income, and occupation-based socioeconomic status (SES) were statistically significant predictors of risk for multiple myeloma. The strongest correlation for risk of developing the disease was with occupation-based low SES. Low SES is associated with many of the environmental factors that may be implicated in multiple myeloma, such as substandard housing, increased exposure to pollutants and infectious agents, reduced access to health care, stress, and poor nutrition (Baris et al., 2000; Koessel et al., 1996).

Increased risk in Black subjects has been associated with nutritionally related factors such as obesity, reduced intake of fish and cruciferous vegetables, and reduced use of vitamin C supplements (Brown et al., 2001). In a previous study, Brown et al. (1997) report no relationship between alcohol and tobacco use and the risk of multiple myeloma.

Continued research is needed to clarify the genetic associations, the links with low SES, occupation, poor nutrition, environmental pollution, inadequate access to appropriate health care, and the development of multiple myeloma.

Immune Dysfunction and Racial Health Disparities

While the causes are elusive, the consensus is that Black Americans are genetically predisposed to developing the immunological disorders outlined above. This underlying predisposition cannot be changed; however, it is severely impacted by modifiable risk factors, which contribute to the disparities in incidence, morbidity, and mortality between Black and White Americans. These modifiable risk factors fall into two interrelated categories: socioeconomic status with the associated environment and inadequate access to appropriate medical care.

Environmental and occupational exposures are clearly linked with higher prevalence of asthma, multiple myeloma, and sarcoidosis. Urbanization carries intrinsic risks associated with poor living conditions and increased exposure to indoor pollutants, including secondhand smoke and debris from vermin and pests. However, it is possible to make improvements to urban housing conditions. Studies have shown that environmentally safe and effective methods exist for the reduction of allergens in inner-city housing units (Eggleston & Arruda, 2001; Eggleston, 1998; Eggleston et al., 1999; Platts-Mills et al., 1991).

Disparities in health-care delivery to Black Americans contribute to the severity of the symptoms and the adverse outcomes of the diseases. Black Americans are diagnosed later in the progress of these diseases, many of which have variable symptoms. These disorders require specialty care, as diagnosis may be difficult and often occurs incidental to routine physical examinations. Late diagnosis and lack of necessary specialty care are a function of financial barriers, which lead to lack of health insurance, inadequate coverage, and reduced accessibility to specialized health care. The implicit consequence of late diagnosis is disease that is more advanced, with greater morbidity, and higher death rates.

For patients who are diagnosed and who receive treatment, disparities may still exist. Physicians, for several reasons, often prescribe lower-quality, less expensive, and less effective drugs in the treatment of Black Americans (Burroughs et al., 2002; Eggleston, 1998; Halterman et al., 2002).

CONCLUSION AND RECOMMENDATIONS

The Black American population suffers disproportionately from the immunological disorders discussed above. Why should this be so, and what can be done to ameliorate the situation? The following are recommendations for reducing the disparities in incidence and severity of immunological disorders, and improving the health of Black Americans.

1. Mandated provision of improved inner-city housing conditions, by enforcing the use of appropriate, environmentally safe methods for the removal of vermin and other agents associated with immune disorders.
2. Regulated control and reduction of occupation-related health hazards.

3. Standard universal health coverage for all citizens that includes an annual physical examination, supports access to specialized care, and provides culturally relevant, easily accessible support groups for affected persons.

4. Promotion of increased awareness in the community and among physicians of the role of race and femaleness as major determinants of the disorders.

5. Inclusion of more Black Americans in studies of the interrelationship between genetics, the environment, and socioeconomic status in the development of these immunological disorders.

Clear identification of the genetic associations and the socioeconomic and the environmental factors that impact genetic predisposition and contribute to more severe outcomes in Black Americans is needed. Once identified, the issues must be addressed in order to reduce the continuing disparities in incidence, morbidity, and mortality in Black Americans with immunological disorders.

REFERENCES

Adebajo, A.O., & Davis, P. (1992). Rheumatology on the Dark Continent: Not as dark as it was. *The Journal of Rheumatology, 19(2)*, 195–197.

Adebajo, A.O., & Davis, P. (1994). Rheumatic diseases in African Blacks. *Seminars in Arthritis and Rheumatism, 24(2)*, 139–153.

Aligne, C.A., Auinger, P., Byrd, R.S., & Weitzman, M. (2000). Risk factors for pediatric asthma. Contributions of poverty, race, and urban residence. *American Journal of Respiratory and Critical Care Medicine, 162(3 Pt.1)*, 873–877.

Bach, J.F. (2002). The effect of infections on susceptibility to autoimmune and allergic diseases. *New England Journal of Medicine, 34(12)*, 911–920.

Baris, D., et al. (2000). Socioeconomic status and multiple myeloma among U.S. Blacks and Whites. *American Journal of Public Health, 90(8)*, 1277–1281.

Baughman, R.P., et al. (2001). Clinical characteristics of patients in a case control study of sarcoidosis. *American Journal of Respiratory and Critical Care Medicine, 164(10)*, 1885–1889.

Benatar, S.R. (1977). Sarcoidosis in South Africa. A comparative study in Whites, Blacks and Coloureds. *South African Medical Journal, 52(15)*, 602–606.

Braun-Fahrländer, C. et al. (2002). Environmental exposure to endotoxin and its relation to asthma in school-age children. *New England Journal of Medicine, 347(12)*, 869–877.

Britton, W. (2001). Hypersensitivity-Type IV. In I. Roitt, J. Brostoff, & D. Male (Eds.), *Immunology* (pp. 371–383). New York: Mosby.

Brodsky, F.M. (2001). Antigen presentation & the major histocompatibility complex. In T.G. Parslow, D.P. Stites, I.T. Abba, & J.B. Imboden (Eds.), *Medical Immunology* (pp. 82–94). New York: Lange Medical Books/McGraw-Hill.

Brown, L.M., et al. (1997). Multiple myeloma among Blacks and Whites in the United States: Role of cigarettes and alcoholic beverages. *Cancer Causes and Control, 8*, 610–614.

Brown, L.M., et al. (2001). Diet and nutrition as risk factors for multiple myeloma among Blacks and Whites in the United States. *Cancer Causes and Control, 12(2)*, 117–125.

Bruce, I.N., & Laskin, C.A. (1997). Sex hormones in systemic lupus erythematosus: A controversy for modern times. *The Journal of Rheumatology, 24(8)*, 1461–1463.

Burroughs, V.J., Maxey, R.W., & Levy, R.A. (2002). Racial and ethnic differences in response to medicines: Towards individualized pharmaceutical treatment. *Journal of the National Medical Association, 94(10 Suppl.)*, 1–26.

Call, R.S., Smith, T.F., Morris, E., Chapman, M.D., & Platts-Mills, T.A. (1992). Risk factors for asthma in inner city children. *Journal of Pediatrics, 121(6)*, 862–866.

Cooke, A. (2001). Regulation of the immune response. In I. Roitt, J. Brostoff, & D. Male (Eds.), *Immunology* (pp. 173–189). New York: Mosby.

Cooper, G.S., et al. (2002). Differences by race, sex and age in the clinical and immunological features of recently diagnosed systemic lupus erythematosus patients in the southeastern United States. *Lupus, 11(3)*, 161–167.

Cooper, W.O., & Hickson, G.B. (2001). Corticosteroid prescription filling for children covered by Medicaid following an emergency department visit for hospitalization for asthma. *Archives of Pediatrics and Adolescent Medicine, 155(10)*, 1111–1115.

Crater, et al., (2001). Asthma hospitalization trends in Charleston, South Carolina, 1956 to 1997: Twenty-fold increase among black children during a 30-year period. *Pediatrics, 108(6)*, E 97.

Crystal, R.G. (2001). Sarcoidosis. In E. Braunwald, A.S. Fauci, D.L. Kasper, S.L. Hauser, D.L. Longo, & J.L. Jameson (Eds.), *Harrison's principles of internal medicine* (pp. 1969–1974). New York: McGraw-Hill, Medical Publishing Division.

Cutolo, M. & Wilder, R.L. (2000). Different roles for androgens and estrogens in the susceptibility to auto-immune rheumatic diseases. [Electronic Version]. *Rheumatic Disease Clinics of North America, 26(4)*.

DeLeo, V., et al. (2002). The effect of race and ethnicity on patch test results. *Journal of the American Academy of Dermatology, 46(2 Suppl)*, S107–112.

Diaz, T., et al. (2000). Medication use among children with asthma in East Harlem. *Pediatrics, 105(6)*, 1188.

Dickel, H., Taylor, J.S., Evey, P., & Merk, H.F. (2001). Comparison of patch test results with a standard series among White and Black racial groups. *Am J Contact Dermat, 12(2)*, 77–82.

Eggleston, P.A. (1998). Urban children and asthma. *Immunology and Allergy Clinics of North America, 18(1)*, 75–84.

Eggleston, P.A., & Arruda, L.K. (2001). Ecology and elimination of cockroaches and allergens in the home. *Journal of Allergy and Clinical Immunology, 107(3 Suppl)*, S422–429.

Eggleston, P.A., Wood, R.A., Rand, C., Nixon, W.J., Chen, P.H., & Lukk, P. (1999). Removal of cockroach allergen from inner-city homes. *Journal of Allergy and Clinical Immunology, 104(4 Pt 1)*, 842–846.

Elford, J., Fitch, P., Kaminski, E., McGavin, C., & Wells, I.P. (2000). Five cases of sarcoidosis in one family: a new immunological link? *Thorax, 55*, 343–344. Retrieved 11/21/2002 from http://thorax.bmjjournals.com/cgi/content/full/55/4/343.

English, J.C., Patel, P.J., & Greer, K.E. (2001). Sarcoidosis. *Journal of the American Academy of Dermatology, 44 (5)*, 725–743.

Floyd, J.L. Thyrotoxicosis. *eMedicine Journal, 3(6)*. 6-21-2002. Retrieved 7/23/2002, from http://www.emedicine.com/radio/topic315.htm.

Gedalia, A., Molina, J.F., Molina, J., Uribe, O., Malagon, C., & Espinoza, L.R. (1999). Childhood-onset systemic lupus erythematosus: A comparative study of African-Americans and Latin Americans. *Journal of the National Medical Association, 91(9)*, 497–501.

Gilliland, B.C. (2001). Systemic sclerosis (scleroderma). In E. Braunwald, A.S. Fauci, D.L. Kasper, S.L. Hauser, D.L. Longo, & J.L. Jameson (Eds.), *Harrison's principles of internal medicine* (pp. 1937–1947). New York: McGraw-Hill.

Goldsby, R.A., Kindt, T.J., & Osborne, B.A. (2000). *Kuby immunology*. New York: W.H. Freeman and Company.

Gould, K.P., & Callen, J.P. (2001) Sarcoidosis. *eMedicine Journal, 2(12)*. Retrieved 7/23/2002 from http://www.emedicine.com/derm/topic381.htm.

Greenwood, B.M., & Wittle, H.C. (1981). *Immunology of medicine in the tropics*. London: Spottiswoode and Ballantyne.

Greidinger, E.L., Flaherty, K.T., White, B., Rosen, A., Wigley, F.M., & Wise, R.A. (1998). African-American race and antibodies to topoisomerase I are associated with increased severity of scleroderma lung disease. *Chest, 114(3)*, 801–807.

Hahn, B.H. (2001). Systemic Lupus Erythematosus. In E. Braunwald, A.S. Fauci, D.L. Kasper, S.L. Hauser, D.L. Longo, & J.L. Jameson (Eds.), *Harrison's principles of internal medicine* (pp. 1922–1928). New York: McGraw-Hill.

Halterman, J.S., et al. (2002). Providers underestimate symptom severity among urban children with asthma. *Archives of Pediatrics and Adolescent Medicine, 156(2)*, 141–146.

Hay, F., & Westwood, O.M.R. (2001). Hypersensitivity-Type III. In I. Roitt, J. Brostoff, & D. Male (Eds.), *Immunology* (pp. 357–369). New York: Mosby.

Hosoda, Y., Yamaguchi, M., & Hiraga, Y. (1997). Global epidemiology of sarcoidosis: What story do prevalence and incidence tell us? *Clinics in Chest Medicine, 18(4)*, 681–694.

Israel, H.L., Gottlieb, J.E., & Peters, S.P. (1997). The importance of ethnicity in the diagnosis and prognosis of sarcoidosis. *Chest, 111(4)*, 839–840.

Janeway, C.A., & Travers, P., with Hunt, S., & Walport, M. (2001). *Immunobiology: The immune system in health and disease.* New York: Current Biology/Garland.

Joseph, C.L.M., Havstad, S.L., Ownby, D.R., Johnson, C.C., & Tilley, B.C. (1998). Racial differences in emergency department use persist despite allergist visits and prescriptions filled for antiinflammatory medications. *Journal of Allergy and Clinical Immunology, 101(4)*, 484–490.

Joseph, C.L.M., Ownby, D.R., Peterson, E.L., & Johnson, C.C. (2000). Racial differences in physiologic parameters related to asthma among middle-class children. *Chest, 117(5)*, 1336–1344.

Julkunen, H.A. (1991). Oral contraceptives in systemic lupus erythematosus: Side-effects and influence on the activity of SLE. *Scand J Rheumatol, 20*, 427–433.

Kajdasz, D.K., Judson, M.A., Mohr, L.C., & Lackland, D.T. (1999). Geographic variation in sarcoidosis in South Carolina: its relation to socioeconomic status and health care indicators. *American Journal of Epidemiology, 150(3)*, 271–278.

Kerdel, F.A., & Moschella, S.L. (1984). Sarcoidosis. *Journal of the American Academy of Dermatology, 11 (1)*, 1–19.

Knight, J.M., Eliopoulos, C., Klein, J., Greenwald, M., & Koren, G. (1996). Passive smoking in children: Racial differences in systemic exposure to cotinine by hair and urine analysis. *Chest, 109(2)*, 446–450.

Koessel, S.L., Theis, M.K., Vaughan, T.L., Koepsell, T.D., Weiss, N.S., Greenberg, R.S., & Swanson, G.M. (1996). Socioeconomic status and the incidence of multiple myeloma. *Epidemiology, 7 (1)*, 4–8.

Kuster, P.A. (1996). Reducing risk of house dust mite and cockroach allergen exposure in inner-city children with asthma. *Pediatric Nursing 22 (4)*, 297–303.

Kuwana, M., Kaburaki, J., Arnett, F.C., Howard, R.F., Medsger, T.A., & Wright, T.M. (1999). Influence of ethnic background on clinical and serologic features in patients with systemic sclerosis and anti-DNA topoisomerase I antibody. *Arthritis Rheumatism, 42 (3)*, 465–474.

Lahita, R.G. (2000). Gender and the immune system. *The Journal of Gender Specific Medicine, 3(7)*, 19–22.

Laing, T.J. et al. (1997). Racial differences in scleroderma among women in Michigan. *Arthritis Rheumatism, 40(4)*, 734–742.

LeRoy, C.E., et al. (1988). Scleroderma (systemic sclerosis): Classification, subsets and pathogenesis. *The Journal of Rheumatology, 15(2)*, 202–205.

Lewis, D.R. et al. (1994). Multiple myeloma among Blacks and Whites in the United States: The role of chronic antigenic stimulation. *Cancer Causes and Control, 5*, 529–539.

Lieu, T.A., Lozano, P., Finkelstein, J.A., Chi, F.W., Jensvold, N.G., & Capra, A.M. (2002). Racial/ethnic variation in asthma status and management practices among children in managed Medicaid. *American Academy of Pediatrics, 109(5)*, 857–865.

Longo, D.L. (2001). Plasma cell disorders. In E. Braunwald, A.S. Fauci, D.L. Kasper, S.L. Hauser, D.L. Longo, & J.L. Jameson (Eds.), *Harrison's principles of internal medicine* (pp. 727–733). New York: McGraw-Hill.

Maliarik, M.J. et al. (1998). Analysis of HLA-DPB1 polymorphisms in African-Americans with sarcoidosis. *American Journal of Respiratory and Critical Care Medicine, 158(1)*, 111–114.

Maliarik, M.J. et al. (2000). The natural resistance-associated macrophage protein gene in African Americans with sarcoidosis. *American Journal of Respiratory Cell and Molecular Biology, 22(6)*, 672–675.

Mannino, D.M., Homa, D.M., Akinbami, L.J., Moorman, J.E., Gwynn, C., & Redd, S.C. *Surveillance for asthma—United States, 1980–1999.* (2002). Division of Environmental Hazards and Health Effects, National Center for Environmental Health: (MMWR 51 (SS01), 1–13. March 29, 2002). Centers for Disease Control. Available at http://www.cdc.gov/mmwr/preview/mmwrhtml/ss5101a1.htm Retrieved 6/26/2002.

Manzi, S. (2001). Epidemiology of systemic lupus erythematosus. *American Journal of Management Care, 7(16 Suppl)*, S474–479.

Mayes, M.D. (1996). Scleroderma epidemiology. *Rheumatic Disease Clinics of North America, 22(4)*, 751–764.

McCarty, D.J., Manzi, S., Medsger, T.A., Ramsey-Goldman, R., LaPorte, R.E., & Kwoh, C.K. (1995). Incidence of systemic lupus erythematosus. Race and gender differences. *Arthritis Rheumatism, 38(9)*, 1260–1270.

Molina, J.F., Molina, J., Garcia, C., Gharavi, A.E., Wilson, W.A., & Espinoza, L.R. (1997). Ethnic differences in the clinical expression of systemic lupus erythematosus: A comparative study between African Americans and Latin Americans. *Lupus, 6*, 63–67.

Newsome, F., & Choudhuri, S.B.G. (1984). Sarcoid in a Nigerian: Geographical variation of the frequency of sarcoid among Blacks considered. *Transactions of the Royal Society of Tropical Medicine and Hygiene, 78*, 663–664.

Odeke, S., & Nagelberg, S.B. (2002). Hashimoto Thyroiditis. *eMedicine Journal, 3(4)*. Retrieved 7/23/2002 from http://www.emedicine.com/MED/topic949.htm.

Okano, Y. (1996). Antinuclear antibody in systemic sclerosis (scleroderma). *Rheumatic Disease Clinics of North America, 22(4)*, 709–729.

Ortega, A.N., & Calderon, J.G. (2000). Pediatric asthma among minority populations. *Current Opinion in Pediatrics, 12(6)*, 579–583.

Petri, M. (1998). The effect of race on incidence and clinical course in systemic lupus erythematosus: The Hopkins lupus cohort. *Journal of American Medical Womens Association, 53(1 winter)*, 9–12.

Platts-Mills, T. (2001). Hypersensitivity-Type I. In I. Roitt, J. Brostoff, & D. Male (Eds.), *Immunology* (pp. 324–343). New York: Mosby.

Platts-Mills, T., Ward, G.W., Sporik, R., Gelber, L.E., Chapman, M.D., & Heymann, P.W. (1991). Epidemiology of the relationship between exposure to indoor allergens and asthma. *International Archives of Allergy and Applied Immunology, 94(1–4)*, 339–345.

Pongracic, J., & Evans, R. (2001). Environmental and socioeconomic risk factors in asthma. *Immunology and Allergy Clinics of North America, 21(3)*, 413–426.

Pottern, L.M., Gart, J.J., Nam, J., Dunston, G., Wilson, J., & Greenberg, R. (1992). HLA and multiple myeloma among Black and White men: Evidence of a genetic association. *Cancer Epidemiology, Biomarkers & Prevention, 1*, 177–182.

Rabin, D.L., Richardson, M.S., Stein, S.R., & Yeager, H. (2001). Sarcoidosis severity and socioeconomic status. *European Respiratory Journal, 18(3)*, 499–506.

Rand, C.S., Butz, A.M., Kolodner, K., Huss, K., Eggleston, P., & Malveaux, F. (2000). Emergency department visits by urban African American children with asthma. *Journal of Allergy and Clinical Immunology, 105*, 83–90.

Rauh, V.A., Chew, G.R., & Garfinkel, R.S. (2002). Deteriorated housing contributes to high cockroach allergen levels in inner-city households. *Environtal Health Perspectives, 110(Suppl 2)*, 323–327.

Roitt, I. (2001). Autoimmunity and autoimmune disease. In I. Roitt, J. Brostoff, & D. Male (Eds.), *Immunology* (pp. 385–415). New York: Mosby.

Roitt, I., Brostoff, J., & Male, D. (1985). *Immunology*. St. Louis: C.V. Mosby Company.

Rosen, F.S. (2001). Primary immunodeficiency. In I. Roitt, J. Brostoff, & D. Male (Eds.), *Immunology* (pp. 303–311). New York: Mosby.

Rybicki, B.A. (1997). Racial differences in sarcoidosis incidence: A 5-year study in health maintenance. *American Journal of Epidemiology, 145(3)*, 234–241.

Rybicki, B.A., et al. (1999). The influence of T cell receptor and cytokine genes on sarcoidosis susceptibility in African Americans. *Human Immunology, 60(9)*, 867–874.

Rybicki, B.A., et al. (2001). Familial aggregation of sarcoidosis. *American Journal of Respiratory and Critical Care Medicine, 164(11)*, 2085–2091.

Sack, K.E., & Fye, K.H. (2001). Rheumatic diseases. In T.G. Parslow, D.P. Stites, A.I. Terr, & J.B. Imboden (Eds.), *Medical immunology* (pp. 401–421). New York: Lange Medical Books/McGraw-Hill.

Sacks, J.J., et al. Trends in death from systemic lupus erythematosus-United States, 1979–1998. *Morbidity & Mortality Weekly Report, 51(17)*, 371–374. May 3, 2002. Centers for Disease Control (CDC). Available at http://www.cdc.gov/mmwr/preview/mmwrhtml/mm5117a3.htm. Retrieved 6/26/2002.

Sanchez-Guerrero, J., Liang, M.H., Karlson, E.W., Hunter, D.J., & Colditz, G.A. (1995). Postmenopausal estrogen therapy and the risk for developing systemic lupus erythematosus. *Annals of Internal Medicine, 122(6)*, 430–433.

Sarcoidosis among U.S. Navy enlisted men 1965–1993. (1997) *MMWR 46(23)*, 539–543., June 13, 1997.

Centers for Disease Control (CDC). Available at http://www.cdc.gov/mmwr/preview/mmwrhtml/0047925.htm. Retrieved 11/6/2002.

Sarpong, S.B., Hamilton, R.G., Eggleston, P.A., & Adkinson, N.F. (1996). Socioeconomic status and race as risk factors for cockroach allergen exposure and sensitization in children with asthma. *Journal of Allergy and Clinical Immunology, 97(6)*, 1393–1401.

Scofield, R.L., & Sadanandan, P. (2001). Arthritis as a manifestation of systemic disease. *eMedicine Journal 2(10)*. Retrieved 7/23/2002 from http://www.emedicine.com/med/topic3099.htm.

Sigal, L.H. (1994). Autoimmune diseases: Systemic and organ specific. In L.H. Sigal & Y. Ron (Eds.), *Immunology and inflammation: Basic mechanisms and clinical consequences* (pp. 599–619). New York: McGraw-Hill. Health Professions Division.

Sigal, L.H., & Ron, Y. (1994). Introduction. In L.H. Sigal & Y. Ron (Eds.), *Immunology and inflammation: Basic mechanisms and clinical consequences* (pp. xxi–xxiv). New York: McGraw-Hill, Health Professions Division.

Smikle, M. et al. (2002). HLA-DRB alleles and systemic lupus erythematosus in Jamaicans. *Southern Medical Journal, 95(7)*, 717–719.

Stevenson, L.A., Gergen, P.J., Hoover, D.R., Rosenstreich, D., Mannino, D.M., & Matte, T.D. (2001). Sociodemographic correlates of indoor allergen sensitivity among United States children. *Journal of Allergy and Clinical Immunology, 108(5)*, 747–752.

Sullivan, K.E. (2000). Genetics of systemic lupus erythematosus. *Rheumatic Disease Clinics of North America, 26(2)*, 103–115.

Terr, A.I. (2001). The atopic diseases. In T.G. Parslow, D.P. Stites, A.I. Terr, & J.B. Imboden (Eds.), *Medical immunology* (pp. 349–369). New York: Lange Medical Books/Division of McGraw-Hill.

Thomas, S.D., & Whitman, S. (1999). Asthma hospitalization and mortality in Chicago. *Chest, 116(4)*, 135–141.

Torrington, K.G., Shorr, A.F., & Parker, J.W. (1997). Endobrachial disease and racial differences in pulmonary sarcoidosis. *Chest, 111(3)*, 619–622.

Walsh, S.J., Algert, C., Gregorio, D.I., Reisine, S.T., & Rothfield, N.F. (1995). Divergent racial trends in mortality from systemic lupus erythematosus. *Journal of Rheumatology, 22(9)*, 1663–1668.

Walsh, S.J., Algert, C., & Rothfield, N.F. (1996). Racial aspects of comorbidity in systemic lupus erythematosus. *Arthritis Care and Research, 9(6)*, 509–516.

Weiss, S.T. (2002). Eat Dirt—the hygiene hypothesis and allergic diseases. *New England Journal of Medicine, 347(12)*, 930–931.

Weller, I. (2001). Secondary immunodeficiency. In I. Roitt, J. Brostoff & D. Male (Eds.), *Immunology* (pp. 313–322). London: Mosby.

Wilson, W.A., Scopelitis, E., & Michalski, J.P. (1984). Association of HLA-DR7 with both antibody to SSA (Ro) and disease susceptibility in Blacks with systemic lupus erythematosus. *Journal of Rheumatology, 11(5)*, 653–657.

CHAPTER 12

Oral Health Status and Disparities in Black Americans

YOLANDA ANN SLAUGHTER AND
JOAN L. GLUCH

INTRODUCTION

The range of oral, dental, and craniofacial diseases and conditions that affect the U.S. population is extensive. There would be scarce dispute that the mouth and face are essential parts of the human body. Yet, there is a tapering consensus regarding the value of oral health care toward maintaining a healthy body. In part, these views are supported by a lack of awareness of the links that exist between oral health conditions and one's overall health status. This perceptual separation of oral health care from general health care not only affects health care decisions on an individual and provider level but also plays a role in health care infrastructure decisions. The saying "put your money where your mouth is" has little merit when comparing the nation's health-care expenditures for medical care services to dental care services (see Figure 12.1).

The first Surgeon General's Report on Oral Health in America released by U.S. surgeon general David Satcher provides a comprehensive description of the interconnectedness of oral health with general health (U.S. Department of Health and Human Services [USDHHS], 2000a). This landmark government publication also proclaims the message that disparities in oral diseases cause needless pain and suffering, adding financial and social costs that diminish quality of life. The report describes oral diseases as a "silent epidemic" that disproportionately affects poor children, the elderly, and members of racial and ethnic minorities, particularly Black Americans.

Public health initiatives such as community water fluoridation have significantly improved the oral health of Americans. The shift in the philosophy of dental care toward an emphasis on prevention has also positively influenced the public's oral health. These advances in dentistry have resulted in a substantial decline in the rates of tooth loss over the past 20 years and reduced dental decay over the past 30 years (Marcus et al., 1996; Evans & Kleinman, 2000). However, these advances mask differences in oral health status among Black Americans. For example, Black Americans experience more dental decay than the national average. At age 2 to 4 years, 22 percent of Black American children have untreated dental decay as compared to 16 percent of children nationwide, and at age 15 years, 29 percent of Black American adolescents have decay as compared to 20 percent of children nationwide, and at age 35 to 44 years, 46 percent of Black American adults have decay as compared with 27 percent of adults nationwide (USDHHS, 2000a).

Figure 12.1
Dental services as a percentage of total U.S. health-care
expenditures by type of service, 1997

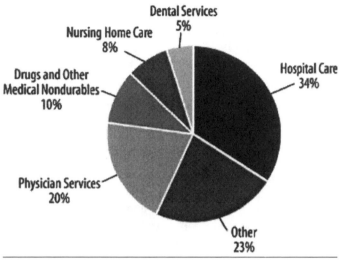

Source: USDHHS, 2000a; USDHHS, 2000b.

To further complicate this issue of disparity, culturally competent, community-based preventive programs are unavailable to substantial portions of the underserved populations (USDHHS, 2000a). To address the problem, Healthy People 2010 presents a comprehensive set of national health objectives and provides a model for developing and implementing health promotion interventions (USDHHS, 2000b). As with health disparities in general, oral health disparities are linked to social, behavioral, environmental, and biological factors. This broader focus on oral health, rather than dental disease, reflects a biopsychosocial model in the causes and prevention of oral diseases and offers many opportunities to promote health at the individual, family, and community level.

THE RELATIONSHIP OF ORAL HEALTH TO OTHER DISEASES

The health of the craniofacial tissues provides a unique opportunity to assess general health status. The mouth has been described as a mirror for the body, and a variety of nutritional disturbances and pathologic findings can be detected from a thorough examination of the head, neck, and mouth. For example, diabetic patients often show increased susceptibility and presence of periodontal diseases, and periodontal problems have been shown to increase complications related to blood glucose and hemoglobin control (Grossi & Genco, 1998; Salvi et al., 1997). Patients with HIV/AIDS and other immunodeficient disorders also are susceptible to more severe forms of periodontal disease and frequently display increased candida (thrush) infections and other oral lesions (Dodd et al., 1991; Klein et al., 1984). Oral complications associated with HIV/AIDS significantly affect general health because they result in mouth pain, loss of appetite, weight loss, and often life-threatening candida (thrush) infections. Recently completed research studies have shown preliminary associations between chronic periodontal infections and premature birth, low birth weight babies, and heart disease (Beck et al., 1998; Genco, 1998; Offenbacher et al., 1996; Offenbacher et al., 1998). To date, none of these studies have examined any disparities along racial lines; however, both diabetes and HIV/AIDS disproportionately affect Black American individuals.

A healthy oral health status goes beyond restoring diseased teeth or replacing missing teeth, and this awareness has the potential to influence perceptions of overall health and well-being on an individual and health-care provider level and can serve to challenge the infrastructure of health care on a societal level. This chapter presents the scope of racial disparities regarding common oral health problems and associated oral-systemic health connections. "Oral Health in America: A Report of the Surgeon General" (USDHHS, 2000a) and Healthy People 2010 (USDHHS, 2000b), provides the framework for discussion. More specifically, the chapter includes a discussion on the following topics: dental caries; tooth loss and edentulism; periodontal disease; and oral cancer.

DENTAL CARIES

Description

Cavities, or dental decay, are popular terms that refer to the most common oral disease, dental caries. Dental caries is a bacterial infection in the hard tooth structures, which are enamel and dentin. Dental caries is initiated by the reaction between bacteria in the plaque biofilm and dietary carbohydrates that form acid directly next to the tooth. Although most people know that the sugar in candy will help cause decay, the sugars in refined carbohydrate foods like juices and potato chips will cause caries also. The acid from the bacterial reaction seeps into the tooth surfaces and demineralizes enamel, beginning inside the tooth surface. Continued acid demineralization destroys tooth enamel and, if left undisturbed, progresses both outward to break through to the tooth surface, causing a cavity, and travels inward to expose the nerve inside the tooth, causing toothache. Saliva in the mouth helps to buffer the acids, and patients with reduced saliva due to illness, injury, or medication usage show higher decay rates (USDHHS, 2000c; Harris & Garcia-Godoy, 1999).

Preventing caries is a multifaceted activity, and approaches at both the community and personal levels have been shown effective in reducing caries experience (Burt & Eklund, 1999). Caries prevention activities at the community level have emphasized fluoridation of public water supplies and dental treatment programs including preventive and therapeutic care, particularly at schools and institutions and educational programs. Caries prevention activities at the personal level involve increasing behaviors in four areas: use of topical fluoride products, such as toothpaste, gels, and mouth rinses; reduction of bacterial biofilm by brushing, flossing, and chemical rinses; reduction of sugar and carbohydrate consumption; and increased visits to the dental office, particularly for application of preventive agents, such as fluoride and sealants. Two promising preventive approaches for both personal and community efforts involve reducing tooth susceptibility by placing pit and fissure sealants to block susceptible tooth grooves and also by providing topical fluoride to remineralize tooth structure and reduce dental decay.

Epidemiology

Dental decay is one of the most common diseases of childhood, and decay experience increases with age through to adulthood. Dental caries is five times more common than asthma and seven times more common than hay fever (USDHHS, 2000b). Although there has been a continued decline in dental caries experience among schoolchildren in the last 50 years, dental caries remains a persistent and significant problem for all children. The majority of children age five to nine (51.6 percent) have at least one tooth with decay, and by age 17, the decay experience rises to 77.9 percent of children. Black children experience higher decay rates than the national average, especially at age 15 and older (USDHHS, 2000b; Vargas et al., 1998; Kaste et al., 1996). Table 12.1 details the dental caries experience of children and adolescents at selected ages based on race and ethnicity, and Table 12.2 pro-

Table 12.1
Dental caries experience for children and adolescents at selected ages

Children and Adolescents, Selected Ages, 1988–94 (unless noted)	Dental Caries Experience		
	21-1a. Aged 2 to 4 Years	21-1b. Aged 6 to 8 Years	21-1c. Aged 15 Years
	Percent		
TOTAL	18	52	61
Race and ethnicity			
American Indian or Alaska Native	76* (1999)	90* (1999)	89* (1999)
Asian or Pacific Islander	DSU	DSU	DSU
Asian	34† (1993–94)	90† (1993–94)	DSU† (1993–94)
Native Hawaiian and other Pacific Islander	DNC	79‡ (1999)	DNC
Black or African American	24	50	70
White	15	51	60
Hispanic or Latino	DSU	DSU	DSU
Mexican American	27	68	57
Not Hispanic or Latino	17	49	62
Black or African American	24	49	69
White	13	49	61
Gender			
Female	19	54	63
Male	18	50	60
Education level (head of household)			
Less than high school	29	65	59
High school graduate	18	52	63
At least some college	12	43	61
Disability status			
Persons with disabilities	DNC	DNC	DNC
Persons without disabilities	DNC	DNC	DNC
Select populations			
3rd grade students	NA	60	NA

DNA = Data have not been analyzed. DNC = Data are not collected. DSU = Data are statistically unreliable. NA = Not applicable. *Data are for IHS service areas. †Data are for California. ‡Data are for Hawaii.

Source: USDHHS (2000a), *Healthy People 2010*, Chapter 21, pp. 12–13.

Table 12.2
Untreated dental decay of children, adolescents, and adults

Children, Adolescents, and Adults, Selected Ages, 1988–94 (unless noted)	Untreated Dental Decay			
	21-2a. Aged 2 to 4 Years	21-2b. Aged 6 to 8 Years	21-2c. Aged 15 Years	21-2d. Aged 35 to 44 Years
	Percent			
TOTAL	16	29	20	27
Race and ethnicity				
American Indian or Alaska Native	67* (1999)	69* (1999)	67* (1999)	67* (1999)
Asian or Pacific Islander	DSU	DSU	DSU	DSU
Asian†	30† (1993–94)	71† (1993–94)	DSU† (1993–94)	DNC
Native Hawaiian and other Pacific Islander	DNC	39‡ (1999)	DNC	DNC
Black or African American	22	36	29	46
White	11	26	19	24
Hispanic or Latino	DSU	DSU	DSU	DSU
Mexican American	24	43	27	34
Not Hispanic or Latino	14	26	19	DNA
Black or African American	22	35	28	47
White	11	22	18	23
Gender				
Female	16	32	22	25
Male	16	25	17	29
Education level (head of household)				
Less than high school	26	44	29	51
High school graduate	16	30	18	34
At least some college	9	25	15	16
Disability status				
Persons with disabilities	DNC	DNC	DNC	DNA
Persons without disabilities	DNC	DNC	DNC	DNA
Select populations				
3rd grade students	NA	33	NA	NA

DNA = Data have not been analyzed. DNC = Data are not collected. DSU = Data are statistically unreliable. NA = Not applicable. *Data are for IHS service areas. †Data are for California. ‡Data are for Hawaii.

Source: USDHHS (2000a), *Healthy People 2010*, Chapter 21, p. 16.

vides data illustrating the number of children and adults with untreated dental decay. However, caution should rule when reviewing these summary charts, because there are no data to indicate the race alone is a factor in differential susceptibility to dental decay. Rather, sociodemographic factors, such as access to care, level of education and income, and attitudes and beliefs, must be considered when analyzing susceptibility to dental decay (Vargas et al., 1998).

Teeth are susceptible to dental decay at any age, and young children are especially vulnerable to early childhood caries (ECC), which is a particularly destructive form of dental decay seen in children between 18 and 36 months of age. Research has associated ECC with transmission of streptococcus mutans bacteria from caregiver's (usually the mother's) saliva that occurs as early as 12 months (Milnes, 1996). ECC has also been termed "baby bottle caries," because it has been associated with feeding practices in which juice, milk, or formula from a bottle is allowed to pool in the mouth overnight. The sugars in these beverages mix with bacteria and produce destructive dental decay, especially around the upper front teeth. ECC has also been associated with blockage of saliva flow during feeding, altered salivary composition due to medication or malnourishment, and arrested tooth development (Milnes, 1996). Between age two and four years, 24 percent of Black children have experienced dental decay, as compared with the national average of 18 percent (USDHHS, 2000a; 2000b; Vargas et al., 1998; Kaste et al., 1996). Many of these children do not receive the dental care that they need, because studies show that 22 percent of Black children have untreated dental decay as compared with the national average of 16 percent (USDHHS, 2000b; 2000c; Vargas et al., 1998; Kaste et al., 1996).

At age 6, the permanent teeth start to erupt into the mouth and continue until the second molars are present in the mouth at age 12, with the third molars variable in their presentation in the mouth. In the past 30 years, the incidence of dental decay in the permanent teeth of children between the ages of 6 and 17 has declined dramatically. However, not all children have shared in these positive health statistics, because oral health status varies based on sociodemographic factors. Dental caries experience and untreated dental decay increase with age, and racial disparities persist. For children age 6 to 8 years, 50 percent of Black children and 51 percent of White children have experienced dental decay, which shows a similar level of disease rates. However, 36 percent of Black children age 6 to 8 years old have untreated dental decay as opposed to 29 percent of the national average, which is a significant disparity. Unfortunately, dental decay progresses over time, so that Black children have more severe dental disease that results in a high level of tooth loss in adulthood. The racial disparity widens as children age, because at age 15, 70 percent of Black children have experienced dental decay as compared with the national average of 61 percent, and 29 percent of Black children have untreated dental decay as compared with the national average of 20 percent (USDHHS, 2000b, 2000c; Vargas et al., 1998; Kaste et al., 1996).

Both dental decay experience and untreated dental decay increases with age, and older adults have the highest rates of dental decay both on the crown and the root surfaces of teeth. For example, 50 percent of men over 65 and women over 75 have decay on at least one root surface. Racial disparities increase into adulthood, with 46 percent of Black adults with untreated dental decay as compared with 27 percent of the national population. However, education plays a more significant role, because only 16 percent of individuals with some college education have untreated dental decay as opposed to 51 percent of individuals with less than a high school education have untreated dental decay (USDHHS, 2000b; National Institute of Dental and Craniofacial Research [NIDCR], 1986).

Comorbidities

For both adults and older adults, the quality and quantity of saliva in the mouth are associated with higher rates of dental decay. Saliva quantity is decreased as a common side effect of many

Table 12.3
Percent of persons aged 65 years of age and older who had a dental visit in the past year by race and educational level, 1997

	Dentate	Edentulous	All Persons
Total			
	70%	18%	54%
Race/ethnicity			
Non-Hispanic White	74	18	57
Non-Hispanic Black	46	17	38
Hispanic	58	22	45
Education			
Less than 12 years	52	16	39
12 years	75	18	57
More than 12 years	82	29	76

Note: Dentate persons have at least one natural tooth.

Source: National Health Interview Survey, 1997; Vargas et al., 2001.

medications, including antidepressants, antihistamines, and antihypertensives and also when radiation to the head and neck destroys salivary gland tissue. Some diseases inhibit or destroy salivary gland function, and unless patients follow strict preventive measures, dental decay rates are high (Harris & Garcia-Godoy, 1999).

TOOTH LOSS AND EDENTULISM

Description

The perception that total tooth loss, or edentulism, is a natural occurrence of the aging process is no longer a prevailing view among Americans. The expectation to retain all or most of one's natural teeth for a lifetime is increasingly plausible. For example, the "Baby Boomer" generation, the first cohort to appreciably benefit from the effects of community water fluoridation and conservative dental treatment, will retain most of their natural dentition with increasing age. Foremost, the shift in dental treatment philosophies from an extraction-based practice to a prevention model has dramatically influenced tooth loss among the American population (Berkey & Berg, 2001). The reasons for tooth loss are not solely linked to the consequences of oral disease, although most teeth are lost due to dental caries and periodontal disease (USDHHS, 2000b). Other correlates include socioeconomic factors, geographic region, individual oral health beliefs regarding the value of retaining natural teeth, and attitudes toward dentistry concomitant with perceptions of dental providers. In turn, these factors influence the use of dental services. (Burt & Eklund, 1999; Tomar, 1999). In 1997, endentulous persons were much less likely to report having visited a dentist in the previous year than were dentate persons, or persons with their natural teeth (Vargas et al., 2001) (see Table 12.3).

Status in the United States

The prevalence of tooth loss and endentulism increases with age and shows distinct cohort effects. Data from national surveys over the past 20 years show the percentage of adults without any teeth

Figure 12.2
The percentage of people without any teeth has declined among adults over the past 20 years

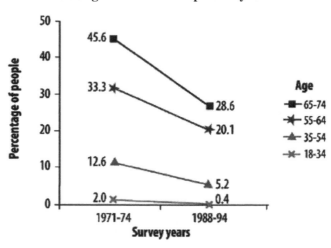

Source: NCHS, 1975; 1996; USDHHS, 2000b.

has consistently declined across age groups (USDHHS, 2000) (see Figure 12.2). These age-cohort differences have, in part, been influenced by technologic advances in restorative dentistry; more positive attitudes toward tooth retention; and third-party payment for dental care (Berkey & Berg, 2001; Burt & Eklund, 1999). Regarding gender, men and women are equally likely to be edentulous (USDHHS, 2000b).

Edentulism is also strongly influenced by socioeconomic level, education level, and geographic region. Data from the 1995–1997 Behavioral Risk Factor Surveillance System (BRFSS) indicate edentulism was more prevalent among persons 65 years and older; more prevalent among persons with less than a high school education than among those with more education; and more prevalent among those without dental insurance than among those who had insurance (Tomar, 1999). Edentulism rates vary by state and region of the country, with higher rates generally seen in the southeastern portion of the United States (Tomar, 1999).

Racial Disparities

Data from NHANES III (years 1988–1991) indicate that the rates of edentulism for adults (aged 18–75+ years) was slightly higher among Whites than Black Americans (Marcus et al., 1996). State-based and national data for 1997 show that edentulism was more prevalent among Black Americans than among Whites aged 65 years and older (Tomar, 1999; USDHHS, 2000b) (see Table 12.4). Although national studies indicate slight variations in the degree of edentulism across age groups, there are variations in tooth retention among White and Black Americans. Whites did not differ from Black Americans in the percentage dentate, or retaining some natural teeth; however, Whites were much more likely to retain all of their natural teeth than Black Americans (Marcus et al., 1996).

CoMorbidities

The prevalence of tooth loss and edentulism increases with age. Edentulism and tooth loss can affect the ability to chew certain foods, which may limit food choices and contribute to undernutrition

Table 12.4

Percentage of persons aged >+65 years who reported having lost all their natural teeth, by selected characteristics

Characteristic	size+	%	(95% CI&)
Sex			
Men	3420	23.6	(+/- 2.0)
Women	6282	24.9	(+/- 1.6)
Age group (yrs)			
65-74	5646	22.9	(+/- 1.6)
>=75	4056	26.7	(+/- 2.0)
Education level			
Less than high school graduate	2437	42.1	(+/- 2.9)
High school graduate	3391	25.1	(+/- 2.2)
Some college	2166	17.1	(+/- 2.2)
College graduate	1662	10.1	(+/- 2.0)
Dental insurance status			
Insured	2670	18.3	(+/- 2.0)
Uninsured	6855	27.0	(+/- 1.4)
Race/Ethnicity			
Non-Hispanic white	8539	24.1	(+/- 1.2)
Non-Hispanic black	641	31.9	(+/- 5.1)
Hispanic	352	18.2	(+/- 5.3)
Other	134	26.2	(+/-12.5)
Cigarette smoking status			
Current, every day	919	41.3	(+/- 4.5)
Current, some days	215	28.9	(+/- 8.0)
Former	3551	25.7	(+/- 2.0)
Never	4983	19.9	(+/- 1.6)
Total	9702	24.4	(+/- 1.2)

Source: Centers for Disease Control and Prevention, Behavioral Risk Factor Surveillance System, 1998; Tomar, 1999.

and weight loss. This consequence can affect one's overall health and is particularly relevant to the frail elderly population. Edentulism also influences elders' decisions to seek preventive dental services, atttibutable to a perceived lack of need for care. The implications are relevant to oral cancer mortality rates, and the association will be discussed in the oral cancer section.

PERIODONTAL DISEASES

Description

Periodontal diseases are infections of the tissues that directly surround and support the teeth and include the gingiva (gum tissue), periodontal ligaments, and alveolar bone. There are two main types of periodontal diseases: gingivitis, which affects the gingiva only, and periodontitis, which affects all of the supporting tooth structures. Most periodontal diseases are caused primarily by specific bacteria that reside in the plaque biofilm that is constantly forming on all mouth surfaces. However, certain health factors, such as taking prescription drugs, the presence of steroid hormones, smoking, and diabetes, increase the risks for periodontal diseases.

Gingivitis

The American Academy of Periodontology has identified two major categories of gingival diseases: dental plaque-induced gingival diseases and non-plaque-induced gingival diseases (AAP, 1999; Armitage, 1999). Dental plaque-induced gingivitis represents an inflammatory response that affects only the gingival tissue and does not include any progressive pathologic changes in the periodontal ligament fibers, bone, or cementum.

Gingivitis is diagnosed by a visual examination of the gingival tissue that reveals redness, enlargement, bleeding, edema, and increase in crevicular fluid. Inflammation confined to the gingiva may persist for extended time periods, especially when local microbial factors continue and host resistance is low. Patients with systemic diseases who experience immunosuppression or a compromised host response may also show an increased incidence of gingivitis. For example, patients with acute leukemia, diabetes, and immunodeficiency diseases should be carefully evaluated for any changes in the periodontal structures (Little & Falace, 1997). The American Academy of Periodontology has identified four types of gingivitis associated with systemic diseases: linear gingival erythema, scorbutic gingivitis, gingivitis associated with hormonal changes, and gingival enlargement (AAP, 1999; Armitage, 1999).

Hormonal changes have long been documented to provoke an exaggerated inflammatory response in the gingiva when microbial plaque is present, most notably prevotella intermedia (Dasanayake, 1998). Although most commonly seen in pregnancy, women with hormonal changes induced by oral contraceptives and puberty will display this exaggerated response, which is thought to be related to the elevated steroid levels in the vascular gingival tissues. Common signs of hormonal gingivitis include red, edematous, enlarged tissues that bleed profusely. Other medications have also been documented to produce inflammatory gingival changes, most notably exaggerated gingival enlargement. These medications include phenytoin (controls seizures), cyclosporin, (controls rejection after transplantation), and nifedipine (calcium channel blocker which controls hypertension) (Little & Falace, 1997).

Periodontitis

Periodontitis is an inflammatory disease characterized by loss of attachment of the tooth to the periodontal structures. Periodontitis is diagnosed from both the clinical examination and radiographic evaluation. Although patients with periodontitis may show signs of gingival inflammation, the key diagnostic sign is loss of alveolar bone and periodontal ligaments that support the tooth. The American Academy of Periodontology has recognized four categories of periodontitis: adult periodontitis, early onset periodontitis, refractory periodontitis, and periodontitis associated with systemic diseases (AAP, 1999; Armitage, 1999).

Epidemiology

Recent epidemiologic research has confirmed that periodontal disease affects a significant number of Americans, with at least 48 percent of adults aged 30 or over affected with some form of periodontal disease (Albandar et al., 1999). Twenty-two percent of these adults were documented to have moderate to severe periodontitis, indicating that the most severe forms were limited to a smaller group. This study documented an increasing prevalence of periodontal disease as individuals age, because 50 percent of the study participants aged 55–90 were found to have some form of periodontitis. The researchers also documented that the differences in periodontal disease in aging were also related to gender. Periodontal disease was found in 35 percent of men younger than 55 and 56 percent of men older than 55 and was found in 23 percent of women younger than 55 and 44 percent of women older than 55 (Albandar et al., 1999).

In addition to age and gender, analysis of racial/ethnic categories revealed differences in prevalence of periodontal diseases. Fifty-one percent of African American adults have gingivitis as compared to 47 percent of White adults. For more destructive periodontal disease, the disparity is greater, with 33 percent of African Americans affected as compared with 20 percent of White adults. When considering the effect of both race and gender, the disparity is still greater, for among men over 55, destructive periodontal disease was documented in 47 percent of White men, 70 percent of African American men, and 59 percent of Mexican American men (USDHHS, Healthy People, 2000b).

Risk Factors

In addition to age, gender, and racial/ethnic status, a number of other categories of risk factors can explain variations in prevalence of periodontal disease among individuals. This section reviews the major risk factors and summarizes key research to support the inclusion of these factors to determine patients' risks for disease (Genco, 1996).

At-Risk Behavior.   In addition to assessing oral hygiene behavior, oral health care professionals should question their patients regarding their use of tobacco, which has been implicated as a major risk factor for periodontal diseases. Although most of the research has focused on smoking, oral health clinicians should include the use of spit tobacco, which has also been associated with perio-dontal diseases (Tomar & Asma, 2000). Recent research has documented that patients who smoke are 2.5 to 6 times more likely to develop periodontal disease and have more rapid progression and greater severity of periodontal disease. An analytic study documented that smoking was ranked second only to age as a risk indicator for periodontal diseases. In addition, smoking has been shown to negatively affect the outcome of regenerative therapy and implant success (Haber et al., 1993).

Dental Visits.   Oral health care providers should also assess their patients' behavior in seeking dental care, because patients who have a history of irregular dental visits has been found to have more attachment loss than patients who make regular dental visits (Grossi et al., 1999). Patients with existing disease and/or risk factors for periodontal diseases should visit the dental office at least every six months, with a more frequent recall interval when active disease is present. When patients return for more frequent evaluation and routine care, periodontal disease can be detected and cured while in the early stages. In addition, health promotion strategies can be used and recommended for at home care during the frequent dental visits. Unfortunately, cumulative progression of infection and tissue loss is difficult to manage and more easily treated in its earliest stages (Harris & Garcia-Godoy, 1999).

Other Emerging Risk Factors.   For many years, the major emphasis in the prevention and control of periodontal disease has focused on behavioral factors in elimination of bacterial plaque almost exclusively. However, research in the last decade has expanded and identified a number of risk factors that may be associated with the progression and severity of periodontal disease, such as genetics, medical conditions, and stress (Genco, 1998; Michalowicz, 1994; Genco, 1999). Oral health-care professionals should assess their patients and alert them to these risks for periodontal disease. Although many of these genetic and medical risk factors cannot be altered, patients can use this information to seek more frequent care for early diagnosis and prompt treatment.

CoMorbidities

Medical risk factors for periodontal disease have received a great deal of publicity lately, which has helped to emphasize the essential role that oral health plays in total health. In a large analytic study, diabetes was ranked third, after age and smoking, in the risks for periodontal disease. However, in a recent study, Moore and colleagues (Moore et al., 1999) found that periodontal disease was not common in a population of Type I diabetics and that the inclusion of additional risk factors (smoking, age and age of diagnosis of diabetes) was more explanatory of the risk for periodontal disease. For example, the odds ratio for periodontal disease in diabetic patients who smoked was 9.73 and for patients who were diagnosed after 8.4 years of age was 3.36 and who were older than 32 years was 3.0. (Moore et al., 1999) Early research studies that have documented a strong link between diabetes and periodontal diseases often used mixed populations of both Type 1 and Type 2 diabetics and may not have controlled variables that we now identify as important, such as smoking and age (Consensus Report, 1999).

Other medical risk factors have included history of cardiovascular diseases and bacterial infections, which have shown early and intriguing associations with the presence and severity of periodontal disease (Beck et al., 1998). Several medications have also been documented to produce inflammatory gingival changes, most notably exaggerated gingival enlargement. These medications include phenytoin (controls seizures), cyclosporin, (controls rejection after transplantation), and nifedipine (calcium channel blocker that controls hypertension). When patients have gingival enlargement, the larger sulcular space is more difficult to clean, and the retention of periodontal pathogens increases the risk for development of periodontal disease. A community-based study indicated that patients with pre-existing periodontal disease had a higher prevalence of gingival enlargement when taking nifedipine than those who had healthy periodontal tissues (Ellis et al., 1999).

Stress.   Stress has been recently identified as a potential factor associated with periodontal disease. Genco and colleagues found that patients who reported a high level of financial stress and who demonstrated poor coping skills had higher levels of attachment loss and bone loss than those with low levels of financial strain. The authors have hypothesized that higher levels of stress and inadequate coping skills alter patients' habits in oral hygiene and dental visits and that these patients may have reduced ability to fight infection due to stress (Genco et al., 1999).

Patients' Oral Condition.   Local factors in the patient's mouth pose additional risks for periodontal diseases. Many patients do not have ideal occlusion, and malposed and missing teeth create problems for patients in thoroughly removing all microbial plaque. In addition, calculus formation and poorly contoured restorations trap plaque and hold bacteria even when patients attempt good oral hygiene. All restorations should be evaluated and restored to functional anatomy in order to maintain periodontal health. Frequent recall visits should be scheduled with patients with malocclusion in order to help reinforce oral hygiene skills and limit the microbial challenge to the tissues. Patients with malocclusion should be carefully evaluated for the presence of any occlusal trauma, which may produce bone loss, especially when preexisting periodontal disease is present.

Although microbial plaque has been implicated as the major etiologic agent for periodontal diseases, research (Genco, 1996) has shed light on the many risks for periodontal diseases that may alter the patient's response to the microbial plaque challenge. Oral health-care providers should assess their patients carefully to determine which risk factors may be affecting the patient's periodontal health status and how these factors can best be eliminated and/or controlled to promote periodontal health.

ORAL AND PHARYNGEAL CANCER

Description

The etiology of oral cancers is multifactorial, including systemic and local factors as well as viral and fungal infections (Erickson, 1997; U.S. Department of Health and Human Services [USDHHS], 2000). Although there appears to be a downward trend of mortality from oral cancers in the United States, there has been little improvement in survival rates for oral cancer during the past several

Figure 12.3
Males have higher incidence rates of oral and pharyngeal cancers than females

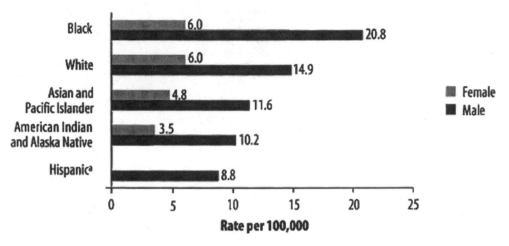

Note: Age adjusted to the 1970 U.S. standard.
[a]Data are unavailable for Hispanic females.

Sources: Adapted from Wingo et al., 1999; SEER Program, 1990–1996, Ries et al., 1999.

decades (Burt & Eklund, 1999; Yellowitz, 1999). There is a lack of awareness among the general population concerning the signs and symptoms of oral cancer and associated risk factors (USDHHS, 2000b; Horowitz et al., 1995; Horowitz & Nourjah, 1996). A national survey showed that only 15 percent of U.S. adults reported ever having had an oral cancer examination (USDHHS, 2000; Horowitz & Nourjah, 1996). Oral cancers occur in sites that lend themselves to early detection by most primary health-care providers (USDHHS, 2000b). Therefore, increasing interdisciplinary partnerships to promote early detection and the public's awareness of the risk factors for oral cancers is needed. Regarding racial differences, oral and pharyngeal cancers pose a particular threat to Black males. There are no differences in incidence rates among Black and White females; however, incidence rates for Black males is 39.6 percent higher than for White males (USDHHS, 2000b; Ries et al., 1999) (see Figure 12.3).

Epidemiology of Oral Cancer in the United States

Oral and pharyngeal cancers are responsible for approximately 8,000 to 9,000 deaths yearly (Greenlee et al., 2000). Oral cancer is the seventh most common cancer in U.S. White males. The incidence and prevalence rates for oral cancer are twice as high in males as compared to females (Greenlee et al., 2000; Burt & Eklund, 1999) (see Figure 12.3). This trend is also evident in oral cancer mortality rates, with males dying at twice the rate than females (Greenlee et al., 2000; Burt & Eklund, 1999). Patients with head and neck cancers have an increased chance of developing a second primary tumor of the upper aerodigestive tract. The five-year survival rate for people with oral and pharyngeal cancers is 52 percent, in part due to only 35 percent of individuals with oral cancers diagnosed at an early stage (USDHHS, 2000b). Just as the incidence rates for oral and pharangeal cancers are higher for Blacks than for Whites, concomitantly, the five-year relative survival rate for Blacks is lower than that for Whites at every stage of diagnosis (USDHHS, 2000b; Ries et al., 1999; Wingo et al., 1999) (see Figure 12.4).

Figure 12.4
At every stage of diagnosis, the five-year relative survival rates for Blacks with oral and pharyngeal cancers are lower than for Whites

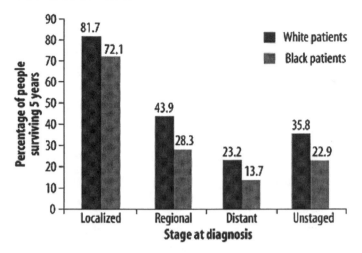

Sources: Adapted from SEER Program, 1989–1995; Ries et al. 1999; USDHHS, 2000b.

Risk Factors

The primary risk factors for oral cancer are tobacco use, including snuff and smokeless tobacco. Cigar and pipe smoking are likely to provide a greater risk than cigarette smoking. The other major factor is alcohol consumption, including current and previous use. The risk for developing oral cancer increases when tobacco and alcohol use are combined. Most lips cancers are associated with sunlight exposure. Viral and fungal factors implicated in oral cancers include infections with herpes simplex type 1, human papilloma virus, and strains of the fungus *Candida albicans* (USDHHS, 2000b). Precancerous or early oral cancer lesions can appear as asymptomatic red, white or red-and-white speckled lesions; as an area of induration or ulceration; or as a result of physical, chemical, or thermal trauma (USDHHS, 2000b).

The most common sites for oral cancers are the tongue, lip, and floor of the mouth. Symptoms to watch for include a sore on the lip or in the mouth that does not heal; a lump on the lip or mouth or throat; unusual bleeding, pain, or numbness in the mouth; a sore throat that does not go away or a feeling that something is caught in the throat; difficulty or pain with chewing or swallowing; swelling in the jaw that causes dentures to fit poorly or become uncomfortable (American Cancer Society, 1997). If an abnormal area has been found in the oral cavity, a biopsy is the only way to know whether it is cancer.

Racial Disparities in Oral Cancer Experience

Older adults (aged 65 to 74) and Blacks disproportionately experience oral cancer. (USDHHS, 2000b; Yellowitz, 1999). The incidence rate is 30 percent higher for Blacks than for Whites and ranks as the fourth most common cancer in the United States among Black males (Kosary et al., 1995; Yellowitz, 1999). Mortality rates for Blacks are generally higher as compared to Whites (Vargas et al., 2001) (see Table 12.5).

Table 12.5
Oral cancer incidence and death rates among persons 65 years of age and older by sex and race, 1993–1997 (rate per 100,000 persons)

Incidence Rate

	Total	Male	Female
All races	44	68	27
White	45	69	28
Black	40	65	21

Death Rates

	Total	Male	Female
All races	14	21	9
White	14	20	9
Black	17	30	9

Note: Rates are age adjusted to the 1970 U.S. standard population.

Sources: Ries et al., 2000; Vargas et al., 2001.

Oral cancers are more likely diagnosed in an early, localized stage among persons who utilize dental services on a routine basis. Oral cancer is found more often in older adults (Yellowitz, 1999), and underutilization of dental services plays a key role in oral cancer disparities. National studies report an increased use of dental services by people aged 65 years and older over the past 20 years; yet, Blacks are less likely than Whites to have visited a dentist during the year (Manski et al., 2001), thus decreasing the likelihood of an early lesion being detected among high-risk elders. Early lesions are usually asymptomatic, and elder Blacks have been shown to be more symptom-related dental care attenders (Kiyak & Miller, 1982), thus increasing the likelihood that oral cancers are detected when the cancer has metastasized (see Figure 12.5).

CoMorbidities

The therapies for oral and pharyngeal cancers cause considerable morbidity that affects physical, functional, as well as social well-being. Problems may include painful ulcers, rampant dental caries, the loss of part of the tongue, lost of taste, loss of chewing ability, difficulty in speaking, pain, and permanent disfigurement (USDHHS, 2000b). These limitations can lead to nutritional deficiencies and weight loss and damage self-esteem. Additionally, facial deformities may cause social embarrassment, social isolation, and depression. If dental professionals increase their efforts to identify early lesions and increase patient awareness so that they reduce their risk behaviors, the morbidity of oral cancer will decline (Yellowitz, 1999).

DETERMINANTS OF ORAL HEALTH DISPARITIES

Healthy People 2010 presents a paradigm of the critical influences that determine the health of individuals and communities (USDHHS, 2000b). These determinants also influence oral health

Figure 12.5
Blacks are less likely to be diagnosed with a localized
oral or pharyngeal cancer than Whites

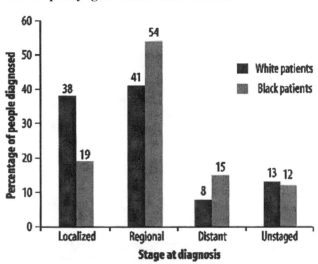

Sources: Adapted from SEER Program, 1989–95, Ries et al., 1999; USDHHS, 2000b.

status, as well as oral health disparities. Specifically, this paradigm provides an understanding of the interrelatedness of oral health with general health and how they impact well-being; and the paradigm provides a framework for developing strategies for health promotion. The following is an overview that highlights the discussed common oral diseases in the context of the determinants of health paradigm and their applicability to oral health disparities (USDHHS, 2000a; USDHHS, 2000b) (see Figure 12.6).

Biology

As a result of population aging, more individuals will be living with multiple systemic conditions. There is growing evidence that periodontal infections are associated with diabetes, heart disease, and stroke. Mechanisms on a biological level include alterations in connective tissue metabolism and host immunological and inflammatory response. These systemic conditions are major causes of morbidity and mortality among Blacks. Among the risk factors for coronary heart disease and stroke are diets that have poor nutritional value. A number of the pharmaceuticals taken to treat these systemic conditions can cause salivary dysfunction (dry mouth) and increase the likelihood of inadequate dietary intakes and increase susceptibility to dental caries.

Behavior and Social Environment

Individual lifestyle habits, attitudes, and cultural values influence oral health status. The attributes of the social environment include cultural customs and beliefs, which are a major influence on the pychosocial effects of dental disease on individuals. Dental care utilization is usually based on "at least one dental visit in the past year," and the lack of dental visits is used as an indicator of unmet health needs. Blacks or individuals with one or more chronic conditions are among those who have higher levels of unmet dental care needs than comparable groups (Mueller et al., 1998; USDHHS,

Figure 12.6
Conceptual framework from Healthy People 2010
for a systematic approach to health improvement

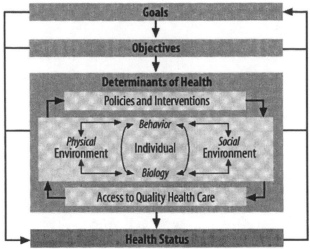

Source: USDHHS, 2000b.

2000b). Functional limitation as a result of systemic conditions are also linked to nonutilization of dental care. Oral health beliefs affect decisions to seek dental care, particularly a lack of perceived need for care. Blacks are more likely to cite "no dental problems" (58.5 percent) as the reason not to frequent dental care services as compared to 44.3 percent for Whites (Bloom et al., 1989; USDHHS, 2000b).

Physical Environment

Individual and community health can be harmed by the physical environment in numerous ways, such as, exposure to toxic substances. A number of signs and symptoms of disease, lifestyle behaviors, and exposure to toxins can be detected in or around the mouth and face. Individuals across age levels who are members of the lower socioeconomic levels disproportionately experience oral diseases (Burt & Eklund, 1999; NCHS, 1996).

Access to Quality Health Care

Barriers to dental care are complex and are linked to social, behavioral, and environmental interactions. Another salient factor is the infrastructure of health care. Federal and state assistance programs are limited regarding oral health services; and reimbursement for dental services is low compared to the usual fee for care. Many older adults lose dental insurance benefits upon retirement. The rates for having private dental insurance are lower for Blacks than for Whites (32.4 versus 41.8 percent) (U.S. Bureau of the Census, 1997). The most vulnerable individuals do not have dental coverage, and the availability of insurance increases access to care. Additionally, racial and ethnic groups are severely underrepresented in the oral health workforce. Increasing diversity among oral care providers may have a positive affect toward decreasing underutilization of dental care services among at-risk populations. Access to dental care, particularly preventive dental services, has been a strong determinant of oral health status. Recent data show that fewer numbers of Black individuals (27 percent) have visited the dentist within the last year than White individuals (47 percent). The same trend is apparent when considering preventive dental care received by children and adolescents. Among those aged 5 to 17 years, Blacks are three times less likely to have dental sealants than Whites (Selwitz et al., 1996; USDHHS, 2000b).

Policies and interventions are discussed within the context of public health strategies in the next section.

PUBLIC HEALTH STRATEGIES TO REDUCE DISPARITIES IN ORAL HEALTH CARE

The research literature contains many examples of policies and interventions that have been effective in promoting oral health. These policies and interventions include efforts designed to prevent dental decay, periodontal disease, and oral cancer. A general intervention that addresses all three oral diseases includes increasing visits to the dentist through a variety of measures. Mandatory dental examinations for school-age children and mandatory oral examinations upon entrance to long-term care facilities ensure that individuals are seen at least once by a dentist but often fall short of comprehensive care due to the complexity of funding and other barriers to care. Increasing funding for oral health services through governmental programs such as Medicaid, EPSDT (Early Periodic Screening, Detection and Treatment), CHIP (Children's Health Insurance Program) and other private programs are critically needed to reduce financial barriers to accessing oral health care. However, even when patients have financing for dental care, nonfinancial barriers such as fear, transportation, and geographic location of dental offices may impact on patients' receiving dental care.

Educational programs completed either with individual patients or in group settings, such as schools, health fairs, or community centers provide the necessary knowledge for health behaviors but may not always result in positive health outcomes. Programs successful in behavior change pair educational activities with skill teaching, motivational sessions, and often incentives to increase the likelihood of behavioral changes.

Preventing dental decay requires a combination of both individual and community efforts. Individual efforts focus on behavioral changes, including increased use of topical fluorides, increasing oral hygiene behaviors and good nutritional patterns, and increasing visits to the dentist. Community-based efforts include water fluoridation, school-based education, and sealant and treatment programs.

Programs to prevent periodontal diseases are most successfully targeted at the individual level and focus on changing individual behavior regarding oral hygiene, including oral hygiene efforts, use of microbial agents and frequent dental visits. Organized community programs to prevent periodontal disease have focused on education, early detection, and referral.

Programs to prevent oral cancer have been targeted at both the individual and community level. Individualized education regarding risk reduction and tobacco cessation have been implemented with moderate success in dental offices. This is, in part, due to limited perceptions on the dentists' part regarding the signs and symptoms of oral cancers and inconsistent practice of oral cancer examinations (Yellowitz, 1999). Tobacco cessation programs have traditionally been the primary approach for reducing the risk for oral and pharangeal cancers (USDHHS, 2000b). Because alcohol reduction also needs to be emphasized, this presents an inability to effectively track the success of prior oral cancer promotion efforts. Community-based approaches for the prevention of oral and pharangeal cancers require intensified developmental efforts (USDHHS, 2000b).

SUMMARY AND RECOMMENDATIONS

"To improve quality of life and eliminate health disparities demands the understanding, compassion, and will of the American people," according to U.S. surgeon general David Satcher. The dental profession alone cannot effectively address the challenge of eliminating oral health disparities. Although many gains have been achieved in promoting and protecting the public's health, there has been relatively little progress across many of the Healthy People 2000 oral objectives. A national public health plan for oral health does not exist. The twenty-first century offers great challenges and great opportunities to improve gaps in oral care for those who need it the most. The oral surgeon general's report recommends a national oral health plan to eliminate health disparities by promoting partnerships among individuals, health-care providers, communities, and policymakers at all levels of society. The following highlights recommendations for action:

• Enhance the public's awareness of the relationship of oral health to general health via ethnically relevant, culturally competent programs.

• Enhance the education of nondental health professionals to oral health diseases and promote interdisciplinary partnerships.

• Inform policymakers to create effective policies that include oral health services in health promotion programs, care delivery systems, and reimbursement schedules.

• Promote evidence-based care by accelerating behavioral and biomedical research, clinical trials, and population-based studies research.

REFERENCES

Albandar, J.M., Brunell, J.A., Kingman, A. (1999). Destructive periodontal disease in adults 30 years of age and older in the United States, 1988–1994. *J Periodontol, 70*, 13–29.

American Academy of Periodontology (AAP). (1996). *Consensus report on periodontal diseases: Epidemiology and diagnosis*. Chicago: American Academy of Periodontology.

American Academy of Periodontology (AAP). (1999). *International workshop for a classification of periodontal diseases and conditions*. Chicago: American Academy of Periodontology.

American Cancer Society (ACS). (1997). *Cancer facts and figures, 1997*. Atlanta: ACS.

Armitage, G.C. (1999). Development of a classification system for periodontal diseases and conditions. *Annals of Periodontology, 4, 1*, 1–6.

Beck, J.D., Offenbacher, S., Williams, R., Gibbs, P., & Garcia, R. (1998). Periodontics: A risk factor for coronary heart disease? *Ann Periodontology, 3*, 127–141.

Berkey, D., & Berg, R. (2001). Geriatric oral health issues in the United States. *International Dental Journal, 51*, 254–264.

Bloom, B., Gift, H.C., & Jack, S.S. (1992). Dental services and oral health: United States, 1989. *Vital Health Stat, 10, 183*, 1–95.

Burt, B.A., & Eklund, S.A. (1999). *Dentistry, dental practice, and the community*, 5th ed. (pp. 267–276). Philadelphia: W.B. Saunders.

Centers for Disease Control and Prevention (1998). Behavioral Risk Factor Surveillance System. Atlanta: USDHHS, CDC.

Dasanayake, A.P. (1998). Poor periodontal health of the pregnant woman as a risk factor for low birth weight. *Annals of Periodontology, 3*, 206–211.

Dodd, C.L., Greenspan, D., Katz, M.H., Westenhouse, J.L., Feigal, D.W., & Greenspan, J.S. (1991). Oral candidiasis in HIV infection: Pseudomembranous and erythematous candidiasis show similar rates of progression to AIDS. *AIDS, 5*, 1339–1343.

Ellis, J.S., Seymour, R.A., Steele, J.G., Robertson, P., Butler, T.J., & Thomson, J.J., (1999). Prevalence of gingival overgrowth induced by calcium channel blocker: A community based study. *Periodontology, 63*, 149–154.

Erickson, L. (1997). Oral health promotion and prevention for older adults. *Dental Clinics of North America, 41*, 727–749.

Evans, C.W., & Kleinman, D.V. (2000). The Surgeon General's report on America's oral health: Opportunities for the dental profession. *Journal of the American Dental Association, 131*, 1721–1727.

Genco, R.J. (1996). Current view of risk factors for periodontal diseases. *Journal of Peridontology, 67* (Suppl.), 1041–1049.

Genco, R.J. (1998). Periodontal disease and risk for myocardial infarction and cardiovascular disease. *Cardiovascular Review Reports, 19*, 34–40.

Genco, R.J. Ho, A.W., Grossi, S.G., Dunford, R.G. & Tedesco, L. (1999) Relationship of stress, distress and inadequate coping behaviors to periodontal disease. *Journal of Periodontology, 70, 7*, 711–723.

Greenlee, R.T., Murray T., Bolden, S., & Wingo, P.A. (2000). Cancer statistics. *CA Cancer J Clin, 50*, 7–33.

Grossi, S.G., & Genco, R.J. (1998). Periodontal disease and diabetes mellitus: A two-way relationship. *Annals of Periodontology, 3*, 51–61.

Grossi, S.G., Zambon, J.J., Ho, A.W., Koch, G. Dunford, R.G., & Machtei, E.E. (1999). Assessment of risk for periodontal disease. I. Risk indicators of attachment loss. *Journal of Periodontology, 65*, 260–267.

Haber, J., Wattles, J., Crowley, M., Mandell, R., Joshipura, K., & Kent, R.I. (1993). Evidence for cigarette smoking as a major risk factor for periodontitis. *Journal of Periodontology, 64*, 16–23.

Harris, N.O., & Garcia-Godoy, F. (1999). Primary Preventive Dentistry. Norwalk: Appleton and Lange.

Health Care Financing Administration. *National health expenditures.* Washington, DC: Health Care Financing Administration.

Horowitz, A.M., & Nourjah, P.A. (1996). Patterns of screening for oral cancer among U.S. adults. *Journal of Public Health Dentistry*, 56, 331–335.

Horowitz, A.M., Nourjah, P.A., & Gift, H.G. (1995). U.S. adult knowledge of risk factors for and signs of oral cancers: 1990. *Journal of the American Dental Association, 126*, 39–45.

Kaste, L.S., Selwitz, R.H., & Oldakowski, R.J. (1996). Coronal caries in the primary and permanent dentition of children and adolescents 1–17 years of age, United States 1988–1991. *Journal of Dental Research, 75*, 631–641.

Kiyak, H.A., Miller, R.A. (1982). Age differences in oral health attitudes and dental service utilization. *Journal of Public Health Dentistry, 41*, 29–41.

Klein, R.S., Harris, C.A., Small, C.B., Moll, B., Lesser, M., & Friedland, G.H. (1984). Oral candidiasis in high-risk patients as the initial manifestation of the acquired immunodeficiency syndrome. *New England Journal of Medicine, 9*, 354–358.

Kosary, C.L., Ries, L.A., Miller, B.A., Hankey, B.F., Harras, A., & Edwards, B.K. (Eds.). (1995). *SEER cancer statistics review. 1973–1992 tables and graphs.* NIH Pub. No. 96-2798. (pp. 17, 34, 542, 355, 361). Bethesda, MD: National Cancer Institute.

Little, J.W., Falace, D.A. (1997). Dental management of the medically compromised patient, 5th ed. St. Louis: Mosby Company.

Manski, R.J., Moeller, J.F., & Maas, W.R. (2001). Dental services: An analyses of utilization over 20 years. *Journal of the American Dental Association, 132*, 655–664.

Marcus, S.E., Drury, T.F., Brown, L.J., & Zion, G.R. (1996). Tooth retention and tooth loss in the permanent dentition of adults: United States, 1988–1991. *Journal of Dental Research, 75*, 684–695.

Michalowicz, B.S. (1994). People at risk for periodontitis—genetic and heritable risk factors. *Journal of Periodontal Research, 65*, 479–488.

Milnes, A.R. (1996). Description and epidemiology of nursing caries. *Journal of Public Health Dentistry, 56*, 38–50.

Moore, P.A., et al. (1999). Type 1 diabetes mellitus and oral health: assessment of periodontal disease. *Journal of Periodontology, 70(4)*, 409–17.

Mueller, C.D., Schur, C.L., & Paramore, L.C. (1998). Access to dental care in the United States. *Journal of the American Dental Association, 4*, 492–437.

National Center for Health Statistics (NCHS). (1975). *First National Health and Nutrition Examination Survey (NHANES I).* Hyattsville, MD: NCHS, U.S. Department of Health and Human Services, Public Health Service, Centers for Disease Control and Prevention.

National Center for Health Statistics (NCHS). (1996). *Third National Health and Nutrition Survey (NHANES*

III) reference manuals and reports [CD-Rom]. Hyattsville, MD: NCHS, U.S. Department of Health and Human Services, Public Health Service, Centers for Disease Control and Prevention.

National Health Interview Survey (1997). Centers for Disease Control and Prevention, National Center for Health Statistics. Office of Analysis, Epidemiology, and Health Promotion. CDC/NCHS, Hyattaville, Maryland.

National Institute of Dental and Craniofacial Research (1986). Department of Health and Human Services, National Institutes of Health, Bethesda, Maryland.

Offenbacher, S., et al. (1996). Periodontal infection as a possible risk factor for preterm low birth weight. *Journal of Periodontology, 67,* 1103–1113.

Offenbacher, S., et al. (1998). Potential pathogenic mechanisms of periodontitis associated pregnancy complications. *Annals of Periodontology, 3,* 233–250.

Ries, L.A., Kosary, C.L., Hankey, B.F., Miller, B.A., Clegg, L., & Edwards, B.K. (Eds.) (1999). *SEER cancer statistics review. 1973–1996.* Besthesda, MD: National Cancer Institute.

Ries, L.A.G., Eisner, M.P., Kosary, C.L., Hankey, B.F., Miller, B.A., Clegg, L., & Edwards, B.K. (Eds.). (2000). *SEER cancer statistics review, 1973–1997.* Besthesda, MD: National Cancer Institute.

Salvi, G.E., Lawrence, H.P., Offenbacher, S., & Beck, J.D. (1997). Influence of risk factors on the pathogenesis of periodontitis. *Periodontol 2000, 14,* 173–201.

Selwitz, R.H., Winn, D.M., Kingman, A., & Zion, G.R. (1996). The prevalence of dental sealants in the U.S. population: Findings from NHANES III-1991. *Journal of Dental Research, 75,* 652–660.

Tomar, S. (1999). Total tooth loss among persons aged greater than or equal to 65 years—selected states, 1995–1997. *CDC MMWR Morbidity Mortality Weekly Report, 48,* 206–210.

Tomar, S., & Asma, S. (2000). Smoking attributable periodontitis in the United States: Findings from NHANES III. *Journal Periodontology, 71,* 743–751.

U.S. Bureau of the Census. (1997). *Health insurance coverage: 1996. Current population reports, P60-199.* Washington, DC: U.S. Department of Commerce.

U.S. Department of Health and Human Services (USDHHS). (2000a). *Oral Health in America: A Report of the Surgeon General—Executive Summary.* Rockville, MD: U.S. Department of Health and Human Services, National Institute of Dental and Craniofacial Research, National Institutes of Health.

U.S. Department of Health and Human Services (USDHHS). (2000b). *Healthy people 2010 (conference edition in two volumes).* Washington, DC: U.S. Department of Health and Human Services.

U.S. Department of Health and Human Services (USDHHS). (2000c). *Healthy people in healthy communities.* Washington, DC: U.S. Department of Health and Human Services.

Vargas, C.M., Crall, J.J., & Schneider, D.A. (1998). Sociodemographic distribution of pediatric dental caries: 1988–1994. *JADA, 129,* 1229–1238.

Vargas, C.M., Kramarow, E.A., & Yellowitz, J.A. (2001). *The oral health of older americans. Aging trends,* No.3. Hyattsville, MD: National Center for Health Statistics.

Wingo, P.A., et al. (1999). Annual report to the nation on the status of cancer, 1973–1996. With a special section on lung cancer and tobacco smoking. *Journal of the National Cancer Institute, 91,* 675–690.

Yellowitz, J.A. (1999). Providing oral cancer examinations for older adults. *CDA Journal of the California Dental Association, 27,* 718–723.

CHAPTER 13

Communication Disorders and African Americans

JOAN C. PAYNE AND
CAROLYN A. STROMAN

INTRODUCTION

The National Institute on Deafness and Communication Disorders (NIDCD) estimates that one of every six Americans suffer from a communication disorder (NIDCD, 2003). In particular, almost 2.7 million Americans have speech impairments, and over 34 million Americans are hearing-impaired (NIDCD, 2002b). Speech, hearing, or language disorders limit one's ability to communicate; this inability to communicate fully can have far-reaching social, economic, and psychological effects for many individuals. Simply put, daily living can be severely compromised for persons who experience communication impairments or disorders.

Data on the prevalence or incidence of communication disorders among African Americans are scarce (Battle, 2002). However, contemporary health prevalence data confirm that African Americans suffer disproportionately from acute and chronic diseases and conditions that can impair speech, hearing, and language. In particular, African American young and old adults are at greatest risk for hypertension and diabetes, which increase their incidences of cerebrovascular accidents (CVAs). African Americans are also disproportionately infected with the human immunodeficiency virus (HIV), which can develop into the full-blown acquired immunodeficiency disease (AIDS). Both asymptomatic and symptomatic expressions of AIDS have been documented to cause strokes and dementia. Finally, some African Americans are also at great risk for brain damage and compromised speech and language from substance abuse.

Repeated strokes can lead to a variably progressive form of dementia called multi-infarct dementia (MID), which compromises language content and pragmatics (Payne, 1997). The prevalence of head injuries from interpersonal violence in African Americans exceeds that of the general population, and traumatic brain injury (TBI) is implicated in cognitive, motor, speech, and language disturbances in children and adults. Sickle-cell disease (SCD), a genetic blood disorder found only in African Americans, presents with complications from sickling crises that can and do interrupt both language and hearing.

In the following sections, speech, hearing, and language disorders in African Americans arising from strokes, dementia, traumatic brain injury, and sickle-cell disease are discussed in greater detail. Attention is given to several critical issues that affect testing and treatment.

ETIOLOGIES OF SPEECH, HEARING, AND LANGUAGE IMPAIRMENTS

Cerebrovascular Accidents and Aphasia

The type of cerebrovascular accident, or stroke, that is most prevalent among older adults is the ischemic stroke, which is largely the result of artherosclerotic vascular and concurrent heart disease. Ischemic stroke is more common in the elderly, males, and African Americans (National Stroke Association, 1996).

Over one million Americans have aphasia, or the reduced ability to use or comprehend words as a result of a stroke primarily due to damage in the left brain hemisphere language areas (Klein, 1995). Many stroke survivors develop both impaired motor speech and aphasia (Morrison & Greeson, 1990). Aphasia is not a disease but a symptom of brain damage. It is estimated that approximately 80,000 persons acquire aphasia each year (NIDCD, 2003).

Prevalence data for aphasia generally do not provide an analysis of incidence by race in the U.S. population. Therefore, it is extremely difficult to report whether an ethnic subgroup is more at risk for aphasia or is more likely to have other specific types of language impairments. However, given the higher rates of hypertension, diabetes, and strokes among African Americans, it is reasonable to assume that African Americans are more at risk for both aphasia and motor speech disorders (Payne, 1977, 1998b).

The aphasias are classified as four major types: expressive, receptive, anomic aphasia, and global (NIDCDS, 2003). Expressive aphasia, the inability to convey thoughts through speech or writing, and the anomic aphasia, which is difficulty in using the correct names for objects, people, places, or events, generally result from more anterior lesions in the brain. Receptive aphasia, difficulty with understanding spoken or written language, is generally thought to be the result of more posteriorly placed lesions. Global aphasia is caused by severe and extensive damage to the language areas of the brain. This form of aphasia is characterized by a significant depression of all language modalities. Speech is typically nonfluent, and comprehension is severely impaired (Mateer, 1989).

Motor speech disorders frequently coexist with aphasia. Dysarthria is an impairment of the ability to form the sounds of the language due to brain damage. In this disorder, several systems may be affected: respiration, phonation, resonation, and articulation. The neurological substrates of dysarthria are caused by damage to the cranial nerves, which are part of the peripheral nervous system, damage to the motor pathways in the cerebrum, and deficiencies of the neurotransmitters acetylcholine and dopamine. Apraxia is a disorder of motor planning thought to be the result of damage to the frontal lobes (Freed, 2000).

Table 13.1 gives a summary of results as reported by the Stroke Data Bank (Foulkes et al., 1988) and the Framingham Study (Gresham, 1979). The most striking findings are the higher frequencies of neurological deficits during the acute period following a stroke and lower frequency of dysarthria and aphasia within 6 to 12 months after. This change is due to rapid recovery of neurological and functional abilities during the first 1 to 3 months poststroke. Some patients continue to improve after that time in visuospatial abilities and memory. However, aphasia and dysarthria persist in some patients even after 6 or more months.

These observations on stroke sequelae are most appropriate for the general population. However, African Americans reportedly return to function much more slowly than Whites (Payne, 1998a). This may be due to the more severe first-time strokes noted in this population (Miles & Bernard, 1992). Motor impairments, for example, from ischemic strokes, were found to be greater in Blacks than in their White cohorts (Horner et al., 1991).

Race, age, and gender effects on stroke and aphasia have been well documented. A number of researchers have examined the effects of age and type of aphasia. Eslinger and Damaisio (1981) observed that there may be aged-related changes in the neurophysiological mechanism subserving

Table 13.1
Neurological deficits following stroke

Neurological Deficit	Acute Stroke Data Bank (Infarctions only)	Chronic Framingham Study (6 or more months)
Right hemiparesis	44	22
Left hemiparesis	37	23
Bilateral hemiparesis	7	3
Ataxia	20	NR
Motor incoordination	NR	NR
Visual-perceptual deficits	32	NR
Aphasia	30	18
Dysarthria	48	16
Sensory deficits	53	24
Cognitive deficits (Memory)	36	NR
Depression	NR	NR
Bladder control	29	NR
Dysphagia	12	NR

NR = Not Reported

Source: Adapted from Gresham et al., 1995, *Post-stroke rehabilitation*, p. 27.

language, such that some types of aphasia would tend to be more prevalent with age, regardless of lesion location. Expressive aphasia incidence peaks between ages 40 and 50. The incidence of receptive aphasia continues to increase until well into old age. Global aphasia is more common in older patients. Receptive aphasia tends to be more debilitating communicatively than expressive aphasia (Payne, 1997).

These findings have particular relevance for African Americans who are diagnosed with hypertension earlier than their White cohorts and, consequently, suffer strokes earlier in age. Gaines and Burke (1995) observed that hypertension is highly associated with strokes in African Americans under 65 years of age. The implications are that younger African Americans will most likely present with more anterior lesions and expressive aphasias. However, unlike their White cohorts, African American women of all ages have the greatest prevalence of strokes and aphasia (Payne, 1997; National Institute on Aging, 1985).

Strokes and AIDS

The Centers for Disease Control report (2002b) that through December 2001, African American males had the highest diagnosed HIV infection cases from birth to age 24 and after age 35 years among all males in the United States. African American females had the highest diagnosed HIV infection rate among females from birth to age 65 years. This means, simply, that African Americans of all ages have the greatest risk for the acquired immunodeficiency syndrome (AIDS) in the United States.

Evidence of cerebrovascular accidents associated with AIDS has been found in varicella-zoster viral encephalitis (VZV). Small and large blood vessel pathology from VZV was found to cause seizures, mental changes, and focal deficits (Amilie-Lefond et al., 1995). In addition, patients with the HIV-associated dementia complex (HAD) frequently develop focal lesions and language disorders as the disease progresses. They may exhibit difficulty understanding spoken language as well as a tendency to misinterpret or mishear what is said. Expressive language problems can also occur, such as word-finding difficulties and slowed or slurred speech. At the end stage, mutism and nonresponsiveness can occur (Bocellari & Zeifert, 1994).

Substance Abuse and Strokes

Cocaine-induced strokes, which have been observed in young adults, have also been reported for middle-aged adults (Wallace, 1993). Although substance abuse may be found in every segment of society, Wallace (1993) observed:

Substance abuse is a risk factor for stroke that appears to disproportionately affect individuals from some segments of the multicultural community . . . some illicit substances have a known deleterious effect on the vascular and nervous systems. Crack, the inhaled form of cocaine, for instance, is a vasoconstrictor that has been reported to cause strokes. (p. 241)

More severe strokes are likely from long-term effects of cocaine-induced strokes and other neuropathies associated with cocaine and polydrug use for older persons who have used these drugs. Although the actual prevalence of cocaine use has declined, medical complications have increased. Reasons for this increase are larger doses, cumulative effects of sustained use, more frequent use, multiple drug use, and more dangerous routes of administration (National Center for Health Statistics, 1994).

The Dementias and Cognitive-Language Impairment

Dementia has two definitions that define the syndrome. The first defines dementia as an acquired, persistent decline of functioning in at least three of the following five domains: language, memory, visuospatial skills, executive function, and personality and mood. Furthermore, memory dysfunction is not required to meet the above criteria, thus allowing the stroke patient with aphasia, depression, and poor executive function—but intact memory—to meet dementia criteria. The second, more traditional definition required impairment in long- and short-term memory with additional decline in at least one other domain, for example, judgment, language, or praxis, that interferes with either occupation, social functioning, or interpersonal relationships (Cummings et al., 1980; APA, 1994).

In this section, three types of diseases that compromise cognitive abilities and therefore language are discussed. Although many diseases cause irreversible dementia, Alzheimer's disease (AD), multi-infarct dementia (MID), and human immunodeficiency virus-dementia complex (HIVD) affect a substantial number of African Americans.

Alzheimer's Disease

Alzheimer's disease, also known as dementia of the Alzheimer's type (DAT), affects persons of all racial and ethnic groups. It is the most frequently diagnosed cause of dementia and is characterized by progressively deteriorating intellectual functioning and language. In AD there is a marked deterioration of semantic knowledge as well as a correlation between the severity of cognitive disorders and the types of language deficits observed. The language disorders associated with dementia have been collectively termed cognitive-language impairments.

Language dissolution during the progression of the disease is in semantics, or the ability to understand and use words. Semantic memory is responsible for categorization, visual imagery, and the conceptualization of steps needed to prepare a meal, get ready for bed, or plan a family reunion. This ability to conceptualize and order associated concepts and propositions is what Bayles (1988) refers to as a schema. Language, therefore, is affected because the conceptual system for semantic memory and discourse cohesion become increasingly impaired as the diseases progresses (Bayles, 1988; Ripich & Terrell, 1988).

Multi-Infarct Dementia

Multi-infarct dementia (MID) is the second most common diagnosis of dementia. MID is caused by repeated focal lesions from strokes and makes up 17 percent of all dementia cases. DAT and MID coexist in another 15 percent of all dementia cases. MID is a loss of intellectual functioning due to significant cerebrovascular disease and repeated infarctions. Multiple infarctions are usually the result of hypertension or arteriosclerosis. MID patients typically have a history of previous strokes, abrupt onset of mental deterioriation, and stepwise course of "patchy" losses of functioning that leads to an uneven and erratic decline (Bayles, 1988; Ripich, 1991; Shadden, 1990). The neurological characteristics include multiple areas of softening of brain tissue and may involve possible pathological alteration in cerebral blood vessels (Baker, 1988).

Results of the New Haven Study (National Institute on Aging, 1985) showed that Black and other non-White males and females had the highest percentages of stroke or brain hemorrhage diagnoses when compared with Whites. There is also evidence of an age effect for stroke diagnoses by ethnicity. White men and women in New Haven reported the highest percentages of stroke after age 80 and non-White men and non-White women reported stroke diagnoses between the ages of 65 and 79. This age differential suggests that younger, non-White male and female patients probably account for a large number of MID cases. The North Carolina Study (Horner et al., 1991) corroborated these findings. Hence, African American older adults are more likely to develop MID at a younger age because of their histories of hypertension and strokes (Baker, 1988).

Table 13.2 provides insight into the types of language deficits that can be expected from MID patients who suffer multiple bilateral, large vessel occlusions, lacuna state, and Binswanger's disease. Lacunes are small cavities of infarcted tissue. Binswanger's Disease is a rare form of infarction that affects the white matter more than the gray and occurs predominantly in the temporal and occipital lobes. The disease is believed to be due to arteriosclerosis of the penetrating arteries in these areas (Payne, 1997). As can be seen from the table, MID can affect the language modalities of reading, writing, and expressive language, as well as speech production, motor planning, word retrieval, and memory.

Human Immunodeficiency Virus-Associated Dementia

In 2002, African Americans accounted for an estimated 54 percent of all new HIV infections (Joint United Nations Programme/World Health Organization, 2002). The human immunodeficiency virus-associated dementia (HIVD) is thought to occur in 20–30 percent of patients diagnosed with AIDS and is estimated to affect up to 60 percent of all individuals in the late stages of HIV disease. Although the life expectancy of AIDS patients has improved because of more sophisticated treatments

Table 13.2
Language and speech disorders associated with MID large vessel occlusion, lacunae state, and Binswanger's disease

Disorder	Language Deficit
Large Vessel Occlusion	
Left Anterior Arteries	Transcortical motor aphasia
Left Middle Cerebral Artery	Aphasia, apraxia, dementia
Right Middle Cerebral Artery	Disturbed emotionally toned speech
Posterior Middle Artery	Angular Gyrus Syndrome (fluent aphasia, alexia with agraphia
Posterior Cerebral Artery	
Left Side	Hemisensory loss, anomia, alexia with agraphia
Lacunae State	Dementia, dysarthria, dysphagia
Binswanger's Disease	Memory impairment

Transcortical motor aphasia: Fluent (expressive) aphasia associated with frontal lobe lesions.

Alexia: Inability to read.

Agraphia: Inability to write.

Anomia: Word-finding difficulty.

Dysphagia: Swallowing disorder.

Source: Adapted from Bayles & Kaszniak, 1987.

for the virus and opportunistic infections, it is estimated that the incidence of neurological complications will increase (McArthur et al., 1993).

HIVD is a subcortical syndrome characterized by abnormalities of cerebral myelin, or diffuse myelin pallor. Diffuse myelin pallor is reduced staining of subcortical and deep white mater by myelin-specific stains. Symptoms include cognitive impairment, specifically memory loss, motor dysfunction, and behavioral abnormalities. Clinical features suggestive of HIVD are demonstrated deficits in frontal lobe tasks and nonverbal memory, ataxia, and slowed limb and eye movement when other factors are accounted for. Memory loss is related to cortical atrophy. Cognitive slowing and ataxia may progress to complete mutism (McArthur et al., 1993).

Traumatic Brain Injury

An estimated 5.3 million Americans currently live with disabilities resulting from traumatic brain injury (Brain Injury Association, 2003). These head-injured individuals have sustained moderate to severe brain injuries resulting in lifelong disabling conditions (Max et al., 1991).

Traumatic brain injury (TBI) is an insult to the brain that is not degenerative or congenital. Rather, TBI is the result of an external physical force that produces a diminished or altered state of consciousness, which causes impaired cognitive abilities or physical functioning.

There are two types of TBI. One is closed head injury (CHI), which is usually caused by the rapid acceleration and deceleration of the head during which the brain is whipped back and forth, thus bouncing off the inside of the skull. The stress of this rapid movement within the cranial vault pulls apart nerve fibers and causes damage to the activated system of neurofibers that send out messages to all parts of the body. The second category of TBI is open or penetrating head injury. This is a visible injury and may be the result of an accident, gunshot wound, or a variety of external factors. This injury is usually located at a focal point in the brain (Brain Injury Association, 1995).

Although assaults and interpersonal violence are the second leading cause of TBIs in the general population (Naugle, 1990), Whitman et al. (1984) found that falls were more prevalent for Whites (31 percent) than for their African American cohorts.

Research on assault-related TBIs across and within ethnocultural groups is relatively sparse. What is known is that personal or family income, employment circumstances, location (urban or suburban), and ethnicity are major factors in the prevalence of TBIs from assaults and interpersonal violence. Head injury epidemiological data provide an incidence rate of 288/100,000, for non-Whites and 194/100,000 for Whites, indicating that non-Whites are approximately 49 percent more likely to suffer head injuries than Whites (Jagger et al., 1984).

It has been suggested that TBI from interpersonal violence produces a posttraumatic stress syndrome in some survivors (Bryant et al., 2000). However, most agree that TBI produces a generalized depressive effect on cognition and language immediately after the injury. The permanence and severity of cognitive, speech, and language deficits are dependent on the severity of the head injury and the length of coma and amnesia (Ommaya, 1995). Persons with open head injuries usually present with language impairments resembling those of poststroke survivors. However, language disorganization rather than categorical linguistic deficits may be the more frequent cause of impaired ability to communicate in closed head injury.

Most persons with CHI demonstrate no language structure problems; however, word retrieval and verbal fluency problems may predominant (Marquardt et al., 1990; Vilkki et al., 1994). Most strikingly, head injury impairs the ability to retrieve syntactic (grammatical) cues. It appears that persons with CHI and persons who have sustained a left cerebral hemisphere infraction are similar in their inability to comprehend syntax (Butler-Hinz et al., 1990). McDonald (1993) also noted that head injury also interferes with language use. Errors in sequencing and inclusion of irrelevant propositions contributed in his investigation of head injury to the disorganized and confusing nature of the language used by CHI subjects to give game directions.

Sickle-Cell Disease

Sickle-cell disease (SCD) is a genetic disease caused by a single amino acid substitution in the ß-chain of hemoglobin. This mutation causes red blood cells to have a sickled shape. It is an autosomal recessive disease that affects approximately 1 in 500 African Americans (Bloom, 1995).

Payne and Stockman (1979) recognized that the sickling of red blood cells impedes or halts blood supply to vital body organs and tissues, including those related to normal speech, language, and hearing functioning. Peters-Johnson and Taylor (1986) suggest that speech and hearing disorders may result from neurological damage associated with a sickle-cell crisis.

It is well established that sickling that occur in any organ, including the brain, and that clinically evident stroke can affect from 6 to 12 percent of patients. The median age at which persons with SCD suffer stroke is 5 years. Those who survive show disturbed learning profiles and psychoemotional problems. Intellectual development is impaired and children perform poorly in school relative to their peers (Cohen, et al., 1994; Cohen et al., 1992).

In children under age 10, the most common cause of stroke is cerebral infarction. Ischemic stroke typically presents with aphasia and impairments in intellectual, motor, and sensory systems. Hemorrhagic stroke, more common with advancing age, is characterized by more generalized phenomena such as coma, headache, and seizures. Recurrent strokes are cumulative, causing greater impairments and a greater likelihood of death (National Institutes of Health, 1995).

Another effect on communication is sensorineural hearing loss. Sensorineural hearing loss is associated with SCD in older children and adults, and may affect up to 40 percent of the population (Gentry et al., 1997). Al-Dabbous and his colleagues (1996) investigated sensorineural hearing loss in a population of SCD patients from 5 to 40 years of age and found a significant correlation between the hearing loss and the onset of the first vaso-occlusive crisis at six years of age or less.

The foregoing material has highlighted how certain diseases can impair speech, language, and hearing among African Americans. The implications that this has for health disparities are discussed below.

ISSUES IN SPEECH, LANGUAGE, AND HEARING FOR AFRICAN AMERICANS

Despite advances in multicultural sensitivity and inclusion, African Americans continue to be an underserved, underresearched population in the speech, language, and hearing literature. This phenomenon occurs in spite of the projection that as the population ages, the likelihood increases that the number of African Americans (and others) with communication disorders, especially hearing, will increase unless appropriate prevention measures are implemented. Specific recommendations for research and practice geared toward reducing health disparities are provided below.

Practice

To reduce health disparities generally, it is necessary for African Americans to participate more fully in all aspects of the health-care system. Likewise, practitioners must be actively involved in advocating for improvements in the quality of health care and treatment for African Americans as a way of reducing the health disparity. Payne (1997) posits that too few African Americans have been included in clinical trials for tests and treatment to make a substantial impact on how assessment and treatment strategies are determined.

For speech and language disorders, a key form of treatment is language therapy. Thus, more African Americans must be motivated to complete language therapy programs in order to receive effective treatment. Payne (1997) offers tips for increasing the number of elderly in language therapy, including providing outpatient rehabilitation in the patient's home instead of a clinical setting and maintaining the same clinicians for the patient.

Speech, language, and hearing professionals must expend more effort on the identification and development of appropriate health intervention strategies to reduce the risk factors associated with communication disorders. For example, community-based intervention and study programs must be designed and implemented that focus on those diseases discussed earlier, including hypertension and diabetes, that indirectly impair speech, language, and hearing.

Relevant evaluation and treatment strategies must be fueled by research. One example of the kind of research that will directly affect how African American stroke survivors will be evaluated and treated in the future is ongoing research that is part of the Howard University Stroke Center. A team of investigators from the medical and behavioral sciences are examining the effects of overexpression of proinflammatory cytokines on neurobehavioral outcomes in acute stroke patients at the Howard University Hospital. These investigators posit that African Americans are living in extremely stressful circumstances in this country and that this stress may be manifested in changes in the immune system. In effect, one investigation turns on whether the overexpression of specific proteins in the immune system compromises poststroke performance on tests of language, memory, and cognition. The implications are that overactivity of some immune system functions may explain why African Americans recover functional skills more slowly than their White cohorts.

In addition to relevant research that has clinical significance, effective treatment approaches for communication impairments in African Americans are highly dependent on whether practitioners correctly identify the disorders. For example, Payne (1997) noted that often disorders in the elderly go unrecognized by their families. As a result, these elders may not receive treatment until the disorder is severe. Thus, in order to improve treatment of speech, language, and hearing disorders in African Americans, practitioners must recognize and correctly identify the specific disorder and similarly educate caregivers of elderly persons.

One exciting development in treating persons with communication disorders is the design and use of new technologies to identify people with speech, language, or hearing disorders and to enhance their communication. For example, a variety of innovative products, including cochlear (inner ear) implants, electronic larynxes, and computer-aided speech devices, is now available for persons with speech and hearing disorders (NIDCD, 2002a). In order to understand and ultimately to contribute to the elimination of health disparities, effort must be made to ensure that African Americans have access to such technologies and devices.

As communication scholars, we are impressed with the promise of e-health (the use of information and communication technology to improve health and health-care services, Eng, 2002). Recent research suggests that technology, especially the Internet, has the potential to provide services that positively influence health attitudes and behaviors (Zarcadoolas et al., 2002). Whenever interactive technologies can help individuals compare speech and hearing treatments and medical options, such technology can be used to remind patients to adhere to treatment and health maintenance plans (Eng & Gustafson, 1999).

Specific emphasis has been placed on expanding patient education programs to increase patients' knowledge of how to best access care, ask the right questions during clinical encounters, and participate in treatment decisions. Preliminary evidence suggests that education through CD-ROM and the Internet can increase the level of patient participation (Institute of Medicine, 2002). In turn, this increased patient participation is expected to significantly enhance the treatment of communication disorders.

The failure of health-care providers to be culturally sensitive has resulted in a number of negative health outcomes in African American patients, particularly patient distrust and patient dissatisfaction with relational aspects of health-care delivery. In addition, cultural and structural barriers to speech, language, and hearing clinical services have prevented many African Americans from seeking or continuing with service providers. These barriers—(1) physical and economic, (2) cultural, (3) institutional, and (4) policy-level—have often deterred persons who may be already too suspicious of the health-care system clinical services to participate in services. Speech, language, and hearing practitioners should look for ways of combining folk models with biomedical models since some African Americans may be more comfortable with choosing alternatives in health beliefs and practices, like folk medicine, religion, and causality related to natural (taking care of one's body) or unnatural illnesses (roots, voodoo) (Payne, 1997). By being aware of culturally preferred modes of treatment and including such preferences in prescribed regimens, health-care providers may increase patients' understanding of prescribed regimens and promote compliance (Stroman, 2000).

Research

In general, researchers must continue the work begun in this volume to identify those factors that contribute to health disparities between African Americans and Whites; researchers must also continue the search for the most efficacious interventions that would reduce and ameliorate the disparities. Specifically in the speech, language, and hearing disciplines, there is a dire need for research on the incidence or prevalence of various types of communication disorders in African Americans. As noted earlier, much of the existing data lacks precise information on the epidemiology of communication disorders in African Americans.

It has been suggested that ethnic minority children are frequently misdiagnosed as language-impaired because culturally appropriate language assessment instruments or procedures are unavailable (Taylor & Peters-Johnson, 1986). Similarly, most standardized aphasia tests are too rigidly constructed to allow for ethnic and cultural differences in language expression and comprehension (Payne, 1997). Valuable information regarding language competence, therefore, is either ignored or not accounted for in therapy (Wallace & Tonkovich, 1998). Hence, there is a need for research that focuses on the development of instruments that are culturally appropriate (e.g., tests that differentiate between language impairment and normal language development in African American children).

In its strategic plan, NIDCD (2002b) recommends that future research "use modern behavior, genetic, imaging and other approaches to precisely define the characteristics of communication disorders in order to optimize clinical diagnosis and intervention" (p. 15). We embrace this suggestion and recommend specifically that communication disorders research related to the Human Genome Project be given high priority.

As has been emphasized throughout this chapter, several diseases are related to communication disorders. Researchers must continue to conduct research that increases our understanding of the development and progression of diseases that contribute to communication disorders, especially hypertension and diabetes.

CONCLUSION

This chapter has demonstrated how chronic diseases such as hypertension and diabetes have disproportionately affected African Americans and have had deleterious effects on their speech, language, and hearing. Research focusing specifically on the elderly has captured the complexity of this symbiotic relationship: elderly adults are most vulnerable to chronic diseases and functional language impairments, particularly with advancing age, because of cardio- and cerebrovascular diseases, cerebrovascular accidents, dementia, progressive neurogenic disorders, and traumatic head injuries (Payne, 1997).

Recommendations, both for practice and research, were provided as a foundation for examining disorders of speech, language, and hearing in African Americans. These recommendations have implications for the identification of communication disorders in African Americans specifically and for the reduction of health disparities generally.

With the combined efforts of practitioners, researchers, and government officials, health disparities can be reduced.

REFERENCES

Al-Dabbous, I.A., Jama, A.H.A., Obeja, S.K., Murugan, A.N.R., & Hammad, H.A. (1996). Sensorineural hearing loss in homozygous sickle cell disease in Quatif, Saudi Arabia. *Annals of Saudi Medicine, 16*, 641–644.

American Psychological Association (APA). (1994). *Diagnostic and statistical manual of mental disorders, fourth edition.* Washington, DC: American Psychiatric Press.

Amilie-Lefond, C., Kleinschmidt-De Masters, B.K., Mahalingam, R., Davis, L.E., & Gilden, D.H. (1995). The vasculopathy of varicella-zoster virus encephalitis. *Annals of Neurology, 37*, 784–790.

Baker, F.M. (1988). Dementing illnesses and Black Americans. In J.S. Jackson (Ed.), *The Black American elderly: Research on physical and psychological health* (pp. 215–233). New York: Springer.

Battle, D.E. (2002). Communication disorders in multicultural populations, 3rd ed. Boston: Butterworth-Heinemann.

Bayles, K.A. (1988). Dementia: The clinical perspective. In H.K. Ulatowska (Ed.), *Aging and Communication: Seminars in Speech and Language, 9*, 143–166.

Bayles, K.A., & Kaszniak, A.W. (1987). The brain and age-related dementing diseases. In K.A. Bayles & A.W. Kaszniak (Eds.), *Communication and cognition in normal aging and dementia* (pp. 27–41). Boston: Pro-Ed.

Bloom, M. (1995). *Sickle cell disease.* Jackson: University of Mississippi Press.

Boccellari, A., & Zeifert, P. (1994). Management of neurobehavorial impairment in HIV-1 infection. In L.S. Zegans & T.J. Coates (Eds.), *The psychiatric clinics of North America: Psychiatric manifestations of HIV disease, 17*, 183–204.

Brain Injury Association. (2003). *Traumatic brain injury.* Washington, DC: Author.

Brain Injury Association. (1995). *Traumatic brain injury.* Washington, DC: Author.

Bryant, R., Marosszeky, J., Crooks, J., Baguley, I., & Gurka, J. (2000). Coping style and post-traumatic stress disorder following severe traumatic brain injury. *Brain Injury, 13*, 175–180.

Butler-Hinz, S., Caplan, D., & Waters, G. (1990). Characteristics of syntactic comprehension deficits following closed head inury versus left cerebrovascular accident. *Journal of Speech and Hearing Research, 33*, 269–280.

Centers for Disease Control (CDC). (2002a). National Center for Chronic Disease Prevention and Health Promotion. Chronic Disease Prevention. *The burden of chronic diseases and their risk factors.* National and State Perspectives, 2002. Atlanta, GA: Author.

Centers for Disease Control (CDC). (2002b). National Center for HIV, STD and TB Prevention. Divisions of HIV/AIDS Prevention. *Survillance Report*, Volume 13, No. 2. Atlanta, GA: Author.

Cohen, A.B., Martin, M.B., &, Silber, J.H. (1992). A modified transfusion program for prevention of stroke in sickle cell disease. *Blood, 79*, 1637–1661.

Cohen, M.J., Branch, W.B., McKie, V.C., Adams, R.J. (1994). Neuropsychological impairment in children with sickle cell anemia and cerebrovascular accidents. *Clinical Pediatrics (Philadelphia), 33*, 517–524.

Cummings, J.L., Benson, D.F., & LaVerne, S. (1980). Reversible dementia: Illustrative cases, definition, and review. *Journal of the American Medical Association, 243*, 2434–2439.

Eng, T.R. (2002). eHealth research and evaluation: Challenges and opportunities. *Journal of Health Communication, 7*, 267–272.

Eng, T.R., & Gustafson, D.H. (1999). Wired for health and well-being: The emergence of interactive health communication. Available at: http://www.health.gov/scipich/pubs/final report.htm.

Eslinger, P.J., & Damaisio, A.R. (1981). Age and type of aphasia in patients with stroke. *Journal of Neurology, Neurosurgery, and Psychiatry, 44*, 377–381.

Foulkes, M.A., Wolf, P.A., Price, T.R., Mohr, J.P., & Hier, D. (1988). The stroke data bank: Design, methods, and baseline characteristics. *Stroke, 19*, 547–554.

Freed, D. (2000). *Motor speech disorders: Diagnosis and treatment.* San Diego: Singular Publishing Group/ Thompson Learning.

Gaines, K., & Burke, G. (1995). Ethnic differences in stroke: Black–white differences in the United States population; SECORDS Investigators. Southeastern consortium on racial differences in stroke. *Neuroepidemiology, 14*, 209–239.

Gentry, B., Davis, P., & Dancer, J. (1997). Failure rates of young patients with sickle cell disease on a hearing screening test. *Perceptual Motor Skills, 2,* 434–436.

Gresham, G.E., et al. (1995). *Post-stroke rehabilitation. Clinical practice guideline, No. 16.* Public Health Service, Agency for Health Care Policy and Research. (AHCPR Publication No. 95-0662). Rockville, MD: U.S. Department of Health and Human Services.

Gresham, G.E., Philips, T.E., Wolf, P.A., McNamara, P.M., Kannel, W.B., & Dawber, T.R. (1979). Epidemiologic profile of long-term stroke disability: The Framingham study. *Archives of Physical Medicine and Rehabilitation, 60,* 487–491.

Horner, R.C., Marchar, D.B., Divine, G.W., & Feussner, J.R. (1991). Racial variations in ischemic stroke-related physical and functional impairments. *Stroke, 22,* 1497–1501.

Institute of Medicine. (2002). Speaking of health: Assessing health communication strategies for diverse populations. Washington, DC: National Academies Press.

Jagger, J., Levine, J.I., Jane, J., & Rimel, R.W. (1984). Epidemiologic features of head injury in a prominantly rural poplation. *Journal of Trauma, 24,* 40–44.

Joint United Nations Programme on HIV/AIDS (UNAIDS)/World Health Organization (2002). AIDS epidemic update. Geneva, Switzerland: Author.

Klein, K. (1995). *Aphasia community group manual.* New York: National Aphasia Association.

Marquardt, T.P., Stoll, J., & Sussman, H. (1990). Disorders of communication in traumatic brain injury. In E.D. Bigler (Ed.), *Traumatic brain injury* (pp. 181–205). Austin, TX: Pro-Ed.

Mateer, C.A. (1989). Neural correlates of language function. In D.P. Keuhn, M.L. Lemme, & J. Baumgartner (Eds.), *Neural bases of speech, hearing and language* (pp. 259–291). Boston: Little, Brown.

Max, W., MacKenzie, E.K., & Rice, D.P. (1991). Head injuries: Costs and consequences. *Journal of Head Injury Rehabilitation, 6,* 76.

McArthur, J.C., et al. (1993). Dementia in AIDS patients: Incidence and risk factors. *Neurology, 43,* 2245–2252.

McDonald, S. (1993). Pragmatic language skills after closed head injury: Ability to meet the informational needs of the listeners. *Brain and Language. 44,* 28–46.

Miles. T.P., & Bernard, M.A. (1992). Morbidity, disability, and health status of Black American elderly: A new look at the oldest old. *Journal of the American Geriatric Society, 40,* 1047–1054.

Morrison, B.J., & and Greeson, A.D. (1990). Curriculum content pertaining to the Black elderly for selected health care professions. In M.S. Harper (Ed.), *Minority aging: Essential curricula content for selected health and allied health professions.* Health Resources and Services Administration, Department of Health and Human Services. (DHHS Publication No. HRS [P-DV-90-4])(pp. 223–268).Washington, DC: U.S. Government Printing Office.

National Center for Health Statistics. (1994). National health discharge survey. DHHS Publication No. PHS 96-1521). Hyattsville, MD: U.S. Department of Health and Human Services.

National Institute on Aging. (1985). *Established populations for epidemiologic studies of the elderly: Resource data book.* U.S. Department of Health and Human Service. Public Health Service., National Institutes of Health (NIH Publication No. 86-2443), Washington, DC: U.S. Government Printing Office.

National Institute on Deafness and Communication Disorders (NIDCD). (2002a). *Aphasia.* NIH Publication No. 97-4257. Rockville, MD: Author.

National Institute on Deafness and Communication Disorders (NIDCD). (2002b). Strategic plan on reducing health disparities. http://www.nidcd.nih.gov/about/plans/strategic/nsrp_02.asp.

National Institute on Deafness and Communication Disorders (2003). *Aphasia.* NIH Publication No. 97-4257. Rockville, MD: Author.

National Institutes of Health. (1995). *Management and therapy of sickle cell disease.* National Heart, Lung, and Blood Institute. National Institutes of Health Publication No. 96-2117. Rockville, MD: Author.

National Stroke Association. (1996). *Stroke/brain attack briefing.* Englewood, CO: Author.

Naugle, R.I. (1990). Epidemiology of traumatic brain injury in adults. In E.D. Bigler (Ed.), *Traumatic brain injury* (pp. 69–103). Austin, TX: Pro-Ed.

Ommaya, A.K. (1995). Head injury mechanisms and the concept of preventive management: A review and critical synthesis. *Journal of Neurotrauma, 12,* 527–546.

Payne, J.C. (1997). *Adult neurogenic language disorders: Assessment and treatment. A comprehensive ethno-biological approach.* San Diego: Singular Publishing Group.

Payne, J.C. (1998a). Culture and stroke sequelae. In *Proceedings of the conference on communication disorders and stroke in African-American and other cultural groups: Multidisciplinary perspectives and research needs.* Bethesda, MD: National Institute on Deafness and Other Communication Disorders.

Payne, J.C. (1998b). Ethnocultural dynamics and acquired aphasia. In M.T. Sarno (Ed.), *Acquired aphasia,* 3d ed. New York: Academic Press.

Payne, J.C., & Stockman, I.J. (1979). Sickle cell disease: Recommendations for research and clinical services in speech pathology and audiology. *Journal of Allied Health and Behavioral Sciences, 2,* 257–264.

Ripich, D.N. (1991). Language and communication in dementia. In D.N. Ripich (Ed.), *Handbook of geriatric communication disorders* (pp. 255–283). Austin, TX: Pro-Ed.

Ripich, D.N., & Terrell, B.Y. (1988). Patterns of discourse cohesion and coherence in Alzheimer's disease. *Journal of Speech and Hearing Disorders, 53,* 8–15.

Shadden, B.B. (1990). Degenerative neurological disorders. In E. Cherow (Ed.), *Proceedngs of the research symposium in communication sciences and disorders and aging.* ASHA Report 19 (pp. 99–113). Rockville, MD: American Speech Language-Hearing Association.

Stroman, C.A. (2000). Explaining illness to African Americans: Employing cultural concerns with strategies. In B. Whaley (Ed.), *Explaining illness: Research, theory, and strategies* (pp. 299–316). Mahwah, NJ: Lawrence Erlbaum.

Taylor, O.L., & Peters-Johnson, C.A. (1986). Speech, language and hearing disorders in Black populations. In O.L. Taylor (Ed.), *Nature of communication disorders in culturally and linguistically diverse populations* (pp. 157–179). San Diego: College-Hill Press.

Vilkki, J., Ahola, K., Holst, P., Ohman, J., Servo, A., & Heiskanen, O. (1994). Prediction of psychosocial recovery after head injury with cognitive tests and neurobehavioral rating. *Journal of Clinical and Experimental Neuropsychology, 3,* 325–338.

Wallace, G.L. (1993). Adult neurogenic disorders. In D.E. Battle (Ed.), *Communication disorders in multicultural populations* (pp. 239–255). Boston: Andover Medical Publishers.

Wallace, G.L., & Tonkovich, J.O. (1998). African Americans: Culture, communication, and clinical management. In G.L. Wallace (Ed.), *Multicultural Neurogenics* (pp. 133–164). San Antonio, TX: Communication Skills Builders.

Whitman, S., Coonley-Hoganson, R., & Desai, B.T. (1984). Comparative head trauma experience in two socioeconomically different Chicago-area communities: A population study. *American Association of Epidemiology, 119,* 570–580.

Zarcadoolas, C., Blanco, M., Boyer, J.F., & Pleasant, A. (2002). Unweaving the Web: An exploratory study of low-literate adults' navigation skills on the World Wide Web. *Journal of Health Communication, 7,* 309–324.

PART III

Lifestyle, Social, and Mental Outcomes

CHAPTER 14

The Life Expectancy of the Black Male: Pressing Issues from the Cradle to the Grave

DONALD R. WARE AND IVOR LENSWORTH LIVINGSTON

INTRODUCTION

On perusing the literature on minority health, it is evident that there is a noticeable increase in the number of authors who have addressed the "plight" of the Black male. For example, mention was made in a past publication of the Black male as an "endangered species" in America (Gibbs, 1998), as well in a recent television broadcast show (UNCTV, 1990). The terms "endangered and embattled" are used to describe the Black (or African American male) simply because he has the shortest life span of all Americans. From the time he is born (i.e., the cradle) until he dies (i.e., the grave), the Black male has a shorter life span than Black females and Whites of both genders.

In 1990, an article in the *New England Journal of Medicine* reported an astounding statistic that "Black men in Harlem were less likely to reach the age of 65 than men in Bangladesh" (McCord & Freeman, 1990, p. 173). Some have questioned "whether the findings in Harlem can be generalized to other areas of poverty in the United States or to other Black communities" (Geronimus et al., 1996, p. 1552). However, although there have been some improvements in the health of Black men, a recent report by the W.K. Kellogg Foundation concluded that "from birth, a Black male on average seems fated to a life so unhealthy that a White man can only imagine it" (Villarosa, 2002).

The Black male's (BM) life expectancy (LE) of 68.2 is usually compared with the other three race/ethnic gender groups' LEs, i.e., the White male (WM = 74.8), the Black female (BF = 74.9), and the White female (WF = 80.0) (Minino et al., 2002). This chapter shows that various conditions (e.g., diseases, including chronic and infectious diseases; poverty; racism; lack of educational and occupational opportunities; living environments, and violence, to only mention a few) individually and collectively place the Black male at-risk to experience, in many cases, premature morbidity and mortality. This being the case, the very existence of the Black male is in jeopardy from the time he is born (and in some cases even when he is in the womb) until the time he dies.

The implications of the Black male's being "endangered" are very important. For example, the Black male who was born in the year 2000, on average, will not long live long enough to fully enjoy the fruits of his labor, if current trends continue. The absence of the male from the Black family unit is a tremendous loss. Not only is economic security threatened, but also family role modeling and leadership as well as spousal companionship are, in many cases, irrevocably compro-

Table 14.1
General demographic characteristics by race and gender for the United States, 2000

Black or African American male population				
	Number		Percent	
Subject	Alone	Alone or in Combination	Alone	Alone or in Combination
Under 5 years	1,424,275	1,607,056	4.1	4.4
5 to 14 years	3,211,993	3,460,037	9.3	9.5
15 to 24 years	2,763,393	2,904,533	8.0	8.0
25 to 34 years	2,451,508	2,548,089	7.1	7.0
35 to 44 years	2,595,486	2,675,956	7.5	7.3
45 to 54 years	1,887,208	1,939,705	5.4	5.3
55 to 64 years	1,057,157	1,083,635	3.1	3.0
65 years and over	1,074,165	1,096,322	3.1	3.0
White American male population				
Under 5 years	6,597,764	7,002,928	3.1	3.2
5 to 14 years	14,521,306	15,163,451	6.9	7.0
15 to 24 years	13,963,980	14,439,498	6.6	6.7
25 to 34 years	14,336,930	14,733,569	6.8	6.8
35 to 44 years	17,176,182	17,525,517	8.1	8.1
45 to 54 years	14,879,139	15,111,657	7.0	7.0
55 to 64 years	9,708,350	9,835,184	4.6	4.5
65 years and over	12,589,543	12,709,392	6.0	5.9

Source: U.S. Census Bureau, Census 2000.

mised. The survival of a race is, in part, defined by its ability to pass on genetic information and culture to the next generation. If this is cut off before it can begin, the makings of genocide, whether it be on the basis of self-destructive behavior or some other causes, can take seed and destroy the vine.

Although the Black male is a relative numerical minority in this country, he is disproportionately burdened by disease. This is especially the case when examining diseases such as hypertension, diabetes, HIV and AIDS, prostate cancer, heart disease, and violence as a public health problem. To further complicate matters, for many African American men, going to the doctor is not something that is readily accepted, and, despite the often fatal consequences, Black men frequently don't seek routine medical intervention (Courtenay, 2000). Because it is difficult to assess the conditions associated with the Black male without having a reference group, in some cases information is presented on the White male (and in other cases, with the Black female) for comparative purposes. For a comparison of selected demographic characteristics of Black males and White males see Table 14.1.

Figure 14.1

Factors influencing the disproportionate incidence of morbidity and mortality among African American males

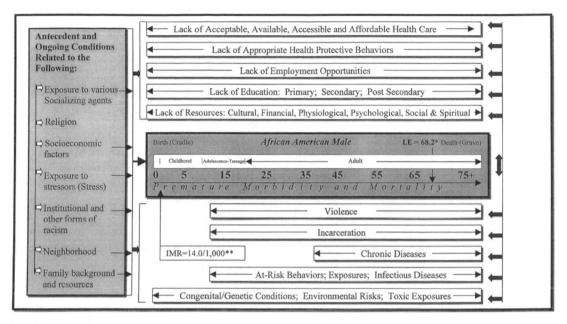

Ivor Lensworth Livingston, 2004.

* Life Expectancy of 68.2 years as of 2000, NCHS, 2002; **Infant Mortality Rate for *all* Blacks.

Focus of the Chapter

Although the multitude of conditions that place the Black male at risk are, in many cases, continuously affecting him as he develops through his life span, the chapter explores the life cycle of the Black male through three basic developmental periods: *childhood years, adolescent and teenage years*, and *adult years*. During each of these periods, which are certainly not mutually exclusive of each other and, therefore, are interconnected, a discussion is presented of selected conditions that he may experience that contributes to his at-risk status (see conceptual model used in Figure 14.1). A discussion is also presented about some prevention strategies that can contribute to efforts in reducing racial and ethnic disparities in health.

CONDITIONS CONTRIBUTING TO AT-RISK STATUS OF THE BLACK MALE: OVERVIEW OF CONCEPTUAL MODEL

Macrolevel and Microlevel Conditions

Any meaningful attempt at explaining the variety of conditions that place the Black male at risk for both premature sickness and death has to fully appreciate the complexity of the factors involved, as well as the dynamic interaction of these conditions. Furthermore, there is a synergistic interaction of these various factors at basically two extreme levels, the "macro," or societal level, and the "micro," or individual level (Anderson et al., 1995; Shepard, 2002; Livingston et al., 2004). The mesolevel, which involves groups (families), falls in the middle between macrolevel conditions and microlevel conditions. Because of space limitations, macrolevel and microlevel conditions are emphasized. Therefore, in order to facilitate a partial and/or selected discussion of the variety of conditions that contribute to the at-risk status of the Black male, a model is used as a conceptual guide.

As seen in Figure 14.1, the selected antecedent and ongoing macro-level conditions all theoretically appear to the left in the model. Because of their wider societal influence, they have the potential of influencing other "derived" (and possibly mediating) macro-level conditions (lack of educational and employment opportunities). They can also influence micro-level conditions (e.g., complying with hypertension and/or diabetes medication, developing a "spiritual" outlook on life), as well. It is important to note from Figure 14.1 that there is ongoing interaction between these antecedent conditions as evidenced by the connected arrows.

Macrolevel conditions are usually antecedent and ongoing in the lives of the individual, and they are very important based on the developmental perspective that guides this chapter. This basic view is that individuals, such as African Americans, are born with a *tabula rasa* (blank slate) and over time through the socialization process (i.e., involving macro-level socialization agents) they acquire a sense of self (e.g., self-identity and racial self-identity). Therefore, as seen in Figure 14.1, these macro-level factors have a direct influence on the various potential health conditions (i.e., those below the "core" in the model), as well as the more structural and possibly mediating conditions (i.e., those above the "core" of the model). An important relationship is the one between these antecedent macro-level conditions and the variety of "resources" (e.g., cultural, physiological, psychological, social and spiritual) the individual acquires as he or she develops and matures from infancy through adolescence to adulthood.

Microlevel conditions are in contrast to the macro-level conditions because they are more modifiable, as they are more under the control of the individual. Examples of micro-level conditions include adhering to the medical regimen of taking blood pressure medication and engaging in other health protective behaviors such as exercising. Most of these health protective behaviors are positively related to improvements in overall health conditions (Courtenay, 2000).

Socializing Agents.   These socializing macro-level agents include the mass media, schools and, at a more personal, or mesolevel, the family. These agents basically teach us about our values that eventually influence behavior (Macionis, 2002) (e.g., those that influence in particular the "positive" health protective that Blacks have to acquire, such as, dietary, sleeping, exercise information). The family continues to be the main source of socialization, especially in the African American community. Through familial socialization, children and adolescents receive (or should receive) the fundamentals regarding values, morals, norms and beliefs and this information is usually transmitted from one generation to the next. Prince (1997) and Warfield-Coppock (1992) concur with Willis (1990), that in the traditional African American family, nurturance and support are associated with Afrocentric instructions of a committed love of the family, mutual respect, communal cooperation and responsibility, and the formation of a racial identity.

Religion.   Religious influences can also be classified as a macrolevel or mesolevel condition depending on the size of the religious establishment involved. Research has shown that the kind of supportive "integrative" interaction African Americans report having with their religious establishments is associated with lower arterial (systolic) blood pressure levels (Livingston et al., 1991).

Socioeconomic Status (SES).   The most basic causes of health disparities are SES disparities (Link & Phelan, 1995). SES has traditionally been defined by education, income, and occupation. However, education is perhaps the most basic SES component since it shapes future occupational opportunities. By earning higher income, a better-educated person gains more ready access to information and resources to promote health (Ross & Wu, 1995). "While SES is clearly linked to morbidity and mortality, the mechanisms responsible for the association are not well understood" (Adler & Newman, 2002, p. 61).

Table 14.2
2003 HHS poverty guidelines

Size of Family Unit	48 Contiguous States and D.C.	Alaska	Hawaii
1	$ 8,980	$11,210	$10,330
2	12,120	15,140	13,940
3	15,260	19,070	17,550
4	18,400	23,000	21,160
5	21,540	26,930	24,770
6	24,680	30,860	28,380
7	27,820	34,790	31,990
8	30,960	38,720	35,600
For each additional person, add	3,140	3,930	3,610

Source: Federal Register, Vol. 68, No. 26, February 7, 2003, pp. 6456–6458.

The poverty guidelines may be formally referenced as "the poverty guidelines updated periodically in the Federal Register by the U.S. Department of Health and Human Services under the authority of 42 U.S.C. 9902(2)."

Whatever the means used to assess SES, it has been reliably associated with a wide range of health problems, including low birth-weight, cardiovascular disease, hypertension, arthritis, diabetes and cancer (Pamuk, 1998; Livingston et al., 2004), all of which are disproportionately seen in the African American population. SES has been conceptualized and measured in a variety of ways. For a comprehensive review of the measurement issues related to social class in general and for implications related to health, see Krieger et al., (1997).

Each year the U.S. Department of Health and Human Services (USDHHS) issues poverty guidelines. These guidelines, which are issued each year in the *Federal Register*, are a simplification of the poverty thresholds, and they are used primarily for administrative purposes—for instance, determining financial eligibility for certain federal programs See Table 14.2 for the HHS Poverty Guidelines. The number of poor African Americans dropped by 600,000 to 9.1 million between 1996 and 1997, while their poverty rate fell from 28.4 percent to 26.5 percent.

For Hispanics, who may be of any race, the number in poverty declined from 8.7 million to 8.3 million, and their poverty rate dropped from 29.4 percent to 27.1 percent. In both years, the poverty rate for Hispanics did not differ statistically from that of African Americans. For comparative purposes, Black males are disproportionately poor compared with their White male counterparts. As seen in at the extreme portions of Table 14.3, there are many more Black males under 18 years (33. percent) and 75+ (37.0 percent) who are under a ratio of income to poverty level of 1.50 compared with their corresponding White counterparts (under 18 years = 16.6 percent 75 + years = 18.4 percent).

There is an important SES–suicide relationship worth mentioning. The stressors experienced by

Table 14.3
Age, sex, and race by ratio of income to poverty level, 2001 (number in thousands)

	Total	Under .50		Under 1.00		Under 1.25		Under 1.50	
		Number	Percent	Number	Percent	Number	Percent	Number	Percent
Black Male									
Total	16,626	1,553	9.3	3,343	20.1	4,456	26.8	5,393	33.4
Under 18 years	5,833	897	15.4	1,735	29.7	2,275	39.0	2,673	44.8
18 to 24 years	1,862	189	10.2	402	21.6	506	27.2	592	31.8
25 to 34 years	2,244	139	6.2	291	13.0	402	17.9	504	22.5
35 to 44 years	2,465	126	5.1	292	11.9	398	16.2	506	20.5
45 to 54 years	2,026	105	5.2	275	13.6	364	18.0	470	23.2
55 to 59 years	640	31	4.8	88	13.8	122	19.1	146	22.7
60 to 64 years	434	21	4.7	84	19.4	117	26.9	139	31.9
65 to 74 years	753	28	3.7	108	14.3	167	22.2	228	30.3
75 years and over	369	16	4.4	67	18.1	105	28.4	137	37.0
White Male									
Total	113,196	3,930	3.5	10,072	8.9	14,101	12.5	18,837	16.6
Under 18 years	28,772	1,511	5.3	3,870	13.4	5,235	18.2	6,765	23.5
18 to 24 years	10,980	545	5.0	1,298	11.8	1,733	15.8	2,331	21.2
25 to 34 years	15,666	464	3.0	1,214	7.8	1,752	11.2	2,447	15.6
35 to 44 years	18,105	497	2.7	1,194	6.6	1,656	9.1	2,228	12.3
45 to 54 years	16,285	463	2.2	911	5.6	1,277	7.8	1,655	10.2
55 to 59 years	6,114	195	3.2	414	6.8	548	9.0	666	10.9
60 to 64 years	4,637	154	3.3	413	8.9	574	12.4	681	14.7
65 to 74 years	7,184	125	1.7	408	5.7	700	9.7	1,062	14.8
75 years and over	5,453	76	1.4	349	6.4	627	11.5	1,002	18.4

Source: U.S. Census Bureau, Current Population Survey, March 2002.

middle-class African American males may account for their pattern of suicide risk. Various studies have found that while SES is inversely related to the suicide rate for Whites, it is positively related to the suicide rate for African American males (Lester, 1998; Fernquist, 2001). One explanation offered for this stress–suicide relationship for African American males is that exposure to discrimination is an added burden faced by middle-class African men. Therefore, these perceptions of discrimination are stressors that can adversely affect physical and mental health (Williams et al., 2003). Another explanation is that African American males' expectations are unfulfilled because their investment in education has not provided the anticipated gains in income, which in turn may produce feelings of alienation (Anderson, 1999).

Exposure to Stressors.   It is reasoned in this chapter that a contributing factor to the stress–health relationship for African Americans is their perception of and negative experiences with the daily realities of both positive (e.g., social support, McNeilly et al., 1996) and negative exogenous factors or stressors (e.g., racism, discrimination and/or low SES conditions or poverty-related experiences, Clark et al., 1999; low SES, Forman et al., 1997). Other macrolevel potential stressors include: poverty, undesirable life events, crowding, crime, noise pollution, discrimination and other hazards or stressors (Baum et al., 1999).

Racism.   A perusal of the literature shows that, irrespective of improvements in the racial and ethnic group attitudes among Whites (Schuman et al., 1985), there still remain "signs" of inequality (Jaynes & Williams, 1989). Examples of racism include examples in the restaurant industry; housing rentals and sales (Yinger, 1995); and hiring practices (Kirschenman & Neckerman, 1991). The exposure to racism can cause anger, distrust, and suspicion in Blacks toward the White society (Thompson, 1994). This anger may manifest itself in some young Black males through chronic frustration, ambivalence, a chronic sense of threat, feelings of relative powerlessness, and stress.

Combined Effect of Antecedent Conditions.   Again, as indicated in Figure 14.1, there is the potential for interaction between these (and other) antecedent conditions. For example, depending on the financial resources of families, as well as their SES, there are certain restrictions placed on the neighborhoods in which they can reside. All of this, in turn, has the potential to influence Black males' values systems (e.g., right versus wrong), daily experiences, and the health protective behaviors they must learn that can serve to benefit their health and lives as they mature and enter adulthood. Low SES can predispose them to a lifestyle that may include substandard housing, unhealthy diet, inadequate education, absence of health insurance, and lack of access to employment opportunities. Additionally, because of relatively low SES (compared to their White counterparts—see Table 14.3), a substantial percentage of the Black population lives in low-income rural or inner-city neighborhoods. In these neighborhoods they are likely to experience high numbers of environmental hazards, including traffic hazards, air pollution, toxic waste, overcrowded housing, and crime (Anderson et al., 1999).

The focal point of Figure 14.1 is at the center, or "core," where the developmental periods of the African American male are highlighted from childhood, through teenage and adolescence, up to the adult years. These are the three periods to be elaborated on later in the chapter. The label of the "endangered" species attached to the Black male (Gibbs, 1998), mentioned before, is aptly depicted in the center of the model. The model illustrates that after birth, through 75+ years, the Black male may experience potential loss of years (or of life) by undergoing premature morbidity and mortality. This occurs as a result of a vast number of reciprocal experiences (see bidirectional arrows in Figure 14.1).

The experiences, which are at the top (e.g., "macro" health care conditions and employment opportunities and "meso" educational opportunities), and run for the entire duration of his life span, are basically the "structural" conditions that, if lacking, can predispose him to early sickness (morbidity) and/or death (mortality). Premature loss of life can begin as early as the first year of life (i.e., infant mortality rate [IMR]), where for all Black infants (irrespective of gender) it is 14.0/1,000 compared to 5.8/1,000 for White infants. Conversely, it can end with premature death, where the mortality rate for Black males was 68.2 years in 2002 (versus 74.8 for White males; 74.9 for Black females; and 80.0 for White females) (Pastor et al., 2002). These experiences contrast with those that are below the core of the model. These conditions (e.g., violence, incarceration, chronic diseases) represent the individual and combined conditions that more directly contribute to the premature morbidity and mortality illustrated at the developmental core of the model.

CHILDHOOD YEARS

Overview

The nation's vital statistics suggest that between ages 1–4 there is a significant difference in death from accidents between Black male children and White male children. According to the National Vital Statistics Report of 2000 (Minino et al., 2002), the top three causes of death in the Black child from age 1–4 are accidents (34 percent), homicide (10.8 percent), and congenital malformations (10.1 percent). In the White male child age 1–4, the top three causes of death are accidents (40.3), malignant neoplasm (15.9 percent), and congenital malformations (9 percent). Homicide (or assault) is the number four cause of death in White males in this age range and constitutes approximately 5.4 percent of deaths. These vital statistics suggest that before the Black male child can reach the age of true self-expression, 45 percent of the deaths in this group will be from accidents or homicide. Clearly, the responsibility of the safety of the child has not been substantially addressed by the supervising parents, siblings, and other responsible adults.

Premature Mortality

Nationally, Black infants are 2.4 times as likely to die as White children (Kozlowski, 2001). In the United States, as well as in other countries, more boys than girls are born each year. However, infant males are more likely to die in their first year of life compared to infant females (NCHS, 2002). Infant mortality, or the death rate among children under one year of age, is basically twice as high for disadvantaged children in the United States versus their more privileged counterparts (Macionis, 2002). As seen in Figure 14.1, the overall infant mortality rate (IMR) for all African Americans is 14.0 per 1,000 (live births) compared to 5.8 per 1,000 for White infants. In a related manner, the neonatal mortality rate (NMR) and postneonatal mortality rate (PMR) for Black infants are 9.5/1,000 and 4.5/1,000, respectively (compared to 3.9/1,000 and 1.9/1,000, respectively, for White infants) (Pastor, et al., 2002).

The Importance of Poverty

It has been seen that the poverty rate among African Americans, which is approximately three times that of their White counterparts, explains, in part, why Black people are more likely to die in infancy (and be associated with a variety of other negative experiences, e.g., violence, illness, and drug abuse) (Hayward et al., 2000). The life expectancy for White children born in 2000 is five years greater than for African American children (77.4 years compared to 71.8) (NCHS, 2001). According to Macaronis, "sex is a stronger predictor of health than race, since African American females outlive males of either race. From another angle, 79 percent of White men but just 62 percent of African American men will live to sixty-five." The comparable figures for women are 87 percent for Whites and 77 percent for African Americans (p. 385).

Unintended Accidents

African American children, like other racial and ethnic groups, are experiencing an increase in unintended accidents, many of which lead to an early death for these children. For example, approximately 1,500 children drown each year in the United States. Studies report that toddlers (and adolescent males) have an increased risk of drowning. Toddlers are drowning more in freshwater sites, like ponds, lakes, and rivers. After 5 years of age, about a third of drowning among African American males are in swimming pools. After age 5, African American males had significantly higher rates of drowning than White males. It has been said that much of this disparity is due to an increased risk of drowning in swimming pools, where rates were 12-15 times higher among African American males than among White males (NIH News Release, 2001).

Lead Poisoning

Although lead poisoning is not on the list for mortality in the early childhood years, it nevertheless has a great impact on the lives of many families. Approximately 4.4 percent of American children ages 1–5 have a blood lead level of at least 10 mcg/dL. This represents just under a million children (890,000) ages 1–5 (Montague, 2000). Lead poisoning may lead to brain and kidney problems. Symptoms include headaches, muscle and joint weakness or pain, tiredness or lethargy, behavioral problems, difficulty concentrating, loss of appetite, metallic taste in the mouth, abdominal pain, nausea or vomiting, or constipation. Concentrations of low-income children in substandard housing have led to low-income and Black children having eight times and five times higher risk of lead poisoning, respectively (Montague, 2000).

ADOLESCENT AND TEENAGE YEARS

Overview

The adolescent and teenage years are crucial for the Black male. As indicated in Figure 14.1, those at risk because of the antecedent (macrolevel and mesolevel) conditions (e.g., poverty, stress, lack of appropriate socializing agents and role models in the family); emerging structural conditions (e.g., lack of appropriate health care, education, and employment opportunities); as well as more personal (micro-level) health protective behaviors, will prematurely become sick and/or die. Such premature sickness and/or death, if not occurring during these years, will, unfortunately, lead over to the next developmental period in young adulthood and, in many cases, later on in life.

By the time the Black male reaches the preteen and teen years, other patterns of death begin to emerge. While accidents continue to be number one in terms of premature death (37.8 percent), homicide rises to number two (10.3 percent), up from number five (3.7 percent) in the 5–9 age range. Malignant neoplasm is at number three (8.3 percent). It is very significant to note that while Black preteens and early teens are being socialized into new roles, suicide enters the top ten causes of death for the first time at number four (6.4 percent). White males in this group suffer from accidents as the number one cause of death with cancer, suicide, and homicide as the next leading causes of death (suicide, 10 percent of the total; homicide, 4.7 percent of the total) (NCHS, 2001).

Suicide

The CDC summarized trends in suicide among Black youth age 10–19 years in the United States during 1980–1995 and indicated that suicidal behavior among all youths has increased. Black youth rates, however, have increased more, although Black youths have historically had lower suicide rates than have Whites. During 1980–1995, the suicide rate for Black youths age 10–19 years increased from 2.1 to 4.5 per 100,000 population. Additionally, among this age group of 15–19-year-olds, firearms use accounted for 72 percent of suicides, followed by strangulation (20 percent). Overall, firearm-related suicides accounted for 96 percent of the increase in the suicide rate for Blacks aged 10–19 years (MMWR, 1998). As of 1995, suicide was the third leading cause of death for Blacks aged 15–19 years, and high school-aged Blacks were as likely as Whites to attempt suicide (Murphy, 2000).

There are many risk factors associated with suicides among youth. Depression, hopelessness, family history of suicide, a previous suicide attempt, and easier access to alcohol have been reported in the past (Garland & Zigler, 1993). Regarding the increase in suicides among Black youth, one explanation has to do with the growth of the Black middle class (Davis, 1980). For example, Black youths in upwardly mobile families are likely to experience stress associated with the new social environments associated with their new socioeconomic status. In a related manner, it has been speculated that the typical risk factors may not adequately predict suicidal behaviors among Black youths. For example, the exposure of other Black youths to poverty, discrimination, and substandard educational opportunities may have negatively influenced their expectations about the future and, therefore, enhanced their resiliency to suicide (Gibbs, 1997).

Mental Health

Factors that affect the mental health of the African American male can begin very early in life (see the various conditions that are likely to impact the developmental experiences of the African American male) (see Figure 14.1). Barbarin (1993) reports on data from the Johns Hopkins Prevention Research Center, which reveal that African American children and adolescents from poor neighborhoods experience a nonclinical and nonreferral depressed mood. This mood manifests itself around age 9. It is suggested to be linked to low self-esteem and morale and the disaffection with education. Chronic poverty and the instability of a secured family life are reported to be contributing factors to this type of depression. It is also reported that frustration surfaces because of dangerous and substandard housing conditions, limited access to medical care, poor nutritional habits and the lack of appropriate safety on playgrounds (Wyatt, 2000).

HIV/AIDS

African Americans are increasingly being disproportionately affected by HIV/AIDS. Although both the infection and the disease are being manifested in the adolescent and teenage years, related, in part, to intravenous drug use and sexual activity, due to the latency period of the virus, an increasing number of AIDS cases are showing up in early adulthood. Although African Americans constitute approximately 12 percent of the U.S. population, they account for about 50 percent of all new HIV infections and about 49 percent of new AIDS cases reported in 2001 (CDC, 2001). It is important to note that the rate of adolescent/adult AIDS cases among African Americans was approximately ten times (76.3/100,000) that of Caucasians (7.9/100,000) and about three times for Hispanics (28.0/100,000). Of the reported HIV cases in 2001 for African American males and females, the numbers were 1,654 and 2,716, respectively. Of the reported AIDS cases for African American males and females the numbers were 1,020 and 1,250, respectively (CDC, 2001).

Some Black males use sex as an escape to get away from family and other personal problems (Gant et al., 1994). However, early sexual activity makes the young Black male susceptible to premature fatherhood and sexually transmitted diseases (STDs). Young Black males appear to have an awareness of AIDS, but some do not believe it can happen to them (Watt, 2000). In an earlier study assessing knowledge and fear of AIDS among college students, Livingston (1990) reported some misconceptions as well as some fear of contracting AIDS.

Lost Opportunities and Lack of Resources

As illustrated in Figure 14.1, the health and related outcomes (e.g., violence, incarceration, chronic diseases, at-risk behaviors) not only are interrelated but are also reciprocally related to the lack of "resource" opportunities located above the core of the model (e.g., lack of desirable health care, health protective behaviors, employment, and education). It is argued that by missing the basic "opportunities" in life, the African American male becomes increasingly marginalized in society, where feelings of alienation, frustration, and/or depression are likely to be experienced. SES is a major contributing factor to such marginalization experiences. In a related manner, one of the more consistent relationships in the literature is the inverse relationship between SES and health (Williams, 2003).

Poverty.   Research suggests that the economic marginalization of African American males (i.e., high unemployment and low wages) is the central determinant of the high rates of female-headed households among African Americans (Sampson, 1987). Whereas in 1960 two-thirds of African American children were living with both parents, in 1999 only 38 percent lived with their parents. This compared with 82 percent for Asian children, 78 percent for non-Hispanic Whites, and 63 percent for American-born Hispanic children (Tucker, 2000). Therefore, the combination of low earnings for African American males and low pay for their female counterparts contributes to high rates of poverty for African American children (Williams, 2003).

Education.   For the Black male, most of the disproportionate health problems he exhibits in late adolescence, early, middle, and late adulthood have to do with his educational attainment in the formative years. According to Reed (1988), Black males face formidable challenges to their educational development. For example, their overall mean achievement scores are below those of other groups in the basic areas; they are more likely to be placed in classes for the educable mentally retarded and for students with learning disabilities than in gifted and talented classes; they are suspended from school more frequently and for longer periods of time than other student groups. Lastly, they complete high school at a lower rate than their Black female counterparts.

In many ways the challenges mentioned above and much more remain as formidable obstacles for the Black male today (Jones & Roberts, 1994). Therefore based on these and other realities, it has been said that frustration, underachievement, or failure often compromise the educational reality of young Black males. It was further suggested that Black males from kindergarten through high school tend to experience substantial feelings of alienation from America's schools. The unfortunate consequences of this reality are major restrictions on the Black male's subsequent economic mobility, which in turn has the potential of leading to high rates of unemployment, crime, and incarceration for a great number of them (Lee, 1991).

Homicide

Dramatic increases in both homicide victimization and offending rates were experienced by young males, particularly young Black males, in the late 1980s and early 1990s. However, during the past few years, homicide victimization rates have dropped for all groups, but, rates are not declining as rapidly as they did in the middle 1990's. For example, in the case of young Black males (ages 14–24), the proportion of offenders begins at 17 percent in 1976 and remains constant until 1987. In 1988 it sharply increases to 22 percent. After peaking at 33 percent in 1993, it decreases to 27 percent in 2000. The proportion of victims who were young Black males begins at 9 percent in 1976 and remains constant until 1985. After 1985 it gradually increases to 18 percent in 1994, and then it decreases to 15 percent in 2000 (BJS, 2002).

Employment, Drugs, Violence, Incarceration, and Related Policy

While each of these four areas is different, as seen in Figure 14.1, they are interrelated. According to McLoyd and Lozoff (2001), the marked increase in American male violence in recent decades coincided with comparable increases in unemployment, the percentage of young African American male high school dropouts with no reported source of income, the use and trafficking of crack cocaine, and decreases in the earnings of young African American males, both absolutely as well as relative to their White counterparts. The death rate from homicide for African American males aged 15 through 24 years has been estimated at 17 times the rate for White males in this age group (Rich & Ro, 2002).

The juvenile arrest records are alarming in the Black community (Tatum, 1996). Tatum cites sources to reveal the national arrest statistics that indicate that young Blacks less than 18 years old account for 30 percent of the part one index crimes (i.e., more serious crimes of murder, battery, and burglary). Young Black males are vulnerable to homicide and *forticide*, committing suicide at the hands of another individual (Majors & Billson, 1992). There is a 1 in 21 chance that a young Black male will be murdered before he reaches his 21st birthday. Furthermore, to add to this travesty is the self-fulfilling prophecy of committing forticide (Wyatt, 2000). Forticide is (Willis, 1990) in other words, consciously allowing yourself to be in the presence of another person that will kill you. According to Willis, young Black males who feel overwhelmed with their daily life situations (see Figure 1, where an emphasis is placed on the various antecedent conditions that can contribute to the outcomes alluded to here) may aggressively put themselves in risky situations where their demise is highly likely to occur.

Many of the above mentioned occurrences can be traced to areas of concentrated poverty created by social policies (Williams & Collins, 2001). At the same time there were a shift in the federal drug policy and a decline in federal spending on drug treatment (McLoyd & Lozoff, 2001). Another factor that exacerbates the situation is the aggressive and discriminatory nature of mandatory sentences given to African American males for alleged drug crimes (Kennedy, 2001). This sentencing activity in essence removes a large portion of the male population from the African American community, which in turn keeps them from providing needed economic and social support to their families (see Figure 14.1). As if things could not get worse, when the African American male is released from prison, a criminal record is a known liability that inhibits the chances of any future, steady gainful employment (Williams, 2003). This cycle of events has the real potential of leading to feelings of marginalization mentioned before, as well as feelings of frustration, anger, and violence and, ultimately, premature morbidity or mortality for the young African American male.

ADULT YEARS: CONDITIONS AND DISEASES AT A GLANCE

Overview

As seen in Table 14.4, as the Black male reaches the age of maturity, diseases of the heart, cancer, and unintentional injuries are the number one, two, and three leading causes of death. These same three causes of death are also similar for White males. While these rates are sex-and race-specific, if age is included, some of these ranked conditions are likely to change; for example, the death rate from homicide for African American males aged 15 through 24 years has been estimated at 17 times the rate for White males in this age group (Rich & Ro, 2002). The exclusion of age in Table 14.4 notwithstanding, it is seen that after the similarity of mortality causes one, two, and three for both Black and White males, some differences emerge. For example, whereas the number five cause of death for Black males is homicide, for Whites the number five cause is chronic obstructive pulmonary disease (COPD). For White males suicide is number seven, and for Black males number seven, is pneumonia.

It is interesting to note that for Black males the number six cause is certain conditions originating in the perinatal period (i.e., before, during and after pregnancy). The ranked position of this cause of death is consistent with the poverty-adverse pregnancy relationship alluded to in the past (Livingston, et al., 2003), as well as the fact that (Black) infant males are more likely to die in their first year of life than infant females (Williams, 2003). In terms of overall life expectancy (see Figure 14.1), on the average, the Black male dies the earliest (68.2), followed by the White male (74.8), the Black female, (74.9), and White female, who lives the longest (80.0) (Murphy, 2000). What follows is an overview of these ten leading causes of death for Black males, as well as some other conditions and activities that contribute to the existing racial/ethnic health disparities.

Heart Disease

Coronary heart disease (CHD) is the leading cause of death in the United States for Americans of African and all other ancestries (Clark et al., 1999). African Americans have the highest overall CHD mortality rate (MR) and the highest out-of-hospital coronary death rate of any ethnic group in the U.S. (Gillum, 1997). Sudden cardiac death, as the initial clinical manifestation of CHD, is considerably higher in African Americans than in Whites (Traven et al., 1996). In many of these studies, sudden coronary death rates have been reported to be as much as three times higher in Black men

Table 14.4
Ten leading causes of death and numbers of deaths, according to sex and race:
United States, 2000

Sex, race and rank order:	2000	
Black males	Cause of Death	Deaths
	All causes	130,138
1.	Diseases of the heart	37,877
2	Malignant neoplasms	25,861
3.	Unintentional injuries	9,701
4.	Cerebrovascular diseases	9,194
5.	Homicide	8,274
6.	Certain conditions originating in the perinatal period	3,869
7.	Pneumonia and influenza	3,386
8.	Chronic liver disease and cirrhosis	3,020
9.	Chronic obstructive pulmonary disease	2,429
10.	Diabetes mellitus	2,010
White males		
	All causes	933,878
1.	Diseases of the heart	364,679
2.	Malignant neoplasms	198,188
3.	Unintentional injuries	62,963
4.	Cerebrovascular diseases	60,095
5.	Chronic obstructive pulmonary disease	5,977
6.	Pneumonia and influenza	23,810
7.	Suicide	18,901
8.	Chronic liver disease and cirrhosis	16,407
9.	Diabetes mellitus	12,125
10.	Atherosclerosis	10,543

Source: Centers for Disease Control and Prevention, National Center for Health Statistics (Hyattsville, MD: National Center for Health Statistics, 2001).

than in White men, even after adjustment for age, SES, and access to care (Clark et al., 1999). The disparities between the Black male and the all other race/ethnic gender categories (i.e., White male and female and the Black female) are relatively pronounced (see Figure 14.2). So pronounced are the CHD disparities, especially between the Black male and the White female and male, that these disparities may be a very important contributor to the overall racial and ethnic disparities in health.

One of the problems Black males have is recognizing the signs of early myocardial attack and reporting to a nearby health facility for proper treatment. Many studies have shown Black people have a significantly higher out-of-hospital mortality rate than other groups (Clark et al., 1999). This could be on the basis of poor recognition of symptoms or poor emergency medical services in the

Figure 14.2
Prevalence of cardiovascular disease, by race/ethnicity

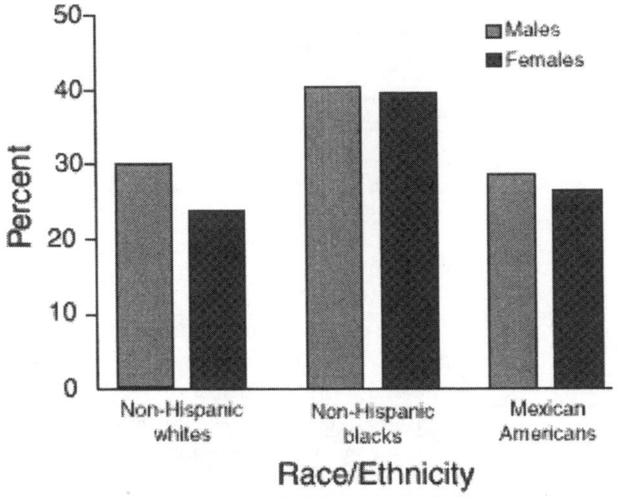

Source: National Health and Nutrition Examination Survey III, 1988–1994, National Center for Health Statistics, CDC (2000).

area. In the area of heart disease, medical science has much to offer. The Institute of Medicine has recently stated that Black Americans are underdiagnosed as having coronary artery disease. This means that many people are dying needlessly each year because they are not being diagnosed properly (Committee on Quality of Health Care in America, 2001).

Coronary Risk Factors.   The prevalence of certain CHD risk factors and clustering of risk factors are greater in African Americans than in the general population (NCHS, 1999). Hypertension, left ventricular hypertrophy (LVH), Type 2 diabetes mellitus, obesity, cigarette smoking and physical inactivity occur more frequently in African Americans (Cutter et al., 1991; Livingston, 1985a, 1985b, 1986/1987). Additionally, the risk of death and other sequelae attributable to some factors (e.g., hypertension, diabetes) is greater for African Americans (Cooper, Liao, & Rotimi, 1996; Livingston, 1991, 1993a, 1993b; Livingston & Ackah, 1992). Hypertension is considered a main risk factor for CHD. Approximately twice as many African American males are hypertensive compared to their White counterparts. Also, they are twice as likely to have moderate hypertension and three times as likely to have severe hypertension (Men's Health Consulting, 2000). Although many factors are associated with the etiology of hypertension, the role stress plays in its etiology was reported in the past (see Livingston, 1985a, 1985b, 1991; Livingston & Marshall, 1991; Livingston et al. 1991).

Cancers

Lung cancer is the deadliest cancer in men. According to the American Cancer Society, tobacco smoking is by far the leading cause of lung cancer. Smoking causes more than 80 percent of lung cancer cases—with the remainder largely attributed to passive exposure to tobacco smoke (American Cancer Society, 1996). Colorectal (colon and rectum) cancer and prostate cancer are also common but when caught early are highly treatable. Prostate cancer is second only to lung cancer in killing men, and African American men develop prostate cancer at a higher rate than men in any other racial or ethnic group. Black men have a 60 percent higher incidence rate of the disease than White men (American Cancer Society, 1996; Feldman & Fulwood, 1999; Weinrich et al., 2000). Research suggests the general barriers to prostrate screening include knowledge, cost, and fear-avoidance; however, for African American men the additional factor of lack of transportation was also mentioned (Weinrich et al., 2000).

Unintentional Injuries

As seen in Table 14.4, unintentional injuries rank as the number three cause of death for both African American and White males. A major contributing factor to unintentional injuries are accidents occurring on the road involving vehicles, at home and/or at work. For college-age men, injuries from accidents are the second leading cause of death (Hoyert et al., 1999).

Minority men tend to be concentrated in jobs that represent risks and high levels of pathogens in the physical environment. Although non-Hispanic men are more likely to be injured in the workplace, African American men are reported to be more likely to die of injuries that occurred in the workplace. A contributing factor to this disproportionate mortality in the workplace is disproportionate exposure African American men have to occupational hazards and carcinogens and, therefore, the resulting diseases (Loomis & Richardson, 1998).

Stroke

Crude rates indicate that stroke is the third leading cause of death, behind heart disease and cancer. It is also the leading cause of serious, long-term disability and accounts for nearly 1 out of 15 deaths in the United States Black men face a higher risk of fatality from stroke than their White counterparts, and, compared with Whites, young African Americans have a twofold to threefold greater risk of stroke. African American men and women have almost twice the death rate due to stroke compared with their White counterparts (Gillum, 1993; Broderick et al., 1998).

Diabetes Mellitus

According to the Centers for Disease Control and Prevention (CDC, 1999), African American males are twice as likely as White men to develop diabetes. As seen in Table 14.2, as a cause of death, it is ranked number ten for African American males and number nine for White males. Overall, the prevalence of diabetes is 70 percent higher in African Americans than in White Americans. The most recent data indicate that approximately 1.5 million African American adults have Type 2 diabetes (Flegal et al., 1991; Clark, 1998). Type 2 diabetes accounts for 90 to 95 percent of diabetes cases and is nearing epidemic proportions, due to people living longer and a greater prevalence of obesity and sedentary lifestyles. The main complications include blindness, amputations, kidney failure, heart attack, stroke, and impotence (USDHHS, 2000).

Interpersonal Violence

As seen in Figure 14.1, violence and incarceration, which could begin on or around the adolescence years (e.g., with juvenile detention/imprisonment), are interrelated and can have an adverse impact on premature morbidity (e.g., wheelchair survivors of gunshots) and mortality of African American men. Interpersonal violence includes various actions as homicide, domestic violence, assault, rape, and suicide. Whereas homicide ranks 13th as a leading cause of death, for African American men it ranks 5th (Livingston, 1994). As mentioned before, forticide is another related problem affecting

African American men. (You may recall that it is basically committing suicide at the hands of another individual [Willis, 1990].)

Incarceration

At year end 2001 there were 3,535 sentenced Black male prisoners per 100,000 Black males in the United States, compared to 1,177 sentenced Hispanic male inmates per 100,000 Hispanic males and 462 White male inmates per 100,000 White males (BJS, 2002). These figures reflect, in part, the effect of institutional racism and individual prejudice as projected by young Black males. Stolen dreams give way to lowered horizons, and a feeling of hopelessness may frequently ensue (Wyatt, 2000).

Rightly or wrongly, once incarcerated, prisoners are placed in unsafe environment where poor medical attention as well as unsafe conditions are prevalent. Prison becomes a place for a death sentence. Unsafe and unrestrained sexual practices lead to HIV, hepatitis, and other unwanted infections. AIDS cases among prison inmates (0.52 percent) is reported to be about four times the rate in the general U.S. population (0.13 percent) (Maruschak, 2002). Given the demographic characteristics of the men who are incarcerated, "it is not surprising that many of the inmates who are infected with HIV/AIDS are young men of color. These numbers exceed the number of Black and Latino males in undergraduate colleges and universities. This is a sad commentary for African Americans and Latinos seeking to live the American dream" (Braithwaite & Arriola, 2003, p. 760).

HIV/AIDS

The rate of HIV infection among minority men is a growing concern, with minority youth being at increased risk. In 2000, HIV/AIDS was the third leading cause of death for African American men between 25 and 34 years (Anderson, 2002). Today, one of the most at-risk groups contracting HIV is young African American men-who-have sex-with-men (MSM). According to the Centers for Disease Control and Prevention's Morbidity and Mortality Weekly Report from June 1, 2001, the prevalence of HIV among African American men (MSM aged 18–22) is almost 15 percent (MMWR, 2001).

Oral Health

Good oral health is important to overall health. Among males with teeth, Mexican Americans (47 percent) and non-Hispanic Blacks (54 percent) are much less likely to have visited the dentist in the past year than are non-Hispanic Whites (68 percentc) (NHANES, 2002). It is important to note the African American males have the highest incidence of oral and pharyngeal cancers (NIH, 2000). "These indicators of poor oral health partly reflect the poor access to dental services experienced by these groups" (Satcher, 2003, p. 707).

Stress.   Stress plays a very important role in the lives of African American men. In the past it has been reported that stress plays a contributing role in the etiology and exacerbation of various diseases associated with African Americans, especially hypertension (Livingston, 1991; 1992a; Livingston & Marshall, 1991). To date, a number of studies have found greater vascular reactivity responses in Blacks than Whites (e.g., Treiber et al. 1990). There is evidence that Blacks have more alpha-adrenergic responses to stress than Whites, with Blacks also exhibiting a blunted beta-adrenergic response. These stronger vascular responses are consistent with observations concerning the natural history of essential hypertension and the fact that Blacks have a higher incidence of hypertension and CHD than age-matched White counterparts (Allen, 2001).

In the case of suicide, it has been reported that stressors (e.g., brought on by discrimination) experienced by middle-class African American males may, in part, account for their pattern of suicide risk (Williams, 2003) and their mental health in general (Williams et al., 2003). Research reveals that unemployment and job insecurity are associated with elevated rates of stress, illness, disability, and mortality. A study in Harlem demonstrated that men who were not employed, who had a history of not having steady work, and who had a history of homelessness were more likely to have hypertension and more likely to smoke than men who worked full-time in steady jobs (Diez-Roux et al., 1999).

PREVENTIVE STRATEGIES AND ALTERNATIVE VIEWS

Overview

While Black men are dying at increasing rates from these chronic diseases, there is hope. Many of these diseases are either preventable or treatable. Many health scientists contend that health behaviors are among the most important factors influencing health and that modifying health behaviors is probably the most effective way to prevent disease. Regular medical exams are critical to the early detection of many potentially fatal diseases, but the willingness to take subsequent action and the availability of care for newly diagnosed problems must also be present. Preventive measures are crucial to the strategy of a long and healthy life. Yet, there are many barriers that interfere with improved life expectancy (see Figure 14.1). A brief mention is made below of some of these barriers.

Immunizations

Immunizations are a hallmark in the prevention strategy. The use of the proper immunizations should be encouraged as part of a general prevention strategy for both young and elder African American populations. These two groups are usually at more risk for infection. One out of four African American children ages 19–35 months did not receive the recommended vaccinations in 1999. Approximately 47 percent of elderly African Americans received the flu vaccine in 1998, compared with 66 percent of elderly Whites. Regarding pneumonia vaccination, in 1998 about 26 percent of elderly African Americans received the vaccine compared with 50 of elderly Whites (HHS Fact Sheet, 2001).

Access to Health Services

Access to medical services continues to be a major deterrent to improved health outcomes. In many cases, access to care is associated with the employment status of individuals. Health insurance, with the exception of those persons who qualify for Medicaid and Medicare, is needed to pay for medical services, and in most cases health insurance policies are tied to people's jobs. Therefore, because African American men have relatively high rates of unemployment, this translates, in part, to low access to medical care. In other cases, while insurance is offered on the job, workers cannot afford it, and in other cases it may not be offered at all based on the kind on work and working relationship that exist (e.g., part-time worker, small business employees). Americans who own less than 200 percent of the federal poverty level (or $27,300 for a family of three) are likely to be uninsured (Kaiser Family Foundation, 2000). Therefore, although employment is important, it is not indicative of adequate access to affordable insurance coverage.

Regarding insurance coverage, men of color are the least insured, with Hispanics (46%) and African Americans (28 percent) having the highest percentages of uninsured workers and Whites having the lowest percentage of uninsured workers (28 percent) (Brown et al., 2000). According to Gornick (2003), analysis of Medicare data revealed three distinct patterns of utilization relative to

White beneficiaries: Black beneficiaries (1) used fewer preventive and health promotion services (e.g., influenza immunization); (2) underwent fewer diagnostic tests (e.g., colonoscopy, surgical procedures as coronary artery grafts); and (c) underwent more of the types of procedures associated with poor management of chronic disease (e.g., partial or lower limb amputations).

Fear and Distrust

It has been well documented that men visit physicians less often than women and utilize significantly fewer health-care services. One reason Black men tend not to go to the doctor is self-perceptions of their role in society. Black men believe in work for the benefit of the family. Often in that process, personal health is sacrificed for the overall good of the family with premature death and disability as outcomes. This happens far too often. It is imperative for Black men to understand that, if personal health and safety become a priority, life can be lengthened and improved. The product of these efforts should be the opportunity to continue to provide for, and remain an important part of, their family's future.

Black men often have fear of knowing the truth about their own health status (Braithwaite & Taylor, 2001). Many will suffer pain without seeking advice or seek medical care very late, frequently in an emergency situation. As a consequence, many Black men further suffer from the penalties of late detection of a condition, as in the case of inoperative cancer of the lung, prostate, or colon.

Distrust of the health source has been historically based on evidence of racial discrimination and the fear of being "guinea pigs" in medical experiments (Thomas & Quinn, 1991; Freimuth et al., 2001). However, such fears were brought dramatically into focus with the unveiling of the abuses of the Tuskegee experiment, as well as more contemporary events. Therefore, Black men have been socialized to be distrustful of the U.S. health-care system because of perceived and actualized racism. To the extent that this fear and distrust inhibit Black men from receiving needed medical care, they contribute, in part, to the wide gap between the life expectancy of White (74.8 years) and Black (68.2 years) men (NCHS, 2002).

CONCLUSIONS

Black males are in danger from before the cradle to the grave. Early mishandling of the male has lead to premature or excess death from highly preventable sources. Death from accidents and homicide are particularly tragic. Deaths by "drive-by" and other preteen and teen violence are other preventable circumstances that contribute to the premature morbidity and mortality illustrated in Figure 14.1. These areas, as well as those listed in the model (see Figure 14.1), must be the areas of concentration in order to provide for adequate and consistent, long-term improvement of the overall life expectancy of Black American males.

In addition, programs that encourage males to discuss health issues in small groups reinforce the health message. Finally, Black American males should be encouraged to have health messages integrated into the overall theme of their religious and other organizations, where health screenings are conducted as is appropriate (see Figure 14.1 as a suggested guide). Males can act as supports to each other. One example where many of the suggestions have been successfully implemented is *The Prince Hall Masons* and *Prince Hall Shriners*. With health promotion activities associated with these organizations, they provide examples of successful health behavior changes, such as dramatic smoking cessation in a matter of years.

ACKNOWLEDGMENTS

I wish to thank Ms. Janis Weaver and Ms. Bridgett Scott for invaluable assistance (Donald R. Ware).

REFERENCES

Adler, N.E., & Newman, K. (2002).Socioeconomic disparities in health: Pathways and policies. *Health Affairs, 21(2)*, 60–76.

African American Men. (2003). Why we do it. Arizona State University. http://www.asu.edu/reslife/aamasu/why_we_do_it.htm.

Allen, M.T. (2001). Cardiovascular reactivity. The Research Network on Socioeconomic Status and Health. Chicago: The John D. and Catherine T. MacArthur Foundation.

American Cancer Society. (1996). Cancer and African Americans. Retrieved February 17, 2003 from www.2cancer.org/siteSearch/aframer.htm

Anderson, E. (1999). The social situation of the Black executive: Black and White identities in the corporate world. In M. Lamont (Ed.), *The cultural territories of race: Black and white boundaries* (pp. 3–29). Chicago: University of Chicago Press.

Anderson, N.B., Bastida, E., Kramer, B.J., Williams, D., & Wong, M. (1995). Panel II: Macrosocial and environmental influences on minority health. *Health Psychology, 14(7)*, 601–612.

Anderson, R.N. (2002). Deaths: Leading causes for 2000. *National Vital Statistics Report, 50(16)*, 1–85.

Barbarin, O.A. (1993). Coping and resilience: Exploring the inner lives of African American children. *Journal of Black Psychology, 19(4)*, 478–492.

Baum, A., Garofalo, J.P. & Yali, A.M. (1999). Socioeconomic status and chronic stress: Does stress account for SES effects on health? *Annals of the New York Academy of Sciences, 896*, 131–144.

Braithwaite, R.L., & Arriola, K.R. (2003). Male prisoners and HIV prevention: A call for action ignored. *American Journal of Public Health, 93(5)*, 759–763.

Braithwaite, R.L., & Taylor, S.E. (2001). Health issues in the Black community, 2nd ed. San Francisco: Jossey-Bass.

Broderick, J., et al. (1998). The greater Cincinnati/Norther Kentucky Stroke Study: Preliminary first-ever and total incidence rates of stroke among Blacks. *Stroke, 29*, 415–421.

Brown, E.R., Ojeda, V.D., Wyn, R., & Levan, R. (2000). *Racial and ethnic disparities in access to health insurance and health care.* Los Angeles: UCLA Center for Health Policy Research and the Henry J. Kaiser Family Foundation.

Bureau of Justice Statistics (BJS). (2002). Homicide trends in the United States. Age, gender and race trends. U.S. Department of Justice Programs, Office of Justice Programs.

Centers for Disease Control (CDC) and Prevention. (1999). National diabetes fact sheet. National estimates and general information on diabetes in the United States. Atlanta, GA: U.S. Department of Health and Human Services.

Centers for Disease Control (CDC) and Prevention. (2001). HIV/AIDS surveillance report, 13(2). Atlanta, GA: U.S. Department of Health and Human Services.

Clark, C. (1998). How should we respond to the worldwide diabetes epidemic? *Diabetes Care, 21*, 475–476.

Clark, L.T., et al. (1999). Coronary heart disease in African Americans. *Heart Disease, 3*, 97–108.

Clarke, R., Anderson, Clark V.R., & Williams, D.R. (1999). Racism as a stressor for African Americans. *American Psychologist, 54(10)*, 805–816.

Committee on Quality of Health Care in America. (2001). Institute of Medicine. Crossing the quality chasm: A new health system for the 21st century. Washington, DC: National Academy Press.

Cooper, R.S., Liao, Y., Rotimi, C. (1996). Is hypertension more severe among U.S. blacks, or is severe hypertension more common? *Annals of Epidemiology, 6*, 173–180.

Courtenay, W.H. (2000). Constructions of masculinity and their influence on men's well-being: A theory of gender and health. *Social Science and Medicine, 50*, 1385–1401.

Cutter, G.R., et al. (1991). Cardiovascular risk factors in young adults. The CARDIA baseline monograph. *Control Clinical Trials, 12*, 1S–25S, 51S–77S.

Davis, R. (1980). Black suicide and the relational system: Theoretical and empirical implications of communal and familial ties. *Research Race Ethnic Relations, 2*, 43–71.

Diez-Roux, A.V., Northridge, M.E., Morabia, A., Bassett, M.T., & Shea, S. (1999). Prevalence and social correlates of cardiovascular disease risk factors in Harlem. *American Journal of Public Health*, 89, 302–307.

Feldman, R., & Fulwood, R. (1999). The three leading causes of death in African America: Barriers to reducing the excess disparity and to improving health behaviors. *Journal of Healthcare for the Poor and Underserved, 10*, 45–71.

Fenz, C. (2002). State health care spending: A systems perspective. *State Coverage Initiatives Issue, 3*, 1.

Fernquist, R.M. (2001). Education, race/ethnicity, age, sex and sucide: Individual-level date in the United States. *Current Research Social Psychology, 3*, 277–290.

Flegal, K., et al. (1991). Prevalence of diabetes in Mexican Americans, Cubans and Puerto Ricans from the Hispanic Health and Nutrition Survey, 1982–1984. *Diabetes Care, 14*, 628–638.

Forman, T.A., Williams, D.R., & Jackson, J.S. (1997). Race, place and discrimination. *Perspectives on Social Problems, 9*, 231–261.

Freimuth V.S., et. al. (2001). African Americans' views on research and the Tuskegee Syphilis study. *Social Science and Medicine, 52(5)*, 797–808.

Gant, L.M., Hwalek, M., & Dix, C. (1994). Increasing responsible sexual behavior among high risk African American adolescent males: Results of a brief, intensive intervention. *Journal of Multicultural Social Work, 3(3)*, 49–58.

Garland, A., & Zigler, E. (1993). Adolescent suicide prevention: Current research and social policy implications. *American Psychologist, 48*, 169–182.

Geronimus, A.T. et al. (1996). Excess mortality among Blacks and Whites in the United States. *New England Journal of Medicine, 335*, 1552–1558).

Gibbs, J.T. (1997). African-American suicide: A cultural paradox. *Suicide Life Threat Behavior, 27*, 68–79.

Gibbs, J.T. (1998). Young Black males in America: Endangered, embittered and embattled. In J.T. Gibbs (Ed.), *Young, Black male in America: An endangered species* (pp. 1–36). Dover, MA: Auburn House Publishing Company.

Gillum, R.F. (1997). Sudden cardiac death in Hispanic and African Americans. *American Journal of Public Health, 87*, 1461–1466.

Gillum, R.F. (1999). Stroke mortality in Blacks: Disturbing trends. *Stroke, 30*, 1711–1715.

Gornick, M.E. (2003). A decade of research on disparities in Medicare utilization: Lessons for the health and health care of vulnerable men. *Journal of American Public Health, 93(5)*, 753–759.

Hayward, M.D., Crimmins, E.M., Miles, T.P., & Yang, Y. (2000). The significance of socioeconomic status in explaining the racial gap in chronic health conditions. *American Sociological Review, 65(6)*, 1162–1194.

Health and Human Services (HHS) Fact Sheet. (2001). Closing the health gap: Reducing health disparities affection African Americans. U.S. Department of Health and Human Services. Retrieved February 17, 2003, from http://www.hhs.gov/news

Hoffman, C. (1998). *Uninsured in America: A chartbook*. Menlo Park, CA: Kaiser Family.

Hoyert, D.L., Kochanek, K.D., & Murphy, S.L. (1999). Deaths: Final data for 1997. National Vital Statistics Reports, 47(19). Hyattsville, MD: NCHS.

Jaynes, G.D., & Williams, R.M. (1989). A common destiny: Blacks and American society. Washington, DC: National Academic Press.

Jones, D.J., & Roberts, V.A. (1994). Black children: Growth, development and health. In I.L. Livingston (Ed.), *Handbook of Black American health: The mosaic of conditions, issues, policies and prospects* (pp. 331–343). Westport, CT: Greenwood Press.

Kaiser Family Foundation. (2000). The uninsured and thir access to health care. Retrieved on February 15, 2003 from, www.kff.org/content/archive/1407.

Kennedy, R. (2001). Racial trends in the administration of criminal justice. In N. Smelser, W.J. Wilson & F. Mitchess (Eds.), *America becoming: Racial trends and their consequences*, vol. 2 (pp. 1–20). Washington, DC: National Academy Press.

Kirschenman, J., &Neckerman, K.M. (1991). We'd love to hire them but . . . : The meaning of race for employers. In C. Jenkins & P.E. Petersen (Eds.), *The urban underclass* (pp. 203–232). Washington, DC: Brookings Institution.

Kozlowski, K. (2001). Black infant survival rate worsens. *Detroit News*.

Kreiger, N. (2000). Discrimination and health. In Berkfman, L.F., & Kawachi, I. (Eds), *Social epidemiology* (pp. 36–75). New York: Oxford University Press, Inc.

Kreiger, N., Williams, D.R., & Moss, N.E. (1997). Measuring social class in U.S. public health research: Concepts, methodologies and guidelines. *Annual Review of Public Health, 18*, 341–378.

Lee, C. (1991). Empowering young Black males. ERIC Clearinghouse on Counseling and Personnel Services. Ann Arbor, MI.

Lee, C.C. (1996). Saving the native son: Empowerment strategies for young Black males. Greensboro, NC: ERIC Counseling and Student Services Clearinghouse.

Lester, D. (1998). *Suicide in African Americans*. Commack, NY: Nova Science.

Link, B.G., & Phelan, J. (1995). Social conditions as fundamental causes of disease. *Journal of Health and Social Behavior, Spec. No*, 80–94.

Livingston, I.L. (1985a). Alcohol consumption and hypertension: A review with suggested implications. *Journal of the National Medical Association, 77*, 129–135.

Livingston, I.L. (1985b). The importance of stress in the interpretation of the race–hypertension association. *Humanity and Society, 9(2)*, 168–181.

Livingston, I.L. (1986/1987). Blacks, lifestyle and hypertension: The importance of health education. *The Humboldt Journal of Social Relations, 14*, 195–213.

Livingston, I.L. (1988a). Co-factors, host susceptibility, and AIDS: An argument for stress. *Journal of the National Medical Association, 80*, 49–59.

Livingston, I.L. (1988b). Stress and health dysfunctions: The importance of health education. *Stress and Medicine, 4(3)*, 155–161.

Livingston, I.L. (1990). Perceived control, knowledge and fear of AIDS among college students: An exploratory study. *Journal of Health and Social Policy, 2(2)*, 47–66.

Livingston, I.L. (1991). Stress, hypertension and renal disease in Black Americans: A review with implications. *National Journal of Sociology, 5(2)*, 143–181.

Livingston, I.L. (1992). The ABC's of stress management—taking control of your life. Salt Lake City UT: Northwest Publishing.

Livingston, I.L. (1993a). Renal disease and Black Americans: Selected Issues. *Social Science and Medicine*, 37(5), 613–621.

Livingston, I.L. (1993b). Stress, hypertension and young Black Americans: The importance of counseling. *Journal of Multicultural Counseling, 2(3)*, 132–142.

Livingston, I.L. (1994). Handbook of Black American health: The mosaic of conditions, issues, policies and prospects. Westport, CT: Greenwood Press.

Livingston, I.L., & Ackah, S. (1992). Hypertension, end-stage renal disease and rehabilitation: A look at Black Americans. The Western Journal of Black Studies, 16, 103–112.

Livingston, I.L., Levine, D.M., & Moore, R. (1991). Social integration and Black intraracial blood pressure variation. *Ethnicity and Disease, 1(2)*, 135–149.

Livingston, I.L. and Marshall, R. (1991). Cardiac reactivity and elevated blood pressure levels among young African Americans: The importance of stress. In D.J. Jones (Ed.), *Prescriptions and policies: the social well-being of African Americans in the 1990s* (pp. 77–91). New Brunswick, NJ: Transaction.

Livingston, I.L., Otado, J. & Warren, C. (2003). Stress, adverse pregnancy outcomes and African American females: Assessing the implications using a conceptual model. *Journal of the National Medical Association*, 95(11), 1103–1109.

Loomis, D., & Richardson, D. (1998). Race and risk of fatal injury at work. *American Journal of Public Health, 88*, 40–44.

Macionis, J.J. (2002). *Society the basics*, 6th ed. Upper Saddle River, NJ: Prentice-Hall.

Majors, R., & Billson, J.M. (1992). Cool pose: The dilemmas of Black manhood in America. New York: Touchstone Books.

Maruschak, L.M. (2002). HIV in prisons, 2000. Washington, DC: U.S. Department of Justice, Bureau of Justice Statistics, Report NCJ 196023.

McCord, C., & Freeman, H. (1990). Excess mortality in Harlem. *New England Journal of Medicine, 322*, 173–177.

McLoyd, V.C., & Lozoff, B. (2001). Racial and ethnic trends in children's and adolescent's behavior and development. In N.J. Smelser, W.J. Wilson, & F. Mitchell (Eds.), *America Becoming: Racial trends and their consequences* (pp. 311–350). Washington, DC: National Academy Press.

McNeilly, M., et al. (1996). The convergent, discriminant, and concurrent criterion validity of the perceived racism scale: A multidimensional assessment of White racism among African Americans. In R.L. Jones (Ed.), *Handbook of tests and measurements for Black Americans* vol. 2, (pp. 359–374). Hampton, VA: Cobb and Henry.

Men's Health Consulting. (2000). African American men's health. Retrieved January 25, 2003. www.menshealth.org/code/afroamer.html

Minino, A.M., Arias, E., Kochanek, K.D., Murphy, S.L., & Smith, B.L. (2002). Deaths: Final data for 2000. *National Vital Statistics Reports, 50(15)*, Hyattsville, MD: National Center for Health Statistics.

MMWR. (1995).Youth risk behavior surveillance—United States, 1995, *Morbidity and Mortality Weekly Report*, 45(SS-4).

MMWR. (1998). Suicide among Black youths—United States, 1980–1995. *Morbidity and Mortality Weekly Report, 47(10)*, 106–193.

MMWR. (2000). HIV and AIDS—U.S. 1991–2000. *MMWR*, 50(21), 430–434.

Montague, P. Lead poisoning: Our children are at risk. TomPaine.com. A Public Interest Journal. Retrieved, 2-17-03. http://www.tompaine.com/feature.cfm/ID/3015

Morris, L.C. (1997). Spirituality and psychosocial competence among African American college students. *Psych Discourse, 28(12)*, 15–21.

Murphy, S.L. (2000). Deaths: Final data for 1998. *National Vital Statistics Report, 49(11)*. Hyattsville, MD: National Center for Health Statistics.

Myer, J.A. (2003). Improving men's health: Developing a long-term strategy. *American Journal of Public Health, 93(5)*, 709.

National Center for Health Statistics (NCHS). (1999). *Health United States 1999 with health and aging chartbook*. Hyattsville, MD: Department of Health and Human Services.

National Center for Health Statistics (NCHS). (2001). *National Vital Statistics Report, 49(8)*. Hyattsville, MD: Department of Health and Human Services.

National Center for Health Statistics (NCHS). (2002). *Health United States with chartbook on trends in the health of Americans*. Hyattsville, MD: Department of Health and Human Services.

National Health and Nutrition Examination Survey (NHANES) III. (2002). National Center for Health Statistics, Center for Disease Control and Prevention, 1988–1994.

National Institutes of Health (NIH). (2000). *Oral health in America: A report of the surgeon general*. Rockville, MD: National Institute of Dental and Craniofacial Research.

National Institutes of Health (NIH) News Release. (2001). *National study examines sites where U.S. children drown*. National Institute of Child Health and Human Development. Bethesda, NIH.

Pamuk, E. (1998). *Socioeconomic status and health chartbook: Health United States, 1998*. Hyattsville, MD: National Center for Health Statistics.

Pastor, P.N., Makuc, D.M., & Xia, H. (2002). *Chartbook on trends in the health of Americans, Health, United States*. Hyattsville, MD: National Center for Health Statistics.

Prince, K.J. (1997). Black family and Black liberation. *Psych Discourse, 28(1)*, 4–7.

Reed, R.J. (1988). Education and achievement of young Black males. In J.T. Gibbs (Ed.), *Young Black and male in America: An endangered species* (pp. 37–96). Dover, MA: Auburn House Publishing Company.

Rich, J.A., & Ro, M. (2002). *A poor man's plight: Uncovering the disparity in men's health*. Battle Creek, MI: The Kellogg Foundation.

Ross, C.E., & Wu, C. (1995). The links between education and health. *American Sociological Review, October*, 719–745.

Sampson, R.J. (1987). Urban black violence: The effect of male joblessness and family disruption. *American Journal of Sociology, 93*, 348–382.

Satcher, D. (2003). Overlooked and underserved: Improving the health of men of color. *American Journal of Public Health, 93(5)*, 707.

Schuman, H., Steeh, C., & Bobo, L. (1985). *Racial attitudes in America*. Cambridge: Harvard University Press.

Shepard, J.M. (2002). *Sociology*. Belmont, CA: Wadsworth/Thomson Learning.

Stevenson, H.C. (1993). Validation of the scale of racial socialization for African American adolescents: A preliminary analysis. *Psych Discourse, 24(12)*, 6–10.

Tatum, B.L. (1996). An analysis of factors contributing to the delinquency of Black youth. *Journal of Black Studies, 26(3)*, 356–368.

The 2003 HHS Poverty Guidelines. (2003). *Federal Register, 68(2)*, 6456–6458.

Thomas, S., & Quinn, S. (1991). The Tuskegee syphilis study, 1932 to 1972: Implications for HIV education and AIDS risk education programs in the black community. *American Journal of Public Health, 81*, 1498–1505.

Thompson, V.L. (1994). A preliminary outline of treatment strategies with African Americans coping with racism. *Psych Discourse, 25(6)*, 6–9.

Traven, N.D., et al. (1996). Coronary heart disease mortality and sudden death among the 35–44 year age group in Allegheny County, Pennsylvania. *Annals of Epidemiology, 6*, 130–136.

Treiber, F.A., et al. (1990). Racial differences in hemodynamic responses to the cold face stimulus in children and adults. *Psychosomatic Medicine, 52*, 286–296.

Tucker, M. (2000). Considerations in the development of family policy for African Americans. In J. Jackson (Ed.), *New directions: African Americans in a diversifying nation* (pp. 162–206). Washington, DC: National Policy Association.

UNCTV. (1990). Black Issues Forum. The black male: An endangered species?

United States Bureau of the Census (2000). *General demographics by race and gender for the United States: 2000*. Redistricting Data (Public Law 94–171). Population Division, U.S. department of Commerce, Washington, D.C.

U.S. Department of Health and Human Services (USDHHS). (2000). *Healthy people 2010*, 2nd ed. *With understanding and improving health and objectives for improving health* 2 vol. Washington, DC: U.S. Government Printing Office.

Villarosa, L. (2002). As Black men move into middle age, dangers rise. *New York Times*, September 23.

Warfield-Coppock, N. (1992). The rites of passage movement: A resurgence of African-centered practices for socializing African American youth. *Journal of Negro Education, 61(4)*, 471–482.

Weinrich, S.P., Reynolds, W.A., Tingen, M.S., & Starr, C.R. (2000). Barriers to prostate cancer screening. *Cancer Nursing, 23*, 117–121.

Williams, D.R. (2003). The health of men: Structures inequalities and opportunities. *American Journal of Public Health, 93(3)*, 724–731.

Williams, D.R., & Collins, C.A. (2001). Racial residential segregation: A fundamental cause of racial disparities in health. *Public Health Reports, 16*, 404–415.

Williams, D.R., Neighbors, H.W., & Jackson, J.S. (2003). Racial/ethnic discrimination and health: Findings from community studies. *American Journal of Public Health, 93*, 200–208.

Willis, J.T. (1990). *Implications for effective psychotherapy with African American families and individuals.* Matteson, IL: Genesis Publications.

Wyatt, S.T. (2000). Identifying factors that affect the development of adolescent African American males. http://www.imgip.siu.edu/HTMLpages/journal/afamdev.html. Retrieved 12/16/2000.

Yinger, J. (1995). Closed doors, opportunities lost: The continuing costs of housing discrimination. New York: Sage.

CHAPTER 15

HIV/AIDS and Sexually Transmitted Diseases

JOHN I. MCNEIL AND KIM M. WILLIAMS

The reduction of health disparities has become a primary focus of the health-care system. The trends seen with human immunodeficiency virus (HIV) over the last two decades especially signify some of the factors contributing to inequities of health care in the United States as well as internationally. As developments in HIV immunology, pharmacology, and virology progressed, many of the health-care gaps widened due to limited developments in health-care policy. Although epidemiological trends indicate overall improvements in the morbidity and mortality of HIV in the United States, these improvements are not evenly distributed to all populations. The goal of this chapter is to look at the epidemiological trends, as well as discussing some of the newer changes in HIV clinical manifestations, treatment, and research, especially as they relate to the health of African Americans.

HIV/AIDS EPIDEMIOLOGICAL TRENDS

The cumulative number of AIDS cases reported in the United States was 816,149 as of December 2001 (CDC, 2001b). Of these cases, adult and adolescent males account for 82 percent. Patients aged 25 to 44 years constitute nearly 75 percent of the total cases. Through the same period, 9,074 pediatric AIDS cases (<13 years in age) were reported to the CDC. Trend data from 1985–2001 indicate substantial increases in the proportion of AIDS cases for African Americans (23 percent to 49 percent) and considerable decreases for Whites (62 percent to 31 percent) (Figure 15.1). Advances in treatments, particularly highly active antiretroviral therapy (HAART) in 1996, have markedly delayed the onset of AIDS and associated deaths (Karon et al., 2001) (Figure 15.2). The CDC estimates that at the end of 2001, 362,857 persons were living with AIDS. Incidence data also reveal regional variations in the distribution of AIDS cases in the United States, with 44 percent of new AIDS occurring in the South followed by 27 percent in the Northeast, 15 percent in the West, and 10 percent in the Midwest as of 2001.

Approximately 40,000 new HIV infections occur each year in the United States, and half of these infections occur among persons less than 25 years in age (CDC, 2001a). A recent report also suggests that an estimated 800,000 to 900,000 persons in the United States are currently living with HIV, and many are unaware that they are infected (Karon et al., 2001). In 2001, 35 states and four U.S.

Figure 15.1
Proportion of AIDS cases by race and year of report, 1985–2001

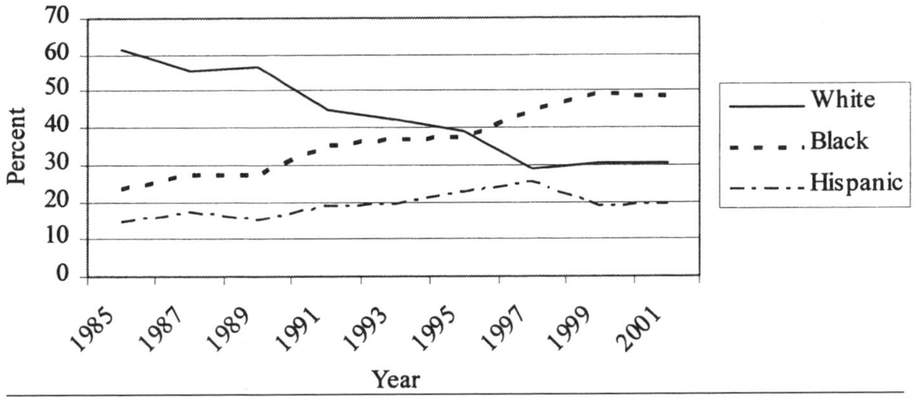

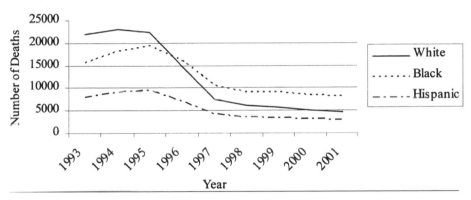

Source: CDC, *HIV/AIDS Surveillance Report* (2001b).

Figure 15.2
Estimated number of deaths of persons with AIDS by race and year of death, 1993–2001

Source: CDC, *HIV/AIDS Surveillance Report* (2001b).

territories had confidential HIV reporting systems in place. Of the 35,032 new HIV cases reported through this mechanism, 68 percent were among men.

African American Trends and Disparities

African Americans continue to be disproportionately affected by HIV/AIDS. Although they constitute 12 percent of the U.S. population, they account for 50 percent of new HIV infections and 49 percent of new AIDS cases reported in 2001 (CDC, 2001b). The rate of adult/adolescent AIDS cases among African Americans (76.3 per 100,000 population) was ten times the rate for Whites (7.9 per 100,000 population) and nearly three times the rate for Hispanics (28.0 per 100,000 population). Racial disparities among women with AIDS were even more disturbing. Of 11,082 AIDS cases reported among all women in the same period, nearly two-thirds (63 percent) were African Ameri-

Table 15.1

HIV[1] and AIDS cases for Blacks, by age at diagnosis and sex and race/ethnicity, reported through December 2001, United States

	Black								
Age	HIV Infection Cases[2]					AIDS Cases			
	Male		Female			Male		Female	
	N	%	N	%		N	%	N	%
Under 5	906	(2)	1,039	(3)		2,165	(1)	2,153	(3)
5-12	244	(<1)	242	(1)		498	(<1)	521	(1)
13-19	1,654	(3)	2,716	(8)		1,020	(<1)	1,250	(1)
20-24	6,271	(11)	5,036	(15)		7,590	(3)	4,844	(6)
25-29	8,729	(16)	5,885	(17)		26,595	(12)	11,876	(14)
30-34	10,637	(19)	6,183	(18)		46,088	(20)	18,055	(21)
35-39	10,249	(19)	5,203	(15)		51,302	(22)	18,351	(22)
40-44	7,485	(14)	3,556	(10)		41,395	(18)	13,221	(16)
45-49	4,479	(8)	2,014	(6)		24,839	(11)	6,922	(8)
50-54	2,288	(4)	984	(3)		12,959	(6)	3,447	(4)
55-59	1,104	(2)	480	(1)		6,987	(3)	1,865	(2)
60-64	543	(1)	271	(1)		3,819	(2)	1,103	(1)
65 or older	523	(1)	258	(1)		3,242	(1)	1,073	(1)
Subtotals	55,112	(100)	33,867	(100)		228,499	(100)	84,681	(100)
Totals	88,981					313,180			

HIV Notes:

[1]Includes only persons reported with HIV infection who have not developed AIDS

[2]From areas with confidential HIV infection reporting (not including: California, Delaware, District of Columbia, Georgia, Hawaii, Illinois, Kentucky, Maine, Maryland, Massachusetts, Montana, New Hampshire, Pennsylvania, Rhode Island, Vermont, Washington, and US dependencies [Puerto Rico].

Source: CDC, *HIV/AIDS Surveillance Report* (2001b).

cans. Moreover, African Americans account for nearly 62 percent of 3,923 pediatric HIV cases reported through December 2001. Table 15.1 shows cumulative HIV and AIDS cases for African Americans by age and sex through 2001. Most notably, a significant proportion of HIV infections were diagnosed in women of childbearing years, as well as men in the same age group (20–39 years). Additionally, given the long latency between initial infection and the onset of AIDS, it is evident that a substantial proportion of infections were acquired while persons were adolescents and young adults.

High-Risk Behaviors

HIV is primarily transmitted through unprotected sexual contact (including vaginal, anal, and oral sex) with an infected partner. The portal of entry for the virus can be the lining of the vagina, vulva, penis, rectum, or mouth. Primary prevention of sexually acquired HIV involves reducing sexual behaviors that place persons at risk. This includes abstaining from sexual intercourse and being in a long-term mutually monogamous relationship with an uninfected partner. Correct and consistent

Figure 15.3
Male adult/adolescent HIV and AIDS cases by exposure category and race through December 2001

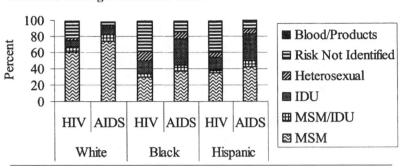

Source: CDC, *HIV/AIDS Surveillance Report* (2001b).

use of condoms when engaging in sexual intercourse can greatly reduce a person's risk for acquiring or transmitting HIV and some STDs (CDC, 2002b).

Transmission of HIV can also occur through sharing contaminated needles and/or syringes used for injection drug use (IDU). Historically, HIV prevention efforts for IDUs have focused on decreasing risk for infection by attempting to dissuade and limit the sharing of drug paraphernalia. Recognizing that not all injectors are willingly able to cease injecting drugs has resulted in interventions that include providing injectors with basic harm reduction supplies (e.g., sterile needles and syringes, condoms, etc.) and improved access to substance treatment programs (VanderWaal et al., 2001).

Mother-to-child transmission of HIV can occur when the infection is spread from an HIV positive woman to her baby during pregnancy, labor and delivery, or breastfeeding. Further, the risk for transfusion-transmitted HIV is very low because of the development of new and more sensitive blood screening tests and treatment (CDC, 2002b).

Reported Risk Exposure

The proportions for adult and adolescent male risk exposure for HIV and AIDS vary significantly by race (Figure 15.3). Men who have sex with men (MSM) remain the predominant risk exposure category for reported HIV and AIDS cases among African Americans, Whites, and Hispanics. However, comparatively more White males identify MSM as the primary risk for HIV and AIDS compared to other racial/ethnic groups. Injection drug use (IDU) is the second highest risk exposure category reported by each of these groups. Heterosexual contact and risk not reported or identified accounts for a substantial number of infections as well. Among African American females, risk for HIV and AIDS is primarily through heterosexual contact (Figure 15.4). The second highest risk category across each racial group for women is IDU. As with African American males, a substantial proportion of cases among women (particularly HIV) did not report or identify risk.

Men Who Have Sex with Men (MSM)

Results of a multisite study of young African American MSM in six U.S. cities found a high incidence of HIV in this population (CDC, 2002c). Recent investigations have also reported increased rates of STDs among African American MSMs and have suggested that relaxing attitudes toward

Figure 15.4
Female adult/adolescent HIV and AIDS cases by exposure category and race through December 2001

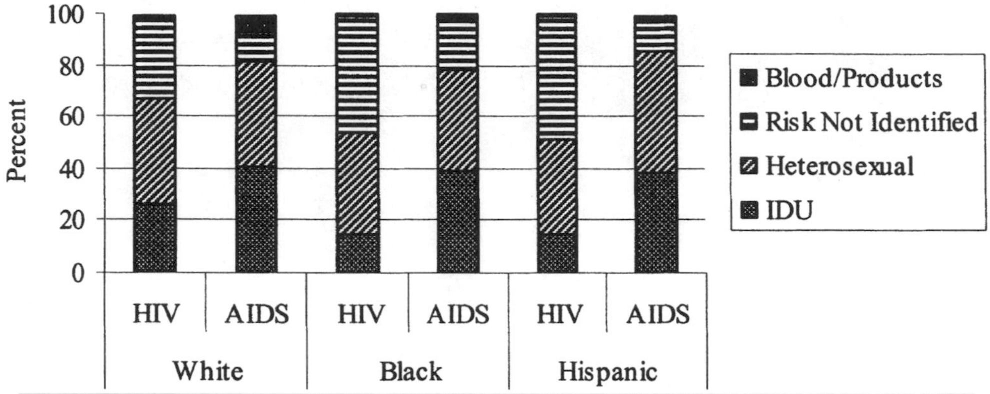

Source: CDC, *HIV/AIDS Surveillance Report* (2001b).

safe sex practices may be supporting a resurgent HIV epidemic among this group (Wolitski et al., 2001). In the African American community there continues to be tremendous stigma surrounding homosexuality. Kraft et al. (2000) reported that African American MSM felt marginal to African American and gay White communities because of perceived homophobia and racism. It is essential that increased dialogue between the African American community and African American MSMs occur to reduce the stigma and negative perceptions of homosexuality. African American MSMs must be intimately involved in designing and implementing HIV prevention interventions. Further, prevention efforts must include outreach to both HIV-infected and -uninfected men, as well as MSM who do not identify as homosexual or bisexual.

Injection Drug Users (IDUs)

Substance abuse, particularly injection drug use, continues to promote the spread of HIV in African American communities. Sharing drug paraphernalia, exchanging sex for drugs, and having a partner who injects drugs are all mechanisms that place people at increased risk for HIV (Nyamathi et al., 1995). Studies have also found that substance use, including alcohol, crack cocaine, and marijuana, contribute to sexual risk taking (Friedman et al., 1992). Reducing drug use and sexual risk behaviors requires comprehensive and collaborative efforts aimed at enhancing knowledge, skills, and support for reducing risk for HIV. For this to occur, HIV and substance use programs must be integrated so as to provide multiple opportunities for prevention and treatment for HIV-infected and -uninfected substance users, as well as their partners. Examinations of the social "roots" of drug use in African American communities must continue as this information is essential to developing effective and appropriate prevention interventions. Also, increasing access to quality substance use treatment programs is a necessary component to reducing the spread of HIV.

Heterosexual Women at Risk

The majority of African American women infected with HIV appear to have acquired the infection through heterosexual contact. Unfortunately, the most effective readily available method for preventing acquisition of HIV is a male-controlled prophylaxis (i.e., male condom). Consequently, men's agreement to consistently and correctly use condoms is essential to reducing women's risk for infection. Wingood and DiClemente (1998) found that African American women whose partners disapproved of using condoms were nearly three and a half times as likely to never use condoms. Feelings of powerlessness experienced by women may result from traditional gender role socialization that typically renders women submissive to their male sexual partners. HIV prevention programs targeting women must address problems resulting from gender-power imbalances. Furthermore, HIV prevention efforts must give increased attention to issues of intimate partner violence, including physical abuse and coercive sex, as well as emotional abuse experienced by many women. Feeling empowered in the ability to reduce risk for HIV is critical if women are to gain more control over sexual encounters. Moreover, effective and acceptable female-controlled barrier contraceptive alternatives must be made widely available.

Adolescents

HIV and STDs continue to represent a major health concern for adolescents. Each year one in four adolescents is infected with an STD. Aside from being biologically more susceptible to HIV and STDs, at-risk youth are more likely to be in short-term relationships, have multiple partners, and have unprotected sex (CDC, 2002a). Results of the 2001 National Youth Risk Behavior Survey (YRBS), a sample of students in grades 9–12 (N=13,601), found that African American adolescents compared to White and Hispanic students were significantly more likely to report having had sexual intercourse, initiating sex before age 13, and having four or more sexual partners. However, African American adolescents were more likely to report using condoms and less likely to report alcohol or drug use at last sexual intercourse compared to their counterparts (CDC, 2002d). Further examinations of the sexual networks of African American adolescents may provide increased understanding of what appear to be discrepant findings in this study. Helping adolescents to reduce sexual risk behaviors and adopt health-promoting behaviors requires comprehensive and collaborative strategies involving families, schools, community-based programs, and STD and HIV prevention programs, as well as substance use programs (Miller et al., 1999). Moreover, improving adolescents' access to, and utilization of, health-care services must become a priority.

SEXUALLY TRANSMITTED DISEASES EPIDEMIOLOGICAL TRENDS

An estimated 15.3 million new cases of STDs are reported each year in the United States, and more than 65 million persons are currently living with an incurable STD (Table 15.2). Many STDs do not produce acute symptoms or apparent signs of infection, thus increasing the likelihood that an undetected infection will be passed on to a sexual partner. Further, untreated STDs can result in damaging and costly outcomes including pelvic inflammatory disease, ectopic pregnancy, chronic pelvic pain, infertility, cancer, and adverse pregnancy outcomes (e.g., neonatal opthalmia, pneumonia, fetal death, physical and mental developmental disabilities) (CDC, 2002a). Correct and consistent use of latex condoms has been shown to be effective in reducing the risk for some STDs (i.e., chlamydia, gonorrhea, and trichomoniasis), including HIV. However, condoms are less effective in protecting against infections that are transmitted through skin-to-skin contact (e.g., herpes [HSV], human papillomavirus [HPV], syphilis) because all exposed areas are not covered (CDC, 2002b).

Surveillance data indicate that minorities, women, and adolescents are disproportionately affected by STDs. However, interpretation of these data is cautioned in view of the fact the data are collected from state and local health departments for persons seeking care in public health facilities. STD cases are more likely to be reported by these facilities as compared to cases diagnosed by private

Table 15.2

Incidence and prevalence of sexually transmitted diseases (STDs)

STD	Incidence (Estimated number of new cases every year)	Prevalence (Estimated # of people currently infected)
Chlamydia	3 million	2 million
Gonorrhea	650,000	Not Available
Syphilis	70,000	Not Available
Herpes	1 million	45 million
Human Papillomavirus	5.5 million	20 million
Hepatitis B	120,000	417,000
Trichomoniasis	5 million	Not Available

Source: Cates (1999).

providers. Presently, the most complete STD data are available for chlamydia trachomatis, gonorrhea and syphilis. Currently, case reporting data is not available for genital herpes simplex virus, human papillomavirus (HPV), nongonococcal urethritis, and trichomoniasis.

African American Trends and Disparities

Chlamydia Trachomatis.   Chlamydia trachomatis is the most commonly reported bacterial sexually transmitted diseases in the United States. In 2001, the overall rate for infection among women (435.2 per 100,000 population) was four times the rate of men (113.9 per 100,000 population). African Americans constitute 41 percent of the 783,242 cases of chlamydia trachomatis reported during the same period. The 2001 rate for African Americans was nearly 10 times greater than the rate for Whites and two and a half times greater than Hispanics (1,114.5, 118.7 and 447.4, per 100,000 population, respectively) (CDC, 2002a). Young African Americans continue to shoulder the burden of this infection. Seventy-five percent of the chlamydia trachomatis cases diagnosed among African Americans were diagnosed in patients 15–24 years in age.

Gonorrhea.   In 2001, 361,705 cases of gonorrhea were reported to the CDC, and African Americans account for 76 percent of this total. Rates in the same year for African Americans were nearly 27 times higher than for Whites and tens times higher than for Hispanics (782.3, 29.4 and 74.2 per 100,000, respectively). In particular, African American adolescents and young adults are at extremely high risk for gonorrheal infections. Compared to other racial and ethnic groups, African American females (15–19 years in age) and African American males (20–24 years in age) had the highest rate of infection compared to all other racial and age groups (3,495.2 and 3,484.0, per 100,000 population, respectively).

Syphilis.   African Americans continue to be disproportionately affected by syphilis infections. Sixty-three percent of the 6,103 primary and secondary syphilis cases reported to the CDC in 2001 occurred among African Americans. The rate for African Americans (11.0 per 100,000 population) was 16 times higher than the rate for Whites (0.7 per 100,000 population), which was a substantial decrease from 1997, when the rate for African Americans was 44 times higher than the rate for Whites.

Relationship between HIV and STDs

HIV is frequently sexually transmitted; therefore STDs and HIV are often seen as comorbidities. The biological mechanism through which STDs may promote transmission of HIV is not yet fully understood. However, data suggest that ulcerative STDs (i.e., syphilis, genital herpes [HSV], chancroid), and nonulcerative or microulcerative STDs (i.e., chlamydia, gonorrhea, trichomoniasis) are associated with increased HIV infectivity and susceptibility (Sullivan et al., 1997). Genital ulcers can serve as direct portals of entry and exit for HIV. Increased susceptibility to HIV can also result from the body's inflammatory response to STDs and the recruitment of HIV target and infected cells (Wasserheit, 1992). Moreover, HIV can affect the clinical presentation of STDs and their treatment outcomes, and in turn, STDs may influence the progression of HIV.

THE RELATIONSHIP BETWEEN HIV, STDS, AND OTHER RELATED CONDITIONS

Comorbidities and HIV

Increasingly, the health-care system is being challenged by the comorbidities present with HIV. Having a behavioral component to its acquisition, HIV is associated with other diseases that are transmitted by similar behavior patterns. For example, the hepatitis viruses such as hepatitis B virus and hepatitis C virus are seen in significant portions of the HIV-infected population. Sexually transmitted disease (STD) clinics are often times comanaging HIV and STDs due to their close affinity. Furthermore, as individuals live longer on high-dosage antiretrovirals, they are faced with complications caused by these agents. For example, diseases such as diabetes, arteriosclerosis, and lipid abnormalities are now taking their toll on these patients. This section discusses several illnesses that must be considered if providers are to be successful in their management of HIV-infected patients.

HIV and Hepatitis.   Hepatitis C virus (HCV) infection is a major comorbidity associated with HIV. Although over 170 million individuals are infected with HCV worldwide, the prevalence of the infection varies from country to country. The highest incidence is seen in the Eastern parts of the globe compared with the Western parts (Memon & Memon, 2002). Ethnic variations also occur with HCV infections, with the incidence being higher in African Americans than in Whites.

The association of HIV and HCV is especially important because it highlights the issues of disparities in HIV care from several vantage points. Although the epidemiological disparity was introduced in the previous paragraph, this represents differences based only on geographic variations. Further disparities that significantly influence treatment outcomes are seen in subtype distributions, access to treatments including liver transplants, and the unavailability of diagnostic procedures to disfranchised patients.

The major risk factors for HCV parallel the risk factors for HIV. Both diseases are predominantly seen in lower socioeconomic groups. The prevalence of hepatitis C virus infection varies in different populations, ranging from as low as 0.6 percent in volunteer blood donors to as high as 80 percent in injection drug users (Yen & Keeffe, 2003). The prevalence is predictable based on the risk factors, including injection drug use, blood product transfusion, organ transplantation, hemodialysis, occupational injury, sexual transmission, and vertical transmission (Yen & Keeffe, 2003).

The seroprevalence rates seen in patients coinfected with HIV and HCV varies depending on their risk factor. Patients who are intravenous drug users have seroprevalence rates between 52 percent and 90 percent. High coinfection seroprevalence rates are also seen in hemophiliacs, 60 percent to 65 percent. Lower seroprevalence rates are seen in men who have sex with men (MSM) and from vertical transmission, 4 percent to 8 percent and 2 percent to 10 percent, respectively (Thomas,

1999). These high seroprevalence rates seen in the coinfected patients has led providers to routinely test for HCV in all patients who are HIV-infected. In fact, screening criteria for HCV includes known HIV infection, a history of IDUs, blood transfusions occurring before July 1992, elevated liver enzymes, hemodialysis, STDs in high-risk settings, and postexposure.

Hepatitis C virus is a flavirus that produces over 10 trillion new virions per day, a much higher number of virions than the 10 billion for HIV per day. It targets hepatocytes and B-lymphocytes. There are six genotypes (1a, 1b, 2, 3, 4, 5, 6) of HCV that vary in their responses to therapy. The predominant subtype seen in the United States and Western Europe is genotype 1a and 1b. Over 90 percent of African Americans infected with HCV have these genotypes.

Patients infected with HCV have a 70 percent chance of developing chronic hepatitis. The association of HIV coinfection does not increase the development of chronic liver disease, acute hepatitis, or fulminant hepatitis, but it does increase the likelihood of liver failure in these patients. Also, there are higher levels of HCVRNA in coinfected patients than in patients infected with HCV alone. The higher viral load of HCV has been postulated as the cause of higher rates of vertical transmission and increases in the rate of sexual transmission of HCV as compared to patients who are not coinfected with HIV.

Unlike hepatitis B, hepatitis C coinfection with HIV-1 may accelerate the progression of HIV (Sabin et al., 1997). The genotype-1 subtype is seen to have a greater impact than the other five genotypes in accelerating HIV progression. In one comparative study of 263 patients infected with HIV alone compared to 166 patients coinfected, the researchers found an 11 percent mortality in the coinfected group versus 7 percent mortality in the group infected with HIV alone (Monja et al., 2001). The coinfected patients also showed higher alanineamino transaminases, 52 U/L versus 35 U/L in the coinfected versus the group infected with HIV alone, respectively.

African American patients coinfected with HIV and HCV do not fully benefit from the treatments available for HCV. Treatment outcomes for HCV have been very poor for African Americans. Forty-five percent of those treated responded to the combination therapy with interferon and ribavirin (Poles & Dieterich, 2000). Further compounding this issue is the large number of African Americans who do not have access to the treatments and liver biopsies required for the proper staging and assessments of the treatment needs. Most patients who receive medications from one of the AIDS Drug Assistance Programs do not have access to interferon and ribavirin. Unfortunately most of these patients are African American patients.

Further compounding the direct complications from HCV/HIV coinfection are the future complications that may develop in those patients who do not have access to care. HCV is a progressive disease that can lead to liver cirrhosis, liver failure, or liver cancer. More than 80 percent of patients infected with HCV will develop chronic liver disease, 20 percent to 30 percent of them will develop cirrhosis after 10 to 20 years, and some develop hepatocellular carcinoma (Hwang, 2001). These complications are often accelerated in patients receiving antiretroviral treatments that affect the liver. However, discontinuing antiretroviral use is not recommended in patients coinfected with the two diseases. Other risks for accelerated cirrhosis include alcohol abuse, other viral infections, and advancements in age.

Further studies including African Americans are needed to elucidate the difference in treatment responses noted between the different ethnic groups. Unfortunately, few African Americans are involved in these studies, and fewer proportions of African American researchers participate in any of these investigations.

Cardiovascular and Endocrine Complications and HIV.   In recent years a variety of metabolic abnormalities and morphologic alterations have been seen in patients infected with human immunodeficiency virus receiving antiretrovirals. Some of these abnormalities include insulin resistance, dyslipidemia, abdominal and dorsocervical fat accumulation, and fat depletion in the extremities and the face. Anecdotal reports suggest that these changes may lead to long-term problems with diabetes, heart disease, and cerebrovascular events in patients. These consequences are complications that disproportionately affect African Americans independently of HIV. For example, African Americans have higher blood pressure and worse complications secondary to hypertension than whites. Type 2 diabetes is also more common and occurs at an earlier age in African Americans as compared to whites (Sherwin, 2000). Consequently, additional emphasis should be placed on screening for diabetes, dyslipidemias, and heart disease in African Americans infected with HIV.

Although the consequences of these metabolic abnormalities seen in African American HIV-infected patients taking antiretrovirals are not specifically known, some investigators have looked at them in the general HIV-infected population. In one large series of patients the prevalence was 21 percent for isolated peripheral atrophy, 17 percent for isolated fat accumulation, 24 percent for mixed syndrome, 23 percent for glucose metabolism alterations, 28 percent for hypertriglyceridemia, and 57 percent for hypercholesterloemia (Saves et al., 2002).

Cardiac involvement may occur in as many as 45 percent to 66 percent of patients infected with HIV (Decastro et al., 1992). Although cardiac involvement includes diseases such as pericardial disease, myocarditis, dilated cardiomyopathy, and endocarditis associated with HIV, coronary artery disease is being seen more recently in the era of protease inhibitor therapy (Passalaris et al., 2000). Specific effects that protease inhibitors may have on the heart include increased insulin resistance, abnormalities in lipid metabolism, and fat redistribution (Sullivan et al., 1998). More recent data suggest that the type of nucleoside reverse-transcriptase inhibitor or protease inhibitor is not constantly associated with these changes. Exposure to stavudine is associated with lipoatrophy, and exposure of ritonavir is associated with hypertriglyceridemia (Saves, 2002).

Dyslipidemia is well described in patients receiving antiretroviral therapy (Sullivan & Nelson, 1997). The lipid abnormality is highly prevalent in patients receiving antiretrovirals. In one clinic the 62 (47 percent) of 133 patients receiving protease inhibitors had lipid abnormalities that met the National Cholesterol Education Program Guidelines intervention criteria (Henry et al., 1998). In another study 56 of 98 (57 percent) protease inhibitor recipients had hyperlipidemia (Behrens et al., 1999). African American HIV-infected patients in the authors' clinic have dyslipidemia at a rate of 75 percent (McNeil unpublished observation). This high prevalence seen in patients on antiretrovirals may eliminate any differences in outcomes contributed by race. However, the increased risks seen in African Americans emphasizes the potential for exacerbating an already existing problem.

Although, type 2 diabetes will develop in a small proportion (1 percent–6 percent) of patients infected with human immunodeficiency virus who are treated with protease inhibitors, a considerable proportion of patients will develop insulin resistance and impaired glucose tolerance (Dube, 2000). Hyperglycemia in association with protease inhibitor use is often also associated with dyslipidemia and abdominal obesity (Dube, 2000). Although differences in race have been elucidated in non-HIV-infected patients, the association with race and antiretroviral use has not been studied.

Psychosocial Issues and HIV.   There is a high prevalence of psychiatric disease seen in patients infected with HIV. In fact, psychiatric disorders can cause an increase in high-risk behavior leading to an increased risk of acquiring HIV. Furthermore, patient nonadherence to antiretroviral use is related to mental illness and substance use disorders (Angelino & Treisman, 2001). Unfortunately, coordinated services including HIV management, case management, and psychiatric care are not always available to minority communities.

A variety of psychiatric disorders are observed in the HIV-infected population. Common ones include major depression, demoralization, bipolar disorder, and substance abuse. Studies have shown the prevalence of major depression in HIV-infected individuals to be in a range of 15 percent to 40 percent (Angelino & Treisman, 2001). One clinic reported that 75 percent of their HIV-infected patients have a substance abuse disorder (Lyketsos et al., 1994). The high prevalence of substance abuse in HIV emphasizes the need for psychiatric services to coexist with medical management services in HIV clinics. Resources should be allocated for these services in minority-HIV-infected clinics.

CLINICAL MANIFESTATIONS, THERAPEUTIC ADVANCES, AND RELATED ISSUES

Clinical Manifestations

During the early years of the HIV epidemic, the treatment of opportunistic infections was the mainstay of HIV care. Evidence that prophylactic therapy was effective for the opportunistic infections was not yet acquired. The incidences of infections such as *Pneumocystis carinii* pneumonia (PCP), disseminated *Mycobacterium avium* complex (MAC) infection, *Cytomegalovirus* retinitis, and toxoplasmosis ranged between 110 and 20 incidences per 1,000 person-years. Subsequently, investigators gathered clinical trial data supporting the effectiveness of prophylaxis for the prevention of these infections (Osmond et al., 1994; Pierce et al., 1996). These data supported the development of guidelines for the prophylaxis of opportunistic infections by the U.S. Public Health Service (USPHS) and the Infectious Diseases Society of America (IDSA) in 1995 and 1997 (working group). Prophylaxis showed a modest improvement in the incidence per 1,000 person-years of opportunistic infections from 330 in 1982 to 300 in 1994.

Current guidelines include recommendations for the use of both primary and secondary prophylaxis. Primary prophylaxis is defined as the prevention of a disease not yet acquired, and secondary prophylaxis is the prevention of the recurrence of a disease that occurred in the patient's past. In both cases patients' immunosuppression places them at increased risk for the development of an opportunistic infection. The opportunistic infections for which prophylaxis are generally recommended are outlined in Table 15.3.

Although opportunistic infections associated with HIV remain an important cause of the complications associated with the disease, the use of highly active antiretrovirals have significantly decreased the incidence of new opportunistic infections and deaths associated with HIV infections (Pallela et al., 1998). Currently, the incidence per 1,000 person-years of all the opportunistic infections is less than 150, a decline from 300 in 1994. These improvements are a direct result of the phenomena of immune reconstitution seen with the use of the antiretrovirals and the suppressive effect that the antiretrovirals have on viral replication that leads to an improvement in CD4 lymphocyte counts. The response is reported to be biphasic with an initial redistribution of cells previously trapped in lymph nodes followed by two to three months of true immunologic recovery (Powderly, 2000).

The evidence for immune reconstitution has led to the development of new guidelines for the prevention of the opportunistic infections. Specifically, the USPHS and IDSA have changed the guidelines to say that primary prophylaxis can now be discontinued in patients whose CD4 cell count has exceeded the threshold for which prophylaxis was initiated for a duration of at least three to six months for PCP, and MAC. The threshold CD4 cell count for discontinuing primary prophylaxis for toxoplasmosis was increased to a level of 200 cells/µL. Secondary prophylaxis can be discontinued for PCP, MAC, toxoplasmosis, and cryptococcosis. Table 15.4 summarizes the criteria for the discontinuation of primary and secondary prophylaxis for the opportunistic infections (USPHS/IDSA 2001).

However, despite the ability to achieve significant improvements in the status of the immune system, the levels of the incidences of the opportunistic infections are leveling off rather than continuing to show a decline. Although, the reasons for this observation are complex, there is evidence

Table 15.3
Summary of opportunistic infections for which prophylaxis is recommended

Primary Prophylaxis	Secondary Prophylaxis
P. carinii*	P. carinii*
Tuberculosis*	T. gondii*
T. gondii*	M. avium*
M. avium*	Cryptococcus*
Varicella zoster*	Histoplasmosis*
S. pneumonia†	Coccidiomycosis*
Hepatitis A & B†	Cytomegalovirus*
Influenzae†	Salmonella bacteremia
* Standard of care † Generally recommended	

that the use of prophylaxis is not being optimized. A 2001 report from the MMWR looking at PCP specifically shows an increasing trend of patients not receiving the appropriate prophylaxis and not being in care. Currently, 45 percent of patients are not in care, an increase from 41 percent between 1993 and 1996. Fourteen percent of patients who are in care meet the criteria for prophylaxis but do not receive any, an increase from 6 percent between 1993 and 1996. Thirty-four percent of patients who are in care meet the criteria and are on prophylaxis, a decline from 44 percent between 1993 and 1996 (CDC, 2001c). Trends also show that the patients who are not in care and who do not receive the appropriate prophylaxis are disproportionately African Americans.

The disproportionate numbers of African Americans initiating an HIV diagnosis at a later stage in the HIV illness suggests that the nadir CD4 cell count is lower than in the white population. However, patients who have different nadir CD4 cell counts pre-highly active antiretroviral therapy (HAART) have no difference in susceptibility to OIs following the immune reconstitution after HAART (Miller et al., 2000), stressing the importance of continuing to get these patients into care regardless of the late stage of the illness.

The changes in the complications of HIV disease, seen with the introduction of HAART, were not a comprehensive decline in all opportunistic infections. For example, the HIV-related pulmonary manifestations have changed over the pre- and post-HAART eras. Although decreases have been noted in the typical OIs such as PCP, and CMV infecting the lung, there was an increase in bacterial pulmonary infections and lymphomas occurring concurrently. One investigator looked at their consultant service over the two eras specified between 1993 and 1995 and 1997 and 2000. They found decreases in PCP and CMV of 37 percent to 18 percent and 7 percent to 4 percent, respectively; however, the changes in pulmonary bacterial infections and non-Hodgkin lymphoma were 30 percent to 48 percent and 3 percent to 16 percent, respectively (Wolff & O'Donnell, 2001).

Many African American HIV-infected patients continue to die from the OIs and continue to be initially diagnosed with HIV at the time of having an OI, late in their illness. The cause of this is multifactorial, representing issues of lack of access to care, the disproportionate numbers of African Americans who receive their care episodically and acutely, the lack of testing being done in the African American communities, and the lack of adequately trained providers who care for African Americans. Health-care providers may confuse patients as they adhere to the changing treatment

Table 15.4
Summary recommendations for the discontinuation of primary and secondary prophylaxis for the opportunistic infections

Disease	Primary Prophylaxis Discontinuation	Secondary Prophylaxis Discontinuation	Recommendations for Discontinuation
PCP	Yes	Yes	CD4 count >200 for $\geq$ 3 months
MAC	Yes	Yes	CD4 count >100 for $\geq$ 3 months CD4 count >100 for $\geq$ 6 months after completing 12 months of MAC therapy and have no symptoms
Toxoplasmosis	Yes	Yes	CD4 count >200 for $\geq$ 3 months CD4 >200 for $\geq$ 6 months if they have completed their initial therapy and have no symptoms
Cryptococcosis	Not Applicable	Yes	CD4 count > 100-200 for $\geq$ 6 months if they have completed their initial therapy and have no symptoms
CMV	Not Applicable	Yes	CD4 count > 100-200 for $\geq$ 6 months in consultation with an ophthalmologist. Consider anatomic location of the lesion, vision in the contralateral eye, and feasibility of regular monitoring

guidelines that incorporate some of the changes noted above and delay treatment to lower CD4 cell counts without offering adequate patient education, support services, and culturally appropriate care settings.

Therapeutic Advances

Highly Active Antiretroviral Therapy.   Highly active antiretroviral therapy (HAART) is the most important aspect of HIV management. Following the introduction of protease inhibitors and the use of potent combination regimens in 1996, the mortality associated with HIV declined to its present level. The goal of successful antiretroviral therapy is achieving maximal viral suppression and immune function reconstitution (Rosenberg et al., 1997).

Despite the significant contribution made by HAART in the management of HIV-infected patients, antiretroviral therapy is often unsuccessful. Several factors have contributed to this challenge, including poor adherence to treatment, limited oral bioavailability, the development of resistant subpopulations of virus, low drug potency, and competing pharmokinetic factors from other drugs. These factors have led to successful virologic and immunologic outcomes in only 50 percent of the patients who take HAART.

Since the introduction of zidovudine in 1987, the pace of new agent approval has been steady. Currently, we have 16 antiretroviral agents available for our use (Table 15.5). Concomitantly increasing with the number of agents was the complexity with which to use them. As a result of the increasing challenge to clinicians, the Department of Health and Human Services and the International AIDS Society-USA Panel have regularly updated recommendations for antiretroviral therapy in adults to assist clinicians in their management of HIV-infected patients.

Guidelines for the Use of HAART.   As noted above, guidelines exist to assist clinicians in the management of their patients and to maximize the long-term benefits of antiretrovirals. There are several versions of these guidelines, including recommendations of the Panel on Clinical Practices for Treatment of HIV Infection by the Department of Health and Human Services and the Henry J. Kaiser Family Foundation and the International AIDS Society–USA panel. These recommendations for the initiation of therapy are summarized in Tables 15.6 and 15.7 (Carpenter et al., 2000: Panel on Clinical Practices for Treatment of HIV Infection, 2002).

Changing therapy is not as simple a decision as initiating therapy and is dependent on the reason for the change. Several reasons exist for changing therapy, including resistance developing to the current regimen, poor adherence to the antiretroviral combination, poor tolerability of the medication, or a complication developing secondary to an unsuspecting comorbidity or drug-drug interaction. Decisions to change therapy are dependent on the close monitoring of patients, including regular review with patients of potential side effects, checking CD4 cell counts and HIV RNA levels regularly, monitoring blood chemistries and hematological profiles, frequent adherence counseling and assessment, and the close monitoring of concomitant medication use.

New Therapeutic Strategies.   Multiple factors are looked at when changing an antiretroviral drug regimen. The regimen must be evaluated from the perspective of the individual patient looking at the resistance profile, possible drug-drug interactions, potency of the new regimen, and tolerability factors unique to the patient. HIV clinicians have developed several strategies that have showed variable success in the treatment of antiretroviral experienced patients over the last several years. These strategies include structured treatment interruptions (STI), intensification of existing regimens, mega-HAART, or potent salvage therapy.

Anecdotal reports exist where antiretroviral treatment has been held for variable periods of time with the intent of reducing drug toxicity and maximally suppressing viremia. This has led to the development of clinical trials for the further study of STI (Papasavvas et al., 2000). However, results have been variable, and this strategy has not experienced widespread use. Historically, many patients have practiced this unsupervised by medical providers, often leading to multiantiretroviral resistant strains of the virus.

The use of intensification techniques in patients who have low levels of viremia (less than 10,000 copies/mm3) without maximal suppression (<50 copies/mm3) is also under study by various clinical trials. This method requires the addition of further antiretrovirals to a regimen that has not shown maximal suppression and there is no evidence of resistance present. However, one can never be absolutely sure that undetectable resistant subpopulations of virus are present, undetectable due to their limited quantity. As a result, this strategy has not experienced widespread use.

Table 15.5
Approved antiretrovirals

Generic name	Brand name	Acronym
Nucleoside reverse transcriptase inhibitors (NRTIs)		
Abacavir	Ziagen	ABC
Didanosine	Videx	ddI
Lamivudine	Epivir	3TC
Stavudine	Zerit	D4T
Zalcitibine	Hivid	ddC
Zidovudine	Retrovir	AZT; ZDV
Nucleotide reverse transcriptase inhibitors		
Tenofovir DF	Viread	TDF
Non-nucleoside reverse transcriptase inhibitors (NNRTIs)		
Delaviridine	Rescriptor	DLV
Efavirenz	Sustivs	EFV
Nevirapine	Viramune	NVP
Protease Inhibitors (PIs)		
Amprenavir	Agenerase	APV
Indinavir	Crixivan	IDV
Lopinavir/ritonavir	Kaletra	ABT-378
Nelfinavir	Viracept	NFV
Ritonavir	Norvir	RTV
Saquinavir	Fortovase/Invirase	SQV

The additional challenge of having virus resistant to multiple drugs from all classes occurs due to the experience of having multiple prior changes. This is one of the biggest challenges facing clinicians who take care of these advanced patients. One strategy used is the introduction of mega-HAART or the use of multiple drugs as high as eight in number. The challenges faced by patients and providers with this strategy are the increased risk of toxicities and reduced tolerability (Montaner, 2000).

Table 15.6
Panel on clinical practices for treatment of HIV infection guidelines for the use of antiretroviral agents in HIV-infected adults and adolescents

Clinical category	Recommendations
Symptomatic infection	Treatment recommended
Asymptomatic AIDS/CD4 count <200 cells/mm3	Treatment recommended
CD4 count 200-350 cells/mm3	Treatment should generally be offered, though controversy exists
CD4 count>350 cells/mm3 and HIV RNA>55,000 (RT-PCR) or >30,000 (bDNA) copies.mL	Some experts would recommend initiating therapy, recognizing that the 3-year risk of developing AIDS in untreated patients is >30%. In the absence of very high levels of plasma HIV RNA, some would defer therapy and monitor the CD4 count and level of plasma HIV RNA more frequently. Clinical outcomes data after initiating therapy are lacking.
CD4 count>350 cells/mm3 and HIV RNA<55,000 (RT-PCR) or<30,000 (bDNA) copies/mL	Many experts would defer therapy and observe, recognizing that the 3-year risk of developing AIDS in untreated patients is<15%.

Although these strategies have shown variable levels of efficacy and subsequently limited widespread use, one strategy has been incorporated into current guidelines due to its proven advantage in the improvement of treatment strategies and ability to measure disease prognosis. This strategy is the use of resistance testing technology in routine care.

Resistance Testing and Viral Failure.   Resistance occurs as a result of point mutations that subsequently lead to the production of virus that does not succumb to the effects of the antiretrovirals. Point mutations occur many times per day in an individual patient's viral population. This phenomenon occurs because of the high rate of replication of the virus in a day (107-108 replication rounds per day). Mutations are introduced at a rate one per one hundred thousand replications. Hence, there are many point mutations occurring each day (Coffin, 1995).

Although antiretroviral adherence is one of the most important factors responsible for the reduction of resistance, the reason for resistance development is multifactorial. Contributions to resistance development include the incomplete suppression of virus in previously infected cells, the presence of latent resistant reservoirs of virus, the recombination of RNA templates in a single HIV virion, and competing pharmokinetics between concomitant drugs present (Grossman et al., 1998; Chun et al., 1997; Moutouh et al., 1996).

Several assays are currently available for the detection of HIV antiretroviral resistance. These assays detect resistance at the genotypic and phenotypic levels. The phenotypic assay measures susceptibility of the virus by determining the concentration of drug that inhibits viral replication in tissue culture. The genotypic assay determines the presence of mutations that are known to produce decreased drug susceptibility (Hanna & D'Aquila, 2001). Although resistance testing is permanently

Table 15.7
Antiretroviral therapy in adults: updated recommendations of the International AIDS Society–USA

Disease stage or risk of clinical progression	Recommendation
Symptomatic infection	Antiretroviral therapy recommended. Acute treatment of a serious opportunistic infection may take precedence (ie, when concomitant therapy would lead to adverse drug-drug interactions)
High risk of clinical progression within 3 years CD4 count<350 cells/mm3 **Or** Plasma HIV RNA>30,000 copies/mL **Or** CD4 count 300-500 cells /mm3 and plasma HIV RNA 5,000-30,000 copies/mL	Treatment generally recommended
CD4 count>500 cells/mm3 and plasma HIV RNA 5,000-30,000 copies/mL	Therapy should be deferred
Low risk of clinical progression within 3 years CD4 count>500 cells/mm3 and HIV RNA<5,000 copies/mL	Disadvantages and risks of therapy should be weighed against potential virologic and clinical benefits. Deferred treatment with continued monitoring is an option.

established in the clinical setting, its full potential has not yet been fully developed. Ongoing research continues to elucidate its full potential.

FUTURE TRENDS

Context of HIV/STD Risk

The reasons African Americans are disproportionately affected by HIV/STDs are complex and multidimensional. Traditionally, approaches to understanding HIV/STD epidemiology have largely been individually based. The principal focus on personal behaviors (i.e., having multiple sex partners, nonuse of condoms, drug use, etc.) has done little to explain or substantively reduce HIV/STD morbidity in the African American community (Aral, 2002). Little attention has been devoted to reconceptualizing HIV/STDs within the context of pervasive economic and social realities that figure prominently in the lives of many African Americans (e.g., racism and discrimination, poverty, poor educational opportunities, deteriorating community structures, lack of access to health care and quality care, etc.) (Cochran & Mays, 1993; Fullilove, 2001). Relative to a myriad of life stressors, including unemployment, lack of quality child care, crime and drugs in the neighborhood, and unavailability of affordable housing, research has indicated that African American women reported less concern about HIV/AIDS (Kalichman et al., 1992).

Role of Culture

Recognizing that African American communities are heterogeneous and consist of many diverse cultural characteristics is essential to tailoring HIV/STD prevention and treatment programs. Culture, defined as a social phenomenon, embodies shared values, beliefs, attitudes, and norms that influence behavior. Unfortunately, research has not adequately addressed the potential interplay between culture and risk for HIV/STDs. Consequently, this devaluing of culture has hindered the development and implementation of culturally competent and sensitive HIV/STD education and prevention programs for the African American community. Randall-David (1994) defines cultural competence as the "ability to work effectively with culturally diverse clients and communities because the individual, agency or system exhibits culturally appropriate attitudes, beliefs, behaviors and policies." As applied to HIV/AIDS prevention and care efforts, it is necessary to have culture situated at the center of all HIV prevention efforts, including education, interventions, and program services.

Recently, the CDC convened a panel of experts to address cultural competence in tailoring HIV/AIDS prevention and treatment services for racial and ethnic minorities. Several macro- and micro-level strategies were proposed and are summarized as follows: (1) commit administrative, financial and programmatic resources to making services and programs culturally appropriate; (2) increase staff development and cultural competence training for those serving affected populations; (3) respond to economic and social contextual factors that influence responses to the HIV epidemic; (4) provide education, interventions and programs in culturally appropriate languages, at appropriate literacy levels, and at locations that are accessible to the community; and (5) ensure that people serving targeted populations share racial/ethnic and/or other background characteristics and (6) possess a positive regard and respect for the targeted community (CDC, 1999).

Despite efforts to alleviate the burden of HIV/STDs in the African American community, results have been hampered by a legacy of distrust between African Americans, government, and the biomedical community. Nearly 70 years after the tragedy of the Tuskegee syphilis study, the longest nontherapeutic experiment on human beings in medical history, many African Americans continue to possess fears of genocide and beliefs that AIDS is an artificially created virus placed in the Black community to exterminate African Americans (Thomas & Quinn, 1991). Recently, in an investigation of 520 African Americans, Klonoff and Landrine (1999) reported that nearly 30 percent held AIDS-conspiracy views and an additional 23 percent were undecided.

Chronic Care Model

The approach to HIV care has changed over the epidemic from emergent care in the first decade, when HAART was not available, to urgent care with the introduction of the nucleoside reverse transcriptase inhibitors. However, these drugs were used as monotherapy, and the impact on the immunologic recovery was limited and transient at best. It was not until the introduction of the protease inhibitors in 1996 that care became transformed to a more chronic format. This transformation occurred because of the impact HAART had on immunologic recovery.

The transformation of the care format introduced new challenges and exacerbated old ones. Prior discussions showed that patients may in general live longer; however, the mortality of African American patients with HIV continues to far exceed that of whites. Long-term toxicities were being introduced as a result of the antiretrovirals exacerbating complications that were already disproportionately seen in the African American community, including heart disease, diabetes, and lipid abnormalities. Resistance to the antiretrovirals was also being introduced. The reasons for resistance have been shown to be multifactorial; however, the inadequate health-care infrastructural support of chronic HIV care promoted nonadherence in disfranchised populations.

In order to achieve success in the treatment of HIV disease as a chronic illness, new approaches will need to be embraced. One approach would be the use of model introduced by Edward Wagner called the chronic care model (Wagner, 1998). The chronic care model was developed for the improvement of health care in a primary care setting focusing on the improvements in six areas, including community resources and policies, health-care organizations, self-management support, delivery system design, decision support, and clinical information systems (Bodenheimer et al., 2002). This model has been used successfully in the areas of diabetes, geriatrics, asthma, congestive heart failure, and cerebral vascular disease. The use of this model in HIV will hopefully improve clinical outcomes.

Changes in HIV-Related Diseases

A retrospective analysis of autopsy data from Mount Sinai Medical Center comparing disease frequencies between the periods 1996 to 2000 versus 1987 to 1995 showed a decrease in the prevalence of pneumocystis carinii pneumonia and Kaposi sarcoma and an increase in the prevalence of cirrhosis and arteriosclerosis (Morgello et al., 2002). Similar data were published by CDC showing changes in the causes of deaths in HIV between 1987 and 1999 (Selik et al., 2002). One author speculated that some of the mortality is not HIV-related but represented side effects from medications in the HAART regimens (Laurence, 2002). Dr. Laurence also described the transformation and challenges of HIV care currently, including a trend toward specialization of HIV care, concomitantly occurring with a departure of many HIV providers away from such care due to low reimbursements. These issues may represent compelling junctures in the future of care to African Americans who may already have limited access to HIV care.

The transformation of the current care model to a chronic model with specialized providers may further disfranchise African American patients unless issues of reimbursement and accessibility are addressed. The Ryan White Care Act has been instrumental in providing care as a last resort to large segments of the African American HIV community. However, further sustainable methods must be developed to address the widening disparities seen with this disease. Disease prevention, health-care policy, clinical care, case management, managed care, and industrial experts must work together to create a health-care infrastructure that will provide affordable equitable care to patients.

Research Focus

HIV has had a remarkable effect on the development of new knowledge in immunology, virology, and drug development. In addition to the challenges of vaccine development, researchers have discovered the complexities of finding new targets for pharmaceutical agents. Currently, agents are being investigated that will inhibit entry into all three steps of the entry of the virus into cells. These steps are attachment, chemokine co-receptor interaction, and fusion. Attachment requires the interaction of the virus with the surface receptors gp-120 and gp41. This then leads to an interaction with one of the available chemokine coreceptors (CCR5, CXCR4), and finally the process of cell membrane fusion with the subsequent incorporation of the virus into the cell. These steps of viral entry into host cells provide potential sites for viral inhibition.

One of the greatest challenges in HIV research has been the development of an AIDS vaccine. Very early in an attempt for a vaccine, researchers realized that an AIDS vaccine would not be successful if based on prior technologies. Vaccines had been thus far been developed as live attenuated, inactivated, or viral proteins. Newer technologies lead to several vaccine candidates based on innovative methods. These include a recombinant gp120 candidate currently in phase III trials, a variety of experimental immunogens, and a combination priming and boosting with a recombinant poxvirus and the recombinant envelope protein respectively (Robinson, 2002). The likelihood of a successful vaccine in the near future is limited. However, the research has helped with the further understanding of viral pathogenesis and the mechanisms of immune protection.

In lieu of a cure or vaccine for HIV and many STDs, the principal means for deterring the spread of infections in the African American community are effectual, tailored, and sustainable behavioral risk reduction efforts. HIV/STD screening, counseling, and referral services are critical for early identification of infection status, as well as prompting modifications in risk behaviors and increasing intent to commence appropriate treatment. Understanding deterrents to engaging in such services by African Americans is sorely needed. Further, for HIV positive persons, attention should be given to increasing awareness of factors facilitating (e.g., social and economic support, mental health services, spirituality) and impeding (e.g., stigma, discrimination) coping with this illness. Issues concerning disclosure of HIV positive status to family and friends, decisions regarding reproductive health and acceptance, and access to treatment must be addressed comprehensively. Moreover, little attention has been given to examining the nature of social, sexual, and drug use networks in the African American community, as well as the plausible interplay between these groups that may contribute to disparate rates of infection. Mounting evidence also points to a need to focus more attention on particularly high-risk groups, for example, persons in correctional settings, victims of sexual trauma and abuse, and persons exchanging sex for money and/or drugs.

CONCLUSION

HIV/AIDS poses one of the greatest challenges to humankind in the new millennium. The chapter looked at the epidemiological disparities seen with the infection, showing the disproportionate numbers of African Americans infected with HIV. The chapter further showed the developments in the field of HIV medicine, including HAART, resistance assays, immune reconstitution, and their effect on the clinical manifestations and opportunistic infections associated with HIV. However, in the face of limiting the progression of the virus, the treatments have exacerbated diseases, such as diabetes, dyslipidemias, and heart disease. Furthermore, the challenge of HIV is not limited to controlling the virus itself but extends to addressing the contemporary inequities of the health-care system. In the publication *Unequal Treatment*, published by the Institute of Medicine, the authors describe the inequities involving participants at several levels including health systems, their administrative and bureaucratic processes, utilization managers, health-care professionals, and patients (Smedely et al., 2003). They then propose that the provision of care should be based on published guidelines and not on financial incentives that disproportionately restrict the care given to minority patients, the proportion of ethnic minorities among health professionals should be increased, and cross-cultural curricula should be integrated early into training of providers.

REFERENCES

Angelino, A.F., & Treisman, G.J. (2001). Management of psychiatric disorders in patients infected with human immunodeficiency virus. *Clinical Infectious Diseases, 33*, 847–856.

Aral, S.O. (2002). Understanding racial-ethnic and societal differentials in STI: Do we need to move beyond behavioral epidemiology? *Sexually Transmitted Infections, 78*, 2–4.

Behrens, G., et al. (1999). Impaired glucose tolerance, beta cell function and lipid metabolism in HIV patients under treatment with protease inhibitors. *Acquired Immunodeficiency Deficiency Syndrome, 13*, F63–70.

Bodenheimer, T., Wagner, E.H., & Grumbach, K. (2002). Improving primary care for patients with chronic illness. *Journal of the American Medical Association, 288*, 1775–1779.

Carpenter, C.C., et al. (2000). Antiretroviral therapy in adults: Updated recommendations of the International AIDS Society-USA Panel. *Journal of the American Medical Association, 283*, 381–390.

Carr, A., et al. (1998). A syndrome of peripheral lipodystrophy, hyperlipidemia, and insulin resistance in patients receiving HIV protease inhibitoprs. *AIDS, 12*, F51–F58.

Cates, W., Jr. (1999). American Social Health Association Panel. Estimates of the incidence and prevalence of sexually transmitted diseases in the United States. *Sexually Transmitted Diseases, 26(4)*, S2–S7.

Centers for Disease Control and Prevention (CDC). (1999). *Cultural competence for program planners, evaluators and researchers*. Atlanta, GA: U.S. Department of Health and Human Services.

Centers for Disease Control and Prevention (CDC). (2001a). *HIV Prevention Strategic Plan through 2005*. Atlanta, GA: U.S. Department of Health and Human Services.

Centers for Disease Control and Prevention (CDC). (2001b). *HIV/AIDS Surveillance Report*, 13 (2). Atlanta, GA: U.S. Department of Health and Human Services.

Centers for Disease Control and Prevention (CDC). (2001c). *HIV/AIDS—United States. Morbidity and Mortality Revew, 50*, 430–434.

Centers for Disease Control and Prevention (CDC). (2002a). *Sexually transmitted disease surveillance, 2001*. Atlanta GA: U.S. Department of Health and Human Services.

Centers for Disease Control and Prevention (CDC). (2002b). *Sexually transmitted disease treatment guidelines 2002*, 51(RR–6).

Centers for Disease Control and Prevention (CDC). (2002c). Unrecognized HIV infection, risk behaviors, and perceptions of risk among young Black men who have sex with men—six U.S. cities, 1994–1998. *Morbidity and Mortality Weekly Report, 51(33)*, 733–736.

Centers for Disease Control and Prevention (CDC). (2002d). Youth risk behavior surveillance—United States, 2001. *Morbidity and Mortality Weekly Report*, 51(No. SS–4).

Chun, T.W. et al. (1997). Presence of an inducible HIV-1 latent reservoir during highly active antiretroviral therapy. *Proceedings of National Academy of Sciences, 94*, 13193–13197.

Cochran, S.D., & Mays, V.M. (1993). Applying social psychological models to predicting. *Journal of Black Psychology, 19(2)*, 142–154.

Coffin, M. (1995). HIV population dynamics in vivo implications for genetic variation, pathogenesis therapy. *Science, 267*, 483–489.

Decastro, S., et al. (1992). Heart involvement in AIDS: A prospective study during various stages of disease. *European Heart Journal, 11*, 1452–1459.

Dube, M.P. (2000). Disorders of glucose metabolism in patients infected with human immunodeficiency virus. *Clinical Infectious Disease, 31*, 1467–1475.

Friedman, S.R., Stepherson, B., Woods, J., Des Jarlais, D.C., & Ward, T.P. (1992). Society, drug injectors, and AIDS. *Journal of Health Care for the Poor and Underserved, 3(1)*, 73–92.

Fullilove, R.E. (2001). HIV prevention in the African-American community: Why isn't anybody talking about the elephant in the room? *AIDScience, 1(7) [online]*.

Grossman, Z., Feinberg, M.B., & Paul, W.E. (1998). Multiple modes of cellular activation and virus transmission in HIV infection: A role for chronically and latently infected cells in sustaining viral replication. *Proceedings of National Academy of Sciences, 95*, 6314–6319.

Hanna, G.J., & D'Aquila, R.T. (2001). Clinical use of genotypic and phenotypic drug resistance testing to monitor antiretroviral chemotherapy. *Clinical Infectious Diseases, 32*, 774–782.

Henry, K., Melrose, H., Huebesch, J., Hermundeson, J., and Simpson, J. (1998). Atrovastatin and gemfribrizil for protease inhibitor related lipid abnormalities. *Lancet, 352*, 1031–1032.

Hwang, S.J. (2001). Hepatitis C virus infection: An overview. *Journal of Microbiological Immunology & Infections, 34*, 227–234.

Kalichman, S.C., Hunter, T.L., & Kelly, J.A. (1992). Perceptions of AIDS susceptibility among minority and nonminority women at risk for HIV infection. *Journal of Consulting & Clinical Psychology, 60(5)*, 725–32.

Karon, J.M., Fleming, P.L., Steketee, R.W., & De Cock, K.M. (2001). HIV in the United States at the turn of the century: An epidemic in transition. *American Journal of Public Health, 9,1(7)*, 1060–1068.

Klonoff, E.A., & Landrine, H. (1999). Do Blacks believe that HIV/AIDS is a government conspiracy against them? *Preventive Medicine, 28(5)*, 451–457.

Kraft, J.M., Beeker, C., Stokes, J.P., & Peterson, J.L. (2000). Finding the "community" in community-level

HIV/AIDS interventions: Formative research with young African American men who have sex with men. *Health Education & Behavior, 27(4)*, 430–41.

Laurence, J. (2002). Changes in HIV-related diseases and the future of HIV medical care. *AIDS Reader, 12*, 283, 287.

Lyketsos, C.G., Hanson, A., Fishman, M., McHugh, P.R., & Triesman, G.J. (1994). Screening for psychiatric morbidity in a medical outpatient clinic for HIV infection: The need for a psychiatric presence. *International Journal of Psychiatry Medicine, 24*, 103–113.

McNeil, J.I Systematic observations in author's clinic. Unpublished observation.

Memon, M.I., & Memon, M.A. (2002). Hepatitis C: An epidemiological review. *Journal of Viral Hepatitis, 9*, 84–100.

Miller, V., et al. (2000). The impact of protease inhibitor-containing highly active antiretroviral therapy on progression of HIV disease and its relationship to CD4 and viral load. *Acquired Immunodeficiency Syndrome, 14*, 2129–2136.

Miller, K.S., Forehand, R., & Kotchick, B.A. (1999). Adolescent sexual behavior in two ethnic minority samples: The role of family variables. *Journal of Marriage & the Family, 61(1)*, 85–98.

Monja, H.K., et al. (2001). Hepatitis C virus infection related morbidity and mortality among patients with human immunodeficiency virus infection. *Clinical Infectious Diseases, 33*, 240–247.

Montaner, J.S.G., et al. (2000). Multidrug rescue therapy (MDRT) in two cohorts of HIV+ ondividuals. 7th Conference on Retroviruses and Opportunistic Infections, San Francisco, January 30–February 2, Abstract 536.

Morgello, S., Mahboob, R., Yakoushina, T., Khan, S., & Hague, K. (2002). Autopsy findings in a human immunodeficiency virus-infected population over 2 decades: Influences of gender, ethnicity, risk factors, and time. *Archives of Pathologic Laboratory Medicine, 126*, 182–190.

Moutouh, L., Corbeil, J., & Richman, D.D. (1996). Recombination leads to the rapid emergence of HIV-1 dually resistant mutants under selective drug pressure. *Proceedings of National Academy of Sciences, 93*, 6106–6111.

Nyamathi, A.M., Lewis, C., Leake, B., Flaskerud, J., & Bennett C. (1995). Barriers to condom use and needle cleaning among impoverished minority female injection drug users and partners of injection drug users. *Public Health Reports, 110(2)*, 166–72.

Osmond, D., Charlebois, C., Lang, W., Shiboski, S., & Moss, A. (1994). Changes in AIDS survival time in two San Francisco cohorts of homosexual men. *Journal of the Americam Medical Association, 271*, 1083–1087.

Pallela, F.J., et al. (1998). Declining morbidity and mortality among patients with advanced human immunodeficiency virus infection. *New England Journal of Medicine, 338*, 853–860.

Panel on Clinical Practices for Treatment of HIV Infection. Guidelines for the use of antiretroviral agents in HIV-infected adults and adolescents. Available at http://www.hivatis.org/guidelines/adult/May23_02/AAMay 23.pdf.

Papasavvas, E., et al. (2000). Enhancement of human immunodeficiency virus type 1-specific CD4 and CD8 T cell responses in chronically infected persons after temporary treatment interruption. *Journal of Infectious Diseases, 182*, 766–775.

Passalaris, D., Sepkowitz, K.A., & Glesby, M.J. (2000). Coronary artery disease and human immunodeficiency virus infection. *Clinical Infectious Diseases, 31*, 787–797.

Pierce, M., et al. (1996). A randomized trial of clarithromycin as prophylaxis against disseminated Mycobacterium avium complex infection in patients with advanced acquired immunodeficiency syndrome. *New England Journal of Medicine, 335*, 384–391.

Poles, M.A., and Dieterich, D.T. (2000). Hepatitis C virus/human immunodeficiency virus coinfection: Clinical management issues. *Clinical Infectious Diseases, 31*, 154–161.

Powderly, W.G. (2000). Prophylaxis for opportunistic infections in an era of effective antiretroviral therapy. *Clinical Infectious Diseases, 31*, 597–601.

Randall-David, E. (1994). *Culturally competent HIV counseling and education.* Washington, DC: Health Resources and Service Administration, Maternal and Child Health Division.

Robinson, H.L. (2002). Viral Vaccines. In N. Nathanson (Ed.), *Viral pathogenesis and immunity* (pp. 187–208). Philadelphia: Lippincott, Williams, and Wilkins.

Rosenberg, E.S., et al. (1997). Rigorous HIV-1 specific CD4+ T cell responses associated with control of viremia. *Science, 278*, 1447–1450.

Sabin, C.A., Telfer, P., Phillips, A.N., Bhagani, S., & Lee, C.A. (1997). The association between hepatitis C virus genotype and human immunodeficiency virus disease progression in a cohort of hemophilic men. *Journal of Infectious Diseases, 175 (1)*, 164–168.

Saves, M., et al. (2002). Factors related to lipodystrophy and metabolic alterations in patients with human immunodeficiency virus infection receiving highly active antiretroviral therapy. *Clinical Infectious Diseases, 34*, 1396–1405.

Selik, T.M., Byers, R.H., Jr., & Dworkin, M.S. (2002). Trends in diseases reported on U.S. death certificates that mentioned HIV infection. *Journal of Acquired Immune Deficiency Syndrome, 29*, 378–387.

Sherwin, R.S. (2000). Diabetes mellitus. In L. Goldman and C. Bennett (Eds.), Cecil *textbook of medicine* (pp. 1263–1284). Philadelphia: W.B. Saunders Company.

Smedley, B.D., Stith, A.Y., and Nelson, A.R. (Eds.). (2003). *Unequal Treatment: Confronting racial and ethnic disparities in health care.* Washington, DC, Board on Health Sciences Policy, Institute of Medicine of the National Academies: National Academies Press.

Sullivan, A.K., Atkins, M.C., & Boag, F. (1997). Factors facilitating the sexual transmission of HIV-1. *AIDS Patient Care & STDs, 11(3)*, 167–77.

Sullivan, A.K., Feher, M.D., Nelson, M.R., & Gazaard, B.G. (1998). Marked hypertriglyceridemia associated with ritonavir therapy. *AIDS, 12*, 1393–1394.

Sullivan, A.K., and Nelson, M.R. (1997). Marked hyperlipidemia on ritonavir therapy. *AIDS, 11*, 938–939.

Thomas, D.L. (1999). Mother–infant hepatitis C transmission: Second generation research. *Hepatology, 29*, 992–993.

Thomas, S.B., & Crouse Quinn, S. (1991). The Tuskegee syphilis study, 1932 to 1972: Implications for HIV education and AIDS risk education programs in the Black community. *American Journal of Public Health, 81(11)*, 1498–1505.

USPHS/IDSA Prevention of Opportunistic Infections Working Group. (1995). USPHS/IDSA guidelines for prevention opportunistic infections in persons infected with human immunodeficiency virus: Disease-specific recommendations. *Clinical Infectious Diseases, 21 (Suppl 1)*, S32–S43.

USPHS/IDSA Prevention of Opportunistic Infections Working Group. (1997). USPHS/IDSA guidelines for prevention opportunistic infections in persons infected with human immunodeficiency virus: Disease-specific recommendations. *Clinical Infectious Diseases, 21(Suppl 3)*, S313–S335.

USPHS/IDSA Prevention of Opportunistic Infections Working Group. (2001). USPHS/IDSA Guidelines for the prevention of opportunistic infections in persons infected with HIV. Avaliable at http://www.hivatis.org. MMWR, 2001.

VanderWaal, C.J., Washington, F.L., Drumm, R.D., Terry, Y.M., McBride, D.C., & Finley-Gordon, R.D. (2001). African-American injection drug users: Tensions and barriers in HIV/AIDS prevention. *Substance Use & Misuse, 36,(6–7)*, 735–55.

Wagner, E.H. (1998). Chronic disease management: What will it take to improve care for chronic illness? *Effective Clinical Practice, 1*, 2–4.

Wasserheit, J.N. (1992). Epidemiological synergy. Interrelationships between human immunodeficiency virus infection and other sexually transmitted diseases. *Sexually Transmitted Diseases, 19(2)*, 61–77.

Wingood, G.M., & DiClemente, R.J. (1998). Partner influences and gender-related factors associated with non-condom use among young adult African American women. *American Journal of Community Psychology, 26(1)*, 29–51.

Wolff, A.J., & O'Donnell, A.E. (2001). Pulmonary manifestations of HIV infection in the era of highly active antiretroviral therapy. *Chest, 120*, 1888–1893.

Wolitski, R.J., Valdiserri, R.O., Denning P.H., & Levine W.C. (2001). Are we headed for a resurgence in the HIV epidemic among men who have sex with men? *American Journal of Public Health, 91*, 883–888.

Yen, T., & Keeffe, E.B. (2003). The epidemiology of hepatitis C virus infection. *Journal of Clinical Gastroenterology, 36*, 47–53.

CHAPTER 16

Infectious Diseases among African Americans

MARIAN MCDONALD, KRISTI R. FULTZ-BUTTS,
HAROLD MARGOLIS, ROBERT W. PINNER, MARIA
CRISTINA RANGEL, KAKOLI ROY, JAY K. VARMA,
CYNTHIA G. WHITNEY, AND MITCHELL L. COHEN

INTRODUCTION

Just 35 years ago it seemed that the United States had finally overcome the scourge of infectious diseases, and public health officials could concentrate on other challenges such as chronic diseases, environmental toxins, and injuries. Antibiotics and immunizations, it was thought, would soon make infectious diseases a thing of the past. But as one scientist had noted prophetically decades before, "However secure and well-regulated civilized life may become, bacteria, protozoa, viruses, infected fleas, lice, ticks, mosquitoes, and bedbugs will always lurk in the shadows ready to pounce when neglect, poverty, famine, or war lets down the defenses" (Zinsser, 1984, p. 14).

Such prophecies became true over the last two decades of the twentieth century as new or reemerging infectious diseases took center stage. The United States and the world faced the challenges of the AIDS epidemic, drug-resistant TB, hepatitis, the West Nile and Ebola viruses, and an ever growing list of new or reemerging diseases that caused death, disability, and social destruction (Centers for Disease Control and Prevention [CDC], 1994, 1998b; Institute of Medicine, 1994).

Certain emerging infections in the United States have particularly affected African Americans, a group that has historically experienced higher rates of infectious diseases as well as other adverse health events (Armstrong et al., 1999; Richardus & Kunst, 2001). In this chapter, we examine some of the disparities in rates of illness and death from infectious agents and attempt to show why African Americans have higher rates of certain infectious diseases and why effective prevention and treatment are often elusive. Given that the burden and impact of certain infectious diseases are so great in the African American community, AIDS and other sexually transmitted diseases are examined in a separate chapter.

In this chapter, we begin by examining the risk factors and conditions that influence the incidence of infectious diseases among African Americans and discuss trends in infectious disease mortality rates among African Americans. We then specifically examine five infectious disease issues—hepatitis, food-borne disease, pneumococcal disease, influenza, and group B streptococcal infections. Each of these diseases has disproportionately impacted African Americans, and, in some instances, there has been remarkable success in addressing disparities that can provide direction for future efforts in other infections and conditions. Although these five diseases are important causes of morbidity and mortality in African Americans, other conditions are associated with significant disparities.

RISK FACTORS AND CONDITIONS FOR INFECTIOUS DISEASES AMONG AFRICAN AMERICANS

Why do African Americans have higher incidences of certain infectious diseases? To answer the question, one must first examine general factors known to affect infectious disease incidence, including housing, food and water supplies, hygiene and sanitation, nutritional levels, and the presence of antibiotics and immunizations. These factors have either influenced the transmission of infectious agents or affected people's susceptibility to infections. As social and economic conditions improved and new treatment and prevention technologies were developed during the twentieth century, rates of transmission fell and host resistance to infection improved. Some of the societal and technologic changes of the twentieth century, however, had unexpected consequences, leading to new infectious diseases and the reemergence of old ones. The Institute of Medicine (1994) has identified six factors as contributing to the emergence of infectious diseases: (1) changes in demographics or behavior influencing the size of populations at risk, such as the aging of the population, which led to the increase in the numbers of persons susceptible to various infections; (2) changes in technology and industry, such as globalization of the food supply: (3) changes in international travel or commerce, which have increased the risk of infectious agents being transmitted; (4) environmental and land use changes, such as deforestation or the growth of megacities in the developing world; (5) microbial adaptation, such as the development of drug resistance or the emergence of new microorganisms (*E. coli* O157:H7); and (6) breakdowns in public health infrastructure, such as a reduction in needed programs or a lack of resources necessary to meet increasing responsibilities.

In the United States, each of these factors contributing to the spread of infectious diseases has disproportionately affected African Americans, largely because they have had less access to the social, economic, and technologic advances of the twentieth century, including quality health care. Factors affecting African Americans can be grouped into general categories of those associated with race, access to medical care, poverty, behavior and culture, and genetics.

Race

Determining what "race" means in general and "Black" or "African American" in particular, as well as who constitutes the African American population, has not always been an easy task. Before 1970, public health data were often stratified only into White race and non-White or "other" race. Thus, aside from containing errors introduced by self-identification of racial group, historical data specific to African Americans are often incomplete or inaccurate.

Inexorably linked to the issue of race has been the impact of racism. In a recent discussion of racism and epidemiology, C.P. Jones (2001) describes three levels of racism—institutionalized, personally mediated, and internalized—and argues that "each can have an impact on health" and that "understanding these three levels is useful to epidemiologists and other public health practitioners for generating hypotheses about the basis of race-associated differences in health outcomes, as well as for designing interventions to eliminate those differences" (p. 300). Jones defines institutional racism as the "differential access to the goods, services, and opportunities of society by race that has been codified in our institutions of custom, practice, and law so there need not be an identifiable perpetrator of any particular injustice." She defines personally mediated racism as "prejudice and discrimination, where prejudice is differential assumptions about the abilities, motives, and intents of others by race, and discrimination is differential actions toward others by race." She defines internalized racism as "acceptance by members of the stigmatized races of negative messages about their own abilities and intrinsic worth."

Access to Medical Care

This construct is particularly useful in understanding the higher rates of infectious disease among African Americans. One aspect of racism, institutional racism, meant that for decades after the Civil War, health-care services provided to African Americans were available only at separate, segregated facilities, where care and resources were often substandard and frequently limited. Such inadequate access to care led to unnecessary illnesses, complications, and deaths. Not until the middle of the twentieth century was the segregated health-care system effectively challenged in the landmark *Simkins vs. Moses H. Cone* case (Reynolds, 1997). Even when services are available, the personally mediated racism of health-care personnel could affect the quality of care and appropriateness of treatment received by African Americans (Nelson, 2002) and internalized racism could impact the seeking of needed medical care.

Poverty.   Poverty remains a condition of life for a disproportionate part of the African American population. This has created impoverishment that stands in sharp contrast to the wealth the country affords many. As W.E.B. Du Bois (1989) noted at the turn of the century, "To be a poor man is hard, but to be a poor race in a land of dollars is the very bottom of hardships" (p. 6).

Poverty has been shown to have a strong correlation with poor health in general and an even stronger correlation with risk for many infectious diseases. Poverty is associated with crowded housing, substandard sanitation, and limited hygiene, all of which promote the transmission of infectious diseases. Poverty also limits people's access to health care, curtailing infectious disease prevention, diagnosis, and treatment. Conversely, concerted efforts to reduce poverty's impact on health through insurance-funding mechanisms have been successful in reducing rates of infectious diseases in target populations (Dowell et al., 2000).

Behavior and Culture.   African Americans are a diverse population of people with multiple cultures, national origins, social classes, and genetic pools. As one commentator notes,

African American life is not a monolith. Black life in the United States is a tapestried reality. Geography, religion, ethnicity, gender, income, occupation, and other factors spark varieties of culture within African American life. There are strong common themes and challenges that help draw Blacks together, but there are equally compelling and necessarily differing paths on that Black folk in the United States take toward our commonalities. (Townes, 1998, p. 50)

Cultural risk factors include modes of communication, food preparation practices, cultural norms regarding sexuality, and attitudes toward health and health-care providers (Logan & Freeman, 2000).

A number of other behavioral factors increase African Americans' vulnerability to infectious diseases and increase the likelihood of such diseases being transmitted. These include inadequate information and misconceptions concerning several sexual activities and risk, high rates of teenage pregnancy, limited reproductive options for women, and behaviors associated with limited economic choices, such as drug use and prostitution to support drug use (White, 1994).

Genetic.   While African Americans are at higher risk for certain genetically based illnesses such as sickle-cell disease, genetic factors have not been shown to account for their elevated rates of infectious diseases. Some observers caution that genetic explanations for racial differences in disease rates, especially for a group as genetically diverse as African Americans, can serve to mask other more important risk factors such as those discussed above (Duster, 1990).

TRENDS IN INFECTIOUS DISEASE MORTALITY

At the beginning of the twentieth century, the estimated life expectancy was 47.6 years for Whites and 33 years for non-Whites. By 1992, life expectancies for Whites and African Americans were 75.8 and 69.6 years, increases of 59 percent and 111 percent, respectively. Much of the increase in life expectancy was the result of decreases in infant mortality rates. In 1900, the chance of an infant dying in the first year of life was 16 percent for Whites and 33 percent for non-Whites. Although in 1992 the infant mortality rate among African Americans was still twice that of Whites, the rates for the two groups had fallen to 1.4 percent and .7 percent, respectively.

Despite these increases in life expectancy among all Americans, the remaining gap in life expectancy between African Americans and Whites has invigorated debates over the effects of race on longevity. The National Institutes of Health (Varmus, 1999) and the Public Health Service (U.S. Department of Health and Human Services, 2000a) have appropriately identified eliminating racial and ethnic disparities in health as major priorities for health research, policy, and practice. While the shorter life expectancy among African Americans has been partially attributed to their lower socioeconomic status, questions remain about the relative roles of environment, socioeconomic, and genetic factors (Davey Smith et al., 1998; Pappas, 1994; Sorlie et al., 1992).

With the recognition of several new and reemerging infectious disease threats, the identification and prevention of infectious diseases have become a top national health priority (CDC, 1998c). However, there have been few studies of racial differences in the trends in infectious disease mortality rates and even fewer studies that include the full range of such diseases or incorporate the impact of socioeconomic status (SES) on such differences (Richardus & Kunst, 2001).

To examine trends in infectious disease mortality rates, the data presented by Pinner et al. (1996) for 1980–1992 were updated to include 1993–1998 (Pinner et al., 2002) (Figure 16.1). U.S. mortality data were extracted from the National Center for Health Statistics multiple cause of death files for 1993 through 1998 (National Center for Health Statistics [NCHS], 1998). Mortality rates were expressed as the number of deaths per 100,000.

In 1998, infectious diseases were the underlying cause of death in 172,505 (7.4 percent) of 2,340,708 deaths in the United States. Overall, infectious diseases ranked as the third leading cause of death in the United States, behind cardiovascular disease and malignancies (Murphy, 2000). While crude mortality rates from infectious diseases increased by 58 percent from 1980 to 1992, they fell slightly from 65 to 64 deaths per 100,000, from 1992 to 1998 (Figure 16.1). This slight fall, however, masked an initial increase, to 71 deaths per 100,000 in 1995, and a sharp drop to 62 deaths per 100,000 in 1997. The estimated age-adjusted death rate, which accounts for changes in the age-distribution of the population, dropped 11 percent, from 1992 to 1998. The infectious disease mortality rate among African Americans increased from 88 deaths per 100,000 in 1992 to 105 deaths per 100,000 in 1995. However, from 1995 to 1998, this trend reversed, and the rate dropped sharply to 76 deaths per 100,000. Among the remainder of the population (White/other), infectious disease death rates rose from 62 to 66 per 100,000 from 1992 to 1995, and then fell back to 62 deaths per 100,000 in 1998 (Table 16.1). After stratifying race by age and gender, Pinner et al. (2002), found the peak in infectious disease death rates in 1995 to be most pronounced among 25- to 44-year-old African American males (206 deaths per 100,000 vs. 45 for that age group as a whole). The mortality rate for this group, however, dropped to 79 deaths per 100,000 by 1998.

The overall percentage difference between mortality rates for African Americans and those for the rest of the U.S. population, however, narrowed from 30 percent in 1997 to just 19 percent in 1998. It is important to note that although the total number of deaths due to infectious diseases increased by 4.0 percent from 1992 to 1998, the proportion of such deaths attributable to HIV dropped by 62 percent, from 20 percent of all infectious disease deaths in 1992 to 7.8 percent in 1998. Consequently, HIV-related deaths dropped from being the number two cause of U.S. deaths from infectious diseases in

Figure 16.1
Infectious disease deaths (rate per 100,000) in the United States

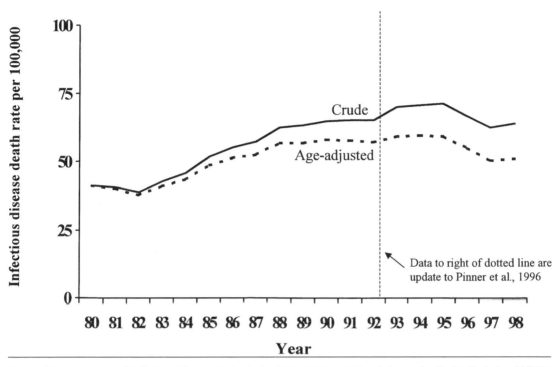

Source: Trends in rates of infectious disease deaths in the United States: National Center for Health Statistics (NCHS), Underlying cause of death data, 1980–1998.

1992 to number four in 1998 (Pinner et al., 2002). This downward trend in HIV-related deaths, which was most pronounced among 25- to 44-year-old males in both race categories, may have contributed to the narrowing disparity between African Americans and Whites in overall infectious disease mortality.

Do SES factors entirely explain the higher mortality rate among African Americans, or does the rate remain higher than that among Whites even if one controls for such factors? To examine this issue, the Multiple-Cause-of-Death Public Use Data Files from the National Health Interview Survey (NHIS) Multiple Cause-of-Death Public Use Data Files that link nine cohorts from NHIS surveys conducted from 1987 to 1994 with the National Death Index for the follow-up period, 1987 through 1997 (NCHS, 1997, 2000) were reviewed. The sample consists of 621,842 adults 18 years or older, 60,659 (9.75 percent) of whom died during the 11 years of follow-up (Table 16.2).

The odds ratios reported in Table 16.2 measure the relative impact of race (African American vs. White) on the probability of dying from various diseases. Three different specifications were estimated to determine whether infectious disease rates remain higher among Blacks even after controlling for demographic factors (age, gender, marital status), SES factors (family income), and other factors associated with SES (education, employment status).

For the overall sample, race was significantly associated with mortality rates, independent of SES, across all disease categories. Controlled for SES and SES-associated factors, African American–White infectious disease mortality differences decreased approximately 32 percent (odds ratio from 1.94 [$p<0.05$] to 1.32 [$p>0.05$]). All-cause mortality ratios decreased by approximately 29 percent after adjusting for the same factors (from 1.77, $p<0.05$ to 1.24, $p<0.05$).

Table 16.1
Infectious disease mortality rates, stratified by gender, race, and age, 1992–1998

	1992	1993	1994	1995	1996	1997	1998
White/Other	61.8	66.1	66.3	66.5	62.6	60.0	62.0
Black	88.4	95.6	101.8	105.0	95.5	78.5	76.4
White Males	67.0	70.6	71.1	70.6	63.1	57.3	57.0
Black Males	117.0	126.0	134.7	138.0	122.2	92.5	86.2
White Females	57.1	61.7	61.5	62.3	62.0	62.6	65.8
Black Females	62.7	68.2	72.0	75.1	71.3	65.7	66.2
Age 0-4 yr: White Males	17.1	14.7	15.5	14.6	14.2	14.2	13.9
Age 0-4 yr: Black Males	49.6	44.4	46.0	38.9	43.6	39.0	40.2
Age 0-4 yr: White Females	13.4	12.5	12.4	11.9	11.2	11.6	11.9
Age 0-4 yr: Black Females	42.8	37.9	38.2	38.0	35.6	32.5	32.9
Age 5-24 yr: White Males	2.8	2.4	2.3	2.2	1.8	1.7	1.5
Age 5-24 yr: Black Males	6.7	6.5	6.5	6.5	5.6	4.3	3.3
Age 5-24 yr: White Females	1.6	1.8	1.6	1.6	1.5	1.5	1.2
Age 5-24 yr: Black Females	4.6	5.7	5.9	6.6	5.0	4.3	4.0
Age 25-44 yr: White Males	49.3	52.0	55.0	53.4	36.0	19.7	16.8
Age 25-44 yr: Black Males	165.3	182.0	202.9	206.0	162.4	95.7	78.8
Age 25-44 yr: White Females	7.2	8.3	9.2	10.0	8.4	6.3	6.1
Age 25-44 yr: Black Females	48.2	54.3	64.5	67.2	58.9	41.9	38.9
Age 45-64 yr: White Males	50.4	51.6	53.8	53.1	44.5	35.5	35.5
Age 45-64 yr: Black Males	171.3	183.8	207.2	218.5	198.7	150.7	145.6
Age 45-64 yr: White Females	19.1	20.6	20.3	20.6	20.3	20.9	20.7
Age 45-64 yr: Black Females	53.0	57.6	66.3	69.6	66.1	62.4	60.5
Age 65-84 yr: White Males	241.8	252.3	243.4	243.9	243.0	248.2	254.7
Age 65-84 yr: Black Males	385.6	395.2	375.3	380.5	381.7	372.0	383.2
Age 65-84 yr: White Females	170.5	178.2	181.0	180.9	183.1	185.4	196.8
Age 65-84 yr: Black Females	229.7	247.7	240.3	247.7	243.1	251.6	266.2
Age ≥ 85 yr: White Males	1814.3	1833.7	1762.5	1708.5	1660.32	1677.22	1710.9
Age ≥ 85 yr: Black Males	1691.4	1715.2	1606.4	1658.2	1655.38	1648.52	1593.6
Age ≥ 85 yr: White Females	1384.6	1469.8	1398.0	1396.9	1380.44	1395.93	1472.3
Age ≥ 85 yr: Black Females	1318.1	1338.5	1272.8	1318.2	1333.38	1342.09	1386.5

Notes:
1. Mortality rates were expressed as the number of deaths per 100,000.
2. Data were extracted from the NCHS multiple-cause-of-death tapes for the years 1992–1998.
3. Deaths due to infectious diseases were identified using the coding scheme established by the *International Classification of Diseases, Ninth Revision (ICD-9)* in conjunction with the Pinner et al. (1996) classification.

Table 16.2
Odds ratios of mortality rates of African Americans versus Whites, with controls for demographic, SES, and SES-relevant factors

Cause of Death	Model 1	Model 2	Model 3
All Causes	1.77*	1.61*	1.24*
Non-infectious Diseases	1.66*	1.54*	1.19
Infectious Diseases	1.94*	1.72*	1.32

Notes:

1. The above results were estimated using data that link eight cohorts from National Health Interview Surveys (NHIS), 1987 to 1994, with the National Death Index, 1987 to 1997, for a maximum of 11 years of follow-up.

2. The data exclude all those below 18 years of age.

3. Odds ratios were estimated using a multivariate logistic regression model, where the dependent variable is the probability of dying from the specified disease, with the following covariates:

Model 1: Age, race, and gender

Model 2: Age, race, gender, education, marital status, employment status

Model 3: Age, race, gender, education, marital status, employment status, and family income

4. The odds ratio measures the effect of the predictor variable on the outcome, after the effects of other predictor variables are controlled for. For example, Model 1 predicts that African Americans were 1.94 times more likely to die from an infectious disease than Whites, after controlling for differences in age and gender.

5. Results reported only if significant: *$P<.05$.

6. The disease classification scheme developed by Pinner et al. (1996) was used to categorize the *International Classification of Diseases, 9th Revision*, codes representing infectious diseases as the underlying cause of death.

In general, significant differences in infectious disease mortality continue to exist between African Americans and Whites in the United States. While the gap narrows when the analysis controls for socioeconomic factors (note that odds ratios are not statistically significantly different from 1.32 in model 3, which controls for multiple SES factors), differences in specific infectious diseases mortality may not be wholly attributable to socioeconomic differences.

VIRAL HEPATITIS

Infection with one of five hepatitis viruses is the most common cause of liver inflammation (hepatitis). Hepatitis viruses were named alphabetically in the order of their characterization: hepatitis A virus (HAV), hepatitis B virus (HBV), hepatitis C virus (HCV), hepatitis D virus (HDV), and hepatitis E virus (HEV). Each represents a different virus family (Margolis et al., 1997).

Modes of transmission and risk factors for infection differ among the respective types of viral hepatitis. HAV and HEV are excreted enterically and transmitted by the fecal-oral route, whereas HBV, HCV, and HDV are blood-borne infections transmitted by percutaneous and permucosal exposure to blood and body fluids.

The consequences of infection vary among the viruses and substantially affect disease burden. Enterically transmitted hepatitis viruses (HAV, HEV) produce an acute, self-limited infection that does not become chronic and does not cause chronic liver disease. Blood-borne hepatitis viruses (HBV, HCV, HDV) produce an acute infection that may be symptomatic or silent and may resolve or become chronic. Aside from the small proportion of patients with acute hepatitis who progress to liver failure, the disease burden for HAV and HEV is primarily related to medical and work loss costs for patients who require hospitalization for acute infection (CDC, 1999a; Margolis et al., 1997); and for HBV, HCV, and HDV, disease burden is related primarily to the medical and work loss costs associated with the consequences of chronic infection—chronic hepatitis, chronic liver disease, or hepatocellular carcinoma (HCC) (Armstrong et al., 2000; Margolis et al., 1997; Margolis et al., 1995).

Prevention and control of viral hepatitis is agent-specific. Safe and effective vaccines are available to prevent HAV and HBV infection, and effective strategies have been implemented to prevent and control these infections (CDC, 1991, 1999a). Because no vaccine exists to prevent HCV infection, the national strategy for prevention and control of hepatitis C is based on testing and counseling of persons at increased risk of infection. Identification of at-risk or HCV-infected persons provides the opportunity to prevent new infections, to prevent further infection transmission, and to reduce the consequences of infection by appropriate medical management (CDC, 1998d, 2002a).

Infection with all of the hepatitis viruses represent major public health problems in the United States, except for HEV, which is primarily found in developing countries of Asia and Africa. The remainder of this discussion is limited to HBV and HCV infection because of their importance in African American communities.

Hepatitis B Virus Infection

Epidemiology.   Worldwide, the prevalence of HBV infection varies widely. The highest endemicity of infection is observed in Asia and Africa, where ≥8 percent of the population has chronic HBV infection, which produces a high disease burden from chronic liver disease and HCC. Prior to infant hepatitis B immunization, the high prevalence of chronic infection in these populations was maintained through infant or early childhood transmission, which occurs either from an infected mother in the perinatal period or during infancy and early childhood from an infected household member or caretaker (Margolis et al., 1997). This pattern of childhood HBV transmission is observed among persons who immigrate to the United States from areas of high HBV endemicity, and infants of foreign-born pregnant women constitute the largest group at risk of perinatal HBV infection (Margolis et al., 1991).

In the United States, approximately 5 percent of the population has been infected with HBV. The prevalence of HBV infection among African Americans is approximately four times higher than among Whites or Mexican Americans; only Asian Americans have a higher prevalence of infection (McQuillan et al., 1999). While foreign-born African Americans have the highest prevalence of HBV infection, compared to Whites and irrespective of place of birth, an increased prevalence of infection is found in all age groups. African Americans older than 40 years of age have the highest prevalence of HBV infection, which appears to be a cohort effect and not due to recent disease acquisition (McQuillan et al., 1999).

Several factors probably account for the increased prevalence of HBV infection among African Americans. Similar to what is observed today, there was probably a high prevalence of chronic HBV infection among persons from Africa who first came to the Americas. Although secular declines in HBV infection prevalence have been observed in some populations that moved from an area of high to low infection endemicity, such declines have primarily been associated with a substantial improvement in socioeconomic status (Margolis et al., 1997).

The age-specific prevalence of HBV infection among African Americans suggests that about 50–60 years ago a shift occurred in the predominant pattern of HBV transmission and went from the majority of infections being acquired among children less than 5 years of age, to most infections being acquired among adolescents and young adults. A significant increase in infection prevalence occurs during early adolescence and occurs earlier among African Americans than among Whites (McQuillan et al., 1999). This increase in HBV infection coincides with the onset of earlier sexual activity in this population and is associated with other sexually transmitted infections (McQuillan et al., 1999). In addition, over the past 20 years of available surveillance data, African Americans have had the highest incidence of acute hepatitis B among adults (Goldstein et al., 2002).

Prior to infant hepatitis B immunization in the United States, African Americans continued to acquire HBV infection during early childhood (Armstrong, Mast, et al., 2001; Watanabe et al., 2000). A recent study of young (17–24-year-old) blood donors found the highest rate of chronic HBV infection among foreign-born Asians, followed by African Americans (Watanabe et al., 2000); infections in both groups presumably being acquired primarily during early childhood.

Among adults, over 50 percent of HBV infections are transmitted by heterosexual or male homosexual activity (~50 percent), followed by injection drug use (~15 percent). Although almost 30 percent of persons have no currently identified risk factors for their acute infection, most had risk factors in the past (Goldstein et al., 2002).

Prevention.   The immunization strategy to eliminate transmission of HBV infection in the United States consists of (1) testing pregnant women to prevent perinatal transmission, (2) infant immunization to prevent early childhood infection and provide protection against infection acquired in later years, (3) catch-up immunization of older children and adolescents, and (4) vaccination of older adolescents and adults with risk factors for infection (CDC, 1991). Hepatitis B vaccine was first included in the childhood immunization schedule in late 1991 and the Vaccines for Children (VFC) program since its inception (CDC, 1996a). High hepatitis B vaccination coverage has been achieved among young children, and little difference in coverage has been found among racial/ethnic groups, although lower overall vaccination rates are found in some large metropolitan areas (CDC, 2002b). In addition, administration of the first dose of hepatitis B vaccine soon after birth and prior to hospital discharge has been shown to significantly improve hepatitis B vaccine series completion and coverage, as well as coverage for other childhood vaccines in a low socioeconomic, predominantly African American population.

The greatest challenge for prevention and control of HBV infection is vaccination of adults in groups at increased risk of infection. Most persons in these risk groups receive health-care services in the public sector, and no national programs cover the cost of hepatitis B vaccine or its administration, which has been shown to be a major barrier to vaccination of adults. Studies have demonstrated the feasibility of sustained immunization of high-risk adults in settings such as clinics for treatment of sexually transmitted diseases (STD), prisons, and substance abuse treatment centers (Goldstein et al., 2002).

Population-based surveillance studies have identified a number of settings where there have been missed opportunities for hepatitis B immunization. Approximately one-third of persons with acute hepatitis B have been previously treated in an STD clinic or have been incarcerated, settings where immunization is currently recommended. African Americans are disproportionately overrepresented among incarcerated populations, a population with a high prevalence of HBV infection (Goldstein et al., 2002). HBV infection has been shown to be transmitted within prisons, and released inmates are at high risk of acquiring infection because of continued high-risk behaviors (CDC, in press). Currently, about 25 state prison systems have some type of hepatitis B immunization program, ranging from vaccination of all incoming inmates to vaccination of inmates requesting this prevention service (CDC, in press). However, until more widespread vaccination of adults occurs, it may take several more decades to fully eliminate transmission of this chronic disease.

Hepatitis C Virus Infection

Epidemiology.   An estimated 1.8 percent of the noninstitutionalized, civilian U.S. population has been infected with HCV (Alter et al., 1999). A higher prevalence of infection is found among African Americans than Whites (3.2 percent vs. 1.3 percent) and 9.8 percent of African American men 40–49 years of age have been infected. Of persons infected with HCV, an estimated 74 percent remain chronically infected (Alter et al., 1999). Chronic HCV infection persists in a higher proportion of African Americans (86 percent) than Whites (68 percent) or Mexican Americans (74 percent). African American males have a higher prevalence of infection than females (98 percent vs. 70 percent), a distinction that is not observed in other racial/ethnic groups. Most persons in the United States are infected with HCV genotype 1 (78 percent) compared to genotype 2 (13 percent). However, African Americans have a higher prevalence of genotype 1 infection (91 percent) than Whites (67 percent) and Mexican Americans (72 percent) (Alter et al., 1999).

Infection prevalence is highest (70–90 percent) among persons with repeated percutaneous exposures to blood or blood products (e.g., injection drug users, hemophiliacs treated with clotting factor concentrates). Moderate infection prevalence (~10 percent) is found among hemodialysis patients and persons who received blood transfusion prior to donor screening. Lower prevalence (2–5 percent) is observed among persons with high-risk sexual practices (e.g., unprotected sex with > two partners in a six-month period) and health-care workers with needlestick exposures (CDC, 1998d).

African Americans and Whites have the same incidence of acute disease, and incidence rates are higher among males than females (Alter, 1997). The major risk factor for HCV infection is injection drug use. Although the number of cases of acute hepatitis C among injection drug users has declined dramatically since 1989, both prevalence and incidence of HCV infection have remained high in this risk group (Alter et al., 1990). Prior to the availability of tests to screen blood donors (1990) for HCV infection and the use of viral inactivation methods for certain blood products (1987), blood transfusions and clotting factor concentrates posed a high risk for infection (Alter et al., 1990).

HCV infection is more rapidly acquired than HBV and HIV infection among injection drug users, because of the higher prevalence of chronic HCV infection in the drug-using population (Garfein et al., 1996; Murrill et al., 2002). Infection is acquired through transfer of blood from shared needles, syringes, and equipment used to prepare drugs for injection. Studies conducted in the 1980s indicated that within five years of initiating injection drug use, 70–90 percent of this population was infected with HCV (Garfein et al., 1996). Although more recent studies suggest this prevalence rate may have declined, the incidence of HCV infection remains high at 10 percent–15 percent per year (Murrill et al., 2002).

Prevention.   Hepatitis C prevention and control efforts seek to reduce both the incidence of new infections and the risk of chronic liver disease in HCV-infected persons. The cornerstone of this prevention strategy is to identify persons with risk factors for infection and provide them counseling and HCV testing (CDC, 1998d, 2002a). Identification of uninfected persons has the potential to change high-risk behaviors through counseling, and substance abuse treatment, when appropriate. Identification of HCV-infected persons has the potential to (1) limit further transmission through counseling, and when indicated, substance abuse treatment; and (2) minimize further liver injury through medical management and when indicated, antiviral treatment and substance abuse counseling and treatment.

HCV testing and counseling are recommended for persons at increased risk for infection (CDC, 1998d) and should be offered in all settings that provide medical and prevention services to high-risk populations (e.g., programs for prevention of HIV/AIDS, drug abuse, and STDs, correctional health programs, and primary and specialty health-care practices). It has been shown that HCV testing and counseling, as well as immunization services, can be integrated into programs that provide prevention services to persons with risk factors for HBV, HCV, and HIV infection. Incarcerated populations, which include a high proportion of African Americans, exemplify the need for hepatitis C prevention activities in their existing health-care services. The prevalence of HCV infection among prison inmates averages about 30 percent (range 15 percent–60 percent) because of the high rate of injection drug use in this population (Ruiz et al., 1999). Currently, a limited number of prisons have begun to screen inmates for HCV infection and provide medical, substance abuse, and counseling services to this population (CDC, in press). Because of the large proportion of incarcerated persons that return to the community each year, viral hepatitis prevention services (testing, counseling, medical evaluation, immunization) should be part of all corrections health programs (CDC, in press).

The effectiveness of counseling, testing, and medical management for the prevention of hepatitis C and its consequences has not been determined in large populations. However, similar prevention strategies have been shown effective for the prevention of HIV/AIDS, another blood-borne viral infection.

FOOD-BORNE DISEASES

Food-borne diseases cause an estimated 76 million illnesses annually in the United States (Mead et al., 1999). Though many of these illnesses go unexplained, about five million illnesses are attributable to bacteria, 31 million to viruses, and 2.5 million to parasites (Mead et al., 1999). Food-borne illnesses represent an ongoing threat to public health, a threat intensified by the globalization of the food supply, the centralization of food processing, the emergence of new pathogens (e.g., *Escherichia coli* O157), an increase in travel and immigration, and an expanding population of elderly and immune-compromised people.

The most common bacterial food-borne pathogens sought in clinical laboratories are, in order, *Campylobacter*, non-Typhoidal *Salmonella, E. coli* O157, *Listeria monocytogenes, Shigella, Yersinia enterocolitica* (YE), and *Vibrio*. Symptomatic infection with these organisms usually causes a syndrome of acute gastroenteritis, which includes nausea, vomiting, abdominal pain, and/or diarrhea (Guerrant et al., 2001). All of these organisms are often transmitted through ingestion of contaminated foods, though other modes of transmission may occur.

Estimating the burden of food-borne disease specifically among African Americans has been challenging. Public health surveillance relies on reports of laboratory-confirmed infection, but most infections are not laboratory-confirmed, and public health case reports often do not include data about an ill person's race or ethnicity. The most reliable population-based estimates for the nation have been derived from CDC's Foodborne Diseases Active Surveillance Network (FoodNet), which collects epidemiologic data, including race and ethnicity, for cases of laboratory-confirmed bacterial and parasitic food-borne infection in all or part of nine U.S. states. In 2000, African Americans had a higher relative risk for infection from one serotype of *Salmonella, S.* Enteritidis, though their overall risk for infection from non-Typhoidal *Salmonella* was no different (CDC unpublished data; Marcus et al., 2002). Risk for infection among African Americans (vs. Whites) was lower for *E. coli* O157 and *Campylobacter*, no different for *Listeria* and *Vibrio*, and higher for *Shigella* and YE (CDC, unpublished data). African Americans were 1.5 times more likely than Whites to become infected with *Shigella* and 6 times more likely to become infected with YE (CDC). Though these findings could result from bias in the surveillance system, other epidemiologic data suggest that there is a real disparity between African Americans and Whites in the rates of illness from these two pathogens.

Shigella

Infection with *Shigella* causes acute gastroenteritis, with symptoms ranging from mild, watery diarrhea to severe, bloody diarrhea. Infection is transmitted through the fecal-oral route, and because infection can occur from exposure to small amounts, *Shigella* is easily spread person to person.

An analysis of surveillance data from 1967 through 1988 demonstrated that the *Shigella* incidence rate in counties with $\geq$ 50 percent African Americans was threefold higher than in counties with

Figure 16.2
Adjusted Y. *entercolitica* incidence, by race and age, FoodNET, 1996–1999

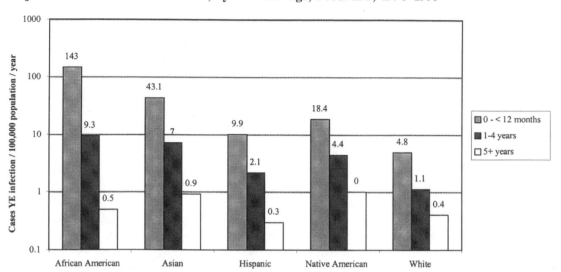

<1 percent African Americans (Lee, Shapiro et al., 1991). Several large community outbreaks of *Shigella* infections have disproportionately affected African Americans (CDC, 1990a). The racial disparity in rates of infections is likely due to social and economic conditions. Outbreaks of *Shigella* among African Americans often occur in poor urban communities, where crowding, poor sanitation, and poor hygiene may facilitate transmission (Lee, Shapiro et al., 1991). In 2001, child-care centers in urban, predominantly African American communities of Ohio were the primary setting of one of the largest outbreaks of *Shigella* infections ever reported in the United States (CDC, unpublished data).

The public health response to *Shigella* infections is focused on preventing outbreaks, and the primary public health intervention involves convincing people to rigorously and consistently wash their hands with soap and water. Reducing the racial disparity in rates of *Shigella* infections depends on educating African American parents and children, as well as child-care staff and urban policy-makers about the importance of hand washing, particularly in high-risk communities.

Yersinia *enterocolitica* (YE)

Infection with YE causes acute gastroenteritis, which may include bloody diarrhea in about half the cases. Acute illness may be accompanied by, or followed by, terminal ileitis, mesenteric adenitis, reactive arthritis, or erythema nodusum (Cover & Aber, 1989). Modes of transmission include exposure to contaminated pork products, ingestion of contaminated foods, contact with sick pets, and transfusion of contaminated blood products (Lee et al., 1990).

In the late 1980s, YE became increasingly recognized as a cause of febrile gastroenteritis in urban African American children. Hospital-based surveillance and population-based surveillance both demonstrated an elevated incidence rate among African Americans, with the highest incidence among African American infants (Lee, Taylor et al., 1991; Ray et al., in press) (Figure 16.2). YE incidence peaks in the winter (November through February), and several outbreaks have occurred in association with the Thanksgiving, Christmas, and New Year holidays (Lee et al., 1990).

One study identified exposure to home-prepared chitterlings as the main risk factor for illness among African American children (Lee, Taylor et al., 1991). Chitterlings, which are boiled pig intestines, are a staple of soul food cuisine and holiday meals in some African American communities. The person preparing chitterlings from raw intestines often spends hours in the home kitchen removing fat and fecal matter prior to boiling the intestines. During preparation, infants in the home are at risk of coming into contact with YE, particularly when their primary caregiver is the same person preparing the food (Lee et al., 1990).

The incidence of YE infections declined dramatically in the United States from 1996 through 2001, but it is unclear why this occurred (CDC, 2002c). Previous efforts at prevention have included targeted education of mothers, grandmothers, and other caregivers during the winter months in predominantly African American communities (CDC, 1990b). Ongoing educational efforts such as this may reduce the disparity in rates of YE infections between African Americans and Whites. Prompt recognition and diagnosis of YE by clinicians, particularly in African American children with febrile gastroenteritis, may improve our understanding of the epidemiology of this important condition and help us identify effective prevention and control strategies.

INFLUENZA

Influenza is a highly contagious acute respiratory disease caused by infection with influenza viruses type A and B. The severity of symptoms, which can be life-threatening, depends on the infected person's age, health status, and prior immunologic experience with antigenically related virus variants. Although all age groups can be affected by influenza, persons 65 years and older, very young children, and persons of any age with underlying cardiopulmonary, metabolic, or renal diseases, cancer, or hemoglobinopathies are at high risk for influenza-related complications and hospitalizations (Barker & Mullooly, 1980; Glezen et al., 2000). The most frequent complication of influenza is pneumonia, especially secondary bacterial pneumonia (Barker, 1986).

Every year, influenza epidemics are responsible for more than 20,000 excess deaths, 110,000 hospitalizations, and more than $12 billion in health-care expenditures in the United States (Barker, 1986; Blackwelder et al., 1982; CDC, 2002d; Glezen et al., 1987; Simonsen et al., 1997; Simonsen et al., 2000). Vaccination with the inactivated influenza vaccine is the primary preventive strategy currently available to reduce the impact of influenza, particularly among elderly adults and persons of any age with high-risk conditions (CDC, 2002d; Gross et al., 1995; Nichol et al., 1994).

Racial and Ethnic Disparities in Influenza Vaccination Rates

The United States established a national goal to vaccinate 60 percent of all high-risk adults by the year 2000 and 90 percent of those 65 years and older by the year 2010 (Public Health Service, 1991; U.S. Department of Health and Human Services, 2000b). However, despite increases in immunization rates for all racial and ethnic groups (Figure 16.3), the year 2000 goal was attained only for adults 65 years and older, but not for adults under 65 years of age with high-risk conditions. According to M.C. Rangel (2002) in 1998, 63 percent of persons 65 years and older but only 32 percent of high-risk adults 18 to 64 years of age reported receiving the influenza vaccine in the prior 12 months. The coverage rate for health-care workers was also very low: only 37 percent of a nationally representative sample of health-care workers reported receiving the influenza vaccine in 1998. Coverage rates in the same year for persons belonging to ethnic minorities were lower than the national goal, and there were significant racial/ethnic differences in coverage rates for persons 65 years or older and for health-care workers. Among persons 65 years or older, non-Hispanic (NH) Whites (66 percent) reported higher vaccination rates than either Hispanics (55 percent, p<0.001) or NH African Americans (48 percent, p<0.001) (Table 16.3). Among health-care workers, the coverage rate in 1998 for NH Whites was 41 percent, compared with 23 percent for NH African Americans (p<0.001)

Figure 16.3
Influenza vaccination coverage among persons 65 years or older by race/ethnicity, National Health Interview Survey, United States, 1989–2001

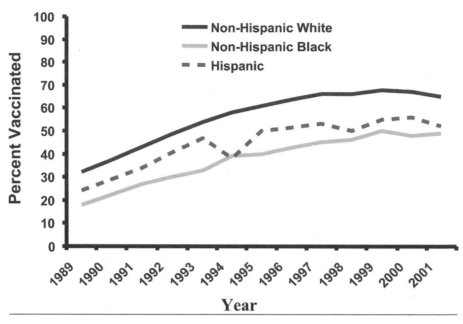

Table 16.3
Influenza vaccination coverage among persons 65 years or older by race/ethnicity, United States, 2000

	Coverage % (CI$_{95}$)	Difference (CI$_{95}$)	P value
Hispanics	55.7 (50.7, 60.6)	10.9	<0.001
Non Hispanic Blacks	48.0 (43.6, 52.5)	18.6	<0.001
Non Hispanic whites	66.6 (65.0, 68.2)	Reference	
Total	64.4 (63.0, 65.9)		

CI$_{95}$ = 95% Confidence limits

and 24 percent for Hispanics (p<0.001). Coverage estimates for 2000 indicate that the racial/ethnic gap has not decreased.

Barriers to Influenza Vaccination

The suboptimal use of influenza vaccine has been attributed to various characteristics of providers, consumers, and health-care systems. A physician's recommendation is the strongest predictor of a person receiving the influenza vaccine, even among people with a negative attitude regarding vaccinations (Ashby-Hughes & Nickerson, 1999; CDC, 1988). Yet some providers do not routinely recommend vaccinations either because they have misconceptions about the effectiveness and safety of the influenza vaccine (Hershey & Karuza, 1997; Nichol & Zimmerman, 2001) or because they do not consider preventive services during busy patient encounters (Schwartz et al., 1991; Williams et al., 1988). Other physician-related factors, such as lack of resources and negative attitudes, that have been associated with low use of other preventive services might also impact the delivery of vaccinations (McKinney & Barnas, 1989; Pachucki et al., 1985; Schwartz et al., 1991).

Patients' attitudes toward preventive services can determine whether these services are accepted or refused (Frank et al., 1985). The results of several studies have shown that erroneous beliefs about the effectiveness or side effects of the vaccine and about vaccinations in general are negatively associated with vaccine acceptance (Armstrong, K. et al., 2001; Frank et al., 1985; CDC, 1999b). For example, in a recent survey conducted among adults 65 years and older in West Philadelphia, investigators found that mistrust regarding the vaccine content, a belief that vaccination is inconvenient and painful, and the prior experience of side effects were negatively associated with having an influenza vaccination (Armstrong, K. et al., 2001).

Health system delivery characteristics are also important determinants of low influenza vaccination coverage. Up to 45 percent of persons at high risk for influenza or who die from influenza were cared for in a health-care institution during the previous year, and 75 percent or more received care in an outpatient clinic without receiving an influenza vaccination (Williams et al., 1988). One way to improve vaccination coverage is for health-care systems to take advantage of these missed opportunities to vaccinate patients.

Strategies to Increase Influenza Vaccination Rates

To improve influenza vaccination coverage among adults, health officials have implemented multiple strategies to increase demand, enhance access, and reduce missed opportunities. These strategies include instituting patient reminder and recall systems (Barton & Schoenbaum, 1990), reducing patients' out-of-pocket vaccine cost (CDC, 1992), offering vaccination services in nontraditional settings (Pearson et al., 1999), implementing standing orders for vaccination (Margolis et al., 1988), and providing educational programs targeted at patients and providers (Pearson & Thompson, 1994; Wuorenma et al., 1994). However, persistent racial disparities in influenza vaccination rates suggest that more specific strategies targeting racial/ethnic minorities are needed. For instance, because elderly African Americans who recall past violations in medical research distrust social institutions and may be reluctant to seek care or accept vaccinations (Corbie-Smith et al., 1999; Gamble, 1997; LaVeist et al., 2000), interventions to increase vaccination rates among them should focus on using culturally sensitive approaches delivered by trusted providers.

Strategies to increase influenza vaccination rates for persons who have contact with the health-care system should emphasize avoiding missed opportunities to vaccinate (Williams et al., 1988). Before the influenza season begins, medical charts should be screened, and those of adults who have an indication for influenza vaccination should be flagged. During the influenza season, reminder/

recall systems should be sent to alert high-risk persons about the need for influenza vaccination (Barton & Schoenbaum, 1990). Vaccinations should be given during a patient's first contact with a health-care provider. Among adults who have limited contact with health-care providers, pharmacies and emergency rooms may be their only contact with the medical system. Therefore, vaccinations should be available at these locations during influenza season (Grabenstein et al., 2001; Pearson et al., 1999).

PNEUMOCOCCAL DISEASE

Streptococcus pneumoniae (pneumococcus) is the primary cause of relatively mild, but common, upper-respiratory infections such as otitis media and sinusitis. Pneumococcus also is the most common cause of severe syndromes such as community-acquired pneumonia and meningitis. Each year in the United States, pneumococcal infections lead to an estimated 3,000 episodes of meningitis, 60,000 episodes of bacteremia, 125,000 hospitalizations for pneumonia, and 7 million episodes of otitis media (Feikin et al., 2000; Robinson et al., 2001; Schuchat et al., 1997). In spite of appropriate therapy, as many as one in three adults with pneumococcal pneumonia and bacteremia will die of his or her illness (Feikin et al., 2000). Over the last decade, pneumococci have become increasingly resistant to antibiotics (Whitney et al., 2000), limiting the number of available treatment options.

Disparity in Disease Burden

The very young and the elderly are at higher risk for pneumococcal disease (Figure 16.4). At all ages, African Americans are at higher risk for disease than Whites; the greatest disparity in disease risk occurs among persons 35–49 years old (Robinson et al., 2001). In this age group, the risk of acquiring invasive pneumococcal disease is five times higher for African Americans than for Whites. In a study of invasive pneumococcal disease in urban Baltimore, researchers found that the vast majority of cases of pneumococcal disease among African Americans occur among those younger than age 65 (Harrison et al., 2000), the age at which routine vaccination against pneumococcal disease is recommended (CDC, 1997). In this Baltimore population, the median age of adults with invasive pneumococcal disease was 27 years younger for African Americans (42 years) than for Whites (69 years). Strategies that focus on improving vaccine delivery to adults 65 years and older will thus do little to prevent the majority of cases among African American adults.

A number of factors are thought to contribute to this disparity in disease risk and median age of those infected. Some underlying conditions that lead to an increased risk for pneumococcal disease, such as HIV disease and diabetes, are more common in African Americans than in Whites (Harrison et al., 2000). Pneumococcal disease is often the first illness associated with HIV infection, and the risk for invasive pneumococcal disease among persons with AIDS is about 50 times the risk among persons without HIV infection (Nuorti et al., 2000). Even among persons with AIDS, however; the risk for invasive pneumococcal disease among African Americans is four times higher than that among Whites, although the overall rate of pneumococcal disease among persons with AIDS has been dropping since the availability of highly active antiretroviral therapy (Nuorti et al., 2000).

Another factor contributing to racial disparities in risk for pneumococcal disease is the very high risk among those with sickle-cell disease, which occurs primarily in African Americans (Zangwill et al., 1996). However, because sickle-cell disease is relatively uncommon, this increased risk does not contribute significantly to the overall difference in disease risk between African Americans and Whites. Penicillin prophylaxis is recommended for children with sickle-cell disease as a means of preventing pneumococcal infections (American Academy of Pediatrics, 2000).

Figure 16.4
Incidence of invasive pneumococcal disease by race and age group

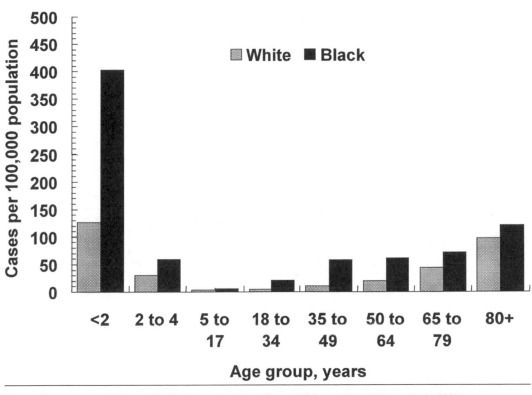

Source: Data are from CDC's Active Bacterial Core Surveillance (ABCs) (1998); Robinson et al. (2001).

Other factors, such as household crowding, inadequate access to health care, and poverty, have been proposed as possible explanations for the higher disease risk among African Americans (Bennett et al., 1992; Breiman et al., 1996; Harrison et al., 2000; Plouffe et al., 1996). In a study of adults without immunocompromising conditions, researchers found that some elevated risk among African Americans persisted after they controlled for other factors such as chronic illnesses, smoking, education level, exposure to children in the household, and income (Nuorti et al., 2000). In Levine et al. (1999), a similar study of risk factors for invasive disease in children under 5 years of age, however, found no racial differences after controlling for other factors. Among persons with HIV infections, African American race was a risk factor for disease after adjusting for severity of HIV disease, therapy, vaccination, and the presence of other chronic illnesses (Dworkin et al., 2001). The extent to which genetic factors associated with African American race could account for some of the disparity in risk for pneumococcal disease has not been explored.

Antibiotic Resistance

African Americans with invasive pneumococcal disease are less likely to have had their illness caused by an antibiotic-resistant strain than are Whites with the invasive disease (Whitney et al., 2000), (Figure 16.5) a finding likely explained by the greater overuse of antibiotics among Whites (Chen et al., 1998; Melnick et al., 1992). This ratio difference in risk for infection with a resistant

Figure 16.5
Proportion of pneumococcal isolates with resistance to penicillin in 1995 and 1998 by race and age group

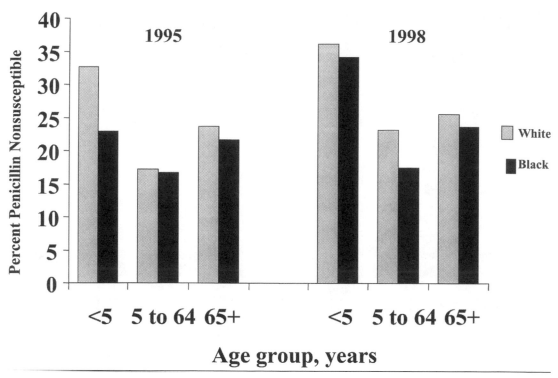

Source: Data are from CDC's Active Bacterial Core Surveillance (ABCs) (1998); Whitney et al. (2001).

strain, however, was greater in 1995 than in 1998, especially among young children (Whitney et al., 2000), suggesting that resistant pneumococcal clones are spreading to more communities in the United States.

Opportunities for Prevention

Vaccines provide the best means for preventing pneumococcal disease. A vaccine that covers 23 of the 90 pneumococcal serotypes has been available since 1983; these 23 serotypes cause over 80 percent of invasive disease (Robinson et al., 2001). The vaccine is recommended for all adults 65 years and older and for persons 2–64 years with certain chronic illnesses or conditions that suppress the immune system (CDC, 1997).

The polysaccharide vaccine has been shown to be effective against invasive disease among persons with intact immune systems (Butler et al., 1993; Shapiro et al., 1991) and cost-effective among persons 65 years and older (Sisk et al., 1997). In spite of this, most people who should have received the polysaccharide vaccine have not received it. According to surveys conducted in 1997, only 46 percent of all adults 65 years or older and only 17 percent of persons 18–64 years old with a vaccine indication had received the vaccine (CDC, 2000c; Holtzman et al., 2000). In 1997, among U.S. adults 65 years or older, vaccine coverage was substantially lower among non-Hispanic Blacks (30 percent) and Hispanics (34 percent) than among non-Hispanic Whites (47 percent) (CDC, 1998b).

The polysaccharide vaccine is less effective among people with immune system disorders such as HIV or AIDS (Breiman et al., 2000; Butler et al., 1993; Dworkin et al., 2001; French et al., 2000), and among Americans with HIV or AIDS, the vaccine seemed to work less well among African Americans than among Whites (Breiman et al., 2000); in a study in Uganda among people with untreated AIDS, the polysaccharide vaccine was actually associated with an increased risk for pneumococcal disease (French et al., 2000). Why the pneumococcal polysaccharide vaccine may work less well among Africans or African Americans with HIV than among Whites with HIV is not yet understood.

Although children less than 2 years of age are at highest risk for pneumococcal disease, most do not develop a protective immune response following vaccination with the pneumococcal polysaccharide vaccine (CDC, 2000b). In early 2000, a new vaccine effective against invasive pneumococcal disease and moderately effective against otitis media and pneumonia was licensed for use in young children (Black et al., 2000; CDC, 2000b; Shinefield & Black, 2000). The vaccine is made of pneumococcal capsular polysaccharide conjugated to a carrier protein; the seven capsular serotypes included in the vaccine cause over 80 percent of the cases of invasive pneumococcal disease among U.S. children (Robinson et al., 2001). CDC's Advisory Committee on Immunization Practices (ACIP) recommends the vaccine for all children less than 2 years of age and for those 2–4 years of age who have certain chronic illnesses or immunocompromising conditions (CDC, 2000b). In addition, ACIP recommends that providers consider vaccination for all children aged 24–59 months but should give priority to those at highest risk: children 24–35 months of age, children of Alaska Native or American Indian descent, African American children, and children who attend group day-care centers. Although earlier vaccine recommendations had included specific recommendations for Alaska Natives, American Indians, and other ethnic groups, these were the first recommendations to suggest that African American children should have higher priority to receive a vaccine because of their higher risk for a particular disease. Use of the new pneumococcal conjugate vaccine provides a real opportunity to reduce the racial disparity in risk for pneumococcal disease among children.

GROUP B STREPTOCOCCAL (GBS) INFECTIONS

GBS infections have been the leading cause of bacterial disease and death among newborns in the United States since their emergence in the 1970s (Schuchat, 1999). Approximately 25 percent of pregnant women are carriers of GBS bacteria; 2 percent of infants born to women who are carriers become infected; and 4 percent to 6 percent of infected newborns die from the infection. The infection is transmitted to newborns either during passage through the birth canal or prior to birth from bacteria that ascend from the mother's lower genital tract into the intrauterine cavity. The rate of disease is higher among infants born to African American women than among infants born to White women (Zangwill et al., 1992). Several research groups examined possible reasons for this difference, including correlations of GBS infection rates with low birth weight, socioeconomic status, maternal GBS colonization, and preterm birth. Most GBS infections among newborns can be prevented by giving antibiotics to women who have been identified as carriers while they are in labor. Until the mid-1990s, there were no coordinated prevention programs in the United States targeted at reducing the burden of GBS disease among newborns, and rates of disease remained high.

Potential for Disease Prevention

In the early 1980s, Boyer and Gotoff (1986) demonstrated that administering antibiotics during labor to women at risk of transmitting GBS to their newborns could prevent invasive disease during an infant's first week of life (i.e., early-onset disease). Despite the recognition by many that this was

Figure 16.6

Invasive group B streptococcal (GBS) disease incidence by age group and race, 1990

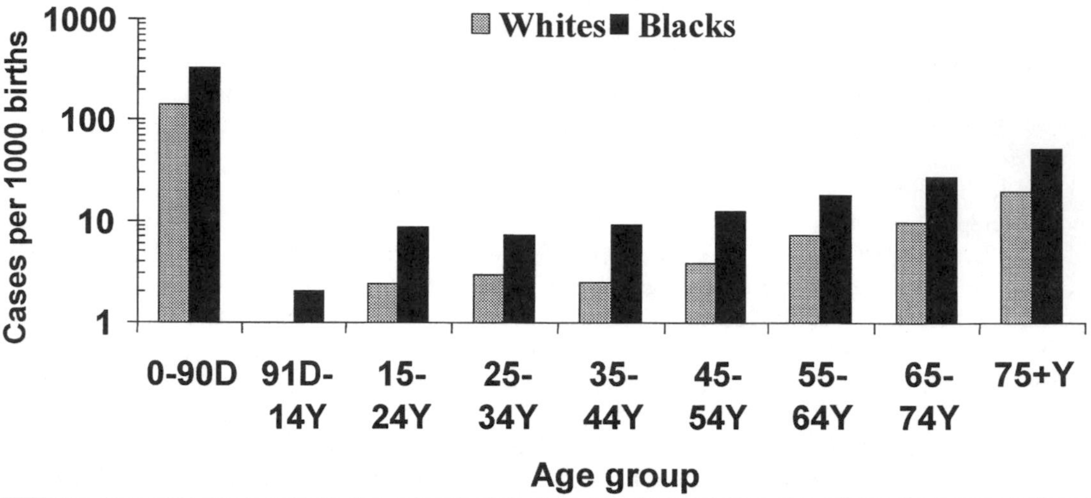

Source: Zangwill et al. (1992).

an effective intervention, the medical community was initially slow to incorporate intrapartum antibiotic prophylaxis into routine care; as a result, during the 1990s, management of pregnant women with GBS was an area of controversy. Parents whose babies had been born with GBS disease formed the Group B Strep Association, which became a strong advocate for educating pregnant women about the risk that GBS poses for newborns and the opportunities for active prevention. As the demand for coordinated prevention grew, CDC, the American Academy of Pediatrics (AAP), and the American College of Obstetricians and Gynecologists (ACOG) released 1996 consensus guidelines recommending strategies for preventing perinatal group B streptococcal disease in newborns (ACOG, 1996; CDC, 1996b; AAP Committee on Infectious Diseases and Committee on Fetus and Newborn, 1997).

Racial Disparities in GBS Rates

Since the emergence of this disease, several studies have revealed that African Americans have a higher incidence than Whites, although no conclusive explanation has been provided for this difference (Figure 16.6). For example, in a study of women giving birth at a Houston hospital from January 1994 to February 1995, Hickman et al. (1999) found that African American women had a significantly higher rate of GBS colonization than White women, an important factor in the higher rates of GBS disease among Black newborns. However, the explanation for this higher colonization rate has not been identified. Another factor associated with the higher rate of early-onset GBS disease among Blacks is the racial disparity in rates of premature births, since children born preterm are at higher risk for GBS disease. According to Fiscella (1996), almost 33 percent of the racial gap in infant mortality rates is attributable to a significantly higher rate of preterm births among African American women. In 1990, the rate of preterm births was more than twice as high among African American women as among White women. The reasons for this racial difference in preterm birthrates are also poorly understood (Fiscella, 1996). Using multivariable analysis of risk factors for early-onset GBS disease, Schuchat et al. (1990) found, however, that the African

Figure 16.7
Incidence of early- and late-onset invasive group B streptococcal (GBS) disease in selected active Bacterial Core Surveillance Areas, 1989–2000, and activities for prevention of GBS disease

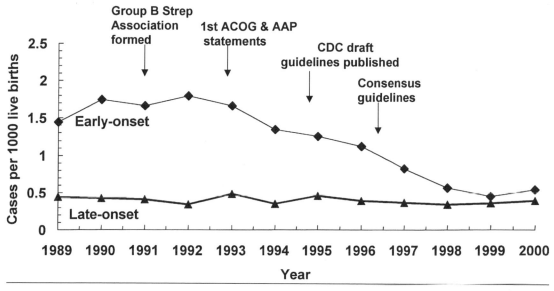

Source: Schrag et al. (2000)

American race was associated with disease risk independent of the risk associated with prematurity or low birth weight.

Decline in GBS Disease Rates

Despite a lack of understanding about what causes racial differences in rates of GBS disease, there has been substantial progress in prevention (Figure 16.7). Survey results have documented declines in the incidence of early-onset disease associated with use of a GBS screening policy (Schuchat et al., 2002), the number of physicians using some GBS prevention method (Watt et al., 2001), and the number of hospitals with new GBS policies (CDC, 2000a; Factor et al., 2000) (Figure 16.8). After active prevention efforts during the 1990s promoted the use of intrapartum antibiotics for high-risk women, incidence of early-onset disease among African American infants, compared with the incidence among White infants, decreased by 75 percent (Schrag et al., 2000) (Figure 16.9). Overall, early-onset GBS disease incidence declined by 70 percent during the 1990s.

Despite progress in the previous decade, GBS remains an important neonatal health concern, with an estimated 1,600 early-onset cases and 80 GBS-related deaths still occurring each year. To identify ways to further reduce the rates of GBS disease among newborns, CDC researchers met with GBS disease-prevention experts in the fall of 2001. Following this meeting, CDC developed a set of revised guidelines for preventing perinatal GBS disease that was jointly issued in 2002 by CDC, ACOG, AAP, and AAFP. The new guidelines, which are based on the results of a recent multistate study (Schrag et al., 2002), recommend universal screening of all pregnant women between 35 and 37 weeks' gestation.

Figure 16.8
Implementation of policies to combat group B streptococcal (GBS) disease, by year

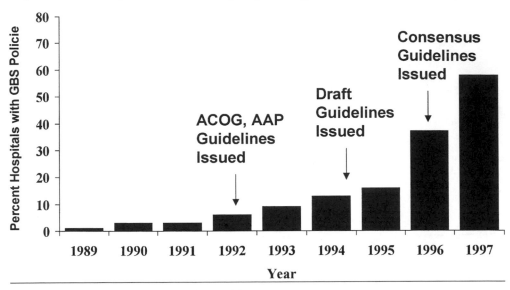

Source: ABCs Hospitals, EIP Network; CDC (1998d).

Figure 16.9
Rate of early-onset group B streptococcal (GBS) disease by race, 1993–1998

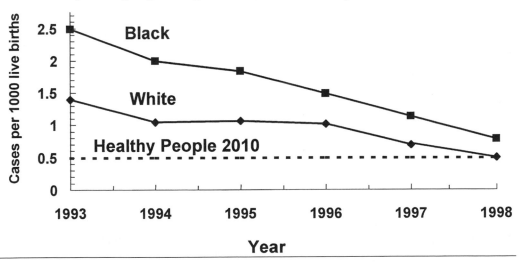

Source: Schrag et al. (2000).

The 75 percent decrease in the racial disparity in GBS rates signifies that intrapartum prophylaxis is an effective means of GBS prevention for all newborns. Therefore, we may not need to completely understand the causes of racial differences in GBS rates in order to eliminate the disparity, as long as the means of prevention is effective and reaches all populations labeled as "at risk."

SUMMARY

This chapter has examined the persistent impact of infectious diseases on African Americans and chosen five disease areas that represent persistent disparities and some successful interventions. These five diseases—hepatitis, food-borne, influenza, pneumococcal, and group B streptococcal—represent only part of the spectrum of infections that disproportionately impact African Americans. For most diseases, the major contributor to disparities is low socioeconomic status, but other factors are likely involved. Better understanding of the relative importance of these risk factors for infectious diseases among African Americans and strategies to address disparities is an important area of additional research.

In each of these disease areas, there have been successes in addressing disparities. In part, these successes have come through identifying critical intervention strategies that target the risk factors influencing the high rate of disease in African Americans. Further improvements will require additional activities that could include (1) improving the conceptual tools needed to understand race and its impact on health and to allow for more accurate surveillance of racial and ethnic minority infectious disease conditions (Jones, 2001); (2) increasing research into the prevalence of, and specific risk factors for, infectious diseases among African Americans (Nelson, 2002; Maxey, 2002); (3) increasing African Americans' participation in health-related research by carefully addressing issues that have created a long-standing mistrust of the health-care system among African Americans (National Medical Association Consensus Paper, 2001a); (4) expanding efforts to increase the ranks of African American public health and health-care personnel (Smedley et al., 2001); (5) ensuring that African Americans have access to the latest health information, vaccines, and treatments; (6) involving African American communities in collaborations with local, state, and federal health-promotion and infectious disease-prevention efforts (Logan & Freeman, 2000); and (7) heightening awareness and increasing risk reduction efforts (National Medical Association Consensus Paper, 2001b).

Understanding the epidemiology of infectious diseases among African Americans can lead to the development of targeted intervention strategies to eliminate racial disparities. African Americans are overdue a respite from the suffering caused by these diseases and are eager for improvements in health. As Langston Hughes said in "History":

> The past has been a mint
> Of blood and sorrow.
> That must not be
> True of Tomorrow

(Hughes, 1980, p. 69)

REFERENCES

Alter, M.J. (1997). Epidemiology of hepatitis C. *Hepatology, 26,* 62S–65S.

Alter, M.J., et al. (1990). Risk factors for acute non-A, non-B hepatitis in the United States and association with hepatitis C virus infection. *Journal of the American Medical Association, 264(17),* 2231–2235.

Alter, M.J., et al. (1999). The prevalence of hepatitis C virus infection in the United States, 1988 through 1994. *New England Journal of Medicine, 341(8),* 556–562.

American Academy of Pediatrics (AAP). (2000). Pneumococcal infections. In L. Pickering (Ed.), 2000 Red Book: Report of the Committee on Infectious Diseases. Elk Grove Village, IL. *American Academy of Pediatrics, 460.*

American Academy of Pediatrics (AAP) Committee on Infectious Diseases and Committee on Fetus and Newborn. (1997). Revised guidelines for prevention of early-onset group B streptococcal (GBS) infection. *Pediatrics, 99(3),* 489–496.

American College of Obstetricians and Gynecologists (ACOG) Committee on Obstetric Practice (1996). Prevention of early-onset group B streptococcal disease in newborns. *ACOG Committee Opinion (No. 173)*.

Armstrong, G.L., Alter, M.J., McQuillan, G.M., & Margolis, H.S. (2000). The past incidence of hepatitis C virus infection: Implications for the future burden of chronic liver disease in the United States. *Hepatology, 31*, 777–782.

Armstrong, G.L., Conn, L.A., & Pinner, R.W. (1999). Trends in infectious disease mortality in the United States during the 20th century. *Journal of the American Medical Association, 281(1)*, 61–66.

Armstrong, G.L., Mast, E.E., Wojczynski, M., & Margolis, H.S. (2001). Childhood hepatitis B virus infections in the United States prior to hepatitis B immunization. *Pediatrics, 108(5)*, 1123–1128.

Armstrong, K., Berlin, M., Schwartz, J.S., Propert, K., & Ubel, P.A. (2001). Barriers to influenza immunization in a low-income urban population. *American Journal of Preventive Medicine, 20(1)*, 21–25.

Ashby-Hughes, B., & Nickerson, N. (1999). Provider endorsement: The strongest cue in prompting high-risk adults to receive influenza and pneumococcal immunization. *Clinical Excellence for Nurse Practitioners, 3(2)*, 97–104.

Barker, W.H. (1986). Excess pneumonia and influenza associated hospitalizations during influenza epidemics in the United States, 1970–1978. *American Journal of Public Health, 76(7)*, 761–765.

Barker, W.H., & Mullooly, J.P. (1980). Influenza vaccination of elderly persons: reduction in pneumonia and influenza hospitalizations and deaths. *Journal of the American Medical Association, 244*, 2547–2549.

Barton, M.B., & Schoenbaum, S.C. (1990). Improving influenza vaccination performance in an HMO setting: The use of computer-generated reminders and peer comparison feedback. *American Journal of Public Health, 80(5)*, 534–536.

Bennett, N.M., Buffington, J., & LaForce, F.M. (1992). Pneumococcal bacteremia in Monroe County, New York. *American Journal of Public Health, 82(11)*, 1513–1516.

Black, S., et al. (2000). Efficacy of heptavalent conjugate pneumococcal vaccine (Wyeth Lederle) in 37,000 infants and children: Results of the Northern California Kaiser Permanente Efficacy Trial. *Pediatric Infectious Disease Journal, 19(3)*, 187–195.

Blackwelder, W.C., Alling, D.W., & Stuart-Harris, C.H. (1982). Association of excess mortality from chronic nonspecific lung disease with epidemics of influenza. Comparison of experience in the United States and in England and Wales, 1968 to 1976. *American Review of Respiratory Disease, 125*, 511–516.

Boyer, K.M., & Gotoff, S.P. (1986). Prevention of early-onset neonatal group B streptococcal disease with selective intrapartum chemoprophylaxis. *New England Journal of Medicine, 314(26)*, 1665–1669.

Breiman, R.F., et al. (2000). Evaluation of effectiveness of the 23-valent pneumococcal capsular polysaccharide vaccine for HIV-infected patients. *Archives of Internal Medicine, 160(17)*, 2633–2638.

Breiman, R., Spika, J.S., Navarro, V.J., Darden, P.M., & Darby, C.P. (1996). Pneumococcal bacteremia in Charleston County, South Carolina: A decade later. *Archives of Internal Medicine, 150*, 1401–1405.

Butler, J.C., et al. (1993). Polysaccharide pneumococcal vaccine efficacy: An evaluation of current recommendations. *Journal of the American Medical Association, 270(15)*, 1826–1831.

Centers for Disease Control and Prevention (CDC). (1988). Adult immunization: Knowledge, attitudes and practices—DeKalb and Fulton Counties, Georgia 1988. *MMWR Morbidity and Mortality Weekly Report, 37(43)*, 657–661.

Centers for Disease Control and Prevention (CDC). (1990a). Current trends community outbreaks of shigellosis—United States. *MMWR Morbidity and Mortality Weekly Report, 3(30)*, 509–513, 519.

Centers for Disease Control and Prevention (CDC). (1990b). Topics in minority health: *Yersinia enterocolitica* infections during the holidays in Black families—Georgia. *MMWR Morbidity and Mortality Weekly Report, 39(45)*, 819–820.

Centers for Disease Control and Prevention (CDC). (1991). Hepatitis B virus: A comprehensive strategy for eliminating transmission in the United States through universal childhood vaccination: Recommendations of the Immunization Practices Advisory Committee (ACIP). *MMWR Morbidity and Mortality Weekly Report, 40 (RR-13)*, 1–25.

Centers for Disease Control and Prevention (CDC). (1992). Medicare influenza vaccine demonstration—Selected states, 1988–1992. *MMWR Morbidity and Mortality Weekly Report, 41(9)*, 152–155.

Centers for Disease Control and Prevention (CDC). (1994). *Addressing emerging infectious disease threats: A prevention strategy for the United States*. Atlanta, GA: U.S. Department of Health and Human Services.

Centers for Disease Control and Prevention (CDC). (1996a). Immunization of adolescents. Recommendations of the Advisory Committee on Immunization Practices, the American Academy of Pediatrics, the American Academy of Family Physicians, and the American Medical Association. *MMWR Morbidity and Mortality Weekly Report, 45(RR-13)*, 1–16.

Centers for Disease Control and Prevention (CDC). (1996b). Prevention of perinatal group B streptococcal disease: A public health perspective. *MMWR Morbidity and Mortality Weekly Report, 45(RR-7)*, 1–24.

Centers for Disease Control and Prevention (CDC). (1997). Prevention of pneumococcal disease: Recommendations of the Advisory Committee on Immunization Practices (ACIP). *MMWR Morbidity and Mortality Weekly Report, 46(RR-08)*, 1–24.

Centers for Disease Control and Prevention (CDC). (1998a). Adoption of hospital policies for prevention of perinatal group B streptococcal disease—United States, 1997. *MMWR Morbidity and Mortality Weekly Report, 47(32)*, 665–670.

Centers for Disease Control and Prevention (CDC). (1998b). Influenza and pneumococcal vaccination levels among adults aged greater than or equal to 65 years—United States. *MMWR Morbidity and Mortality Weekly Report, 47(38)*, 797–802.

Centers for Disease Control and Prevention (CDC). (1998c). *Preventing emerging infectious diseases. A strategy for the 21st century.* Atlanta, GA: U.S. Department of Health and Human Services.

Centers for Disease Control and Prevention (CDC). (1998d). Recommendations for prevention and control of hepatitis C virus (HCV) infection and HCV-related chronic disease. *MMWR Morbidity and Mortality Weekly Report, 47(RR-19)*, 1–39.

Centers for Disease Control and Prevention (CDC). (1999a). Prevention of hepatitis A through active or passive immunization: Recommendations of the Advisory Committee on Immunization Practices (ACIP). *MMWR Morbidity and Mortality Weekly Report, 48 (RR-12)*, 1–37.

Centers for Disease Control and Prevention (CDC). (1999b). Reasons reported by Medicare beneficiaries for not receiving influenza and pneumococcal vaccinations—United States, 1996. *MMWR Morbidity and Mortality Weekly Report, 48(39)*, 556–890.

Centers for Disease Control and Prevention (CDC). (2000a). Hospital-based policies for prevention of perinatal group B streptococcal disease—United States, 1999. *MMWR Morbidity and Mortality Weekly Report, 49(41)*, 936–940.

Centers for Disease Control and Prevention (CDC). (2000b). Prevention of pneumococcal disease among infants and young children: Recommendations of the Advisory Committee on Immunization Practices. *MMWR Morbidity and Mortality Weekly Report, 49 (RR-9)*, 1–35.

Centers for Disease Control and Prevention (CDC). (2000c). Use of standing orders programs to increase adult vaccination rates. *MMWR Morbidity and Mortality Weekly Report, 49(RR-1)*, 15–26.

Centers for Disease Control and Prevention (CDC). (2002a). National Center for Infectious Diseases. National hepatitis C prevention strategy Web site, http://www.cdc.gov/hepatitis

Centers for Disease Control and Prevention (CDC). (2002b). National, state, and urban area vaccination coverage levels among children aged 19–35 months—United States, 2001. *MMWR Morbidity and Mortality Weekly Report, 51(30)*, 664–666.

Centers for Disease Control and Prevention (CDC). (2002c). Preliminary FoodNet data on the incidence of foodborne illnesses—selected sites, United States. *MMWR Morbidity and Mortality Weekly Report, 51(15)*, 325–329.

Centers for Disease Control and Prevention (CDC). (2002d). Prevention and control of influenza: Recommendations of the Advisory Committee on Immunization Practices (ACIP). *MMWR Morbidity and Mortality Weekly Report, 51(RR-3)*, 1–31.

Centers for Disease Control and Prevention (CDC). (in press). Prevention and control of infections with hepatitis viruses in correctional settings. *MMWR Morbidity and Mortality Weekly Report.*

Chen, F.M., Breiman, R.F., Farley, M., Plikaytis, B., Deaver, K., & Cetron, M.S. (1998). Geocoding and linking data from population-based surveillance and the U.S. Census to evaluate the impact of median household income on the epidemiology of invasive *Streptococcus pneumoniae* infections. *American Journal of Epidemiology, 148*, 1212–1218.

Corbie-Smith, G., Thomas, S.B., Williams, M.V., & Moody-Ayers, S. (1999). Attitudes and beliefs of African-Americans towards participation in medical research. *Journal of General Internal Medicine, 14(9)*, 537–546.

Cover, T.L., & Aber, R.C. (1989). *Yersinia enterocolitica. New England Journal of Medicine, 320*, 16–24.

Davey Smith, G., Neaton, J.D., Wentworth, D., & Stamler, R. (1998). Mortality differences between Black and White women in the U.S.A.: The contribution of income and other risk factors among men screened for MRFIT. *Lancet, 351(9107)*, 934–939.

Dowell, S.F., Kupronis, B.A., Zell, E., & Shay, D.K. (2000). Mortality from pneumonia in children the United States, 1939 through 1996. *New England Journal of Medicine, 342 (19)*, 1399–1407.

Du Bois, W.E.B. (1989). *The souls of Black folk*. New York: Bantam.

Duster, T. (1990). *Back door to eugenics*. New York: Routledge.

Dworkin, M.S., Ward, J.W., Hanson, D.L., Jones, J.L., Kaplan, J.E., & the Adult and Adolescent Spectrum of HIV Disease Project. (2001). Pneumococcal disease among HIV-infected persons: Incidence, risk factors, and impact of vaccination. *Clinical Infectious Diseases, 32(5)*, 794–800.

Factor, S.H., Whitney, C.G., Zywicki, S.S., & Schuchat, A. (2000). Effects of hospital policies on the 1996 group B streptococcal consensus guidelines. *Obstetrics and Gynecology, 95(3)*, 377–382.

Feikin, D.R., et al. (2000). Mortality from invasive pneumococcal pneumonia in the era of antibiotic resistance, 1995–1997. *American Journal of Public Health, 90(2)*, 223–229.

Fiscella, K. (1996). Racial disparities in preterm births: The role of urogenital infections. *Public Health Reports, 111*, 104–113.

Frank, J.W., Henderson, M., & McMurray, L. (1985). Influenza vaccination in the elderly. Determinants of acceptance. *Canadian Medical Association Journal, 132*, 371–375.

French, N., et al. (2000). 23-valent pneumococcal polysaccharide vaccine in HIV-1-infected Ugandan adults: Double-blind, randomized and placebo controlled trial. *Lancet, 355(9221)*, 2106–2111.

Gamble, V.N. (1997). Under the shadow of Tuskegee: African Americans and health care. *American Journal of Public Health, 87(11)*, 1773–1778.

Garfein, R.S., Vlahov, D., Galai, N., Doherty, M.C., & Nelson, K.E. (1996). Viral infections in short-term injection drug users: The prevalence of the hepatitis C, hepatitis B, human immunodeficiency, and human T-lymphotropic viruses. *American Journal of Public Health, 86(5)*, 655–661.

Glezen, W.P., Decker, M., & Perrotta, D.M. (1987). Survey of underlying conditions of persons hospitalized with acute respiratory disease during influenza epidemics in Houston, 1978–1981. *American Review of Respiratory Disease, 36*, 550–555.

Glezen, W.P., Greenberg, S.B., Atmar, R.L., Piedra, P.A., & Couch, R.B. (2000). Impact of respiratory virus infections on persons with chronic underlying conditions. *Journal of the American Medical Association, 283(4)*, 499–505.

Goldstein, S.T., et al. (2002). Incidence and risk factors for acute hepatitis B in the United States, 1982–1998: Implications for vaccination programs. *Journal of Infectious Diseases, 185(6)*, 713–719.

Grabenstein, J.D., Guess, H.A., Hartzema, A.G., Koch, G.G., & Konrad, T.R. (2001). Effect of vaccination by community pharmacists among adult prescription recipients. *Medical Care, 39(4)*, 340–348.

Gross, P.A., Hermogenes, A.W., Sacks, H.S., Lau, J., & Levandowski, R.A. (1995). The efficacy of influenza vaccine in elderly persons. A meta-analysis and review of the literature. *Annals of Internal Medicine, 123(7)*, 518–527.

Guerrant, R.L., et al. (2001). Practice guidelines for the management of infectious diarrhea. *Clinical Infectious Diseases, 32(3)*, 331–350.

Harrison, L.H., Dwyer, D.M., Billmann, L., Kolczak, M., & Schuchat, A. (2000). Invasive pneumococcal infection in Baltimore, MD—implications for immunization policy. *Archives of Internal Medicine, 160*, 89–94.

Hershey, C.O., & Karuza, J. (1997). Delivery of vaccines to adults: Correlations with physician knowledge and patient variables. *American Journal of Medical Quality, 12*, 143–150.

Hickman, M.E., Rench, M.A., Ferrieri, P., & Baker, C.J. (1999). Changing epidemiology of group B streptococcal colonization. *Pediatrics, 104(2)*, 203–209.

Holtzman, D., Powell-Griner, E., Bolen, J., & Rhodes L. (2000). Behavioral Risk Factor Surveillance System Coordinators. State—and sex-specific prevalence of selected characteristics—Behavioral Risk Factor Surveillance System, 1996 and 1997. *MMWR Morbidity and Mortality Weekly Report, 49*, 1–39.

Hughes, Langston. (1980). *The panther and the lash. Poems of our times*. New York: Knopf.

Institute of Medicine. (1994). *Emerging infections: Microbial threats to health in the United States*. Washington, DC: National Academy Press.

Jones, C.P. (2001). Invited commentary: "Race," racism, and the practice of epidemiology. *American Journal of Epidemiology, 154(4)*, 299–304.

LaVeist, T.A., Nickerson, K.J., & Bowie, J.V. (2000). Attitudes about racism, medical mistrust, and satisfaction with care among African American and white cardiac patients. *Medical Care Research and Review, 57(Supp 1)*, 146–161.

Lee, L.A., Gerber, A.R., & Lonsway, D.R. (1990). *Yersinia enterocolitica* O:3 infections in infants and children associated with the household preparation of chitterlings. *New England Journal of Medicine, 322*, 984–987.

Lee, L.A., Shapiro, C.N., Hargrett-Bean, N., & Tauxe, R.V. (1991). Hyperendemic shigellosis in the United States: A review of surveillance data for 1967–1988. *Journal of Infectious Diseases, 164*, 894–900.

Lee, L.A., Taylor, J., & Carter, G.P. (1991). *Yersinia enterocolitica* O:3: An emerging cause of pediatric gastroenteritis in the United States. *Journal of Infectious Diseases, 163*, 660–663.

Levine, O.S., Farley, M., Harrison, L.H., Lefkowitz, L., McGeer, A., & Schwartz, B. (1999). Risk factors for invasive pneumococcal disease in children: A population-based case-control study in *North American Pediatrics, 103*, E28.

Logan, S.L., & Freeman, E.M. (Eds.). (2000). *Health care in the black community: Empowerment, knowledge, skills, and collectivism*. Binghamton, NY: Haworth Press.

Marcus, R., et al. (2002, March). Age, ethnic and racial disparity in *Salmonella* serotype *enteritidis* (SE): FoodNet. International Conference on Emerging Infectious Diseases. Atlanta, GA.

Marcus, R., et al. (2004). Dramatic Decrease in the Incidence of Salmonella Serotype Enteritidis (SE) Infections in Five FoodNet Sites: 1996–1999. *Clinical Infectious Diseases* (in press).

Margolis, H.S., Alter, M.J., & Hadler, S.C. (1991). Hepatitis B: Evolving epidemiology and implications for control. *Seminars in Liver Disease, 11*, 84–92.

Margolis, H.S., Alter, M.J., & Hadler, S.C. (1997). Viral hepatitis. In A.S. Evans & R. Kaslow (Eds.), *Viral infections of humans: Epidemiology and control*, 4th ed., pp. 363–418. New York: Plenum.

Margolis, H.S., Coleman, P.J., Brown, R.E., Mast, E.E., Sheingold, S.H., & Arevalo, J.A. (1995). Prevention of hepatitis B virus transmission by immunization. An economic analysis of current recommendations. *Journal of the American Medical Association, 274(15)*, 1201–1208.

Margolis, K.L., Lofgren, R.P., & Korn, J.E. (1988). Organizational strategies to improve influenza vaccine delivery. A standing order in a general medicine clinic. *Archives of Internal Medicine, 148*, 2205–2207.

Maxey, R. (2002). NMA addresses health care disparities. Consensus statement. *Journal of the National Medical Association, 94(8)*, 747–748.

McKinney, W.P., & Barnas, G.P. (1989). Influenza immunization in the elderly: Knowledge and attitude do not explain physician behavior. *American Journal of Public Health, 79(10)*, 1422–1424.

McQuillan, G.M., Coleman, P., Kruszon-Moran, D., Moyer, L.A., Lambert, S.B., & Margolis, H.S. (1999). Prevalence of hepatitis B virus infection in the United States: The National Health and Nutrition Examination Surveys, 1976–1994. *American Journal of Public Health, 89(1)*, 14–18.

Mead, P.S., et al. (1999). Food-related illness and death in the United States. *Emerging Infectious Diseases, 5(5)*, 607–625.

Melnick, S.L., Sprafka, J.M., Laitinen, D.L., Bostick, R.M., Flack, J.M., & Burke, G.L. (1992). Antibiotic use in urban Whites and Blacks: The Minnesota Heart Survey. *Annals of Pharmacotherapy, 26*, 1292–1295.

Murphy, S.L. (2000). Deaths: Final data for 1998. *National Vital Statistics Reports, 48(11)*.

Murrill, C.S., et al. (2002). Age-specific seroprevalence of HIV, hepatitis B virus, and hepatitis C virus infection among injection drug users admitted to drug treatment in 6 U.S. cities. *American Journal of Public Health, 92(3)*, 385–387.

National Center for Health Statistics (NCHS). (1997). *National Health Interview Survey, Years 1986–1994*. Hyattsville, MD: National Center for Health Statistics. U.S. Department of Health and Human Services.

National Center for Health Statistics (NCHS). (1998). *Vital Statistics Mortality Data, Multiple Cause Detail, 1993–1998*. Hyattsville, MD: National Center for Health Statistics. Public use tape contents and documentation package.

National Center for Health Statistics (NCHS). (2000). *National Health Interview Survey Multiple Cause-of-Death Public Use Data Files, 1986–94 Survey Years, Dates of Death 1986–1997.* Hyattsville, MD: National Center for Health Statistics. U.S. Department of Health and Human Services.

National Medical Association Consensus Paper. (2001a). *Biomedical research.* National Colloquium on African American Health.

National Medical Association Consensus Paper. (2001b). *Promoting prevention of viral hepatitis in the African American community.* National Colloquium on African American Health.

Nelson, A. (2002). Unequal treatment: Confronting racial and ethnic disparities in health care. *Journal of the National Medical Association, 94(8),* 66–668.

Nichol, K.L., Margolis, K.L., Wuorenma, J., & Von Sternberg, T. (1994). The efficacy and cost effectiveness of vaccination against influenza among elderly persons living in the community. *New England Journal of Medicine, 331(12),* 778–784.

Nichol, K.L., & Zimmerman, R. (2001). Generalist and subspecialist physicians' knowledge, attitudes, and practices regarding influenza and pneumococcal vaccinations for elderly and other high-risk patients: A national survey. *Achives of Internal Medicine, 161(22),* 2702–2708.

Nuorti, J.P. (2000). Cigarette smoking and invasive pneumococcal disease. *New England Journal of Medicine, 342(10),* 681–689.

Nuorti, J.P., Butler, J.C., Gelling, L., Kool, J.L., Reingold, A.L., & Vugia, D.J. (2000). Epidemiologic relation between HIV and invasive pneumococcal disease in San Francisco County, California. *Annals of Internal Medicine, 132(3),* 182–190.

Pachucki, C.T., Lentino, J.R., & Jackson, G.G. (1985). Attitudes and behavior of health care personnel regarding the use and efficacy of influenza vaccine. *Journal of Infectious Diseases, 151,* 1170–1171.

Pappas, G. (1994). Elucidating relationships between race, socioeconomic status, and health. *American Journal of Public Health, 84(6),* 892–893.

Pearson, D., Jackson, L.A., Winkler, B., Foss, B., & Wagener, B. (1999). Use of an automated pharmacy system and patient registries to recruit HMO enrollees for an influenza campaign. *Effective Clinical Practice, 2(1),* 17–22.

Pearson, D.C., & Thompson, R.S. (1994). Evaluation of Group Health Cooperative of Puget Sound senior immunization program. *Public Health Reports, 109,* 571–578.

Pinner, R.W., et al. (1996). Trends in infectious disease mortality in the United States. *Journal of the American Medical Association, 275(3),* 189–193.

Pinner, R.W., Roy, K., & Shoemake, H. (2002). *Mortality from Infectious Diseases in United States, 1993–1998.* Unpublished manuscript.

Plouffe, J., Breiman, R., Facklam, R., & the Franklin County Pneumonia Study Group. (1996). Bacteremia with *Streptococcus pneumoniae*: Implications for therapy and prevention. *Journal of the American Medical Association, 275(3),* 194–198.

Public Health Service. (1991). *Healthy People 2000: National Health Promotion and Disease Prevention Objectives-Full Report with Commentary.* U.S. Department of Health and Human Services Publication No. (PHS) 91-50213. Washington, DC: U.S. Department of Health and Human Services, Public Health Service.

Rangel, M.C. (2002). Racial and ethnic disparities in influenza vaccination. [dissertation]. Chapel Hill: University of North Carolina at Chapel Hill.

Ray, S.M., et al. (in press). Population-based surveillance for *Yersinia enterocolitica* infection: Higher risk of disease in infants and minority populations. *Clinical Infectious Diseases.*

Reynolds, P.P. (1997). Hospitals and civil rights, 1945–1963: The case of Simkins v Moses H. Cone Memorial Hospital. *Annals of Internal Medicine, 126(11),* 898–906.

Richardus, J.H., & Kunst, A.E. (2001). Black–White differences in infectious disease mortality in the United States. *American Journal of Public Health, 91(8),* 1251–1253.

Robinson, K.A., et al. (2001). Epidemiology of invasive *Streptococcus pneumoniae* infections in the United States, 1995–1998: Opportunities for prevention in the conjugate vaccine era. *Journal of the American Medical Association, 285(13),* 1729–1735.

Ruiz, J.D., et al. (1999). Prevalence and correlates of hepatitis C virus infection among inmates entering the California correctional system. *Western Journal of Medicine, 170(3),* 156–160.

Schrag, S., et al. (2000). Group B streptococcal disease in the era of intrapartum antibiotic prophylaxis, *New England Journal of Medicine, 342(1)*, 15–20.

Schrag, S.J., et al. (2002). A population-based comparison of strategies to prevent early-onset group B streptococcal disease in neonates. *New England Journal of Medicine, 347(4)*, 233–239.

Schuchat A. (1999). Group B streptococcus. *Lancet, 353(9146)*, 51–56.

Schuchat, A., et al. (1990). Population-based risk factors for neonatal group B streptococcal disease: Results of a cohort study in metropolitan Atlanta. *Journal of Infectious Diseases, 162*, 672–677.

Schuchat, A., et al. (1997). Bacterial meningitis in the United States in 1995. *New England Journal of Medicine, 337(14)*, 970–976.

Schuchat, A., Roome, A., Zell, E.R., Linardos, H., Zywicki, S., & O'Brien, K.L. (2002). Integrated monitoring of a new group B streptococcal disease prevention program and other perinatal infections. *Maternal and Child Health Journal, 6(2)*, 107–114.

Schwartz, S.J., Lewis, C.E., Clancy, C., Kinosian, M.S., Radany, M.H., & Koplan, J.P. (1991). Internists' practices in health promotion and disease prevention: A survey. *Annals of Internal Medicine, 114(1)*, 46–53.

Shapiro, E.D., et al. (1991). The protective efficacy of polyvalent pneumococcal polysaccharide vaccine. *New England Journal of Medicine, 325*, 1453–1460.

Shinefield, H.R., & Black, S. (2000). Efficacy of pneumococcal conjugate vaccines in large scale field trials. *Pediatric Infectious Disease Journal, 19(4)*, 394–397.

Simonsen, L., Clarke, M.J., Williamson, G.D., Stroup, D.F., Arden, N.H., & Schonberg, L.B. (1997). The impact of influenza epidemics on mortality: Introducing a severity index. *American Journal of Public Health, 87(12)*, 1944–1950.

Simonsen, L., Fakuda, K., Schoenberger, L.B., & Cox, N.J. (2000). The impact of influenza epidemics on hospitalizations. *Journal of Infectious Diseases, 181(3)*, 831–837.

Sisk, J.E., et al. (1997). Cost-effectiveness of vaccination against pneumococcal bacteremia among elderly people. *Journal of the American Medical Association, 278*, 1333–1339.

Smedley, B.D., Stith, A.Y., & Colburn, L. (2001). *The right thing to do, the smart thing to do: Enhancing diversity in health professions.* Summary of the Symposium on Diversity in Health Professions in honor of Hebert W. Nickens, M.D. Washington, DC: National Academy Press.

Sorlie, P., Rogot, E., Anderson, R., Johnson, N.J., & Bacllund, E. (1992). Black–White mortality differences by family income. *Lancet, 340*, 346–350.

Townes, E.M. (1998). *Breaking the rain of death: African American health issues and a womanist ethic of care.* New York: Continuum.

U.S. Department of Health and Human Services. (2000a). *Healthy People 2010. Objectives: Draft for public comment.*

U.S. Department of Health and Human Services. (2000b). *Healthy People 2010*, 2d ed. With understanding and improving health and objectives for improving health. 2 vols. Washington, DC: U.S. Government Printing Office.

Varmus, H.E. (1999). Statement before the House and Senate Appropriations Sub-committees on Labor, Health and Human Services, and Education, February 23–24.

Watanabe, K.K., Williams, A.E., Schreiber, G.B., & Ownby, H.E. (2000). Infectious disease markers in young blood donors. *Transfusion, 40(8)*, 954–960.

Watt, J.P., Schuchat, A., Erickson, K., Honig, J.E., Gibbs, G., & Schulkin, J. (2001). Group B streptococcal disease prevention practices of obstetrician-gynecologists. *Obstetrics and Gynecology, 98(1)*, 7–13.

White, E.C. (Ed.). (1994). *The Black women's health book.* Seattle: Seal Press.

Whitney, C.G., et al. (2000). Increasing prevalence of multidrug-resistant *Streptococcus pneumoniae* in the United States. *New England Journal of Medicine, 343(26)*, 1917–1924.

Williams, W.W., Hickson. M.A., Kane, M.A., Kendal, A.P., Spika, J.S., & Himman, R. (1988). Immunization policies and vaccine coverage among adults. The risk of missed opportunities. *Annals of Internal Medicine, 108(4)*, 616–625.

Wuorenma, J., Nichol, K., & Vonsternberg, T. (1994). Implementing a mass influenza vaccination program. *Nursing Management, 25*, 81–88.

Zangwill, K.M., Schuchat, A., & Wenger, J.D. (1992). Group B streptococcal disease in the United States,

1990: Report from a multistate active surveillance system. In CDC Surveillance Summaries, November 20, 1992, *MMWR Morbidity and Mortality Weekly Report, 41(No. SS-6)*, 25–32.

Zangwill, K.M., Vadheim, C.M., Vannier, A.M., Hemenway, L.S., Greenberg, D.P., & Ward, J.I. (1996). Epidemiology of invasive pneumococcal disease in southern California: Implications for the design and conduct of a pneumococcal conjugate vaccine efficacy trial. *Journal of Infectious Diseases, 174*, 752–759.

Zinsser, H. (1984). *Rats, lice and history* (3d ed.). London: Routledge.

CHAPTER 17

Forms of Violence and Violence Prevention

LE ROY E. REESE, ALEXANDER E. CROSBY, LA MAR HASBROUCK, AND LEIGH A. WILLIS

Issues related to the disproportionate public health burden experienced by African Americans with respect to morbidity and premature mortality on a number of health indicators have been the subject of a number of volumes in this series. Here we discuss violence-related morbidity and mortality in the African American community and what is known about the scope of its occurrence and its preventability. With an emphasis on the prevention of violence-related mortality (death) and morbidity (injury), we use the public health approach to construct this chapter. In this vein, our chapter provides descriptive data on homicide, assault victimization, and suicide in the United States to illustrate the magnitude of the problem of violence on the health and life expectancy of African Americans. We discuss what is known about how risk and protective factors influence behaviors leading to fatal and nonfatal violent injuries, describe intervention and prevention strategies to reduce the burden of violent victimization on African Americans, and consider strategies for disseminating and implementing what has been learned (Figure 17.1).

HOMICIDE AND ASSAULT

Homicide as a cause of excess deaths among Blacks, especially Black males, compared to Whites has been well documented (USDHHS, 1985; CDC, 1989). Homicide has historically been the leading cause of death for Blacks in the 15–24 and 25–34 year age groups, and this pattern continues today (USDHHS, 2002). The impact of homicide on the overall health of Blacks was revealed in a recent study by the Centers for Disease Control (CDC) and Prevention that found homicide to be a significant contributor to the six-year difference in the life expectancy for Blacks and Whites. After heart disease and cancer, the leading contributors to the difference, homicide was the next largest contributor to the life expectancy gap, accounting for nearly 10 percent of the variance (CDC, 2001). The findings of this study underscore the importance of addressing homicide and other antecedent forms of nonfatal violence among Blacks for reducing the overall disparity in health between Blacks and Whites.

Influence on Life Expectancy

According to a recent CDC study (2001) using data from the National Center for Health Statistics for 1998, Whites lived 6.2 years longer than Blacks. Homicide accounted for 0.6 years (9.7 percent)

Figure 17.1
The public health approach to prevention

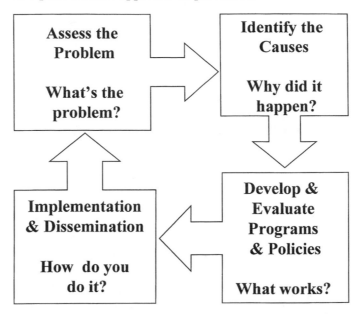

Figure 17.2
Number of years difference in LE between Blacks and Whites, by cause of death and sex, United States, 1998

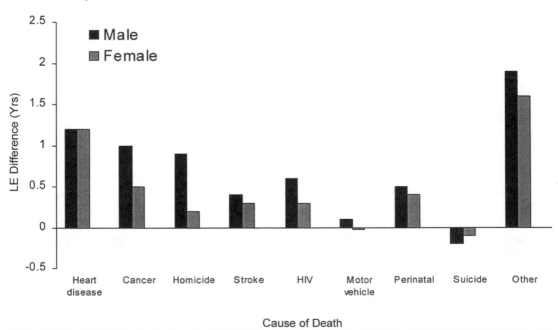

Source: National Center for Health Statistics, CDC Mortality Tapes, 1998.

Figure 17.3
Homicide rates by race and sex of victim, United States, 1990–1999

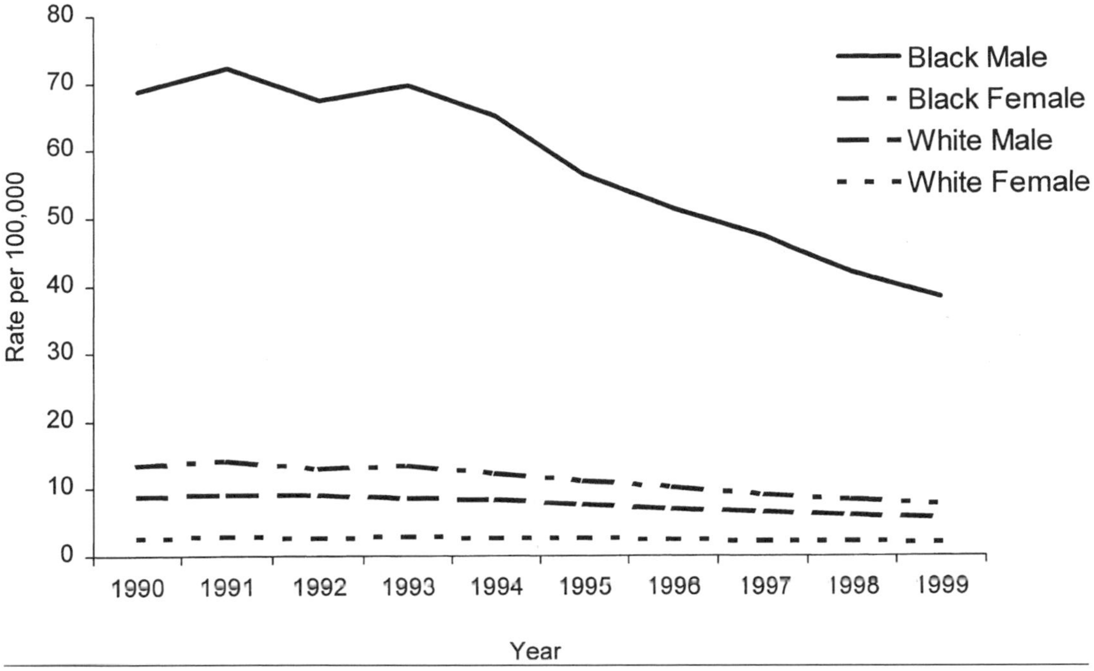

Note: Analysis include Black and White only.

Source: National Center for Health Statistics, CDC Mortality Tapes, 1998.

of the difference in life expectancy, despite accounting for less than 1 percent of the total deaths for the U.S. population in 1998. For males, homicide accounted for 0.9 years (14.1 percent) of the 6.4 years difference in life expectancy. For females, the contribution of homicide to the 4.4-year life expectancy gap was less, 0.2 years or 4.5 percent (Figure 17.2). Important reasons for the disproportionate influence of homicide on life expectancy are that homicide primarily affects persons in their second and third decade of life, whereas death from heart disease and cancer primarily affects persons in their fifth and sixth decade of life. In addition, the mortality burden from homicide on Blacks is much greater than for Whites. Death rates from homicide are sixfold greater for Blacks, as compared to Whites.

Age, Race, and Sex Differences

In 1999, there were 17,287 total homicide deaths in the United States. Of these deaths 6,339 (37 percent) were Black males and 1,435 (8 percent) were Black females. Throughout the period reported 1990–1999, Black males had the highest death rates, followed by Black females, White males, and White females, who had the lowest death rates (Figure 17.3).

Figure 17.4 shows homicide rates by age, race, and sex in 1999. The highest rates were among persons aged 15 to 34 years, with peak rates for the 15–24 and 25–29 year age groups, regardless of race or sex. However, the rates among young persons were particularly high for Black males. The mortality rate ratio for Black–White deaths among persons 20–29 years was 8:1 in 1990 and decreased only slightly to 7:1 in 1999.

The media have historically highlighted the extremely high rate of homicide found among young

Figure 17.4
Homicide rates by race and sex of victim, United States, 1999

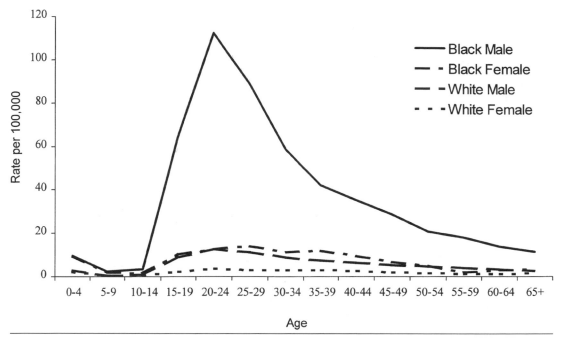

Note: Analysis include Black and White only.

Source: National Center for Health Statistics, CDC Mortality Tapes, 1998.

Black males. While this is alarming, it is important to recognize that homicide rates for Blacks are greater than those for Whites in nearly all age groups for both sexes. These include young adult females, infants of both sexes, and the elderly. Figure 17.4 shows that the Black–White homicide gap, although most pronounced at the young adult age range, extends throughout the life span. For example, Black children under 1 year of age and elderly Black persons ≥ 65 years become victims of homicide at rates three times those of their White counterparts.

Homicide by Law Enforcement Action

Another important type of homicide death is by legal intervention, or homicide by a law enforcement agent committed "in the line of duty." Legal intervention homicide, often referred to as justifiable homicide, accounts for a relatively small proportion of all homicide deaths each year. There were 379 legal intervention homicides in 1998, corresponding to 2 percent of the 18,272 homicide deaths that year. Blacks, who make up 13 percent of the U.S. population, accounted for 34 percent of these deaths. Overall, Blacks become victims of homicide due to law enforcement action at rates nearly four times those of Whites. Black males between the ages of 20 to 39 years have the highest rates.

The gap in legal intervention death rates between Blacks and Whites has decreased dramatically since the late 1960s, when the gap was about 10:1; however, the gap has remained constant over the past decade. Reasons for the closing of the gap may be related to improved training of police, community policing models, better research, more restrictive policies by police agencies regarding

Figure 17.5
Percentage of homicides in young adults (20–39 years) by relationship between victim and offender and by race,* United States, 1999

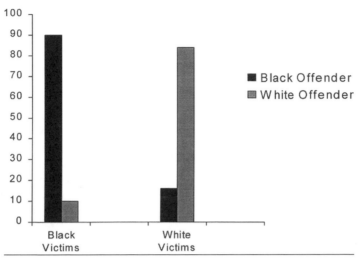

*In cases where race of both victim and offender is known.

Source: FBI Supplemental Homicide Report, 1999.

the use of lethal force, heightened community surveillance, and other factors. It is unclear why the fourfold mortality rate has remained stable over the past decade. However, this persistent and unexplained disparity does little to bolster relations between law enforcement and the Black community.

Firearms, Victim–Offender Relationships, and Other Patterns

Weapon choice plays a significant role in determining the outcome of a violent altercation. Firearms are obviously the more lethal method for the perpetration of violence compared to other commonly used methods (e.g., knife, club). The decade between 1983 and 1993 was marked by an epidemic of homicide and other violent behaviors. This upsurge in homicides was tied to an increased use of firearms in the commission of violent acts. Likewise, the decrease in homicide rates seen from 1994 to 1999 can be explained largely by a decline in the use of firearms in homicide and other violent acts. In 1999, 64 percent of all homicides involved the use of a firearm; the majority of these were committed with a handgun. Among Black victims, 73 percent involved the use of a firearm. This compares to 58 percent of all homicides among Whites.

Fatal violence is not usually a random act. It is more often the terminal end of an escalating interpersonal dispute that has occurred between two people who know each other. In 1999, about half (48 percent) of victims were killed by someone they knew: family members (10 percent) or acquaintances (38 percent). Because close contacts and intimates are more likely to be of the same racial/ethnic group, victims and offenders are usually the same race/ethnicity. Data in Figure 17.5 show that 91 percent of all young Black victims 20 to 39 years were killed by a Black offender. This compares with 84 percent of young White adults who were killed by White offenders. The media's emphasis on the phenomenon of "Black-on-Black" murder, while accurate, is misleading because it presents only a partial explanation of the same-race, same-ethnicity relationships that exist across all groups.

Nonfatal Assault Victimization

Similar to patterns seen for homicide, violent crime rates have continued to decline since 1994. There were approximately 7.4 million violent crimes experienced by Americans age 12 and older in 1999, according to a national survey by the U.S. Department of Justice (Rennison, 2000). This represented a 10 percent decline in the overall rate of violent crime (e.g., rape or sexual assault, aggravated assault, simple assault, and robbery) from 1998. However, Blacks did not experience a similar decline in their rates from 1998 and, along with males, continued to be victims of violent crime at rates greater than those of Whites and persons of other ethnic groups. The rate of violent victimization for Blacks remained stable at 42 per 1,000 persons in 1999. This rate is compared to 32 Whites, and 25 persons of other ethnic groups per 1,000 that were victimized during this time. The gap in violent victimization between Blacks and Whites was greatest for robbery (8 compared to 3 per 1,000 persons) and aggravated assault (11 compared to 6 per 1,000 persons).

In general, younger people had the highest rates of violent victimization. Among persons age 25 and older, rates decreased with age. About half (54 percent) of violent victims knew the offender(s). Other important patterns noted in the national survey was that violent victimization varied with income and marital status. Higher annual household incomes were associated with lower violent victimization rates, and those who never married were the most likely to be victims of violent crime (Rennison, 2000). These factors must be taken into account when explaining the higher rates of violent victimization among Blacks compared to other groups. For example, Blacks are more likely than Whites to have poorer households and are less likely to be married, as compared to Whites (see "Risk Factors").

School Violence

During the peak of the violence epidemic in the early 1990s, a number of myths emerged including the concern that there was a new violent breed of young people, "superpredators." These superpredators were depicted as youth, often Black males, responsible for, or capable of, random acts of violence without remorse. Such myths have been supplanted by public concern for the safety of schools following a series of high-profile school shootings that occurred in the late 1990s. Recent studies, however, have shown that schools are relatively safe when compared to rates of community violent victimization (Brener et al., 1999; Anderson et al., 2001).

Overall, there have been declines in fighting and weapon carrying among school-aged adolescents between 1991 and 1997, and fatal injuries on school campus (or at a school-associated event) is a rare event. However, despite these encouraging trends, Blacks (along with males and those attending urban schools) are at greater risk for being killed or injured at school than others. Blacks were more than five times likely to have been murdered in a school-associated event compared to Whites (Anderson et al., 2001). A similar pattern was seen for nonfatal, violence-related behavior among high school students. Blacks were twice as likely to carry a gun, be involved in a fight, and be threatened or injured with a weapon on school property compared to Whites (Brener et al., 1999).

Risk and Protective Factors for Interpersonal Violence

Violence in its various forms has had a long, enduring, and disproportionate impact on the African American community beginning with the enslavement of Africans in this country (Ani, 1994; Reese et al., 2002). More recently, the impact of this phenomenon has continued, although its manifestation has changed. Whereas historically violence had been perpetrated against Blacks by non-Blacks, the last several decades has seen a significant increase in Black-on-Black violence (Jenkins & Bell, 1994).

As discussed elsewhere in this volume, violence and interpersonal violence in particular have had a devastating impact on African American males. To illustrate this point, in 2000, there were 4,939 deaths in the United States for persons between the ages of 15 and 24. These deaths were caused by homicides, where 2,501, or 50 percent, of these victims were African American males. The rates of these homicides are more than eight times the representation of African Americans in this age cohort (CDC, 2002). What these data and other data reported here suggest is that efforts to reduce health disparities must also include efforts to reduce the premature mortality and morbidity caused by violence in the African American community.

In this section, we discuss some of what is known about risk and protective factors for interpersonal violence and the developmental nature of certain risk factors. In discussing risk factors for interpersonal violence, it is important to be clear at the outset that identifying certain behaviors, living conditions, or life experiences as a causal factor for either perpetrating, or being victimized by, violence cannot be determined at this time. Instead, the factors discussed here can increase the probability of being directly impacted by violence as either a victim, perpetrator, or both. Indeed, the vast majority of African American youth and young adults who are exposed to many of these risk factors never engage in aggressive or violent behavior. Equally important, ethnicity is not a risk factor for violence, as suggested by others, although it may be a risk "marker" for violence as discussed in the Surgeon General's Report on Youth Violence (USDHHS, 2001). Last, exposure to multiple risk factors can increase the cumulative risk that a person may be at for violence given the reciprocal nature of many risk factors (Jessor & Jessor, 1977).

Contextual Experiences.   Other factors important to accurately understanding "risk" for violence are embedded within contextual and developmental considerations and are specific to the individual, families, and peer groups (Bronfenbrenner, 1979; Berkman & Kawachi, 2000). By developmental, we mean that certain factors may have a more pronounced effect earlier in life (e.g., childhood) and other factors have a greater effect at later developmental stages (e.g., adolescence) (Dahlberg & Potter, 2001). There are also risk factors that generalize across different developmental stages. For example, exposure to, and witnessing, violence increases a person's risk for engaging in violent behavior regardless of developmental stage (Osofsky, 1999).

Again, to fully understand the influence of context and developmental stage, many of the risk factors discussed here, while typically manifesting in children and adolescents, have implications for different forms or violence (e.g., intimate partner violence, child abuse, and elder abuse) observed during adulthood (Menard, 2001). For example, in a longitudinal analysis of youth and their social experiences who were followed into adulthood, Menard (2001) found that early violent victimization and perpetration created heightened risk for later perpetration of violent behavior into adolescence and young adulthood.

As a full discussion of all the contextual and ecological factors affecting violence is beyond the scope of this volume, it is important to note that the influence of certain contextual factors in a given social ecology may explain some of the variance in the disproportionate experience of violence by African Americans. For example, recent census data indicate that despite representing only 12 percent of the U.S. population, African Americans represent 23 percent of the population living in poverty (U.S. Census Bureau, 1999). Ecological influences related to the occurrence of violence include income inequality, the availability of health and social support resources, underemployment, and social cohesion and capital (Kawachi & Berkman, 2000). Wilson (1987) describes in detail how such factors work together to create an ecology in which the poor and ethnic minorities are systemically put at risk for a number of adverse health outcomes including violence. As an example, Sampson et al. (1997) report data in which higher levels of social cohesion among neighbors were associated with lower levels of violence and conversely lower levels of social cohesion were associated with greater community violence. These investigators report that such findings can potentially be enhanced when structural inequalities within communities are simultaneously addressed, suggesting the interrelatedness of these factors. Such considerations are critical to accurately understanding violence and its occurrence given that beyond its impact on the broader African American community, violence has had a more concentrated impact on poor African Americans.

While difficult to quantify, we assert that the macro-level experience of discrimination as a function of ethnicity has influenced the experience of violence by African Americans. Some scholars have discussed how the stress associated with experiences of discrimination influences the overall quality of life for African Americans and their experience with health issues such as cardiovascular disease, mental health, alcoholism, and violence (Clark et al., 1999). Other stress-related factors that can cumulatively manifest at a macro or societal level for African Americans include underemployment and undereducation. Labor statistics have historically demonstrated higher rates of underemployment and income inequality among African Americans (Wilson, 1987, 1996). Additionally, recent empirical evidence has demonstrated a relationship between academic achievement and homicide. Specifically, African Americans' rates of academic achievement are related to their risk for homicide, revealing that lower levels of academic achievement have a positive relation to greater risk for homicidal victimization (Reese & Crosby, 2002).

The Surgeon General's Report on Youth Violence (see USDHHS, 2001) gives a thorough review of different risk factors and their relative effect on violence, although not specifically for African Americans. We highlight here some of the more prominent risk factors. The brief review offered here is organized around family- and individual-level factors given the preceding discussion of contextual factors.

Family and Developmental Experiences.   As discussed earlier, developmental stage is an important consideration to understanding individual risk factors. For example, early involvement in aggressive behavior (Farrington, 1991) and early evidence of belief systems supportive of aggressive behavior (Guerra et al., 1995) have a greater impact on younger children than adolescents and young adults. Longitudinal studies have also demonstrated that youth who engage in aggressive behavior at younger ages tend to be more likely to persist in that behavior and go on to escalate to more violent behavior than youth who initiated such behavior at older ages (Thornberry et al., 1995). For adolescents, delinquent peer groups (e.g., gangs) can create risk for aggressive and violent behavior (Dahlberg & Potter, 2001; Howell, 1998). In addition, adolescents who experience isolation and rejection from their peers can be at greater risk for violence (USDHHS, 2001).

There are a multitude of family risk factors for violence, many of which diminish in their influence once young people reach adolescence, where peer groups have a greater influence (see Reese et al., 2000). Among the more influential risk factors include parents who are engaged in antisocial and criminal behavior and model that behavior in front of their children. Additionally, parents who use harsh and inconsistent discipline practices (Wells & Rankin, 1988) create greater risk for violent behavior in their children. The effect of harsh or violent discipline practices is that it can teach youth that the way to handle problems is through the use of force and violence. These are behaviors that youth subsequently model in their interactions with peers and later in life without intervention. Child abuse and neglect have also been demonstrated to influence aggressive and acting-out behavior in youth (USDHHS, 1998). Families whose socioeconomic position is characterized by poverty can be at greater risk for violence, although the income inequality and disproportionate poverty observed in the African American community have historical antecedents in U.S. society (Wilson, 1987).

Empirical investigations on protective factors for violence have been limited, although this area of violence prevention has been identified as a priority area for prevention research and practice (USDHHS, 2001). Some have reasoned that protective factors effectively represent the opposite of known risk factors while simultaneously suggesting such explanations can be overly simplistic. While a reasonable and attractive hypothesis, this argument lacks empirical support and the fact that significant numbers of youth and adults are exposed to a variety of risk factors and never engage in violent behaviors suggests there may be other processes at work. In the absence of empirical evidence, what are offered here are factors believed to provide a "buffer" against violence perpetration and victimization.

At an individual level, attitudes informed by positive cognitive processes and social experiences can be a direct mediator of behavior and have shown potential to be a protective factor against violence (USDHHS, 2001). Specifically, having an attitude unsupportive of violence and other delinquent behavior can decrease the influence of other risk factors. Similarly, associating with peers with similar prosocial attitudes can serve a protective function. For example, Jagers (1997) suggests that attitude toward violence and other risk behaviors is influenced by socialization. Also for African Americans, socialization that occurs in a milieu affirms the cultural integrity of people of African descent, which in turn promotes nonviolent attitudes (see also Jessor et al., 1998). Being female would appear to serve some protective function, considering that males, particularly African American males, are disproportionately victimized by violence.

Family-related protective factors include positive and nurturing relationships. People living in families characterized by emotional support and fair treatment tend to have a greater repertoire of effective coping and problem-solving skills (Masten & Coatsworth, 1998). In families where parents model prosocial attitudes and behaviors for their children, there is a higher likelihood of those behaviors also manifesting in children, particularly young children. Schools and communities in which people feel safe, experience a positive attachment, and have adequate health and social resources also tend to provide a buffer against violence.

Preventive Interventions

Interventions that have demonstrated sustained empirical evidence in preventing violence are limited and have largely focused on youth. In addition, there has been an emphasis on school-based interventions in part due to a decade of rare, albeit tragic, high-profile, school-associated shootings and violent assaults. Recent national studies highlight the infrequency of school and school-associated homicides and serious assault when compared to rates of community homicide and assault rates. These studies provide data demonstrating that less than 1 percent of all youth homicides occur at schools or at school-associated events (Kachur et al., 1996; Anderson et al., 2001).

Preventive interventions tend to be organized as either *universal, indicated,* and *targeted,* with universal interventions having a *primary prevention orientation.* Indicated or *secondary prevention* approaches are oriented toward persons who have shown some evidence of being at risk for violence or other health-compromising behavior. Targeted or *tertiary interventions* focused on persons who have demonstrated clear evidence of the targeted risk behavior or a history of such behavior. The lines of demarcation in these types of interventions are not always clear as some intervention can have elements of each prevention model. Additionally, interventions can vary in their focus. For example, some interventions target individual-level behavior, others focus on changing a social ecology in an effort to influence behavior, and still others take a combined person-in-context approach wherein the focus is on the individual and the environment. There is some evidence that person-in-context approaches may be more effective in influencing behavior and attitude (see Catalano et al., 1998; see also USDHHS, 2001 for a complete review). A brief overview is offered here as examples of these interventions. Also, where available, evidence is presented of the effectiveness of these interventions with African Americans.

One example of a primary prevention program that encompasses aspects of secondary prevention is the Home Nurse Visitation Program, where the focus is on the individual within the context of family ecology. Visitation programs send nurses to the homes of pregnant women where there is reason to think the pregnancy may be at risk for developmental challenges, frequently a precursor to behavior difficulties. Home visitation programs provide health care and health education to expectant mothers. The goals of these programs include improving health outcomes for infants, reducing the likelihood of child maltreatment and improving family functioning (Olds et al., 1998). The program is designed to serve low-income women considered at risk and experiencing their first pregnancy. Nurses work with mothers during the pregnancy and the first two years of the child's life to address concerns affecting the child, while simultaneously helping the mother develop her coping and problem-solving skills. In one longitudinal, evaluation study with 1,100 participants where 92 percent were African American women, the results were revealing. The results showed significantly fewer reports of child maltreatment from those in the study or program, as compared to women not participating in the program. Mothers who reported more social support also report lower rates of smoking (in Olds et al., 1998). The children of these women also had significantly fewer arrests, lower rates of drug use, fewer sexual partners, and fewer behavior problems at age 15 when compared to nonparticipants.

On the other end of the continuum is multisystemic therapy (MST), a tertiary or targeted intervention focusing on youth engaged in delinquent behaviors, including aggressive and violent behavior. This intervention attempts to affect the social-ecology of the youth in the form of the family by building on the strengths of the family while also attending to those areas that need improvement (Henggeler et al., 1998). The treatment model of this program is based on empirically evaluated interventions and takes individually based and family-based interventions to construct a treatment approach inclusive of the individual needs of the youth as they exist within the context of a variety of family constellations (e.g., single parent, two-parent) and social condition (e.g., poverty). Evaluations have been with ethnically diverse youth engaged in a variety of delinquent behavior, including violence. In one four-site-randomized control trial, results showed significant decreases in arrests, out-of-home placements, and improved family functioning. At two- and four-year follow-up, participants showed sustained effects of the intervention (Henggeler et al., 1998).

SELF-DIRECTED VIOLENCE

The Epidemiology of Suicide and Related Behaviors

Injury from self-directed violence, including suicidal behavior, is a major public health problem in the United States (Institute of Medicine, 2002) and throughout the world (WHO, 1996; Krug et al., 2002). In the United States, suicide has ranked among the 12 leading causes of death since 1975. In 1999, suicide was the eleventh leading cause of death overall in the United States, responsible for 29,199 deaths; it was the third leading cause of death among people aged 15 to 24 years; fourth among people aged 25 to 44 years; and eighth among those aged 45 to 64 years (Hoyert et al., 2001). Though suicide is a problem among youth and young adults, overall rates of death due to suicide continue to be highest among persons aged 65 years and older (Stevens et al., 1999).

The number of completed suicides reflects only a small portion of the impact of suicidal behavior. Many more people are hospitalized due to nonfatal suicide attempts than are fatally injured. Additionally, an even greater number of patients who are treated in ambulatory settings are not treated at all for injuries due to suicidal acts when compared to those patients who are hospitalized (Rosenberg et al., 1987). The comparative descriptions of suicidal ideation and behavior show some important differences; for example, the rate of suicide in males is higher than that in females, but studies of suicidal thoughts and suicide attempts routinely show females with higher rates (USPHS, 2001). Prior studies have shown a high prevalence of nonfatal suicidal behavior among adults. The National Hospital Ambulatory Medical Care Survey estimated 387,000 visits to U.S. hospital Emergency Departments for self-directed violence in 2000 (McCaig & Ly, 2001). Other research indicates that over 70 percent of people who attempt suicide never seek health services (Diekstra, 1987). As a result, prevalence figures based on health records substantially underestimate the societal burden of suicide.

Injuries and deaths resulting from self-directed violent behaviors represent a substantial drain on the economic, social, and health resources of the nation. The human and economic costs of suicide are enormous; one study estimated the total economic burden of suicide in the United States in 1995 to be $111.3 billion (Miller et al., 1999). Compounding these costs are the unquantifiable costs of loss of life and the emotional trauma experienced by surviving family, friends, and communities that are affected by each person's attempted or completed suicide (Crosby & Sacks, 2002).

Despite the widespread impact of self-directed violence in the United States, the problem has frequently been viewed as primarily a problem affecting European American males (Davis, 1979) and the affluent (Earls et al., 1990). Among non-European Americans, only the incidence of suicide among Native Americans has been widely noted (USDHHS, 1986). There are several reasons for studying suicidal behavior among a variety of minority populations in the United States. One, it is a leading cause of premature death and injury within these populations. Two, since European American suicide deaths represent over 90 percent of the U.S. national total (Kachur et al., 1995), the national rates and many of the risk and protective factors studied reflect patterns among that population and not necessarily those of African Americans. In this section we characterize the problem of self-directed violence and its prevention among African Americans using the public health approach.

Problem Description

The total number of suicides among African Americans (unless otherwise noted, figures cited for African Americans represent those for non-Hispanic African Americans) in the United States increased slightly by 2.4 percent during the study period, from 1,879 in 1990 to 1,924 in 1999. However, the age-adjusted suicide rate for this group declined (17.8 percent) over the same period. In 1990, the age-adjusted suicide rate was 7.15 deaths per 100,000 population (all rates are per 100,000 population). The rate peaked at 7.21 in 1994, then fell to 5.88 by 1999.

Suicide was the sixteenth leading cause of death, overall, in 1999 for African Americans and was among the 10 leading causes of death for several age groups in this population (Table 17.1). For African Americans aged 20–29, suicide was the 3rd leading cause of death behind homicide and unintentional injury. African American adolescents and young adults have the highest number and the highest rate of suicide of any age group of African Americans.

Years of potential life lost before the age of 75 (YPLL-75), which measures premature mortality, is another way of defining the burden of a health problem on the population. By calculating the years difference between the individual's death and age 75, this technique weighs more heavily those conditions that cause the death of children, adolescents, and young adults. In terms of YPLL-75, suicide was the tenth leading cause of YPLL for African Americans in 1999. It accounted for 73,667 years of potential life lost, which represents approximately 1.8 percent of YPLL-75 for all causes of death and was preceded in rank by the following causes in order from 1 to 9: heart disease, cancer, unintentional injury, conditions of the perinatal period, homicide, AIDS, stroke, diabetes mellitus, and congenital anomalies.

Age Trends

Among those aged 15–39 years, rates declined from 1990 to 1991 (10.5 to 10.2), then increased from 1991 to 1994 (10.2 to 11.3), and have declined over recent years 1994 to 1999 (11.3 to 8.8).

Table 17.1

Ten leading causes of death among African Americans by age groups, United States, 1999

rank	<1	1-4	5-9	10-14	15-19	20-24	25-34	35-44	45-54	55-64	65+	Total
1	Short gestation 1836	Uninten. injuries 428	Uninten. injuries 392	Uninten. injuries 309	Homicide 1117	Homicide 1635	Homicide 2122	Heart disease 3506	Malig. neopl. 7749	Malig. neopl. 12322	Heart disease 53883	Heart disease 77713
2	Congenital anomalies 994	Homicide 151	Malignant neoplasms 84	Malignant neoplasms 95	Uninten. injuries 764	Uninten. injuries 930	Uninten. injuries 1738	AIDS 3154	Heart disease 7448	Heart disease 11346	Malignant neoplasm 37077	Malig. neopl. 61409
3	SIDS 827	Cogen. anomalies 137	Homicide 65	Homicide 80	Suicide 176	Suicide 287	AIDS 1479	Malig. neopl. 3049	AIDS 2057	Cerebrova. accid. 2269	Cerebrova. accid. 13750	Cerebrova.a ccid. 18731
4	Maternal preg. Complic. 486	Heart Dis. 49	Congenital anomalies 49	Congenital anomalies 56	Malig. neopl. 136	Heart Disease 208	Heart Disease 913	Uninten. injuries 2245	Uninten. injuries 1903	Diabetes mell. 2136	Diabetes mell. 7757	Uninten. injuries 12533
5	Resp. distress 362	Malignant neoplasms 47	Heart Dis. 32	Chronic Low Resp Dis 47	Heart Disease 128	Malig. neopl. 178	Malig. neopl. 660	Homicide 1305	Cerebro. accid. 1662	Chronic Low Resp Dis 1085	Chronic Low Resp Dis 5620	Diab. mell. 11830
6	Placenta Cord memb. 349	Pneumonia & Influ 40	AIDS 26	Heart Dis. 45	Congenital anomalies 42	AIDS 109	Suicide 497	Cerebro. accid. 808	Diabetes mellitus 1219	Unintent. injuries 1047	Nephritis 4655	Chronic Low Resp Dis 7840
7	Uninten. inj. 103	Perinatal period 29	Chronic Low Resp Dis 19	Suicide 29	Chronic Low Resp Dis 36	Anemias 51	Diabetes mellitus 160	Diabetes mellitus 502	Liver disease 905	Nephritis 879	Pneum. & Influ. 4253	AIDS 7751
8	Bacterial sepsis 249	Anemias 20	Anemias 17	Anemias 16	Anemias 23	Chronic Low Resp Dis 42	Cerebro. accid. 149	Liver disease 453	Nephritis 615	Septicemia 716	Septicemia 4006	Homicide 7536
9	Atelectasis 179	Chronic Low Resp Dis 18	Benign neoplasms 12	AIDS 15	AIDS 21	Congenital anomalies 40	Chronic Low Resp Dis 140	Suicide 430	Homicide 557	Liver disease 691	Hypertens. 2612	Nephritis 6659
10	Circulatory system dis. 175	AIDS 17	Pneumonia & Influ. 8	Cerebrova. accident 12	Cerebro. accid. 18	Pneum. & Influ. 35	Anemias 139	Nephritis 310	Chronic Low Resp Dis 556	AIDS 613	Uninten. injuries 2514	Pneum. & Influ. 5794

During the same period, 1990–1999, rates among middle-aged adults aged 40–64 years showed a decline (7.8 to 5.9). Among the oldest age groups, aged 65 and older, the rates also showed a general decline, 7.5 in 1991 to 5.7 in 1999.

Age-Specific Suicide Rates

During the 1990s, as in previous decades, young adults aged 20–39 years had the highest rates, and children, the lowest. Suicide rates for several other age groups changed substantially, however. Similar to national rates among older adolescents, rates for African American adolescents aged 15–19 increased during the 1980s and early 1990s. However, rates for African American youth demonstrated a sharper increase than national rates during 1981–1994, rising by 174.3 percent (from 3.5 to 9.6); since then, 1994–1999, they have declined by 38.5 percent (9.6 to 5.9).

The rates among the majority of African American young and middle-aged adults followed a similar pattern during the 1990s. The rates peaked in the early to mid-1990s usually 1992, 1993 or 1994, then declined through 1999, the exception being those aged 35–39 years, who followed the pattern except for a slight increase from 1998 to 1999.

Among older adults, aged 65 years and older, there was more fluctuation in suicide rates. This may have been due to the small number of deaths due to suicide; the range was from approximately 60 deaths among those aged 65–69 years to about 20 among the 80–84 age group and the 85 and older age group. However, the general pattern for these groups was a decline from 1990 to 1999. The pattern for those aged 70–74 years demonstrated a decline from 1990 to 1992 (8.6 to 6.4), increase from 1992 to 1995 (6.4 to 8.7), then a decline from 1995 to 1999 (8.7 to 5.1).

Race/Ethnicity and Age Group–Specific Suicide Rates

There are five major race/ethnicity groups examined in this study: European American non-Latino, African American non-Latino, Latino, Asian-Pacific Islander, and Native American. The last group includes both American Indians and Alaskan Natives. Examining the patterns of suicide rates by age group along with race/ethnicity demonstrates two general patterns (Figure 17.6). Among three groups, European American non-Latinos, Latinos, and Asian-Pacific Islanders, the rates are low among children, have a sharp rise during adolescence and young adulthood, remain relatively level during middle-age, then show the highest rates among those aged 65 years and older. In contrast, suicide rates among the other two groups, African Americans non-Latinos and Native Americans, are low among children but have the highest rates among adolescents and young adults; the rates then decline for middle-aged adults and have relatively low rates among those aged 65 years and older.

In each of the racial and ethnic groups, suicide rates were higher for males than for females, but the male to female ratio differs among these groups. In 1999, the age-adjusted suicide rate for European American non-Latino males (20.3) was four times higher than the rate for European American non-Latino females. Among African Americans non-Latinos, the rate was six times higher for males (10.8) than for females (1.7). Among Native American non-Latinos, the male to female ratio was 2.7 to 1 (21.6 and 5.2, respectively), and among Asian or Pacific Islander Non-Latinos, it was 4.2 to 1 (10.1 and 3.7, respectively). Finally, among Latino groups, suicide was five times more common for males (10.6) than for females (1.9).

Marital Status

Suicide rates differ by marital status among persons aged 25 years or older. In 1999, for males, married persons had the lowest rates (9.5), followed by those who were divorced (16.9), then never-

Figure 17.6

Suicide rates by ethnicity and age group, United States, 1995–1999

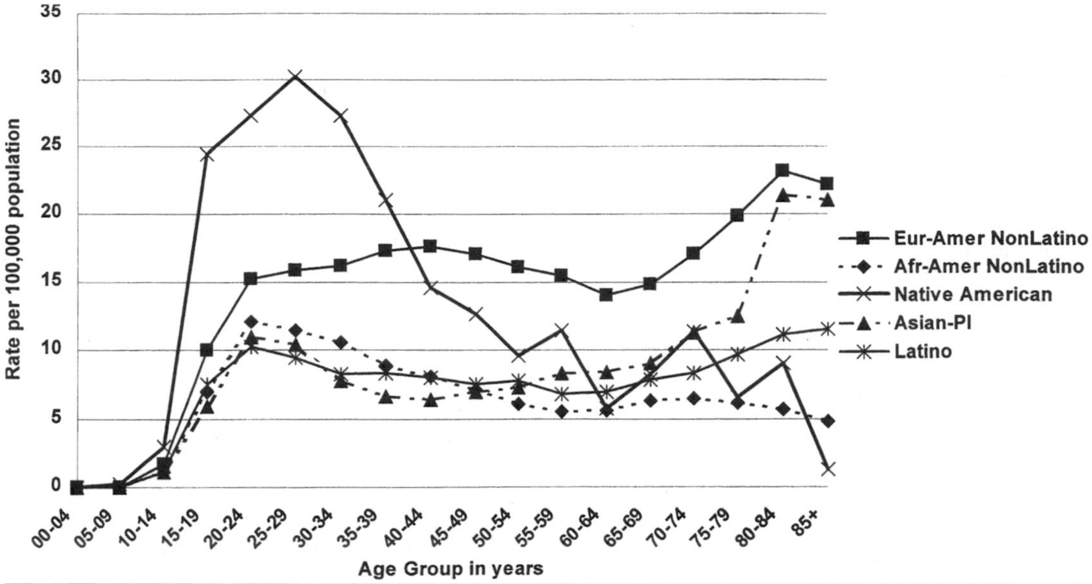

Source: Centers for Disease Control and Prevention (CDC) mortality data, 2002.

married individuals (17.1), with the highest rates among widowed persons (20.2). During the same year for females, the lowest rates were among those widowed (1.5) and married (1.5), followed by never-married (2.6), and the highest rates occurred among divorced persons (3.3).

Method of Suicide

Firearms were the leading method used in suicides among African Americans in the United States during the 1980s and early 1990s. Firearms were the method used in 57.8 percent of all suicides in 1999. The next most commonly reported methods were suffocation (19.3 percent), poisoning (9.9 percent), and falls (4.0 percent). Other, or unspecified means, accounted for 13 percent of all suicides in 1999. The methods of suicide in 1999 varied by sex. Among African American males, firearms accounted for the majority of suicides (61.8 percent), followed by suffocation (20.2 percent), poisoning (6.9 percent), then other methods. Firearms were also the principal means of suicide used by African American females (35.7 percent), followed by poisoning (26.5 percent), suffocation (14.6 percent), then other methods.

Geographic Variation

Examining age-adjusted suicide rates for the period 1990–1998 varied substantially across states, from 13.2 in Nevada and New Mexico, to 5.0 in New Jersey (Figure 17.7). There were several states (Alaska, Hawaii, Idaho, Maine, Montana, New Hampshire, North Dakota, South Dakota, Utah, Vermont, and Wyoming) with a small number of suicides among African Americans. The rates in these states may be unstable and should be used with caution. The age-adjusted U.S. average suicide rate

Figure 17.7
Age-adjusted suicide rates among African Americans by state, United States, 1990–1998

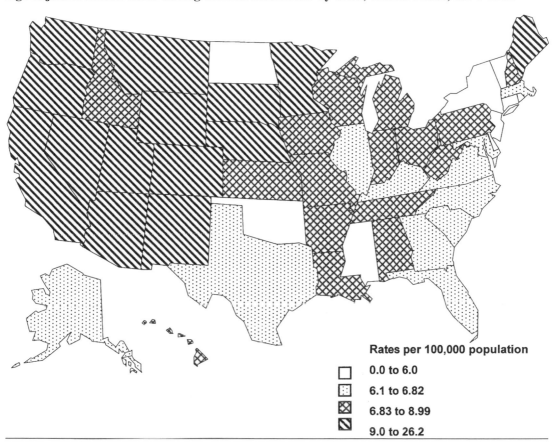

Rates per 100,000 population

☐ 0.0 to 6.0

⊡ 6.1 to 6.82

⊠ 6.83 to 8.99

◩ 9.0 to 26.2

Source: Centers for Disease Control and Prevention (CDC) mortality data, 2002.

for non-Latino African Americans was 6.8. Suicide rates in the western states were generally higher than those in the South and Northeast.

Morbidity

Only within the past 20 years have nationally representative statistics been available for suicidal thoughts and behavior among adolescents in the United States. Since 1990, one assessment tool that has been used is the Youth Risk Behavior Surveillance System (YRBSS). The YRBSS is a school-based measure of health risk behaviors (including suicidal thoughts and behavior) among high school students, using a self-report questionnaire. Since 1991, the survey has been conducted biennially. In each of the surveys, students answered four questions about seriously considering suicide; making a suicide plan; attempting suicide; and making a medically treated suicide attempt during the 12 months preceding the survey. In 2001, African American high school students reported the following: seriously considered suicide: males 9.2 percent, females 17.2 percent; made a suicide plan: males 7.5 percent, females 13.0; attempted suicide: males 7.5 percent, females 9.8 percent; attempted suicide which required medical attention: males 3.6 percent, females 3.1 percent (Grunbaum et al., 2002).

Figure 17.8
Overlap of spheres of influence for suicidal behavior

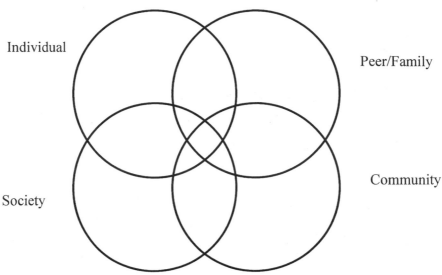

The National Electronic Injury Surveillance System (NEISS), developed by the Consumer Product Safety Commission (CPSC), was adapted in July 2000 to include all types and external causes of nonfatal injuries treated in U.S. hospital Emergency Departments (EDs). The NEISS has a nationally representative sample of U.S. hospital EDs. Overall, self-inflicted injury rates were highest among adolescents and young adults, particularly females. Most (90 percent) self-inflicted injuries were the result of poisoning or being cut/pierced with a sharp instrument, and 60 percent were probable suicide attempts. During 2000, an estimated 22,703 African Americans were treated in the United States for nonfatal self-inflicted injuries (rate of 64.3 per 100,000 population). Among African American females, 12,575 were seen for these injuries (rate of 67.8 per 100,000); for males, 10,128 (rate of 60.4 per 100,000). These difference were not statistically significant (Ikeda et al., 2002).

Risk and Protective Factors for Suicide

Similar to other violent injuries and many health behaviors, self-directed violence results from an interaction of risk and protective factors that exist on multiple levels. One way of examining these factors is by using the social-ecological model. In our review of suicidal risk and protective factors for African Americans, we divide the factors into four interrelated levels: societal; community (e.g., school, neighborhood, religious institution); close interpersonal (e.g., family, peer group); and individual (Figure 17.8). These factors are dynamic, and their influence depends on when they occur in a person's life and under what particular circumstances. Some of the following factors have been empirically tested among African Americans, but many are only theorized to have a connection to suicidal behavior (Table 17.2).

Prevention Strategies

The majority of strategies for preventing suicidal behavior have traditionally focused on high-risk individuals using a clinical mental health model. However, an interdisciplinary prevention model has been increasingly utilized for the prevention of suicidal behavior. This model focuses attention on

Table 17.2
Risk and protective factors for suicidal behaviors among African Americans

Level	Factor	Description	Empirical (E) or theoretical (T)	Risk (R), Protective (P), Uncertain (U)
Societal				
	Availability of Lethal Means	Ease of access to highly lethal object (e.g., firearm, toxic gas or chemical, elevated place) by vulnerable individual (Joe and Kaplan 2001; Griffith and Bell, 1989)	E	R
	Racism and Discrimination	May contribute to hopelessness or alternatively survival solidarity (Earls, Escobar and Manson, 1990; Davis, 1980)	T	U
	Media Influence/ Exposure	May cause vulnerable persons to imitate destructive behavior (Poussaint and Alexander, 2000; Williams, Molock, & Kimbrough)	T	R
	Geography	State variation in suicide rates shows higher rates in Western region (Hawkins, Crosby & Hammett, 1994; Lester, 1991)	E	R
	Utilization of or access to mental health services	Lack of access or avoidance of mental health workers or staff has shown differing effect (Kung, Liu & Juon, 1998; Borowsky et al., 2001; Nisbet, 1996)	E	U
	Unemployment	Decreases social ties to others (Seiden, 1972; Lester, 1991)	E	R
	Acculturation/ Alienation/Social mobility	Recent historical and demographic developments have resulted in increased mobility, decreased social cohesion and increased psychological vulnerability (Wilson, 1987; Gibbs, 1988; Anderson, 1990)	T	R
Community				
	Religiosity/Spirituality	Belief that suicide is morally wrong factor may also offer social support and social integration (Early & Akers, 1993; Robbins, West & Murphy, 1977)	E	P
	Incarceration	Increased rates among incarcerated individuals, this population also has disproportional representation of African American males (Haycock 1989)	T	R
	Social support	Traditional reliance on collective efficacy (Swanson and Breed, 1976; Juon and Ensminger,1997)	E	P
	Social isolation	Loss of attachments can lead to vulnerability to adverse health outcomes (Hickman, 1984; Smith and Carter, 1986 ; Willis et al., 2002; Baker 1994)	E	R
Close Interpersonal				
	Marital Status	Marriage has a protective effect (Davis and Short, 1977; Stack 1996)	E	P
	Family dysfunction	Marital discord, parental neglect, or early childhood loss of or separation from parent/caretaker (Kaslow et al, 2000; Lyon, Benoit and O'Donnell, 2000; Marietta 1999; Richters & Martinez 1993)	E	R
	Family cohesion	Perceptions of family adjustment and attachment are especially protective for adolescents (Borowsky, Ireland, and Resnick, 2001; Topol and Reznikopff, 1982; Nisbet 1996)	E	P
	Exposure to interpersonal violence	Witnessing or being victimized by interpersonal violence (Price, Dake and Kucharewski, 2001; Richters and Martinez 1993)	E	R
	Family history of suicidal behavior	Social learning may promote imitative behavior (Pfeffer, 1989; Roy, 1983).	T	R
	Victim of child maltreatment	Long-term effects associated with health problems (Dube et al, 2001)	T	R
	Flexibility of family roles	May allow for improved adjustment to adverse circumstances (Gibbs, 1997)	T	P
Individual				
	Age	Adolescents and young adults have highest rates (CDC, 1998; Frederick, 1984; Rutledge, 1990)	E	R
	Sex	Males have higher rate of completed suicide, females have higher rates of nonfatal behavior (Kachur, Potter, James, and Powell, 1995; Grunbaum et al, 2002; Ikeda R et al, 2002)	E	U
	Alcohol or other substance use disorders	Substances vary including alcohol, heroin, cocaine (Frederick et al, 1973; Smart 1980; Lester & Beck, 1975; Murphy, Wetzel and Robinson 1992; Borowsky, Ireland and Resnick, 2001; Jones 1997; Juon and Ensminger 1997; Marzuk, Tardiff & Leon 1992)	E	R
	Psychiatric disorders	Disorders include anxiety disorder, conduct disorder, personality disorder, depression, post traumatic stress disorders (PTSD), schizophrenia and panic disorders (Feldman & Wilson, 1997; Frierson and Lipman, 1990; Kirk and Zucker, 1979; Rotheram-Borus, 1993; Walter and Vaughan, 1995; Palmer, 2001; Poussaint & Alexander, 2000)	E	R
	Aggression & Delinquency	Some at-risk populations may share factors related to self-directed and interpersonal violence (Hendin, 1978)	T	R
	Socio-economic status (SES) (e.g., education, income)	Studies differ some indicate higher SES are at increased risk, other studies show the opposite (Lester, 1991; Stack, 1998)	E	U
	Hopelessness	Lack of prospect for the future has been shown to be a strong risk factor for suicidal behavior (Kiev and Anumonye, 1976; Durant, Mercy, Simon, and Hammond, 1998)	E	R
	Witness or victim of interpersonal violence	Intimate partner victimization increases risk for non-fatal suicidal behavior among adult African-American females (Thompson, Kaslow, and Kingree, 2002)	E	R

how certain populations are chosen and employs the terms universal, selective, and indicated to refer to the groups (Gordon, 1983).

Universal strategies, including population-based programs, may have a greater impact on decreasing mortality over those focused on individuals. They may be able to lower the risk of adverse health outcome for an entire population and potentially prevent more cases than strategies that target a small number of high-risk persons (Rosenman, 1998). Universal strategies can include media campaigns (Shanahan et al., 2000; Reinholdt et al., 2000; Washington State Department of Health, 1995) that seek to provide information, modify negative social norms, or create an environmental change. Other prevention strategies aim to reduce access to means, such as firearms (Loftin et al., 1991; Ludwig & Cook, 2000); self-poisoning (Gunnel et al., 1997; Bowles, 1995); gas (Kreitman, 1976; Marzuk et al., 1992) or high places (Marzuk et al., 1992).

Some efforts have lowered access to proximal risk factors for suicidal behavior like alcohol misuse (Birckmayer & Hemenway, 1999). Universal programs can also include modification of potentially hazardous portrayal's of suicide (primarily news) by media (Sonneck et al., 1994; Annenberg Public Policy Center et al., 2002). Many school-based programs have used a universal approach with awareness and skills training projects (CDC, 1992; White & Jodoin, 1998). These programs are designed to educate the participants about suicide and available resources and teach various skills (e.g., decision-making or social skills).

Several types of strategies operating at the selective level have been used for suicide prevention. Examples include screening programs that identify and assess at-risk groups (CDC, 1992). Programs using a gatekeeper training model instruct participants to identify and refer persons at risk for suicidal behavior. Those who are trained can be school staff, community members, or physicians (White & Jodoin, 1998; Rutz et al., 1989). Another type of selected program offers support and skills training (Eggert et al., 1995). Hot lines and crisis centers may also be categorized as selective. There are scant studies that have evaluated these strategies, and those that have reach inconsistent findings (Mishara & Daigle, 2001).

Although several intervention strategies can be used, most notable among these strategies include clinical or medical interventions (Haynes, 1991; American Academy of Child and Adolescent Psychiatry, 2001); family support training; skill-building support groups for high-risk individuals (Thompson et al., 2001); case management; and referral resources for crisis intervention and treatment (Linehan, 1997). Included in this category would be programs that address suicidal behavior prevention among those who are incarcerated (Hayes, 1995).

Several organizations have utilized integrated approaches. While these are challenging to design, execute, and evaluate, as activities occur on multiple levels of prevention, they may have the best chance of success (Litts et al., 1999; Serna et al., 1998). There are also programs designed to address other health problems that have potential for reducing suicidal behavior. These programs, though not "suicide-specific," may apply to a range of "suicide-inclusive" factors (e.g., factors that may relate to several health issues like early antisocial behavior, substance abuse, or child maltreatment) (Durlak & Wells, 1997; National Health and Medical Research Council and Department of Health and Aged Care, 1999). Interventions for suicide-inclusive factors have the promise to bring a wider range of health benefits, in that they may reduce more than one adverse outcome.

Despite the recent attention African Americans suicide has received, there are few interventions that address the phenomenon specifically in that population. The few programs that exist have been primarily community-based, meaning that individuals in the community have control and ownership of the program. One such program was carried out by the Youth Mediation Corps (YMC), based in Jamaica, New York. The program focuses on providing resources to community youth to address suicide and had two goals: (1) to assess the problem of African American male suicide and (2) to inform the community about the rising rate of suicide in the African American community.

SUMMARY

Self-directed violence is one of the leading causes of death and disability among African Americans, especially youth, and is an important public health problem. Self-directed violence is a complex event that warrants significantly more surveillance and etiological research to inform the development of prevention programs for African Americans. By identifying patterns of suicide and suicidal behavior specific to African Americans, progress can be made in reducing its occurrence. The public health approach provides an organized way for developing, implementing, and evaluating suicide prevention efforts among African Americans.

Dissemination and Implementation

Improving the health of our communities in general and African American communities in particular relies on people determining that health issues are a high priority. The greater the support for a given health issue and related health policy, the better its opportunity to receive the necessary resources to be effective. The shaping of effective health policy involves three areas: the development of a scientific base, the development of political will, and the development of social strategy (Richmond & Kotelchuk, 1983). Dissemination involves informing the public about the importance of self-directed and interpersonal violence as a public health problem, its risk and protective factors, and the preventability of the problem. A public that understands the issue is more likely to mobilize the political will to deal with the topic (USPHS, 1999). Communities and organizations working in the African American community have called for, or developed, policies to address self-directed and interpersonal violence, demonstrating that in some measure violent victimization and perpetration are garnering attention (WHO, 1996; USPHS, 2001; Metha et al., 1998).

Implementation refers to widespread adoption of evaluated programs or the core elements of effective prevention practice. In order for incidents of violence to dramatically decline in the African American community, organizations need to have information on what is known about violence as well as evaluated programs. Health communication and education effort help inform the work of policymakers, public health practitioners and researchers, and our constituents. Such communications assist in making better decisions about which programs or elements of programs can be implemented and integrated for the participants (Satcher, 1998; Potter et al., 1995).

CONCLUSIONS

Suggesting that interpersonal and self-directed violence is a serious public health problem in the African American community is an understatement. Beyond the obvious public health burden that morbidity and mortality from intentional injury represent, its implications for the overall health and future of the African American community exceeds the space afforded here. Besides the obvious cost of violence including years of potential life lost, disability, health care, and other related costs, other costs have impacted the stability, cohesion, and further development of the African American community. Including among these costs are the numbers of men available to their children and families; lost economic productivity; and lost potential leadership in community and civic arenas.

Efforts to reduce the impact of violence go well beyond the reach of school or community-based prevention efforts. As this chapter has pointed out, many of the most critical factors influencing the occurrence of violence are embedded within the social, economic, and educational structures of our society, particularly as they influence the African American community. To effect meaningful and lasting change, it will be necessary to cause change within these structures, change that will require a societal commitment, human and fiscal resources, and sustained effort. For example, observation of trend data reflects that during the economic prosperity of the 1990s, unemployment of African Americans was at an all-time low; at the same time there was a downward trend in homicide and serious assaults among African Americans (Blumstein & Wallman, 2000). During this same period, there were also increases in the numbers of African American youth completing high school and going on to college. While the empirical relations between these more macro-level variables and violence have not been examined in great detail, there is promising research in this area (see Reese & Crosby, 2002).

Methodologically, emergent disciplines such as social epidemiology are needed to appropriately contextualize violence and focus violence prevention efforts. In addition, there is greater need for longitudinal studies that examine the sustained effects of "packaged" violence prevention programs. The continued positive effects of some of these programs at six-month and one-year intervals are important and encouraging yet insufficient to attest to their lasting impact in the most underresourced and affected communities. Equally important to evaluations of violence prevention programs is the need to factor in health economic data. During periods of economic unrest, fiscal allocations for prevention programs often decrease, and some of the most promising interventions are prohibitively expensive if implementation of these programs is contingent upon the resources of poorer communities and their school districts. Last, a leading zeitgeist of prevention practice in the last decade has focused on the need for "culturally competent and responsive" interventions in an effort to reduce the morbidity and mortality of violence among African Americans and other ethnic minority groups (see Bell & Mattis, 2002; Cunningham et al., 2002). We argue that as efforts to prevent interpersonal violence are advanced, appropriate attention should be given to the theoretical, practical, and evaluative relevance of contemporary prevention and health promotion efforts with African Americans. These efforts must be contextualized by the historical and contemporary experiences of African Americans in the United States.

NOTE

Unless otherwise noted, the source of all mortality data is the Centers for Disease Control and Prevention's Multiple Cause of Death data and rates were calculated for 1990–1999 using population data from the U.S. Bureau of the Census.

REFERENCES

American Academy of Child and Adolescent Psychiatry. (2001). Summary of the practice parameters for the assessment and treatment of children and adolescents with suicidal behavior. *Journal of American Academy of Child and Adolescent Psychiatry, 40*, 495–499.

Anderson E. (1990). *Streetwise: Race, class, and change in an urban community*. Chicago: University of Chicago Press.

Anderson, M., et al., (2001). School-associated violent deaths in the United States, 1994–1999. *Journal of the American Medical Association, 286*, 2695–2702.

Ani, M. (1994). *Yurugu: An African-centered critique of European cultural thought and behavior*. Trenton, NJ: Africa World Press.

Annenberg Public Policy Center, Centers for Disease Control and Prevention, National Institute of Mental Health, Office of the Surgeon General, Substance Abuse and Mental Health Administration, American Foundation for Suicide Prevention, American Association for Suicidology. (2002). Reporting on suicide: Recommendations for the media. *Suicide and Life-Threatening Behavior, 32*.

Baker, F.M. (1994). Suicide among ethnic elderly: A statistical and psychosocial perspective. *Journal of Geriatric Psychiatry, 27*, 241–264.

Bell, C.C., & Mattis, J. (2002). The importance of cultural competence in ministering to African American victims of domestic violence. *Violence Against Women, 6*, 515–532.

Berkman, L.F., & Kawachi, I. (2000). A historical framework for social epidemiology. In L.F. Berkman and I. Kawachi (Eds.), *Social epidemiology* (pp. 3–12). New York: Oxford.

Birckmayer J. & Hemenway D. (1999). Minimum-age drinking laws and youth suicide, 1970–1990. *American Journal of Public Health, 89*, 1365–1368.

Blumstein, A. & Wallman, J. (2000). The recent rise and fall of American violence. In A. Blumstein & J. Wallman (Eds.), *The crime drop in America* (pp. 1–13). New York: Cambridge.

Borduin, C.M., Henggeler, S.W., Blaske, D.M., & Stein, R. (1990). Multisystemic treatment of adolescent sexual offenders. *International Journal of Offender Therapy and Comparative Criminology, 35*, 105–114.

Borowsky, I.W., Ireland, M., & Resnick, M.D. (2001). Adolescent suicide attempts: Risks and protectors. *Pediatrics, 107*, 485–493.

Bowles J.R. (1995). Suicide in Western Samoa: An example of a suicide prevention program in a developing country. In R.F.W. Diekstra et al. (Ed.), *Preventive Strategies on Suicide* (pp. 173–206). Leiden and Brill. Netherlands.

Brener, N.D., Simon, T.R., Krug, E.G., & Lowry, R. (1999). Recent trends in violence-related behaviors among high school students in the United States. *Journal of the American Medical Association, 282*, 440–446.

Bronfenbrenner, U. (1979). The ecology of human development: Experiments by design and nature. Cambridge: Harvard University Press.

Catalano, R.F., Berglund, M.L., Ryan, J.A.M., Lonczak, H.C., & Hawkins, J.D. (1998). Positive youth development in the United States: Research findings of positive youth development programs. U.S. Department of Health and Human Services, National Institute for Child Health and Human Development. Washington, DC.

Centers for Disease Control and Prevention. (CDC). (1989). Differences in death due to injury among blacks and whites, 1984. *Journal of the American Medical Association, 261*, 214–216.

Centers for Disease Control and Prevention. (CDC). (1992). Youth Suicide Prevention Programs: A Resource Guide. Atlanta, GA: CDC.

Centers for Disease Control and Prevention. (CDC). (1998a). Suicide among Black youth—United States, 1980–1995. *MMWR, 47*, 193–196.

Centers for Disease Control and Prevention. (CDC). (1998b). Influence of homicide on racial disparity in life expectancy, United States, 1998. *MMWR, 50*, 780–783.

Centers for Disease Control and Prevention. (2002). Web-based injury statistics query and reporting system [Online]: National Center for Injury Prevention and Control, Centers for Disease Control and Prevention. Available from URL: www.cdc.gov/ncipc/wisqars

Clark, R., Anderson, N.B., Clark, V.R., & Williams, D.R. (1999). Racism as a stressor for African Americans. *American Psychologist, 54*, 805–816.

Crosby, A.E., & Sacks, J.J. (2002). Exposure to suicide: Incidence and association with suicidal ideation and behavior. *Suicide and Life-Threatening Behavior, 32*, 321–328.

Cunningham, P.B., Foster, S.L., & Henggeler, S.W. (2002). The elusive concept of cultural competence. *Children's Services: Social, Policy, Research, and Practice, 5*, 231–243.

Dahlberg, L.L., & Potter, L.B. (2001). Youth violence: Developmental pathways and prevention challenges. *American Journal of Preventative Medicine, 20*, 3–21.

Davis, R. (1979). Black suicide in the seventies: Current trends. *Suicide and Life Threatening Behavior, 9*, 131–140.

Davis, R. (1980). Suicide among young Blacks: Trends and perspectives. *Phylon, 41*, 223–229.

Davis, R., & Short, J.P. (1977). Dimensions of Black suicide. *Suicide and Life Threatening Behavior, 8*, 161–173.

Diekstra, R.F.W. (1987). Epidemiology of attempted suicide in the EEC. In J. Wilmott & J. Mendlewicz (Eds.), *New trends in suicide prevention* (pp 1–16). New York: Karger.

Dube, S.R., Anda, R.F., Felitti, V.J., Chapman, D.P., Williamson, D.P., & Giles, W.H. (2001). Childhood abuse, household dysfunction, and the risk of attempted suicide throughout the life span. *Journal of the American Medical Association, 86*, 3089–3096.

Durant, T.M., Mercy, J.A., Simon, T.R., & Hammond, W.R. (April, 1998). Racial differences in hopelessness as a risk factor for near-lethal suicide. Presented at the 47th annual Epidemic Intelligence Service Conference of the Centers for Disease Control and Prevention, Atlanta, GA.

Durlak, J.A., & Wells, A.M. (1997). Primary prevention mental health programs for children and adolescents: A meta-analytic review. *American Journal of Community Psychology, 25*, 115–152.

Earls, F., Escobar, J.I., & Manson, S.M. (1990). Suicide in minority groups: Epidemiologic and cultural perspectives. In S.J. Blumenthal & D.J. Kupfer (Eds.), *Suicide over the life cycle: Risk factors, assessment, and treatment of suicidal patients* (pp. 571–598). Washington, DC: American Psychiatric Press.

Early, K.E. & Akers, R.L. (1993). "It's a White thing": an explanation of beliefs about suicide in the African-American community. *Deviant Behavior, 14*, 227–296.

Eggert, L.L., Nicholas, L.J., & Owen, L.M. (1995). *Reconnecting youth: A peer group approach to building life skills*. Bloomington, IN: National Educational Service.

Farrington, D.P. (1991). Childhood aggression and adult violence: Early precursors and later-life outcomes. In D.J. Pepler & K.H. Rubin (Eds.), *The development and treatment of childhood aggression* (pp. 5–29). Hillsdale, NJ: Lawrence Erlbaum.

Feldman, M., & Wilson, A. (1997). Adolescent suicidality in urban minorities and its relationship to conduct disorders, depression and separation anxiety. *Journal of the American Academy of Child Adolescents and Psychiatry, 36*, 75–84.

Frederick, C.J. (1984). Suicide in young minority group persons. In H.S. Sudak, A.B. Ford, & N.B. Rushforth (Eds.), *Suicide in the young* (pp. 31–44). Boston: John Wright/ PSG.

Frederick, C.J., Resnik, H.L., & Wittlin, B.T. (1973). Self-destructive aspects of hard core addiction. *Archives of General Psychiatry, 28*, 579–585.

Frierson, R.L., & Lippmann, S.B. (1990). Attempted suicide by Black men and women: An 11 year study. *Journal of Kentucky Medical Association, 88*, 287–292.

Gibbs, J.T., (1988) Conceptual, methodological, and sociocultural issues in Black youth suicide: Implications for assessment and early identification. *Suicide and Life Threatening Behavior, 18*, 73–89.

Gibbs, J.T. (1997). African-American suicide: A cultural paradox. *Suicide and Life Threatening Behavior, 27*, 131–140.

Gordon, R. (1983). An operational classification of disease prevention. *Public Health Reports, 98*, 107–109.

Griffith, E.H., & Bell, C.C. (1989). Recent trends in suicide and homicide among Blacks. *Journal of the American Medical Association, 262*, 2265–2269.

Grunbaum, J.A., Kann, L., Kinchen, S.A., Williams, B., Ross, J.G., Lowry, R., & Kolbe, L. (2002). Youth Risk Behavior Surveillance—United States, 2001. In Surveillance Summaries, June 28, 2002. *MMWR, 51(No. SS-4)*, 1–62.

Guerra, N.G., Huesman, L.R., & Hannish, L. (1995). The role of normative beliefs in children's social behavior. In N. Eisenberg (Ed.), *Review of personality and social psychology, 15*, 140–158. Thousand Oaks, CA: Sage.

Gunnel, D., Hawton, K., Murray, V., Garnier, R., Bismuth, C., Fagg, J., & Simkin, S. (1997). Use of paracetamol for suicide and non-fatal poisoning in the UK and France: Are restrictions on availability justified? *Journal of Epidemiology and Community Health, 51*, 175–179.

Hawkins, D.F., Crosby, A.E., & Hammett, M. (1994). Homicide, suicide, and assaultive violence: The impact of intentional injury on the health of African-Americans. In I. Livingston (Ed.), *Handbook of Black American health* (pp 169–189). Westport, CT: Greenwood Press.

Haycock, J. (1989). Race and suicide in jails and prisons. *Journal of the National Medical Association, 81*, 405–411.

Hayes, L.M. (1995). *Prison suicide: An overview and guide to prevention*. Mansfield, MA: National Center on Institutions and Alternatives.

Haynes, M.A. (1991). Suicide prevention: A U.S. perspective. In R.B. Goldbloom & R.S. Lawrence (Eds.), *Preventing disease: Beyond the rhetoric*. New York: Springer-Verlag.

Hendin, H. (1978). Suicide: The psychosocial dimension. *Suicide and Life Threatening Behavior, 8*, 99–117.

Henggeler, S.W. Mihalic, S.F., Thomas, & Timmons-Mitchell J. (1998). *Blueprints for violence prevention: Multisystemic therapy*. Boulder: C&M Press.

Hickman, L.C. (1984). Descriptive differences between Black and White suicide attempters. *Issues in Mental Health Nursing, 6*, 293–310.

Howell, J.C. (1998). Promising programs for youth gang violence prevention and intervention. In R. Loeber & D.P. Farrington (Eds.), *Serious and violence juvenile offenders: Risk factors and successful intervention*. Thousand Oaks, CA: Sage.

Hoyert, D.L., Arias, E., Smith, B.L., Murphy, S.L., & Kochanek, K.D. (2001). Deaths: Final Data for 1999. National Vital Statistics Reports, 49, no. 8. Hyattsville, MD: National Center for Health Statistics.

Ikeda, R., Mahendra, R., Saltzman, L., Crosby, A., Willis, L., Mercy, J., Holmgren, P., & Annest, J.L. (2002). Nonfatal self-inflicted injuries treated in hospital emergency departments—United States, 2000. *MMWR, 51*, 436–438.

Institute of Medicine, Goldsmith, S.K., Pellmar, T.C., Kleinman, A.M., & Bunney, W.E. (Eds.). (2002). *Reducing suicide: A national imperative.* Washington, DC: National Academy Press.

Jagers, R.J. (1997). Afrocultural integrity and the social development of African American children: Some conceptual, empirical, and practical considerations. In R.J. Watts & R.J. Jagers (Eds.), *Manhood development in urban African Americans.* New York: Haworth Publishing.

Jenkins, E.J., & Bell, C.C. (1994). Violence among inner-city high school students and post-traumatic stress disorder. In S. Friedman (Ed.), *Anxiety disorders in African Americans.* New York: Springer.

Jessor, R., & Jessor, S.L. (1977). *Problem behavior and psychological development: A longitudinal study of youth.* San Diego: Academic Press.

Jessor, R.J., Turbin, M.S., & Costa, F.M. (1998). Risk and protection in successful outcomes among disadvantaged adolescents. *Applied Developmental Science, 2,* 923–933.

Joe, S., & Kaplan, M.S. (2001). Suicide among African-American men. *Suicide and Life Threatening Behavior, 31,* 106–121.

Jones, G.D. (1997). The role of drugs and alcohol in urban minority adolescent suicide attempts. *Death Studies, 21,* 189–202.

Juon, H.S., & Ensminger, M.E. (1997). Childhood, adolescent, and young adult predictors of suicidal behaviors: A prospective study of African-Americans. *Journal of Child Psychology & Psychiatry & Allied Disciplines, 38,* 553–563.

Kachur, S.P., et al. (1996). School-associated violent deaths in the United States, 1992–1994. *Journal of the American Medical Association, 275,* 1729–1733.

Kachur, S.P., Potter, L.B., James, S.P., & Powell, K.E. (1995). Suicide in the United States, 1980–1992. Atlanta: Centers for Disease Control and Prevention. Violence Surveillance Summary Series, No. 1.

Kaslow, N.J., Thompson, M.P., Brooks, A., & Twoomeym, H. (2000). Ratings of family functioning of suicidal and nonsuicidal African-American women. *Journal of Family Psychology, 14,* 585–599.

Kawachi, I., & Berkman, L.F. (2000). Social cohesion, social capital, and health. In L.F. Berkman & I. Kawachi (Eds.), *Social epidemiology.* New York: Oxford.

Kiev, A., & Anumonye, A. (1976). Suicidal behavior in a Black ghetto. *International Journal of Mental Health, 5,* 50–59.

Kirk, A.R., & Zucker, R.A. (1979). Some sociopsychological factors in attempted suicide among urban Black males. *Suicide and Life-Threatening Behavior, 9,* 76–86.

Kreitman N. (1976). The coal gas history: United Kingdom suicide rates, 1960–1971. *British Journal of Preventive and Social Medicine, 30,* 86–93.

Krug, E.G., Dahlberg, L.L., Mercy, J.A., Zwi, A., & Lozano, R. (Eds.). (2002). World report on violence and health. Geneva: WHO.

Kung, H.C., Liu, X., & Juon, H.S. (1998). Risk factors in Caucasians and in African-Americans: A matched case-control study. *Social Psychiatry and Psychiatric Epidemiology, 33,* 155–161.

Lester, D. (1991). Mortality from suicide and homicide for African-Americans in the U.S.A.: A regional analysis. *Omega: Journal of Death and Dying, 22,* 219–226.

Lester, D., & Beck, A. (1975). Attempted suicide in alcoholics and drug addicts. *Journal of Studies on Alcohol, 35,* 162–164.

Linehan, M.M. (1997). Behavioral treatments of suicidal behaviors: Definitional obfuscation and treatment outcomes. In D.M. Stoff and J.J. Mann (Eds.), *The neurobiology of suicide: From the bench to the clinic* (pp. 302–328). New York: New York Academy of Sciences.

Litts, D.A., Moe, K., Roadman, C.H., Janke, R., & Miller, J. (1999). Suicide prevention among active duty air force personnel—United States, 1990–1999. *MMWR, 48,* 1053–1057.

Loftin, C., McDowell, D., Wiersma, B., & Cottey, T.J. (1991). Effects of restrictive licensing of handguns on homicide and suicide in the District of Columbia. *New England Journal of Medicine, 325,* 1615–1620.

Ludwig, J., & Cook, P.J. (2000). Homicide and suicide rates associated with implementation of the Brady Handgun Violence Prevention Act. *Journal of the American Medical Association, 284,* 585–591.

Lyon, M.E., Benoit, M., O'Donnell, R.M., Getson, P.R., Silber, T., & Walsh T. (2000). Assessing African-American risk for suicide attempts: Attachment theory. *Adolescence, 35,* 121–134.

Marietta, A.A. (1999). Interpersonal violence and suicidal behavior in midlife African-American women. *Journal of Black Studies, 29,* 510–522.

Marzuk, P.M., Leon, A.C., Tariff, K., Morgan, E.B., Stajic, M., & Mann, J.J. (1992). The effect of access to lethal methods of injury on suicide rates. *Archives of General Psychiatry, 49*, 451–158.

Masten, A.S., & Coatsworth, J.D. (1998). The development of competence in favorable and unfavorable environments: Lessons from research on successful children. *American Psychologist, 53*, 205–220.

McCaig, L.F., & Ly, N. (2001). National Hospital Ambulatory Medical Care Survey: 2000 Emergency Department summary. *Advance data from vital and health statistics*, no. 326. Hyattsville, MD: National Center for Health Statistics.

Menard, S. (2001). *Short and long term consequences of violent victimization*. Center for the Study of the Prevention of Violence, Boulder, CO: Institute for Behavioral Sciences.

Metha, A., Weber, B., & Webb, L. (1998). Youth suicide prevention: A survey and analysis of policies and efforts in the 50 states. *Suicide and Life-Threatening Behavior, 28*, 150–164.

Miller, T., Covington, K., & Jensen A. (1999). Costs of injury by major cause, United States, 1995: Cobbling together estimates in measuring the burden of injuries. In S. Mulder & E.F. van Beeck (Eds.), *Proceedings of a conference in Noordwijkerhout* (pp. 23–40). Amsterdam: European Consumer Safety Association.

Mishara, B., & Daigle, M. (2001). Helplines and crisis intervention services: Challenges for the future. In D. Lester (Ed.), *Suicide prevention resources for the millennium* (pp. 153–171). Philadelphia: Brunner-Routledge.

Murphy, G.E., Wetzel, R.D., Robins, E., & McEvoy, L. (1992). Multiple risk factors predict suicide in alcoholism. *Archives of General Psychiatry, 49*, 459–463.

National Health and Medical Research Council and Department of Health and Aged Care. (1999). National Youth Suicide Prevention Strategy—Setting the evidence-based research agenda for Australia. Department of Health and Aged Care, Commonwealth of Australia, Canberra.

Nisbet, P.A. (1996). Protective factors for suicidal Black females. *Suicide and Life-Threatening Behavior, 26*, 325–341.

Olds, D.L., Hill, P.L., Mihalac, S.F., & O'Brien, R.A. (1998). Blueprints for violence prevention: Prenatal and infancy home visitation by nurses. Boulder, CO: C&M Press.

Osofsky, J.D. (1999). The impact of violence on children. *The Future of Children, 9*, 33–49.

Palmer, C.J. (2001). African-Americans, depression and suicide risk. *Journal of Black Psychology, 27*, 110–122.

Pfeffer, C.R. (1989). Family characteristics and support systems as risk factors for youth suicidal behavior. In USDHHS, *Report of the Secretary's Task Force on Youth Suicide*, Vol. 2, *Risk factors for youth suicide* (pp. 71–87). Washington, DC: U.S. Government Printing Office.

Potter, L., Powell, K.E., & Kachur, S.P. (1995). Suicide prevention from a public health perspective. *Suicide and Life-Threatening Behavior, 26*, 82–91.

Poussaint, A.F., & Alexander, A. (2000). Lay my burden down: Unraveling suicide and the mental health crisis among African-Americans. Boston: Beacon Press.

Price, J.H., Dake, J.A., & Kucharewski, R. (2001). Assets as predictors of suicide attempts in African-American inner-city youths. *American Journal of Health Behavior, 25*, 367–375.

Reese, L.E., & Crosby, A.E. (May 2002). Examining the relationship between educational attainment and homicide: United States 1991–1998. Paper presentation at the World Injury Conference, Montreal, Canada.

Reese, L.E., Vera, E.M., & Hasbrouck, L. (2002). Examining the impact of violence on ethnic minority youth, their families, and community: Issues for prevention practice and science. In Bermol, G., J.E. Trimble, A.K. Burlew, & F.T. Leong (Eds.), *Handbook of racial and ethnic minority psychology* (Chaft 22, pp. 465–484). Newbury Park, CA: Sage.

Reese, L.E., Vera, E.M., Simon, T.R., Ikeda, R.M. (2000). The role of families and care givers as risk and protective factors in preventing youth violence. *Clinical Child and Family Psychology, 3*, 61–77.

Reinholdt, N.P., Mehlum, L., & Ystgaard, M. (2000). There's help for just about everything: Evaluation of the Petre campaign 1999. *Suicidologi, 1*, 19–21.

Rennison, C.M. (2000). Criminal victimization 1999: Changes 1998–99 with trends 1993–99. Bureau of Justice Statistics National Crime Victimization Survey. U.S. Department of Justice (NCJ 182734).

Richmond, J.B., & Kotelchik, M. (1983). Political influences: Rethinking national health policy. In C.H. McGuire, R.P. Foley, A. Gorr, & R.W. Richards (Eds.), *Handbook of the health professions education.* San Francisco: Jossey-Bass.

Richters, J.E., & Martinez, P. (1993). The NIMH community violence projects 1. Children as victims of and witnesses to violence. *Psychiatry, 56,* 7–21.

Robbins, L., West, P.A, & Murphy, G.E. (1977). The high rate of suicide in older White Men: A study testing ten hypotheses. *Social Psychiatry, 12,* 1–20.

Rosenberg, M.L., Gelles, R.J., Holinger, P.C., Zahn, M.A., Stark, E., Conn, J.M., Fajman, N.N., & Karlson, T.A. (1987). Violence: Homicide, assault and suicide. In R.W. Amler & H.B. Dull (Eds.), *Closing the Gap: The burden of unnecessary illness* (pp. 164–178). New York: Oxford University Press.

Rosenman, S.J. (1998). Preventing suicide: What will work and what will not. *Medical Journal of Australia, 169,* 100–102.

Rotheram-Borus, M.J. (1993). Suicidal behavior and risk factors among runaway youths. *American Journal of Adolescent Research, 150,* 103–107.

Roy, A. (1983). Family history of suicide. *Archives of General Psychiatry, 40,* 971–974.

Rutledge, E.M. (1990). Suicide among Black adolescent and young adults. In D.W. Stiffman & L.E. Davis (Eds.), *Ethic issues in adolescent mental health* (pp. 339–351). Newbury Park, CA: Sage.

Rutz, W., von Knorring, L., & Walinder, J. (1989). Frequency of suicide on Gotland after systematic postgraduate education of general practitioners. *Acta Psychiatrica Scandinavica, 80,* 151–154.

Sampson, R.J., Raudenbush, S.W., & Earls, F. (1997). Neighborhoods and violent crime: A multilevel study of collective efficacy. *Science, 177,* 918–924.

Satcher, D. (1998). Bringing the public health approach to the problem of suicide. *Suicide and Life-Threatening Behavior, 28,* 325–327.

Seiden, R. (1972). Why are suicides of young Blacks increasing? *Health Services and Mental Health Administration, 87,* 3–8.

Serna, P, May, P., & Sitaker, M. (1998). Suicide prevention evaluation in a Western Athabaskan American Indian Tribe—New Mexico, 1988–1997. *MMWR, 47,* 257–261.

Shanahan, P., Elliott, B., & Dahlgren, N. (2000). Review of public information campaigns addressing youth risk-taking: A report to the National Youth Affairs Research Scheme. Sandy Bay, Tasmania, Australia: Australian Clearinghouse for Youth Studies.

Smart, R.G. (1980). Drug abuse among adolescents and self-destructive behavior. In E. Sneidman (Ed.), *The many faces of suicide* (pp. 170–186). New York: McGraw-Hill.

Smith, J.A., & Carter, J.H. (1986). Suicide and Black adolescents. *Journal of the National Medical Association, 78,* 1061–1064.

Sonneck, G., Etzersdorfer, E., & Nagel-Kuess S. (1994). Imitative suicide on the Viennese subway. *Social Science and Medicine, 38,* 453–457.

Stack, S. (1998). Education and risk of suicide: An analysis of African-Americans. *Sociological Focus, 31,* 295–302.

Stack, S. (1996). The effect of marital integration on African-American suicide. *Suicide and Life Threatening Berhavior, 26,* 405–414.

Stevens, J.A., Hasbrouck, L., Durant, T.M., Dellinger, A.M., Batabyal, P.K., Crosby, A.E., Valluru, B.R., Kresnow, M., & Guerrero, J.L. (1999). Surveillance for injuries and violence among older adults. In CDC Surveillance Summaries. *Mortality and Morbidity Weekly Report, 48,* 27–50.

Swanson, W.C., & Breed, W. (1976). Black suicide in New Orleans. In E.S. Shneidman (Ed.), *Suicidology* (pp. 99–128). New York: Grune & Stratton.

Thompson, E.A., Eggert, L.L., Randell, B.P., & Pike, K.C. (2001). Evaluation of indicated suicide risk prevention approaches for potential high school dropouts. *American Journal of Public Health, 91,* 742–752.

Thompson, M.P., Kaslow, N.J., & Kingree, J.B. (2002). Risk factors for suicide attempts among African-American women experiencing recent intimate partner violence. *Violence and Victims, 17,* 283–295.

Thornberry, T.P., Huizinga, D., & Loeber, R. (1995). The prevention of serious delinquency and violence: Implications from the program of research on the causes and correlates of delinquency. *Sourcebook on juvenile offenders* (pp. 213–237). Washington, DC: U.S. Department of Justice.

Topol, P., & Reznikoff, M. (1982). Perceived peer and family relationships, hopelessness and locus of control as factors in adolescent suicide attempts. *Suicide and Life Threatening Behavior, 12*, 1143–1150.

Uniform Crime Reporting Program data. Supplementary homicide reports 1999 [electronic data tapes].

U.S. Census Bureau. (1999). *Poverty in the United States*. Washington, DC: U.S. Department of Commerce, Economics and Statistics Administration.

U.S. Department of Health and Human Services (USDHHS). (2002). Vital statistics mortality data, underlying cause of death, 1999. [Machine-readable data tapes]. Hyattsville, MD: USDHHS, National Center for Health Statistics.

U.S. Department of Health and Human Services (USDHHS). (2001). Youth Violence: A Report of the Surgeon General. Rockville, MD: USDHHS.

U.S. Department of Health and Human Services (USDHHS), Children's Bureau. (1998). Child maltreatment 1996: Reports from the states to the national child abuse and neglect data system. Washington, DC: U.S. Government Printing Office.

U.S. Department of Health and Human Services (USDHHS). (1986). Report of the Secretary's Task Force on Black and Minority Health, Vol. 1: Executive Summary. Washington, DC: U.S. Government Printing Office.

U.S. Department of Health and Human Services (USDHHS). (1985). Report of the Secretary's Task Force on Black and Minority Health. Bethesda, MD: USDHHS.

U.S. Public Health Service (USPHS). (2001). National Strategy for Suicide Prevention: Goals and objectives for action. Washington, DC: USDHHS.

U.S. Public Health Service (USPHS). (1999). The Surgeon General's Call to Action to Prevent Suicide. Washington, DC: USDHHS.

Walter, H.J., Vaghan, R.D., Armstrong, B., & Krakoff, R. (1995). Sexual, assaultive, and suicidal behaviors among urban minority junior high school students. *Journal of the American Academy of Child and Adolescent Psychiatry, 34*, 73–80.

Washington State Department of Health. (1995). Youth suicide prevention plan for Washington state. Olympia: Washington State Department of Health.

Wells, L.E., & Rankin, J.H. (1988). Direct parental controls and delinquency. *Criminology, 26*, 263–285.

White, J., & Jodoin, N. (1998). "Before-the-fact" interventions: A manual of best practices in youth suicide prevention. Vancouver, British Columbia, Canada: British Columbia Ministry for Children and Families.

Williams, S., Molock, S., & Kimbrough, S. (1996). Glamorized suicide and their contagious effects: Are Black Americans at risk? In J. McIntosh (Ed.), 29th Annual Conference of American Association of Suicidology (pp. 129–130). St. Louis, MO.

Willis, L.A., Coombs, D., Cockerham, W.C., & Frison, S.L. (2002). Ready to Die: A postmodern interpretation of the increase of African-American adolescent male suicide. *Social Science and Medicine, 55*, 907–920.

Wilson W.J. (1987). *The truly disadvantaged: The inner city, the underclass, and public policy*. Chicago: University of Chicago Press.

Wilson, W.J. (1996). *When work disappears: The world of the new urban poor*. New York: Vintage Books.

World Health Organization (WHO). (1996). Prevention of suicide: Guidelines for the formulation and implementation of national strategies (document ST/SEA/245). New York: United Nations.

CHAPTER 18

Unintentional Injuries: The Burden, Risks, and Preventive Strategies to Address Diversity

CHRISTINE M. BRANCHE,
ANN M. DELLINGER, DAVID A. SLEET,
JULIE GILCHRIST, AND SARAH J. OLSON

Unintentional injury is one of the most important public health problems facing the United States, claiming over 97,500 lives each year. Unintentional injury has been the leading cause of death for all persons in the United States ages 1 to 34 years for more than a decade. In 1999, unintentional injury was the third leading cause of death among African Americans (CDC, 2001). Death rates attributed to unintentional injuries (what many people describe as "accidents," e.g., motor vehicle crashes, fires and burns, drowning, falls, etc.) vary by age and race and ethnicity. Examining unintentional injury death rates (per 100,000 population) by age and race for 1990–1998, we see that rates are higher for African Americans than for White Americans in almost every decade of life except ages 9 to 20 years and after age 70 years (Figure 18.1). In fact, the unintentional injury death rate for African American children from birth through age 9 years is almost twice that of White American children, and the rate is close to one and a half times greater for African Americans ages 40 years and older. American Indians and Alaska Natives have the highest unintentional injury death rates of all race and ethnic groups through age 70 years (CDC, 2001).

The need for hospitalization may be an indication of injury severity, with the most severe injuries warranting an overnight hospital stay. For every death, there are about 17 persons who are hospitalized and another 200 who are seen in Emergency Departments due to injury (CDC, 2001). For persons under age 65 years, hospitalization rates for African American males are about twice those for White males. Among children, African Americans have rates that are about twice those of their White counterparts, and differences narrow with increasing age (data from Fingerhut & Warner, 1997, as quoted in Institute of Medicine (1999).

Emergency Department data from the combined 1992–1995 National Hospital Ambulatory Medical Care Survey (NHAMCS) indicate that the overall age-adjusted injury visit rate for African Americans was 1.3 times the rate for Whites, although the magnitude of the disparity differed by age and sex. Differences of note included persons ages 25–44 years, for whom the Emergency Department injury visit rates for African American males (26.7 per 100,000 persons) exceeded the rates for other groups; it was about 1.4 times the rates for White males and African American females and 2.3 times the rate for White American females (CDC, 1998).

Many factors influence individual risks for injury, including general health and wellness, lifestyle, environment, risk-taking behavior, use of personal protective equipment, mood, and attitudes. Many

Figure 18.1
Unintentional injury death rates per 100,000 population, United States, 1990–1998

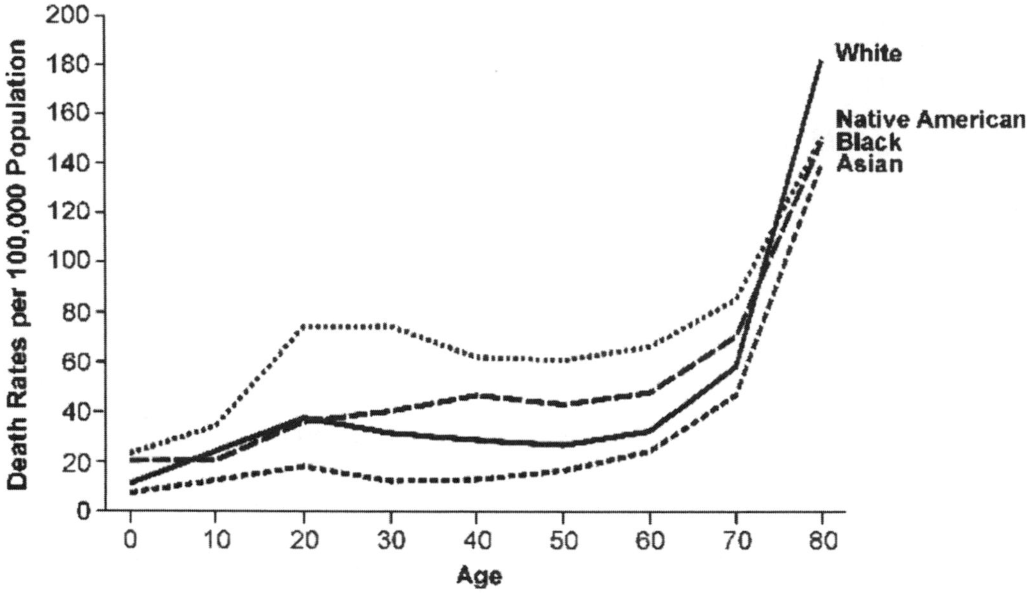

Source: CDC (2001).

injuries are heavily influenced by social factors such as social norms and the behavior of others (Rothengatter & Vaya, 1997). We know from the science of injury prevention that injuries and events that cause injury are not random events—they are predictable, and most are preventable. Changing human behavior, modifying products, and changing environments present three key opportunities for reducing injuries and their consequences. Using terms such as *injury prevention* rather than *accident prevention* helps make clear the potential for preventing such events (Sleet & Branche-Dorsey, 1997).

MOTOR VEHICLE INJURIES

Motor vehicle injuries are the leading cause of unintentional injury death among African Americans (CDC, 2001). Each year more than 40,000 people of all races are killed, and three million are nonfatally injured in crashes (NHTSA, 2001a). Overall, crash-related death rates differ by race. Generally, American Indian/Alaskan Natives have the highest rates, and Asian/Pacific Islanders have the lowest rates; death rates are similar for African American and White Americans (16.2/100,000 age-adjusted population among African Americans vs. 15.6/100,000 age-adjusted population among Whites in 1999) (CDC, 2001). However, overall rates mask differences by age, sex, and type of victim.

African American children ages birth to 9 years have higher motor vehicle-related death rates than White children. This difference is most pronounced for children under 5 years (7.3/100,000 population among African American children vs. 3.9/100,000 population among White children). Males have higher death rates than females; African American males have death rates nearly three times that of African American females. The highest death rates among African American males and females occur among those in their 20s and those ages 75 years and older. There are also differences by type of victim (i.e., vehicle occupant, pedestrian, bicyclist, motorcyclist). Although African Americans and Whites have similar death rates among vehicle occupants, bicyclists, and motorcyclists, African American pedestrians have higher deaths rates than White pedestrians (3.5/100,000 age-adjusted population among African Americans vs. 2.0/100,000 age-adjusted population among Whites). More than 1,000 pedestrian deaths a year occur among African Americans (CDC, 2001).

Risk Factors

Deaths due to motor vehicle-related injury are not randomly distributed in the population. Patterns and contributing causes of death from crashes vary by many factors including race, age, amount of exposure to the traffic environment, socioeconomic status, and alcohol (drinking and driving and/or riding with a driver who has been drinking). In an analysis of the relationship of race and other demographic and risk factors among persons killed in motor vehicle crashes, Mayrose and Jehle (2002) found that young males, African Americans, and passengers were less likely to be wearing their seat belts than females, White Americans, and drivers. Baker et al. (1998) looked at risk of motor vehicle-related deaths to children and teenagers two different ways, by population and by exposure to the traffic environment. They found that race differences per 100,000 population were minor, but per billion vehicle miles of travel, death rates were highest among African American children (14 per billion vehicle miles for African Americans vs. 8 for Hispanics vs. 5 for Whites). Braver (2001) found education level was a stronger determinant of motor vehicle occupant deaths than race or ethnicity. In the same analysis, after controlling for socioeconomic status, African American drivers with high school degrees or more education were less likely to have high blood alcohol concentrations than White drivers of the same gender and educational level; however, these differences were not statistically significant.

Preventive Strategies

Effective injury prevention strategies apply equally to African Americans and White Americans, most notably seat belts and child restraint devices (e.g., child safety seats, booster seats). Research shows that lap/shoulder belts, when used, reduce the risk of fatal and serious injury to front-seat passenger car occupants by 45 to 50 percent. Child safety seats reduce fatal injury by 71 percent for infants and by 54 percent for toddlers (NHTSA, 2001b). However, not all persons use these devices consistently. Information from the 1997 Behavioral Risk Factor Surveillance System, a nationwide household telephone survey of adults, found that 63 percent of African Americans reported always using their seat belts versus 70.1 percent of Whites. In addition, African Americans were slightly less likely to report that a child in their household used an appropriate restraint when riding in a car (82 percent for African Americans vs. 87 percent for Whites) (CDC, 1997). In the Youth Risk Behavior Surveillance System, a school-based survey of students in the 9th through 12th grades, 23 percent of African American and 16 percent of White students reported that they had rarely or never worn seat belts when riding in a car or truck driven by someone else. However, White students were more likely to report drinking and driving in the previous 30 days (15 percent of White students compared to 8 percent of African American students). Proportions for students who reported riding with a driver who had been drinking in the previous 30 days were similar (34 percent for African American students versus 32 percent for White American students) (CDC, 2000).

Recent systematic reviews of the scientific literature found that seat belt laws increased observed use by 33 percent and reduced fatal injuries by 9 percent. Enhanced law enforcement increased belt use by 16 percent and reduced fatalities from 7 percent to 15 percent (Dinh-Zarr et al., 2001). Moreover, primary laws (a driver can be stopped for a seat belt violation alone) were found to be more effective than secondary laws (a driver must be stopped for another reason) in increasing belt use and reducing fatalities (Dinh-Zarr et al., 2001). Wells et al. (2001) found that in cities with primary belt laws, there were no differences in belt use by race or ethnicity; in cities with secondary laws, African Americans were less likely than Whites or Hispanics to be belted. Seat belt use remains one of the most important preventive strategies for African Americans. Ellis et al. (2000) estimated that if all African Americans buckled their seat belts, 1300 lives would be saved and 26,000 injuries would be prevented.

RESIDENTIAL FIRE-RELATED INJURIES

Fires and burns are the fourth leading cause of unintentional injury death among African Americans (CDC, 2001). Each year there are approximately 400,000 residential fires in the United States, killing nearly 3,600 people, 300 of whom are African American. Eighty percent of all fire deaths nationwide occur in the home. In addition, almost 16,000 fire-related injuries occurred. Residential fires result in direct property damage of roughly $5 billion a year. In 1994 and in 1998, unintentional residential fire mortality rates were highest among the youngest and oldest Americans; among males; among African Americans; and among persons living in the South (CDC, 2001).

Risk Factors

Elderly populations are at particular risk of death from residential fire, and, in this age group, African Americans are five times more likely to die than their White American counterparts. In examining the U.S. residential fire death rates by race, rates were highest in African Americans and Native Americans in every age category (CDC, 2001). Poverty, differences in the rates of smoking, and medical conditions that reduce the chances of escape in a fire are factors for fire and burn injuries in the United States (Branche-Dorsey et al., 1994). While nationally, African Americans had the highest average annual residential fire and burn mortality rates during 1994–1998, this was not the case in every region of the United States. African Americans had the highest age-adjusted residential fire and burn death rates in the South (3.6/100,000) and Northeast (2.7/100,000). Interestingly, the lowest race-specific regional incomes were associated with the highest race-specific regional fire death rates: midwestern Native Americans had the lowest per capita income ($7,615) and the highest fire mortality rate (4.57 deaths/100,000 population/year), and southern African Americans had the second lowest average per capita income ($7,874) and the second highest fire mortality rate (3.63/100,000).

Preventive Strategies

In high-risk populations, smoke alarm installation and education programs can reduce deaths by 80 percent (Mallonee et al., 1996). Working smoke alarms increase the chance of surviving a fire by 50 percent (Ahrens, 2001). A working smoke alarm plus a residential sprinkler system can increase a person's chance of surviving a fire by 97 percent. From one study, we know that for $1 invested in a smoke alarm program, including installation, about $3 in medical costs and $27 in lost productivity costs are saved (Haddix et al., 2001).

DROWNING

About 4,000 people drown in the United States each year, and drowning is the second leading cause of injury death among children ages 1 to 14 years. An estimated 5,700 Emergency Department visits occur annually related to drowning or near-drowning events. More than 40 percent of these require admission to the hospital, compared with a 4 percent admission rate for all other injury visits (CDC, 2001). While drowning rates have declined steadily over the last two decades (CDC, 2001), they continue to be disproportionately high among children under 5 years (3.1/100,000 population in 1999) and adolescents and young adults ages 15 and 24 years (1.9/100,000 population in 1999) (CDC, 2001). Overall, the U.S. drowning rates for African Americans are 1.4 times those of White Americans; however, the relationship varies by age. Among infants and children under 1 year, the rate for African Americans is 2.3 times that of White Americans; among children ages 10 to 14 years, the rate is five times higher; and for adults, the rate is 1.25 higher (CDC, 2001).

Risk Factors

Risk factors for drowning differ by age group and include the type of water source, lapses in supervision of children, inadequate barriers, and the use of alcohol, among others. Drowning in young children usually occur in water sources around the household, including bathtubs, buckets, toilets, or swimming pools and spas (Brenner et al., 2001). Children can drown quickly and silently, even where many adults are present. Sixty percent of drownings among infants occur in bathtubs, and almost 50 percent of drownings in toddlers and preschoolers occur in swimming pools. Brief lapses in adult supervision caused by chores, socializing, phone calls, or other distractions have been implicated in most drowning incidents among young children (Present, 1987).

Many factors such as differences in household makeup (e.g., number and ages of children and adults) and the environment (e.g., presence of or access to swimming pools) may be responsible for the racial differences in drowning rates in these two groups. Among children age 5 to 14 years, drownings are common in pools or natural bodies of water. In pools, the drowning rate in this age group for African Americans is eight times higher than in White Americans. In natural bodies of water, it is 2.5 times that of Whites. These differences may be due in part to differences in early exposures in and around recreational water, such as access to ponds or backyard swimming pools (Schuman et al., 1977). There may be sociocultural differences in the choices made for young children's recreational activities. As these children reach ages where they are more independent and may not be supervised as closely, they may encounter aquatic situations for which they have not been prepared (Brenner et al., 2001).

Among adolescents and adults, drowning occurs most often during swimming, wading, and boating in natural bodies of water, frequently with alcohol use as a contributing factor (Branche-Dorscy et al., 1994; Howland et al., 1996; Smith et al., 2001). In this age group, more than three-quarters of drownings where the location is known occur in natural bodies of water such as lakes, rivers, and oceans (CDC, 2002). A survey on self-reported swimming ability in U.S. adults aged 18 years and older noted that 62 percent of African Americans reported limited swimming ability, while 32 percent of White Americans responded similarly (Gilchrist et al., 2000). While the drowning rates among African American and White American adults are similar, little is known about boating and swimming activities, regardless of race. If African Americans choose to engage less often in aquatic activities, their true drowning rates (per exposure) might actually be much higher than reported here.

Preventive Strategies

With fewer epidemiologic studies in its history, the field of drowning prevention is not as mature scientifically as other areas in unintentional injury. Several public health strategies may reduce the risk for drowning, including public education regarding the need for supervision, elimination of hazards, and environmental changes. Additionally, policies encouraging training in first aid, swimming instruction, water safety training, and alcohol restriction at aquatic sites may be beneficial.

Drowning prevention requires multiple approaches, depending on age, location, and circumstances. Persons caring for small children must be aware that all bodies of water are dangerous and need to vigilantly supervise young children around all household and outdoor water sources to help prevent drownings. All adults who have young children in their care should be trained in cardiopulmonary resuscitation (CPR) and basic first aid (AAP, 1994). Appropriate supervision, however, is only one necessary component. Limiting access to hazardous water sources is always prudent where small children are present. This would include promptly draining bathtubs and buckets, fencing backyard pools to separate the pool from the yard and house, and fencing the yard to limit access to natural water hazards (e.g., ditches or ponds). The use of personal floatation devices when children are around the water is also recommended. Swimming skill may play a role in preventing drownings in older children and adolescents (AAP, 2000).

While there remain many gaps in our understanding of risk and preventive factors in drowning among adolescents and adults, some additional prevention strategies should be considered, including improving swimming skill, avoiding the use of alcohol, and avoiding high-risk, water-related activities. Federal agencies continue to call for research in drowning prevention to guide programs (CDC, 2002; Brenner, 2002). This includes information regarding differing risk and protective factors and differing aquatic habits between African American and White Americans.

FALL INJURIES AMONG OLDER ADULTS

Among persons 65 years and older, falls are the leading cause of injury death and the most common cause of nonfatal injuries and hospital admissions for trauma (CDC, 2001; Murphy, 2000; Alexander et al., 1992). In 1999, more than 10,000 older adults died from fall-related injuries, and in 2000, 1.6 million seniors were seen in Emergency Departments for fall injuries (CDC, 2001). One of every three older Americans—about twelve million seniors—fall each year (Hornbrook et al., 1994; Hausdorff et al., 2001), and the likelihood of falling increases sharply with age. For both fatal and nonfatal injuries among persons age 65 or more years, African Americans are at second highest risk after White Americans (CDC, 2001).

Of all fall-related injuries, hip fractures not only cause the greatest number of injury deaths but lead to the most severe health problems and reduced quality of life. Hip fracture rates increase exponentially with age for both sexes (Samuelson et al., 2002). The impact of hip fractures is significant in terms of quality of life and medical costs. Medicare costs for hip fractures are about $3 billion annually. Among hip fracture survivors, up to 25 percent remain institutionalized a year after their fracture (Magaziner et al., 2000). This contributes to the fear of falling and loss of independence, which are great concerns among older adults. Salkeld and colleagues (2000) reported that in a randomized, controlled trial of older women age 80 or more years who had previously fallen, 80 percent said that they would rather be dead than experience the loss of independence and quality of life from a bad hip fracture and admission to a nursing home.

Risk Factors

We know what the major risk factors are for older adult falls for all races. These can be grouped into two categories: personal risks and environmental risks. Personal risks include being female (Baker et al., 1992; Tromp et al., 1998); having experienced a fall previously (AGS, 2001); weakness in the lower extremities (AGS, 2001; Lord et al., 1993); taking more than four medications or using psychoactive medications (Tinetti & Speechley, 1989; Ray & Griffin, 1990; Lord et al., 1993; Cumming, 1998); vision problems (Ivers et al., 1998; Lord et al., 2001); a history of chronic disease

(Tinetti et al., 1986; Dolinis et al., 1997; Northridge et al., 1995); and physical limitations such as difficulty in walking (Koski et al., 1996).

Environmental risk factors may play a role in about half of all home falls (Nevitt et al., 1989). Common environmental fall hazards include lack of stair railings or grab bars, slippery or wet floors, poor lighting, and tripping hazards in walkways (Connell, 1996; Northridge et al., 1995; Gill et al., 1999). Such risk factors may be exacerbated in substandard housing facilities.

Preventive Strategies

As with other injuries, multiple strategies are important to consider for effective prevention of fall-related injuries. Several strategies addressing personal risks have documented evidence of effectiveness in older adult populations. A regular exercise program that increases lower body strength and improves balance is key (Campbell et al., 1999; Judge et al., 1993). Tai chi, for example, has been shown to reduce fall risk by almost 50 percent (Wolf et al., 1996). A regular review of the prescription and over-the-counter medications taken by older adults by a health-care provider or pharmacist is recommended. Tranquilizers, sleeping pills, and antianxiety drugs, in particular, should be evaluated by the physician and reduced in number (Ray & Griffin, 1990). Regular vision examination and correction have been shown to aid in reducing falls (Lord et al., 2001; Ivers et al., 1998). While calcium with vitamin D is critical at all ages for maintaining healthy bones and preventing osteoporosis, calcium intake through diet or supplements may not be adequate for older adults to prevent bone loss or reduce hip fractures; prescription medications for osteoporosis may be more effective (Stevens, 1997).

Experts on environmental risk factor strategies recommend installing grab bars, especially next to the toilet and the tub or shower; and improving lighting in the home, especially between the bedroom and bathroom (e.g., night-lights). Removing tripping hazards, such as clutter and electrical cords in walkways and throw rugs, and fixing loose or uneven steps and stairs are recommended (Lord et al., 2001; Tideiksaar, 1986).

DISPARITIES IN RATES OF UNINTENTIONAL INJURY

African Americans have higher rates of unintentional injury than do White Americans due to a variety of causes. Among children ages 14 and younger, African Americans are almost twice as likely to die from unintentional injuries compared to White Americans. Overall, the rates of motor vehicle-related fatalities, the leading cause of unintentional injury, are comparable for these races. If the differences in rates are not occurring in motor vehicle injuries, then the differences must be due to factors related to fire-related injuries, drowning, and other types of unintentional injuries. It would appear that race is the causal factor, but is race really causing these differences in rates? We do not think so. We contend, then, that the differences that we observe among African American and other groups for fatal and nonfatal unintentional injury are not attributable to race per se but to other causes.

A key issue in explaining the differences is poverty and all that is associated with it: poorer living conditions, access to quality recreational activities, and access to home improvement programs that install safety devices (e.g., installation of smoke alarms, grab bars). In part, racial differences in injury rates have been attributed to the greater proportion of African Americans living below the poverty level (U.S. Department of Commerce, 1986). Low-income areas are associated with higher unintentional injury death rates (Baker et al., 1992). Such areas experience inadequately designed and maintained roads, older vehicles, poorly maintained residences, and less adequate emergency and medical care (Baker et al., 1992). Wise et al. (1985) found that fire death rates were less related to racial differences than to income differences. Furthermore, Fullilove and

Fullilove (1995) showed that neighborhood deterioration (e.g., building abandonment and loss of housing units) and a concentration of poor people occurred after a series of catastrophic fires in New York City.

Cultural differences must also be considered in understanding differences in fatal and nonfatal injury rates among racial and ethnic groups. Cultural factors affect parenting practices, transportation alternatives, home safety practices, conditions of living (e.g., where one lives, the type of home, the kind of neighborhood, and the income level of the census tract), choices in recreation, lifestyle factors, and risk-taking behaviors. The increased drowning rate that we observe in African American teenagers and adults, for example, may reflect socioeconomic and/or cultural differences in exposure to residential swimming pools among very young children (Branche-Dorsey et al., 1994). These cultural factors affect injury exposures, and exposures affect risk.

Prevention strategies proceed from a better understanding of exposures, risks, and target populations. The strategies need not be tailor-made to be effective in preventing injury but can be adapted from prevention efforts designed for other health conditions. Over the years, visiting nurse programs, well-child visits, and similar health programs have been examined by injury prevention specialists to determine if these health programs can be used to add home inspections, injury prevention education, and home/residence amelioration (Kitzman et al., 1997). These have been successful avenues for introducing injury prevention strategies directly to populations that need them, principally persons living at lower income levels, who are often also African Americans. These programs provide an opportunity to target injury prevention education and interventions to persons who need them immediately. Such opportunities are diminishing as state and local health-care dollars dwindle. In fact, state health programs can be prohibited from adding non-health-care delivery to home visits.

Injury prevention programs targeted at populations at high risk for selected injuries always include African Americans but depend almost exclusively on the public sector for their funding. As such, these programs are subject to shifting political priorities. Private sector-sponsored programs are helpful and spread the responsibility of good corporate citizenship but are subject to the funding priorities of the donor organization. Injuries will continue to occur, so the prevention strategies available to stem the tide must be plentiful and consistently available. Hence, injury prevention needs long-term solutions with commensurate resources that are not dependent on shifting funding priorities. Drafting solutions for this broader problem requires active commitment and debate among the public and private sectors and representatives of communities served.

Legislation and other policy solutions carry with them a permanence that is less vulnerable to shifting priorities. For example, laws requiring small children to travel in automobiles only when seated in a child safety seat can be found in all 50 states. From time to time, public debate has occurred over the size or age of the child whom the laws should cover, but not on the general principle of protecting children in automobiles. With such legislation in place, both private and public sector funding opportunities have been used to make child safety seats more widely available and to increase their correct use. If families cannot afford one, hospitals often will equip families with child safety seats and instruct them on proper use for the ride home when the newborn is discharged. These programs have strong evidence of effectiveness (Zaza et al., 2001). Nongovernment organizations also sponsor programs that distribute seats to low-income families. Distribution programs like these would not be as widely available without the supporting legislation.

Unintentional injuries are a leading cause of premature death among African Americans. While the pattern of these injuries can be described, the underlying causes are less well understood. Future research should be directed to better understand the causes. Solutions, whether through programs or policies, require researchers to work collaboratively with religious and community leaders and advocacy groups to design, promote, and evaluate prevention strategies that address the unintentional injury problem among African Americans.

NOTE

The authors would like to thank Tim Groza, M.P.A., for his assistance in preparing this manuscript.

REFERENCES

Ahrens, M. (2001). *U.S. experience with smoke alarms and other fire alarms.* Quincy, MA: NFPA.

Alexander, B.H., Rivara, F.P., & Wolf, M.E. (1992). The cost and frequency of hospitalization for fall-related injuries in older adults. *American Journal of Public Health, 82, (7),* 1020–1023.

American Academy of Pediatrics (AAP). (1994). The pediatrician's role in advocating life support courses for parents (RE9424). *AAP News.* Available from URL: www.aap.org/policy/570.html. [Access date September 27, 2002].

American Geriatrics Society (AGS), British Geriatrics Society, and the American Academy of Orthopaedic Surgeons Panel on Falls Prevention. (2001). Guideline for the prevention of falls in older persons. *Journal of the American Geriatrics Society, 49,* 664–672.

Anonymous. (2000). Swimming programs for infants and toddlers. Committee on Sports Medicine and Fitness and Committee on Injury and Poison Prevention. American Academy of Pediatrics. *Pediatrics, 105(4 Pt 1):* 868–870.

Baker, S.P., Braver, E.R., Chen, L., Pantula, J.F., & Massie, D. (1998). Motor vehicle occupant deaths among Hispanic and Black children and teenagers. *Archives of Pediatric and Adolescent Medicine, 152,* 1209–1212.

Baker, S.P., Ginsburg, M.J., Li, G., & O'Neill, B. (1992). *The Injury Fact Book,* 2d ed. New York: Oxford University Press.

Branche-Dorsey, C.M., Chorba, T.L., Greenspan, A.I., & Russell, J.C. (1994). Unintentional injuries: The problems and some preventive strategies. In I.L. Livingston (Ed.), *Handbook of Black American health.* Westport, CT: Greenwood Press.

Braver, E.R. (2001). *Race, Hispanic origin, and socioeconomic status in relation to motor vehicle occupant death rates and risk factors among adults.* Arlington, VA: Insurance Institute for Highway Safety.

Brenner, R.A. (2002). Childhood drowning is a global concern: Prevention needs a multifaceted approach. *British Medical Journal, 324,* 1049–1050.

Brenner, R.A., Trumble, A.C., Smith, G.S., Kessler, E.P., & Overpeck, M.D. (2001). Where children drown, United States, 1995. *Pediatric, 108,(1),* 85–89.

Campbell, A.J., Robertson, M.C., Gardner, M.M., Norton, R.N., & Buchner, D.M. (1999). Falls prevention over 2 years: A randomized controlled trial in women 80 years and older. *Age and Aging, 28,* 513–518.

Centers for Disease Control and Prevention (CDC). (1997). *Behavioral Risk Factor Surveillance System Survey Data.* Atlanta, GA: U.S. Department of Health and Human Services, Centers for Disease Control and Prevention.[Accessed July 2002].

Centers for Disease Control and Prevention (CDC). (1998). Injury visits to hospital emergency departments: United States, 1992–95. *Vital and Health Statistics, DHHS Pub No. (PHS) 98-1792,* Hyattsville, MD.

Centers for Disease Control and Prevention (CDC). (2000). Youth Risk Behavior Surveillance—United States, 1999. *Morbidity & Mortality Weekly Report, 49 (SS05),* 1–96.

Centers for Disease Control and Prevention (CDC). (2001). Web-based Injury Statistics Query and Reporting System (WISQARS) [Online]. (2001). National Center for Injury Prevention and Control, Centers for Disease Control and Prevention (producer). Available from URL: www.cdc.gov/ncipc/wisqars. [Access dates: September 14, 2001, February 2002, July 16, 2002, August 27, 2002].

Centers for Disease Control and Prevention (CDC). (2002). Data from the National Electronic Injury Surveillance System-All Injury Program operated by the U.S. Consumer Product Safety Commission. Atlanta, GA: Centers for Disease Control and Prevention, National Center for Injury Prevention and Control.

Connell, B.R. (1996). Role of the environment in falls prevention. *Clinics in Geriatric Medicine, 12,* 859–880.

Cumming, R.G. (1998). Epidemiology of medication-related falls and fractures in the elderly. *Drugs and Aging, 12,* 43–53.

Dinh-Zarr, T.B., et al. (2001). Task Force on Community Preventive Services. Reviews of evidence regarding interventions to increase the use of safety belts. *American Journal of Preventive Medicine, 21, (4S)*, 48–65.

Dolinis, J., Harrison, J.E., & Andrews, G.R. (1997). Factors associated with falling in older Adelaide residents. *Australian & New Zealand Journal of Public Health, 21*, 462–468.

Ellis, H.M., Nelson, B., Cosby, O., Morgan, L., Haliburton, W., & Dew, P. (2000). Achieving a credible health and safety approach in increasing seat belt use among African Americans. *Journal of Health Care for the Poor and Underserved, 11*, 144–150.

Fingerhut, L.A., Warner M. (1997). *Injury Chartbook, Health, United States, 1996–97*. Hyattsville, MD: National Center for Health Statistics.

Fullilove, R.E., & Fullilove, M.T. (1995). Community disintegration and public health: A case study of New York City. In *Assessing the Social and Behavioral Science Base for HIV/AIDS Prevention and Intervention: Workshop Summary*. Washington, DC: Institute of Medicine, 99–100.

Gilchrist, J., Sacks, J.J., & Branche, C.M. (2000). Self-reported swimming ability in U.S. adults, 1994. *Public Health Reports, 115(2–3)*: 110–111.

Gill, T.M., Robison, J.T., Tinetti, M.E., & Williams, C.S. (1999). A population-based study of environmental hazards in the homes of older persons. *American Journal of Public Health, 89*, 553–556.

Haddix, A.C., Mallonee, S., Waxweiler, R., & Douglas, M.R. (2001). Cost effectiveness analysis of a smoke alarm giveaway program in Oklahoma City, Oklahoma. *Injury Prevention, 7*, 276–281.

Hausdorff, J.M., Rios, D.A., & Edelber, H.K. (2001). Gait variability and fall risk in community-living older adults: A 1-year prospective study. *Archives of Physical Medicine and Rehabilitation, 82*, 1050–1056.

Hitzman, H., et al. (1997). Effects of prenatal and infancy home visitation by nurses on pregnancy outcomes, childhood injuries, and repeated childbearing: A randomized controlled trial. *Journal of the American Medical Association, 278*, 644–652.

Hornbrook, M.C., et al. (1994). Preventing falls among community-dwelling older persons: Results from a randomized trial. *The Gerontologist, 34*, 16–23.

Howland, J., Hingson, R., Mangione, T.W., Bell, N., & Bak, S. (1996). Why are most drowning victims men? Sex differences aquatic skills and behaviors. *American Journal of Public Health, 86(1)*: 93–96.

Institute of Medicine. (1999). *Reducing the burden of injury: Advancing prevention and treatment*. Washington, DC: National Academy Press, p. 51.

Ivers, R.Q., Optom, B., Cumming, R.G., Mitchell, P., & Attebo, K. (1998). Visual impairment and falls in older adults: The Blue Mountains eye study. *Journal of the American Geriatrics Society, 46*, 58–64.

Judge, J.O., et al. (1993). Balance improvements in older women: effects of exercise training. *Physical Therapy, 73*, 254–62, 263–5.

Kitzman H., Olds, D.L., Henderson, C.R., et al. (1997). Effect of prenatal and infancy home visitation by nurses on pregnancy outcomes, childhood injuries, and repeated childbearing: A randomized controlled trial. *Journal of the American Medical Association, 278*, 644–652.

Koski, K., Luukinen, H., Laippala, P., & Kivela, S.L. (1996). Physiological factors and medications as predictors of injurious falls by elderly people: A prospective population-based study. *Age and Aging, 25*, 29–38.

Lord, S.R., Caplan, G.A., & Ward, J.A. (1993). Balance, reaction time, and muscle strength in exercising and nonexercising older women: a pilot study. *Archives Physical Medicine and Rehabilitation, 74*, 837–839.

Lord, S.R., Sherrington, C., & Menz, H.B. (2001). *Falls in older people: Risk factors and strategies for prevention*. Cambridge: Cambridge University Press.

Magaziner, J., et al. (2000). Recovery from hip fracture in eight areas of function. *Journal of Gerontology: Medical Sciences, 55A*, M498–M507.

Mallonee, S., et al. (1996). Surveillance and prevention of residential-fire injuries. *New England Journal of Medicine, 335*, 27–31.

Mayrose, J., & Jehle, D.V.K. (2002). An analysis of race and demographic factors among motor vehicle fatalities. *Journal of Trauma Injury, Infection, and Critical Care, 52*, 752–755.

Murphy, S.L. (2000). Deaths: Final data for 1998. *National Vital Statistics Reports, vol. 48, no. 11*. Hyattsville, Maryland: National Center for Health Statistics.

National Highway Traffic Safety Administration (NHTSA). (2001a). *Traffic Safety Facts 2000: A compilation of motor vehicle crash data from the Fatality Analysis Reporting System and the General Estimates System*. Department of Transportation publication No. HS-809-337. Washington, DC: Author.

National Highway Traffic Safety Administration. (2001b). *Traffic Safety Facts 2000, Occupant Protection*. Department of Transportation publication No. HS-809-337. Washington, DC: Author.

Nevitt, M.C., Cumming, S.R., Kidd, S., & Black, D. (1989). Risk factors for recurrent non-syncopal falls: A prospective study. *Journal of the American Medical Association, 261*, 2663–2668.

Northridge, M.E., Nevitt, M.C., Kelsey, J.L., & Link, B. (1995). Home hazards and falls in the elderly—the role of health and functional status. *American Journal of Public Health, 85*, 509–515.

Present, P. (1987). *Child drowning study: A report on the epidemiology of drownings in residential pools to children under age five*. Washington, DC: U.S. Consumer Product Safety Commission, Directorate for Epidemiology.

Ray, W., & Griffin, M.R. (1990). Prescribed medications and the risk of falling. *Topics in Geriatric Rehabilitation, 5*, 12–20.

Rothengatter, T., Vaya, E.C. (Eds). (1997). *Traffic and transport psychology: Theory and application*. Oxford: Elsevier Science.

Salkeld, G., Cameron, I.D., Cumming, R.G., Easter, S., Seymour, J., Kurrle, S.E., & Quine, S. (2000). Quality of life related to fear of falling and hip fracture in older women: A time trade off study. *British Medical Journal, 320*, 341–346.

Samelson, E.J., Zhang, Y., Kiel, D.P., Hannan, M.T., & Felson, D.T. (2002). Effect of birth cohort on risk of hip fracture: Age-specific incidence rates in the Framingham Study. *American Journal of Public Health, 92*, 858–862.

Schuman, S.H., Rowe, J.R., Glazer, H.M., & Redding, J.S. (1977). Risk of drowning: An iceberg phenomenon. *JACEP, 6*, 139–143.

Sleet, D.A., & Branche-Dorsey, C.M. (1997). Injury risks and prospective medicine: The role of education and behavior change. *Proceedings of the Society for Prospective Medicine*. Atlanta, GA.

Smith, G.S., Keyl, P.M., Hadley, J.A., Bartley, C.L., Foss, R.D., Tolbert, W.G., & McKnight, J. (2001). Drinking and recreational boating fatalities: A population-based case-control study. *Journal of the American Medical Association, 286(23)*, 2974–2980.

Stevens, J.A. (1997). The association of calcium intake and exercise with hip fracture risk among older adults [Dissertation]. Atlanta, GA: Emory University.

Tideiksaar, R. (1986). Preventing falls: Home hazard checklists to help older patients protect themselves. *Geriatrics, 41*, 26–28.

Tinetti, M.E., & Speechley, M. (1989). Prevention of falls among the elderly. *New England Journal of Medicine, 320*, 1055–1059.

Tinetti, M.E., Williams, T.F., & Mayewski, R. (1986). Fall risk index for elderly patients based on number of chronic disabilities. *American Journal of Medicine, 80*, 429–434.

Tromp, A.M., Smit, J.H., Deeg, D.J.H., Bouter, L.M., & Lips, P. (1998). Predictors for falls and fractures in the Longitudinal Aging Study Amsterdam. *Journal of Bone Mineral Research, 13*, 1932–1939.

U.S. Department of Commerce. (1986). *Bureau of the Census, Current population report*. (Series P-60 No. 152.) Characteristics of the population below the poverty level, 1984. Washington, DC: Author.

Wells, J.K., Williams, A.F., & Farmer, C.M. (2001). Seat belt use among African Americans, Hispanics, and Whites. Insurance Institute for Highway Safety, Arlington, VA.

Wilkins, K. (1999). Health care consequences of falls for seniors. *Health Reports, 10*, 47–55.

Wise, P.H., Kotelchuck, M., Wilson, M.L., & Mills, M. (1985). Racial and socioeconomic disparities in childhood mortality in Boston. *New England Journal of Medicine, 313*, 360–366.

Wolf, S.L., Barnhart, H.X., Kutner, N.G., McNeely, E., Coogler, C., & Xu, T. (1996). Reducing frailty and falls in older persons: An investigation of tai chi and computerized balance training. Atlanta FICSIT Group. Frailty and Injuries: Cooperative Studies of Intervention Techniques. *Journal of the American Geriatrics Society, 44*, 489–497.

Zaza, S., Sleet, D.A., Thompson, R.S., Sosin, D.M., & Bolen, J.C. (2001). Task Force on Community Preventive Services. Reviews of evidence regarding interventions to increase use of child safety seats. *American Journal of Preventive Medicine, 21 (4S)*, 31–47.

CHAPTER 19

Illicit Drug Use and Adverse Consequences: Impact on Black Americans

HOWARD D. CHILCOAT AND
JAMES C. ANTHONY

INTRODUCTION

The issue of health disparities in health outcomes related to illicit drug use is rather complex. Certainly, there is an appearance that Black Americans are more adversely affected by involvement in illicit drug use than Whites, as well as members of many other minority groups (McCaffrey, 1997). However, the appearance of greater problems related to drug use in African American communities might be due to greater visibility of drug sales rather than drug use and dependence (Saxe et al., 2001). On the other hand, there is considerable evidence that Black Americans are more likely to experience a variety of negative health outcomes related to drug use, such as HIV infection among injecting drug users, compared to other racial/ethnic groups.

In order to understand the extent and nature of health disparities related to drug use, it is necessary to examine a variety of aspects of illicit drug use. These outcomes range from initiation to the harmful consequences of drug use, including drug dependence, medical consequences such as HIV infection, and legal consequences such as incarceration. In this chapter, we use data from population-based surveys to probe for epidemiologic evidence of disparities in drug use outcomes and explore etiologic mechanisms that might account for differences by race/ethnicity. We further explore evidence that Blacks might be more adversely affected by the consequences of drug use through examination of evidence from additional sources, such as emergency room visits and criminal justice records.

EPIDEMIOLOGIC EVIDENCE

As a basis for understanding the extent to which Blacks might be more adversely affected by the health consequences of drug use, we examine the distribution of drug use outcomes by race/ethnicity, using data from national surveys of drug abuse. We compare prevalence of drug use outcomes by race/ethnicity in order to examine the extent to which disparities might exist, with the understanding that race per se is not likely to have a direct causal influence on these disparities.

Reliance on population surveys of drug abuse, which collect information based on respondents' self-reports of drug use and related behaviors, is essential for understanding the nature and scope of illicit drug use and the differences that exist between racial/ethnic groups. Despite potential errors and biases that can emerge in estimates based on survey data, which we consider below, these studies provide important data and substantial advantages over other data collection approaches, including the use of bioassays (Harrison, 1997).

A significant concern regarding prevalence estimates based on survey data is grounded on the reliance on respondents' self-reports of drug use. Studies such as the National Household Survey on Drug Abuse (NHSDA) use structured interviews, which require responses to scripted questions about the respondent's use of drugs and related behaviors. Although there may be random sources of error in self-reports of drug use, systematic bias in responding, such as underreporting of drug use, is a more critical issue. To reduce the underreporting of sensitive behaviors, major population-based surveys have striven to develop instruments that maximize the validity of self-reports. Confidentiality of responses is assured, and respondents are presented with a Federal Certificate of Confidentiality. In addition, recent technical advances have helped assure respondents that their responses will be kept confidential. One example of advancement in data collection is the use of computer-assisted self-interviewing (CASI) instruments, which has been adopted by the NHSDA and has been shown to increase the likelihood of positive self-reports of sensitive behaviors (Turner et al., 1998). Despite the concern about the threat of underreporting of drug use, a number of studies have supported the validity of self-reported data (Harrison, 1997). In fact, self-reports have distinct advantages over other sources of data for drug use. For example, there has been increased interest in the use of bioassays as valid indicators of drug use, including analysis of blood, urine, hair, sweat, and saliva. While these methods are often touted as "gold-standards" as measures of drug use, their utility is limited. In addition to the barriers to collecting and analyzing large numbers of bioassays in population-based studies with sample sizes exceeding 50,000 people, biological measures are limited by the half-life of the substance to be assayed (e.g., in blood samples), or the nature of the sample, such as the length of an individual's hair (Wish et al., 1997). In order to obtain needed information about the history and course of drug use across an individual's life span, it will be necessary to obtain valid self-reports.

Although it is important to maximize the accuracy of responses about drug use and related behaviors, a particular threat in the study of health disparities due to drug abuse is differential underreporting across racial/ethnic groups. For example, it is possible that, due to suspicion that responses will not be kept confidential, Blacks are more likely to underreport drug use than Whites. This would tend to underestimate the difference in prevalence of drug use if in fact one did exist. While there is no specific evidence that differential underreporting occurs across racial/ethnic groups, it is important to interpret the findings based on survey data in light of the potential limitations and sources of bias.

Although data are available from a number of population-based studies, in this report, we focus on findings from the National Household Survey on Drug Abuse (NHSDA, now named the National Survey of Drug Use and Health [NSDUH]). The NHSDA is conducted annually by the Office of Applied Studies (OAS) at the Substance Abuse and Mental Health Services Administration (SAMHSA, 2001). The NHSDA has provided prevalence estimates of drug use for the household population of the United States since 1979. The NHSDA was carried out approximately every three years through the 1980s and has been conducted annually since 1990. Sample sizes have increased more than tenfold since the study's inception, with sample sizes exceeding 50,000 respondents since 1999. The sample universe of the NHSDA consists of the civilian, noninstitutionalized population of the United States aged 12 and older, including residents of noninstitutional group quarters such as college dormitories, group homes, shelters, rooming houses, and civilians dwelling on military installations (SAMHSA, 2001). Incarcerated individuals are not eligible for inclusion in the NHSDA,

Table 19.1
Lifetime prevalence of any illicit drug use, marijuana, cocaine, crack cocaine, and heroin

Race/Ethnicity	Any Illicit Drug	Marijuana	Cocaine	Crack	Heroin
12+ years old					
African American	36.1	31.4	7.5	3.6	2.1
White	41.3	36.8	12.4	2.3	1.2
Hispanic	30.1	24.5	8.9	1.8	1.1
12-17 years old					
African American	24.2	14.2	0.5	0.0	0.1
White	27.4	19.2	2.6	0.6	0.4
Hispanic	27.5	19.0	3.9	1.0	0.3
18-25 years old					
African American	44.9	39.5	3.3	0.5	0.2
White	56.2	50.7	13.0	3.5	1.8
Hispanic	39.1	33.7	10.7	2.3	1.5
26-34 years old					
African American	46.7	40.8	8.4	3.3	1.1
White	57.7	53.0	17.8	4.3	1.1
Hispanic	33.3	27.6	12.4	2.3	1.5
35+ years old					
African American	33.3	30.5	10.1	5.5	3.4
White	37.2	33.4	12.7	1.9	1.2
Hispanic	26.2	21.3	8.3	1.5	1.2

Source: National Household Survey on Drug Abuse (2000).

but released prisoners currently in the general population are eligible. Through the use of a complex sample design and sample weighting, prevalence estimates of drug use in the household population of the United States can be generated.

Findings

Initially, we set out to compare the prevalence of use of any illicit drug, as well as important classes of drugs, using data from the 2000 NHSDA (SAMHSA, 2001). Lifetime use for a specific drug or class of drugs, such as cannabinoids, is ascertained through a single item, "Have you ever, even once, used marijuana or hashish?" Recent use, such as use in the year or month prior to interview is assessed by a follow-up question, "How long has it been since you last used marijuana or hashish?" Since lifetime use captures use that has occurred at any point in a respondent's lifetime, lifetime users include those who used in the past but no longer use, as well as chronic users and those with a recent onset of use. Recent use includes individuals who are new users (e.g., starting in the past year or month) and chronic users whose use persists.

As shown in Table 19.1, the prevalence of use of any illicit drug among African Americans (35.5 percent) is intermediate between that for Whites (41.5 percent) and Hispanics (29.9 percent). Prevalence of recent use (past year) is nearly identical across these racial/ethnic groups (Table 19.2). While this information suggests that Black Americans are no more likely to have ever used illicit drugs in their lifetime or recently than Whites, a more detailed examination is required to understand the nature of health disparities related to drug use. To shed more light on this issue, we start by

Table 19.2
Past-year prevalence of any illicit drug use, marijuana, cocaine, crack cocaine, and heroin

Race/Ethnicity	Any Illicit Drug	Marijuana	Cocaine	Crack	Heroin
12+ years old					
African American	11.0	8.7	1.3	0.8	0.1
White	11.3	8.6	1.5	0.3	0.2
Hispanic	10.1	6.6	1.7	0.3	0.1
12-17 years old					
African American	15.1	9.3	0.4	0.0	0.0
White	19.6	14.5	1.8	0.3	0.3
Hispanic	17.8	12.8	2.6	0.6	0.2
18-25 years old					
African American	25.1	22.0	1.6	0.2	0.0
White	30.8	26.5	5.2	0.8	0.5
Hispanic	19.8	15.3	3.9	0.6	0.2
26-34 years old					
African American	12.6	10.2	1.1	0.5	0.0
White	15.1	11.6	2.3	0.4	0.1
Hispanic	9.8	5.9	2.2	0.4	0.0
35+ years old					
African American	5.6	4.3	1.6	1.2	0.2
White	5.8	3.9	0.6	0.1	0.1
Hispanic	4.3	1.7	0.4	0.1	0.1

Source: National Household Survey on Drug Abuse (2000).

comparing the prevalence of use of selected drugs of abuse, specifically marijuana, cocaine, and heroin, across racial/ethic groups over time and across age groups.

In Table 19.1, we compare the prevalence of drug use by race/ethnicity for four different age groups. These are standard age groups typically used in reports of NHSDA findings, and they generally differentiate important developmental stages with respect to drug use. Adolescence (age 12–17 years) is a period in which individuals begin to experiment with drug use and patterns of drug use begin to emerge (Wagner & Anthony, 2002). Initiation of use typically begins in this age group, but problems related to drug use are more likely to occur later. Early adulthood (ages 18–25) is an important stage in which individuals make many important transitions and changes in roles (e.g., from school to workplace, moving away from parents' home to college dorms, armed services, or living on their own). It is also a period when patterned drug use is more likely to become established and drug use disorders (abuse and dependence) are most likely to emerge (Wagner & Anthony, 2002). Ages 26–34 represent a period of entrenchment in adult roles in which illicit drug use tends to cease or diminish. Drug use is least likely to occur (either onset of new use or persistence of prior use) later in adulthood (ages 35+). Comparisons of the prevalence of drug use by race/ethnicity across these age groups can provide useful clues for understanding health disparities for drug use outcomes.

ANY ILLICIT DRUG USE

Across all age groups, the lifetime prevalence of any illicit drug use is lower for African Americans than for Whites and estimates for Hispanics are lower than for both Whites and Black Americans

(Table 19.1). Nonetheless, prevalence of lifetime illicit drug use is quite high in all racial ethnic groups. Approximately one-quarter of Blacks, Whites, and Hispanic adolescents have tried an illicit drug at least once. About one-half of Black and White young adults and one-third of Hispanics (18–25 years old and 26–34 years old) have tried an illicit drug in their lifetime. The difference in prevalence between adolescents and young adults reflects the fact that older individuals have accumulated more time in which to initiate drug use. Because onset of illicit drugs is unlikely to occur later in adulthood, there is little increase in lifetime prevalence of drug use for the 25–34-year-olds versus 18–25-year-olds. On the other hand, it is likely that the lower prevalence of drug use among those 35+ years old relative to younger adults is due to cohort differences since many of those at the older end of this age range never initiated illicit drug use.

Marijuana

The patterns of racial/ethnic differences in prevalence of marijuana use across age groups are similar to those observed for any illicit drug use. Such a finding is expected since marijuana is used by nearly all of those who report the use of any other illicit drug. The largest relative difference in prevalence of lifetime and past-year use of marijuana for Blacks compared to Whites and Hispanics was found among adolescents. White adolescents were about 50 percent more likely to have used marijuana in the year prior to interview than Blacks. For other age groups, past-year use was very similar for Blacks and Whites.

Cocaine

Estimates of the prevalence of cocaine are based on the use of all forms of cocaine, including powder and crack cocaine. Racial/ethnic differences in lifetime prevalence of cocaine use are more marked than those observed for marijuana—for the population 12+ years old, Whites were nearly twice as likely to have used cocaine than Blacks. For adolescents (12–17 years old), the lifetime prevalence of cocaine use was five times that of Blacks (2.6 percent vs. 0.5 percent). The relative difference in prevalence for Whites versus Blacks diminished with increasing age (Table 19.1)— there was a threefold difference in lifetime prevalence of cocaine use for Whites compared to Blacks in the 18–25-year-old age group, a twofold difference for 25–34-year-olds, and nearly equal prevalence in the 35+-year-old-group. This pattern of findings was also observed for more recent use (past year), with Whites more likely to use in all age groups except older adults (35+ years old).

Crack cocaine is one of the few drugs for which the prevalence is higher for Blacks versus other racial/ethnic groups. Since the emergence of the crack epidemic in the 1980s, the prevalence of cocaine use has been higher for Black Americans relative to Whites and Hispanics (Lillie-Blanton et al., 1993; Chilcoat & Schutz, 1995). This disparity has been maintained through 2000, although the relative difference in prevalence of crack use has diminished over time (Figure 19.1). Although the lifetime prevalence of crack use has remained relatively stable for Blacks, there has been an increase in prevalence for Whites and Hispanics. These trends in lifetime prevalence of use must be interpreted in light of several considerations. First, it is important to keep in mind that lifetime use reflects use at any time in a respondent's lifetime, and we would expect lifetime prevalence to change little from year to year. However, an influx of new users in a given year would cause an increase in lifetime prevalence. Conversely, a loss of previous users in a given year (e.g., if large numbers of crack users died due to overdoses or other causes) would result in a decrease in lifetime prevalence.

Given that crack was introduced to the population relatively recently and because it is likely that the increase of new users would exceed the decrease in previous users, it is expected that lifetime prevalence in the population should increase over time. In general, this is the trend that is observed

Figure 19.1
Lifetime prevalence of crack cocaine use by race/ethnicity: U.S. population 12+ years old

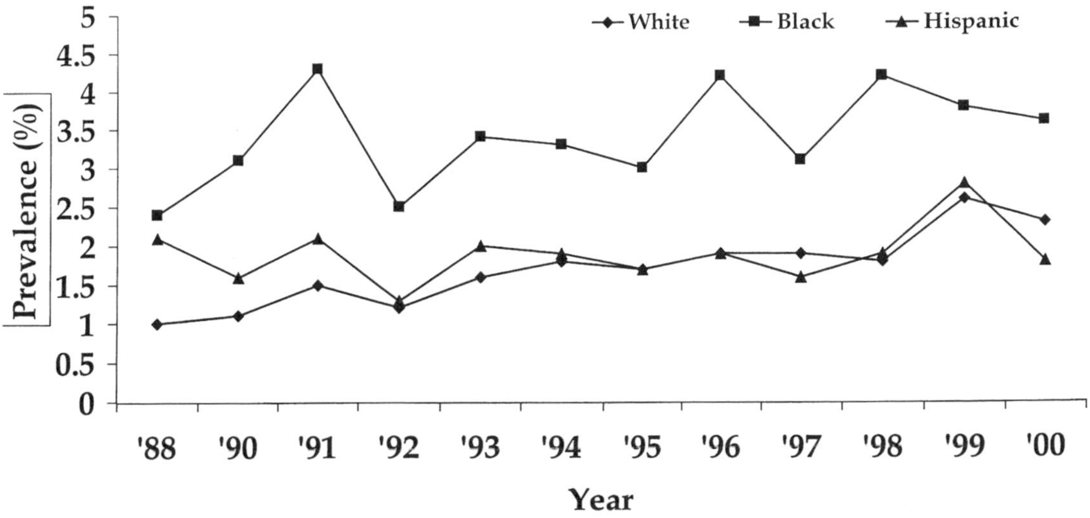

Source: National Household Survey on Drug Abuse, 1988–2000.

in Figure 19.1, with a few exceptions. These exceptions could be due to variation from year to year due to sampling error. Even if there is no measurement error due to the assessment of crack use, the mean for a sample selected any given year is likely to deviate from the true population mean. The extent of this deviation is a function of sample size. The relatively large sample size for the NHSDA, especially in recent years, helps minimize this error. A second consideration is that trends can vary due to measurement and methods used in survey implementation. While there is a substantial effort made to maintain the consistency of methods used each year, changes in instrumentation and sampling design can be a source of error and, potentially, bias.

Taking these considerations into account, one explanation for the narrowing of the racial/ethnic gap in lifetime crack use might be greater increases in onset use of crack among Whites and Hispanics, relative to Blacks. To explore this possibility further, we compare recent use of crack cocaine, that is, use occurring in the past year (Figure 19.2a). Some caution must be applied when interpreting these data due to the relatively low prevalence of recent crack use in the population, which would result in some instability in prevalence estimates (sample mean $+/-$ standard error). Nonetheless, some interesting trends are evident. Although prevalence of recent use has remained relatively constant across the period from 1988 to 2000 for Whites and Hispanics, there were a decreasing trend for Blacks and a dramatic drop in prevalence in 1999 and 2000.

A comparison of trends across age groups (Figures 19.2b–19.2e) sheds more light on patterns of use over time. In all age groups, there has been a decrease in the past-year prevalence of crack use among Blacks through the 1990s to 2000, whereas prevalence was relatively constant or increasing for Whites and Hispanics. It is notable that crack use currently is at virtually nondetectable levels for Black adolescents (Figure 19.2b), decreasing from a level of 1 percent in the early 1990s. Prevalence of recent crack use among Whites and Hispanics has been relatively constant. These results are consistent with ethnographic reports of crack use, which indicate that African American youth have negative attitudes toward crack use, even among those involved in the sale and distribution of crack (Dunlap & Johnson, 1992). For young adults (18–25 years old), the prevalence of crack use among Black Americans has decreased dramatically, declining from 2.5 percent in 1990 to less than

Figure 19.2a
Past-year prevalence of crack cocaine use by race/ethnicity: U.S. population 12+ years old

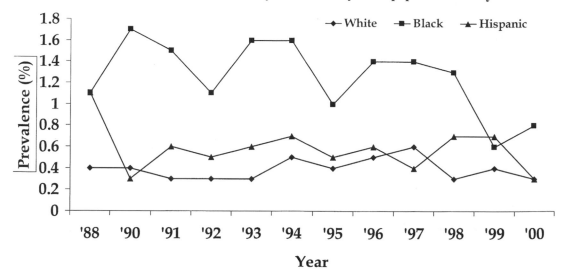

Source: National Household Survey on Drug Abuse, 1988–2000.

Figure 19.2b
Past-year prevalence of crack cocaine use by race/ethnicity: U.S. population 12–17 years old

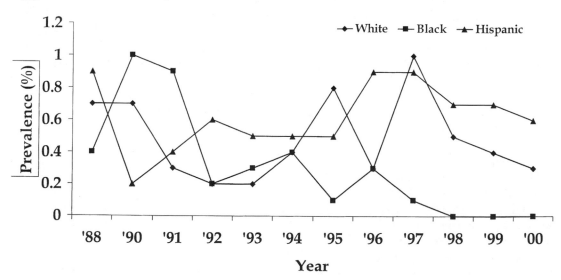

Source: National Household Survey on Drug Abuse, 1988–2000.

Figure 19.2c
Past-year prevalence of crack cocaine use by race/ethnicity: U.S. population 18–25 years old

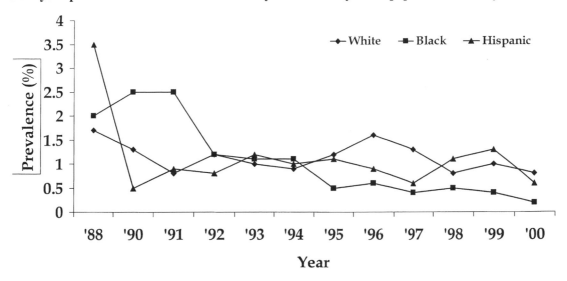

Source: National Household Survey on Drug Abuse, 1988–2000.

Figure 19.2d
Past-year prevalence of crack cocaine use by race/ethnicity: U.S. population 26–34 years old

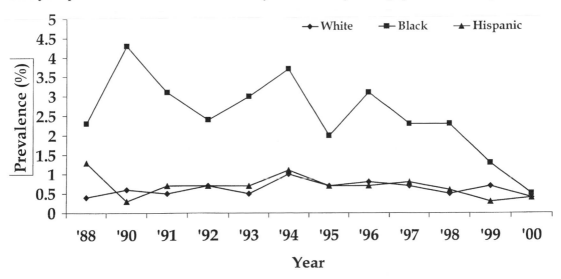

Source: National Household Survey on Drug Abuse, 1988–2000.

Figure 19.2e
Past-year prevalence of crack cocaine use by race/ethnicity: U.S. population 35+ years old

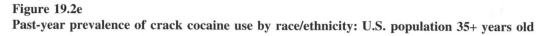
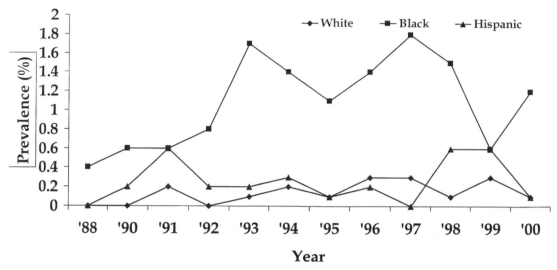

Source: National Household Survey on Drug Abuse, 1988–2000.

0.25 percent in 2000. In contrast, past year prevalence for Whites and Hispanics have remained relatively steady, around 1 percent.

Perhaps the most interesting change in trends in crack use has occurred among 25–34-year-olds. There has been a marked decrease in past-year prevalence of crack use among Blacks, whereas prevalence estimates for Whites and Hispanics have remained constant. As a result, the rather large racial/ethnic disparities in crack use observed in the early 1990s have dissipated, as indicated by the latest available data from the 2000 NHSDA. Blacks were several times more likely to be recent users of crack cocaine throughout the early to mid-1990s, with 3 to 4 percent of African Americans 26–34-year-olds reporting recent crack use versus less than 1 percent of Whites and Hispanics throughout this period. The relative difference in prevalence of crack use diminished throughout the late 1990s, and most recent estimates indicate nearly identical prevalence of recent crack use across these three major racial/ethnic groups. Disparities in crack use remain among the oldest age group (35+ years old). Prevalence of recent crack use in this age group increased among Black Americans through the 1990s, peaking at nearly 2 percent in 1997, whereas prevalence for Whites and Hispanics remained below 0.6 percent.

These data on trends in crack use point to a potential cohort effect that merits further investigation. There is clear evidence that the cohort of African Americans who were young adults in their mid-20s to mid-30s was the population most susceptible to crack use as availability became more widespread. Many of these individuals initiated the use of crack at an age at which new onset of drug use becomes less common (Chilcoat & Schutz, 1995). Involvement with social roles, such as marriage, parenthood, and employment, is associated with a reduction in drug use in young adulthood (Chilcoat & Breslau, 1996; Kandel & Raveis, 1989). At the same time, crack use never increased among African American youth, whom many suspected as being a particular vulnerable population. Additional research investigating the factors that influenced the increase of crack use among African American young adults is necessary to understand the crack epidemic of the last decade and could help prevent epidemics in future generations as new (and existing) drugs become available (Chilcoat, 1994).

A closer examination into racial/ethnic disparities in crack cocaine use provides useful clues about the burden of drug use among African Americans. Lillie-Blanton et al. (1993) conducted a study using data from the 1988 NHSDA to probe the meaning of racial/ethnic differences in the prevalence of crack use. Specifically, they compared respondents living within the same neighborhoods to test whether the observed racial/ethnic disparities in crack use persisted once neighborhood was held constant. Findings from this study indicated that the odds of crack use were nearly identical for Blacks, Whites, and Hispanics once neighborhood was taken into account. A subsequent study (Chilcoat & Schutz, 1995) replicated this finding using data from the 1990 NHSDA and also found that African American young adults (25–34-year-olds) had higher odds of crack use than their White and Hispanic counterparts, even when neighborhood was held constant. Although the inferences from these studies can be applied only to neighborhoods in which Blacks, Whites, or Hispanics live together, it points to the importance of neighborhood as a potential influence on crack use. Specifically, drug distribution patterns can have an important influence on the availability of crack use in urban, primarily African American neighborhoods. In addition, there might be shared attitudes or cultural factors that influence drug use in these neighborhoods.

Heroin

Overall, African Americans are approximately twice as likely to have ever used heroin compared to Whites or Hispanics. However, racial/ethnic differences in heroin use vary considerably by age group. For younger age groups (12–17 and 18–24), lifetime prevalence of heroin use is several times higher for Whites than African Americans. There is no difference in prevalence of heroin use by race/ethnicity among 25–34-year-olds. For older adults (35+ years-old), the pattern in prevalence of heroin use reverses, with African Americans in this age group nearly three times more likely to have ever used heroin than Whites or Hispanics. Lifetime prevalence for older African American adults was 3.4 percent versus 1.2 percent for Whites and Hispanics. Nearly 5 percent of African American males in this age group reported ever using heroin. Although prevalence of past-year heroin use is too low to yield reliable estimates, it appears that very few lifetime users in this age group continue to use heroin.

Racial/ethnic disparities in heroin use are more evident when focusing on urban areas. In a longitudinal study of children born in Baltimore in the early 1960s who participated in the Pathways to Adulthood study (Hardy et al., 1997) and were followed up when they were 27 to 33 years old, 17 percent of African Americans reported ever using heroin versus 7 percent for Whites in the sample (Windham, 2002). Nearly half of the lifetime heroin users maintained their use for several years and were still using as they entered mid-adulthood. Findings from this study point to the need for research designed to detect regional and neighborhood variation in drug use, particularly with respect to understanding health disparities in drug use. While data from national samples such as the NHSDA yield useful information about drug use in the United States as a whole, they are limited in their ability to provide information about drug use in specific localities where there might be high prevalence of drug abuse.

Other Drugs

For other major drugs of abuse, including hallucinogens, misuse of prescription drugs, and inhalants, prevalence of use for African Americans is one-third to one-half that for Whites (data not shown). These differences are even more pronounced at younger ages. For example, although there is a sharp peak in past-year use of hallucinogens around age 19 for Whites, there is no such peak for African American youth, whose level of use is almost undetectable (Chilcoat & Schutz, 1996).

Data from the 2000 NHSDA show that one-quarter of White 18–25-year-olds have used a hallucinogen in their lifetime (25.2 percent) versus 5.1 percent for African Americans.

Although many African Americans are adversely affected by abuse of these drugs, it is apparent that the bulk of health disparities in drug use are accounted for by marijuana, heroin, and cocaine, particularly in the form of crack cocaine. It is somewhat of a paradox that African American youth appear to be at reduced risk for drug use, given that they are believed to possess more risk factors for use (Vega et al., 1993; Ellickson & Morton, 1999; Gil et al., 2002). The reduced risk of drug use does not appear to be maintained as African American youth enter young adulthood, at which time they are more likely to engage in use of crack and heroin.

Drug Dependence

In previous sections, we focused on use of various drugs. However, of greater public health concern than use per se is the development of problems of drug dependence. Drug dependence is defined by the *Diagnostic and Statistical Manual of Mental Disorders* (DSM-IV) (APA, 1994) as the presence of a constellation of cognitive, behavioral, and physiological symptoms indicating the use of a drug or drugs despite significant drug-related problems. The pattern of repeated self-administration may result in tolerance, withdrawal, and compulsive drug use behavior.

The diagnostic criteria for drug dependence as specified in DSM-IV are as follows: a maladaptive pattern of drug use, leading to clinically significant impairment or distress, as manifested by three (or more) of the following, occurring at any time in the same 12-month period: (1) tolerance, as defined by either of the following: (a) a need for markedly increased amounts of the drug to achieve intoxication or desired effect or (b) markedly diminished effect with continued use of the same amount of the drug; (2) withdrawal, as manifested by either of the following: (a) the characteristic withdrawal syndrome for the drug or (b) the same (or closely related) drug is taken to relieve or avoid withdrawal symptoms; (3) the drug is often taken in larger amounts or over a longer period than was intended; (4) there is a persistent desire or unsuccessful efforts to cut down or control drug use; (5) a great deal of time is spent in activities necessary to obtain the drug, use the drug, or recover from its effects; (6) important social, occupational, or recreational activities are given up or reduced because of drug use; (7) drug use is continued despite knowledge of having a persistent or recurrent physical or psychological problem that is likely to have been caused or exacerbated by the drug.

The NHSDA measured the presence of symptoms of drug dependence occurring in the past year for individual drugs. In Table 19.3, we present findings for past-year dependence of any illicit drug, marijuana, and cocaine by age group. Although African Americans were less likely to use any illicit drug than Whites, they were more likely to qualify for a diagnosis of drug dependence. This difference was most pronounced at later ages—for respondents 35+ years old, African Americans were nearly three times more likely to have past-year drug dependence than Whites (1.3 percent vs. 0.5 percent). Marijuana accounted for the largest portion of drug dependence and followed the same pattern of racial/ethnic differences as observed for any illicit drug. Prevalence of past-year cocaine dependence was low for all racial/ethnic groups but was significantly higher for African Americans compared to Whites and Hispanics. As was the case for any illicit drug, the most pronounced differences by race/ethnicity were found for older adults (35+ years old) in which prevalence was several times higher for African Americans versus Whites and Hispanics (0.8 percent vs. 0.1 percent and 0.0 percent, respectively), although the small numbers of dependent individuals in this age group limits the reliability of these estimates. Prevalence of cocaine dependence for African Americans in this age group was higher than that for any race/ethnicity in any age group. This observation is consistent with findings for use of crack cocaine and heroin, which indicate that there is a subgroup

Table 19.3
Past-year dependence of any illicit drug use, marijuana, and cocaine. Estimates provided for U.S. population and among those who have ever used the drug

Race/Ethnicity	All Respondents			Users of Specified Drugs		
	Any Illicit Drug	Marijuana	Cocaine	Any Illicit Drug	Marijuana	Cocaine
12+ years old						
African American	1.8	1.1	0.6	5.0	3.6	8.1
White	1.2	0.7	0.2	2.9	1.9	1.7
Hispanic	1.2	0.8	0.2	3.8	3.2	1.8
12-17 years old						
African American	1.7	1.4	0.0	7.0	10.1	5.1
White	2.5	1.9	0.2	9.2	9.9	7.5
Hispanic	2.6	2.1	0.3	9.6	11.1	8.6
18-25 years old						
African American	4.3	3.8	0.4	9.6	9.7	12.2
White	3.8	2.6	0.6	6.8	5.1	4.5
Hispanic	2.1	1.7	0.3	5.4	5.0	3.0
26-34 years old						
African American	1.3	0.8	0.5	2.9	1.9	6.2
White	1.3	0.7	0.3	2.2	1.3	1.9
Hispanic	0.7	0.2	0.3	2.0	0.8	2.1
35+ years old						
African American	1.3	0.4	0.8	3.8	1.3	8.2
White	0.5	0.2	0.1	1.5	0.6	0.9
Hispanic	0.6	0.3	0.0	2.1	1.2	0.2

Source: National Household Survey On Drug Abuse (2000).

of individuals experiencing drug use and problems related to use at an age at which individuals typically have terminated their drug use.

We extended this analysis of the prevalence of drug dependence, restricting the sample to include only drug users. In this way, it was possible to focus on the transition to dependence once drug use has started. Because the NHSDA only measures symptoms of drug dependence that occur in the year prior to interview, those who are drug-dependent are likely to be either new-onset cases of drug dependence (most likely for younger users) or chronically dependent over extended periods of time (most likely for older users). Nonetheless, this analysis allows a test of the hypothesis that minorities, particularly African Americans, are more likely than Whites to experience adverse consequences of drug use. The findings depicted in Table 19.3 provide support for this hypothesis. For any drug dependence, African Americans are more likely to report recent dependence than Whites for all age groups except the youngest. Most striking were the findings for cocaine dependence—8.1 percent of African American cocaine users met criteria for past-year cocaine dependence compared to only 1.7 percent and 1.8 percent White and Hispanic cocaine users, respectively. This disparity in cocaine dependence was observed for all age groups with the exception of the youngest group of cocaine users. These findings provide support for the hypothesis that African Americans are more likely than Whites to experience adverse effects of drug use once use begins. The relatively small number of heroin users and smaller number of respondents with dependence in the NHSDA limits our ability to conduct a parallel analysis for heroin. Certainly, the findings from Windham (2002) point to the need for epidemiologic studies of the impact of heroin use in urban African American populations.

HEALTH CONSEQUENCES OF DRUG USE AND ABUSE

Consistent with findings for drug dependence, there is a large body of evidence that there are large disparities in the adverse consequences of drug use, in which minorities, particularly African Americans, have an excess of health and other problems related to their drug use (Estrada, 2002). The adverse consequences of drug use are limited not to health outcomes, such as infectious disease due to injection drug use, but also to negative social outcomes, such as drug-related arrests.

HIV/AIDS Prevalence

Americans are disproportionately affected by HIV/AIDS in the United States, accounting for nearly one-third of all AIDS cases and 46 percent of HIV infection in men (CDC, 2000). This disparity was higher for women, as 57 percent of AIDS cases and 68 percent of HIV infection were accounted for by African American women. Only 9 percent of AIDS cases for White non-Hispanic males are related to injecting drug use, compared to 34 percent of cases among African Americans. Among women, the proportion of AIDS cases related to injecting drug use was similar across racial/ethnic groups—ranging from 40 to 42 percent for Hispanics, Blacks, and Whites. These findings are particularly striking when examined in light of epidemiologic findings on injecting drug use. Although results from the 2000 NHSDA indicate that there are nearly 15 times more White than African American injecting drug users, there are three times more cases of AIDS related to injecting drug use in African Americans versus Whites (CDC, 2000).

Similar evidence of health disparities among injecting drug users have been found for Hepatitis B and Hepatitis C virus infection (HBV and HCV) (Estrada, 2002). An epidemiologic study of injecting drug users found that African Americans were three times as likely to be HBV-infected than White injecting drug users, even when duration of drug use and patterns of drug use were taken into account (Levine et al., 1995). Differences have also been found for HCV, indicating that minority injecting drug users are more likely to be infected than White IDUs (Zeldis et al., 1992; Levine et al., 1994).

Emergency Room Visits

The Drug Abuse Warning Network (DAWN), operated by the Substance Abuse and Mental Health Services Administration (SAMHSA) Office of Applied Studies, is a surveillance system to track mentions of drug use linked to episodes of emergency care. Data are abstracted from records of participating hospital emergency rooms, recording whether there is a mention of use of an illegal drug. Mentions are recorded regardless of whether drug use played a causal role leading to the emergency room visit. In recent years, there has been an effort to systematize sampling of participating facilities to provide a nationally representative sample for projections to the entire nation.

In 2000, Whites accounted for 58 percent of DAWN hospital Emergency Department visits, compared to 21 percent for Black Americans (Table 19.4); however, Blacks accounted for the largest proportion of visits with a mention of cocaine than any other racial/ethnic group. Blacks accounted for 43 percent of visits for cocaine versus 34 percent for Whites. There was also an excess of emergency room visits with mentions of heroin and PCP for Blacks versus Whites relative to their proportion of DAWN visits. There was a proportionate number of mentions of marijuana use, and Blacks had less than expected mentions for LSD, amphetamine, and methamphetamine.

Drug-related Arrests

Although African Americans account for only 13 percent of drug users (past month) in the United States, they account for more than half (56 percent) of all drug offenders in state prisons (King &

Table 19.4

Comparison of race/ethnicity distribution for total DAWN hospital emergency episodes with race/ethnicity distribution for selected drug mentions, 2000

Selected Drug Mention	Race/Ethnicity		
	White	Black	Hispanic
Percentage of Total DAWN ER episodes	57.5	21.4	10.9
Percentage of ER drug mention			
Heroin/morphine	40.5	32.6	15.8
Methadone	67.9	10.4	8.6
LSD	72.6	6.3	9.7
PCP/PCP combinations	42.1	35.1	12.5
Cocaine	34.2	43.4	13.6
Marijuana/hashish	50.8	27.4	12.2
Amphetamine	63.9	5.6	15.4
Methamphetamine/speed	63.7	6.2	16.1

Source: Drug Abuse Warning Network, 2000. Substance Abuse and Mental Health Services Administration (2001).

Mauer, 2002). Three-quarters of these offenders were arrested for drug or nonviolent offenses, including drug possession and trafficking, and the majority of those involved in drug trafficking would be considered "low-level" dealers, whose arrest would have little impact on drug marketing activity. These data point to an important adverse consequence of drug use that extends beyond typical health consequences. The impact of incarceration for drug-related offenses extends beyond drug offenders to their families and communities (Iguchi et al., 2002). Drug offenders who are released from prison have limited access to resources, such as health and housing benefits, education, and employment opportunities, which places them at risk for remission of drug use and recidivism. Treatment and rehabilitation have been recommended for nonviolent drug offenders as alternatives to incarceration (Iguchi et al., 2002), and there appears to be growing public support for alternative sanctions (Peter D. Hart Research Associates, 2002).

SUMMARY

The observed patterns of racial/ethnic disparities in drug use raise a number of issues regarding causal influences on drug use. As data from the NHSDA and other sources indicate, there is clear evidence that African American youth are less likely to be involved in the use of any drug relative to their White counterparts. On the other hand, drug use and its adverse consequences are higher among older African American adults, particularly those 35+ years old. There is little reason to suspect that genetic factors can account for these differences (Buka, 2002), and it is necessary to probe social environmental factors that account for these disparities.

The patterns and trends in the prevalence of crack cocaine use in the U.S. population can provide some clues in understanding the social environmental influences that lead to disparities in drug use. Because crack cocaine became available only in the 1980s, it provides an excellent opportunity to examine the diffusion of drug use in the population. Within a few years after introduction of crack cocaine, use surged among African American adults. By 1990, 8 percent of African American 26–34-year-olds had used crack cocaine, and over half of these users had used in the past year. At the same time, use among younger African Americans was considerably lower and was almost nonexistent among youth. Recent data based on treatment admissions in 2000 in several major U.S. cities indicate that the majority of those admitted for treatment with cocaine as the primary drug of abuse are over 35 years old (NIDA, 2003). African Americans in this age group (35+) currently maintain the highest prevalence of crack cocaine use relative to any age group for Blacks, Whites, and Hispanics. It is important to understand why use of crack and indicators of problem drug use remain so high among this group of older African American adults.

Despite widespread availability of cocaine, the prevalence of crack cocaine use among African Americans 26–34 years old is a fraction of that of their counterparts a decade ago. Further research is needed to determine whether younger cohorts will experience the same patterns of risk exhibited by their older counterparts. Drug use prevention efforts typically have targeted children and adolescents. Findings from this report suggest that greater intervention efforts be shifted to young adults among Black Americans. Increased understanding of the mechanisms that have placed older Black Americans at increased risk for drug use outcomes is imperative for reducing health disparities in a variety of adverse outcomes of drug use.

REFERENCES

American Psychiatric Association (APA). (1994). *Diagnostic and Statistical Manual of Mental Disorders*, 4th ed. Washington, DC: American Psychiatric Association.

Buka, S.L. (2002). Disparities in health status and substance use: Ethnicity and socioeconomic factors. *Public Health Reports, 117*, S118–S125.

Centers for Disease Control and Prevention (CDC). (2000). HIV/AIDS surveillance report, 12.

Chilcoat, H.D. (1994). The war on drugs (letter). *New England Journal of Medicine, 331*, 126.

Chilcoat, H.D., & Breslau, N. (1996). Alcohol disorders in young adulthood: Effects of transitions into adult roles. *Journal of Health and Social Behavior, 37, 339–349.*

Chilcoat, H.D., & Schutz, C.G. (1995). Racial/ethnic and age differences in crack use within neighborhoods. *Addiction Research, 3*, 103–111.

Chilcoat, H.D., & Schutz, C.G. (1996). Age-specific patterns of hallucinogen use in the U.S. population: An analysis using generalized additive models. *Drug and Alcohol Dependence, 43*, 143–153.

Dunlap, E., & Johnson, B.D. (1992). The setting for the crack era: Macro forces, micro consequences (1960–1992). *Journal of Psychoactive Drugs, 24*, 307–321.

Ellickson, P.L., & Morton, S.C. (1999). Identifying adolescents at risk for hard drug use: Racial/ethnic variations. *Journal of Adolescent Health, 25*, 382–395.

Estrada, A.L. (2002). Epidemiology of HIV/AIDS, hepatitis B, hepatitis C, and tuberculosis among minority injection drug users. *Public Health Reports, 117*, S126–S134.

Gil, A.G., Vega, W.A., & Turner, R.J. (2002). Early and mid-adolescence risk factors for later substance abuse by African Americans and European Americans. *Public Health Reports, 117*, S15–S29.

Hardy, J.B., et al. (1997). Self-sufficiency at ages 27 to 33 years. Factors present between birth and 18 years that predict educational attainment among children born to inner-city families. *Pediatrics, 99*, 80–87.

Harrison, L. (1997). The validity of self-reported drug use in survey research: An overview and critique of research methods. In L. Harrison, & A. Hughes, A. (eds.), *The validity of self-reported drug use: Improving the accuracy of survey estimates*. National Institute on Drug Abuse Research Monograph 167. Washington, DC: U.S. Government Printing Office, pp. 17–36.

Iguchi, M.Y., London, J.A., Forge, N.G., Hickman, L., Fain, T., & Riehman, K. (2002). Elements of well-being affected by criminalizing the drug user. *Public Health Reports, 117*, S146–S150.

Kandel, D.B., & Raveis, V.H. (1989). Cessation of illicit drug use in young adulthood. *Archives of General Psychiatry, 46*, 109–116.

King, R.S., & Mauer, M. (2002). Distorted priorities: Drug offenders in state prisons. The Sentencing Project. Available from URL: http://www.sentectingproject.org/news/state_priorities.pdf.

Levine, O.S., Vlahov, D., & Nelson, K. (1994). Epidemiology of hepatitis B virus infections among injecting drug users: Seroprevalence, risk factors, and viral interactions. *Epidemiology Review, 16*, 418–436.

Levine, O.S., Vlahov D., Koehler, J., Cohn, S., Spronk, A.D., Nelson, K.E. (1995). Seroepidemiology of hepatitis B virus in a population of injecting drug users. *American Journal of Epidemiology, 142*, 331–341.

Lillie-Blanton, M., Anthony, J.C., & Schuster, C.R. (1993). Probing the meaning of racial/ethnic group comparisons in crack cocaine smoking. *Journal of the American Medical Association, 269*, 993–997.

McCaffrey, B.R. (October 5, 1997). Race and drugs: Perception and reality. *Washington Times*, B4.

National Institute on Drug Abuse (2003). Epidemiologic Trends in Drug Abuse, Volume II: Proceedings of the Community Epidemiology Work Group, December 2002. NIH Publication Number 03-5365, Rockville, MD: National Institute on Drug Abuse.

Office of Applied Studies, Substance Abuse and Mental Health Services Administration. (2001). Summary of findings from the 2000 National Household Survey on Drug Abuse (DHHS Publication No. SMA 01-3549, NHSDA Series H-13). Rockville, MD: Substance Abuse and Mental Health Services Administration, Office of Applied Studies. Also available at http://www.samhsa.gov/oas/nhsda.html.

Peter D. Hart Research Associates. (2002). Changing public attitudes toward the criminal justice system. Results of a telephone survey of 1,056 U.S. adults and six focus groups, May–December 2001, conducted for Open Society Institute, www.soros.org.

Saxe, L., Kashudin, K., Beveridge, A., Livert, D., Tighe, E., Rindskopf, D., Ford, J., & Brodsky, A. (2001). The visibility of illicit drugs: Implications for community-based drug control strategies. *American Journal of Public Health, 91*, 1987–1994.

Substance Abuse and Mental Health Services Administration (2001). Drug Abuse Warning Network. Annual Emergency Department Data 2000. DAWN Series D-18. DHHS Publication Number (SMA) 01-3532, Rockville, MD: SAMHSA.

Substance Abuse and Mental Health Services Administration (SAMHSA). (2001). Preliminary Estimates from the 2000 National Houschold Survey on Drug Abuse. Washington, DC: U.S. Government Printing Office.

Turner, C.F., Ku, L., Rogers, S.M., Lindberg, L.D., Pleck, J.H., & Sonenstein, F.L. (1998). Adolescent sexual behavior, drug use, and violence: Increased reporting with computer survey technology. *Science, 280*, 867–873.

Vega, W.A., Zimmerman, R.S., Warheit, G.J., Apospori, E., & Gil, A.G. (1993). Risk factors for early adolescent drug use in four ethnic and racial groups. *American Journal of Public Health, 83*, 185–189.

Wagner, F.A., & Anthony, J.C. (2002). From first drug use to drug dependence: Developmental periods of risk for dependence upon marijuana, cocaine, and alcohol. *Neuropsychopharmacology, 26*, 479–488.

Windham, A. (2002). Pathways to problem drug use: The role of early maternal nurturing (doctoral dissertation). Johns Hopkins University, Baltimore.

Wish, E.D., Hoffman, J.A., & Nemes, S. (1997). The validity of self-reports of drug use at treatment admission and at follow-up: Comparisons with urinalysis and hair assays. In L. Harrison and A. Hughes (Eds.), *The validity of self-reported drug use: Improving the accuracy of survey estimates*. National Institute on Drug Abuse Research Monograph 167. Washington, DC: U.S. Government Printing Office, pp. 200–226.

Zeldis, J., Jain, S., Kuramoto, I., Richards, C., Sazama, K., Samuels, S., Holland, P.V., & Flynn, N. (1992). Seroepidemiology of viral infections among intravenous drug users in northern California. *Western Journal of Medicine, 156*, 30–35.

CHAPTER 20

African Americans and Alcohol Use: Implications for Intervention and Prevention

FREDERICK D. HARPER, TERESA GRANT, AND
KIMBERLY N. MONTGOMERY

This chapter examines the drinking patterns and behaviors of African Americans as well as social and health disparities of African Americans compared to Whites and other U.S. ethnic groups. In addition, the chapter examines risk factors for alcohol problems and etiological explanations of alcohol use, abuse, and nonuse among African Americans. Moreover, strategies and recommendations are presented for diagnosis, therapeutic intervention, and prevention of alcoholism and alcohol-related health and social problems.

DRINKING PATTERNS AND BEHAVIORS

National surveys and community studies of drinking behaviors by ethnicity tend to indicate that African American adults have a lower rate of alcohol use in the previous year and a lower rate of heavy alcohol use in the previous month when compared to the general U.S. population (Jones-Webb, 1998; Substance Abuse and Mental Health Services Administration [SAMHSA], 1998). Furthermore, African American women and youth have lower rates of drinkers, heavy drinkers, and problem drinkers when compared to their Native American Indian, Latino/a, and White counterparts (Epstein et al., 1998; National Institute on Alcohol Abuse and Alcoholism [NIAAA], 1997; SAMHSA, 1998). Nevertheless, Asian Americans demonstrate the lowest rates of drinkers, heavy drinkers, and problem drinkers, that is, as compared to other non-White ethnic groups, White Americans, and the general U.S. population (NIAAA, 1997). As regard to men, Black males have similar to lower rates of drinkers and heavy drinkers when compared to White males; however, Black males have a higher level of problem drinkers (Herd, 1994; NIAAA, 1997).

SOCIAL AND HEALTH DISPARITIES

Although African Americans have lower to similar rates of drinkers and heavy drinking compared to the general U.S. population and most U.S. ethnic groups (except Asian Americans), surveys suggest that African Americans tend to have a higher rate of alcohol-related social and health problems when compared to a national sample of the U.S. population (Caetano & Clark, 1998; Herd,

1994; NIAAA, 1997). The following list delineates some of the alcohol-related social and health disparities for African Americans:

1. African American males tend to have a higher rate of cirrhosis than White males, a liver disease that is strongly associated with alcoholism or frequent heavy drinking (NIAAA, 1997).

2. Declining health in a significant proportion of middle-age African American men is often exacerbated by heavy drinking (NIAAA, 2000). Moreover, African Americans, in general, are more likely than White Americans to engage in heavy drinking and problem drinking during their 30s and 40s, that is, as regard to age (Dawkins & Harper, 1983; Herd, 1990).

3. Socioeconomic predictors that put African American females at risk for fetal alcohol syndrome or fetal alcohol effects include (a) three or more children, (b) unmarried status, (c) heavy drinking with a partner, (d) low socioeconomic status, and (e) level of heavy drinking and frequency of heavy-drinking episodes (NIAAA, 2000).

4. White Americans are more likely to have alcohol-related road accidents than African Americans (Cohall & Bannister, 2001; NIAAA, 2000).

AT-RISK AFRICAN AMERICAN GROUPS

Compared to White males and females in general, African American males are at greater risk for alcohol-related social and health problems (Herd, 1994; NIAAA, 1997). African American males are much more likely to be a victim or perpetrator of alcohol-related homicides or to suffer from alcohol-related health problems such as alcoholism and liver disease. Moreover, African American males are at risk for diseases that are exacerbated by frequent episodes of heavy drinking, for example, hypertension, diabetes, heart disease, and certain types of cancer or malignant neoplasms (Cohall & Bannister, 2001; NIAAA, 1997). African American males who have arrests for alcohol-related criminal offenses and who are consistently unemployed are also at risk for alcoholism or alcohol-related problems (Caetano & Clark, 1998; Herd, 1990).

Although African American women, in general, are not at risk for alcoholism and problem drinking, certain subgroups of African American women who may be at risk include the persistently homeless, African American women who drink heavily with a group or a partner, and those who suffer from depression and posttraumatic syndrome (Cohall & Bannister, 2001; Dawkins & Harper, 1983).

African American college students on White campuses have a lower rate of drinkers and binge drinkers as compared to their White and Hispanic counterparts; however, their drinking rate is higher than that of their noncollege African American cohorts of comparable age, 18–25, and it is higher than the drinking rate of their counterparts at traditionally African American colleges (NIDA, 1995; Williams & Newby, 1993). Moreover, there is empirical evidence that Black Greeks on predominantly African American college campuses drink and binge less frequently than Black Greeks on predominantly White college campuses and that Black Greeks, in general, drink and binge less frequently than their White counterparts (Presley et al., 2002). Based on college drinking behaviors, it appears that African Americans on White college or university campuses are more at risk for alcohol abuse and alcohol problems when compared to their age cohorts on Black college campuses (Wechsler et al., 1994). Williams and Newby (1993) define alcohol problems of college students as including alcohol-induced academic problems, conflicts with the opposite sex, and other social problems related to campus life.

Several studies indicate that college athletes tend to have higher rates of drinkers than college nonathletes (Hildebrand et al., 2001; Selby et al., 1990). According to the National College Athletic Association (2001), alcohol was found to be the number one socially used drug by college athletes. Selby et al. (1990) note that team atmosphere among athletes contributes to group binge drinking, especially during the off-season, and that athletes tend to increase their drinking by as much as 50 percent during the off-season. Although one national survey of college athletes (Anderson et al., 1991) found Black college athletes to have a lower rate of drinkers than their White counterparts, there was also an indication that drinking by Black athletes had increased at a faster rate than White athletes, since 1985, suggesting an increasing risk for alcohol problems.

In general, African American students on White college and university campuses are at greater risk for drinking problems as compared to African American students on Black college or university campuses (Williams & Newby, 1993). In part, the risk factors for African Americans students on White campuses may be associated with racial isolation and White indifference, racial bias and conflicts, loneliness, and depression.

ETIOLOGY OF ALCOHOLISM AND ALCOHOL-USE PATTERNS

In planning ethnoculturally appropriate intervention and prevention, one should have some understanding not only of who is at risk but also of the etiological causes that are associated with alcohol-related behaviors and problems of African Americans. Jones-Webb (1998) posits, "Variables such as age, social class, church attendance, drinking norms, and coping behaviors may be important in understanding differences in drinking and drinking problem rates among African Americans and Whites" (p. 263). In addition to Jones-Webb's etiological variables, especially as related to African Americans, one cannot overlook influential etiological factors such as race and racism, gender, and geographic context. The fact that a large proportion of African Americans are subject to racism and racial bias, are members of lower-income strata, and reside in urban geographic areas all tend to play a role toward influencing heavy drinking and problem drinking among certain socioeconomic sectors of the African American community. In addition, the prevalence of liquor stores or alcohol outlets in African American residential communities contributes to the accessibility of alcohol and, therefore, a cultural tendency by some African Americans in those communities to drink as a way of life. Furthermore, gender and culture-specific gender role seem to play a significant part in distinguishing the high rate of abstention among African American women.

Explaining Alcohol Use

In developing an etiological model of explaining alcohol use versus nonuse by African Americans, Harper (1986) conceptualized the following hypotheses:

Hypothesis 1 (Historical Reasons).   Historical patterns of alcohol use during slavery and racial segregation in the United States have had an intergenerational influence on weekend, group, and heavy drinking by some African Americans and abstention by others. For example, on some White plantations during American slavery, African slaves were encouraged to drink heavily on the weekend as a social outlet from the toils of slavery, while on other plantations, Black slaves were not allowed to drink alcohol at all for fear they would lose control and either rebel violently or escape to freedom. Moreover, prior to the mid-1960s, racial segregation in the United States limited recreational and social opportunities for African Americans, causing some of them to resort to alcohol use at house parties and in nightclubs and taverns. While some African Americans took the path of alcohol use as entertainment, others took the route of involvement in fundamental Protestant churches that preached abstention from any alcohol use and thus influenced or reinforced nondrinking behaviors. In addition, the Black Muslim movement in the United States has emphasized nondrinking for both its members and the Black community in general.

Hypothesis 2 (Social Reasons).   Unlike all-White or predominantly White residential neighborhoods, liquor outlets are often located in African American residential communities, especially in

African American urban and rural neighborhoods. Moreover, there is social expectation or peer influence to drink in specific ethnocultural contexts such as house parties, celebration events, public group drinking (e.g., by the homeless and/or unemployed), and at some athletic and recreational functions. In these respects, the accessibility of alcohol and social expectations to drink have influenced African American drinking behaviors.

Hypothesis 3 (Psychological Reasons).   Heavy drinking is a means of psychologically escaping the painful and unhealthy realities of racism and racial discrimination or of escaping unpleasant emotions and painful experiences of life in general. For African Americans, heavy drinking is also a means of dealing with multifaceted stress, for example, stress that is related to challenges of poverty, negative racial bias, the fear of community or domestic violence, and past traumatic experiences.

Hypothesis 4 (Economic Reasons).   African Americans, especially men, may drink heavily because of economic and employment problems that include unemployment, underemployment, unstable employment, and racial discrimination in employment, as well as racial discrimination in job promotion, compensation or salary, and job dismissal. By the same token, economic problems can contribute to alcohol abuse that are not related to racial discrimination or racial bias, for example, economic losses that result from gambling.

As regard to Harper's fourth hypothesis on economic reasons for heavy drinking and problems drinking, Welsing (1991) reports that large numbers of African American males engaging in alcohol and other drug abuse are tied directly to the "severely crippled" African American family structure, a circumstance that is often brought about by a racist society that systematically denies African American males the same opportunities as White males to achieve and, thus, to assume their rightful functional roles as husbands and fathers. In general, there is still a significant proportion of African Americans who are locked into poverty and locked out of educational, employment, and career advancement opportunities, which creates a great deal of stress that can lead to alcohol abuse as an escape mechanism.

In terms of the large proportion of African American women who do not drink, as compared to White females, this phenomenon can be explained partially by African American females' historic commitment and responsibility to parenting (which is antithetical to alcohol abuse), their high commitment to work and career achievement, their active involvement in the church or other religious or faith-based activity, and an attitude that money and time cannot be wasted on drinking.

DIAGNOSIS, ASSESSMENT, AND THERAPEUTIC INTERVENTION

This section addresses alcohol-related diagnosis, assessment, and intervention or treatment strategies for African American alcoholics or those with alcohol-related problems. Within this chapter, the term intervention is used interchangeably with the concept of treatment.

Ethnic-Specific Assessment and Diagnosis

Prior to treatment or an intervention plan, there is usually some kind of intake interview or process in order to assess or diagnose the alcohol-related disorder or problem of the client (or patient). If the client is diagnosed to be an alcoholic or to be dependent on, or addicted to, the drug alcohol, then detoxification is the usual first step prior to the beginning of treatment. Detoxification, of course, is a process for the purpose of getting the alcoholic client off the drug alcohol and through the withdrawal phase of the alcohol addiction to a sober state of being free from alcohol dependency and a daily craving or metabolic need for alcohol. Furthermore, detoxification is the precursor to counseling, alcoholism treatment, or a comprehensive intervention plan.

Proper assessment and diagnosis of possible alcohol problems or disorders should entail obtaining information about the African American client's medical history, educational background, employment history, legal problems, alcohol/substance abuse behaviors and history, family and social history, psychological behaviors, close relationships, cultural background, and spiritual history. Ascertaining information in these areas is valuable for understanding the individual client or patient, making an appropriate diagnosis or assessment of the problem, and developing the most appropriate treatment plan. In order to screen for alcohol problems, some treatment or mental health centers employ self-report or interview instruments such as the Michigan Alcoholism Screening Test (MAST) or the Addiction Severity Index (ASI) (Lewis et al., 2002); however, these assessment tools have to be interpreted from an ethnic or cultural perspective based on the nature of the items or questions and the nature of the responses of African American clients to these assessment items.

A diagnostic classification is not necessary for acquiring a clinical understanding of the African American client's drinking problems, manifestations, contexts, and motivations; nevertheless, some mental health centers and treatment centers may require a diagnosis for the purpose of third-party payment or because of requirements by local government or a private agency. If a diagnostic tool such as the *Diagnostic and Statistical Manual of Mental Disorders* (DSM-IV) is used (American Psychiatric Association, 1994), the counselor should be careful to take into consideration the ethnic, cultural, and psychosocial dynamics as well as the overall circumstances and contexts of the African American drinker or alcohol abuser. In delineating standards for culturally or ethnically competent diagnosis, Guindon and Sobhany (2001) state, "The goals of diagnosis are to (a) identify mental health problems, (b) recognize factors contributing to and maintaining these identified problems, (c) select and implement optimum courses of intervention, and, when needed, (d) revise intervention strategies to meet the needs of the client" (p. 270).

INTERVENTION OR TREATMENT APPROACHES

The following discussion includes ethnocultural approaches and perspectives for intervention or treatment with African American alcoholics or clients who have alcohol-related problems.

African American–Centered Intervention

African American–centered intervention refers to intervention, treatment, and counseling strategies that are sensitive to, and appropriate for, the cultural ways and psychosocial conditions of the African American client. During therapeutic intervention, the clinical practitioner (counselor, psychologist, social workers, or case manager) should be aware and address the role and dynamics of the African American family, faith groups or spirituality, close interpersonal relationships, need for employment or adequate employment, and racial unfairness and racially traumatic experiences.

Harper (2001) presents the following considerations for working with African American alcoholics or African Americans who have problems with alcohol use or heavy drinking: (a) ethnic-sensitive assessment and diagnosis of alcohol-related problems or disorders, (b) a preference for intervention programs that are located in African American communities, (c) an understanding of, and sensitivity to, African American culture as well as the diversity within the African American culture, (d) the involvement of African American counselors where and when possible, (e) cultural competence and commitment of helping practitioners, and (f) the establishment of accessible Alcoholics Anonymous (AA) groups in the African American community or the use of ethnically diverse AA groups with a predominantly African American membership when possible. If African American or ethnically mixed AA groups cannot be identified, White or predominantly White AA groups should be recommended and used, as long as such groups are accepting and therapeutically supportive of African American alcoholics.

Counseling African American Alcoholics.   When it comes to counseling, the following are strategies or skills that are useful in working with African American alcoholics and alcohol abusers, that is, based on interviews of counselors who represented a diverse array of alcoholism treatment programs throughout the United States that served a significant percentage of African American clientele (Harper, 1979; Harper & Saifnoorian, 1991):

1. Outreach counseling—reaching out to counsel African American clients within their natural environments and eventually recruiting them into health care, alcoholism treatment, counseling, or referral for social or medical services.

2. Family counseling—involving the African American alcoholic or problem drinker's family members; counseling the entire family and securing services, resources, and jobs for the family or family members as needed.

3. Group counseling—working with African American alcoholics and alcohol abusers in small groups to assist with interpersonal problems, intrapersonal conflict, and personal concerns as well as provide support for recovery from alcoholism (Harper, 1984).

4. Action-oriented or directive counseling approaches—employing cognitive-behavioral therapy, reality therapy, or transcendent counseling. Transcendent counseling is an existential, cognitive-behavioral counseling theory that focuses on changing the heavy drinking lifestyle of the client by changing thoughts that drive life choices and by getting the client to focus on existential meaning in life other than drinking (Harper & Stone, 1999, 2003).

5. Appropriate and timely referral to agencies—referring the African American client to helping agencies for health, social, and alcohol-related services and assistance. Also, the recruitment of clients from agencies for treatment or counseling, for example, from the court/prison system, unemployment agencies, and from the ranks of the homeless alcoholics or public inebriates. There should be a significant counseling effort to place the chronically unemployed, African American client into meaningful jobs and/or to refer the client for job placement or job training opportunities.

An Afrocentric Approach

The Afrocentric paradigm, developed by Robinson and Howard-Hamilton (1994), is a model that can assist the therapist who works with African American clients who have alcohol-related problems or an alcohol-related diagnosis. This model enables the client to progress toward developing effective interpersonal relationships and a positive self-image. Moreover, it enables clients to establish direction and meaning in their lives. The paradigm utilizes the seven principles of Kwanzaa (Official Kwanzaa Web site, 2002): (a) *Umoja* (unity with African people; also, solidarity and harmony in the African American community), (b) *Kujichagulia* (self-determination and the defining of self), (c) *Ujima* (collective work and responsibility: building and maintaining "our" community together; establishing a connectedness with others in terms of meaningful work toward a common destiny), (d) *Ujamaa* (cooperative economics: economically building and maintaining our own community), (e) *Nia* (purpose that benefits self and the collective community), (f) *Kuumba* (creativity, imagination, and ingenuity), and (g) *Imani* (faith).

Robinson and Howard-Hamilton's (1994) paradigm also incorporates the resistance modality of Robinson and Ward (1991), which has two orientations: the liberation/empowerment orientation and the survival/oppression orientation. These therapeutic themes may be used to promote psychological liberation from racism and movement toward racial empowerment and self-determination for the African American client. Robinson and Howard-Hamilton's Afrocentric paradigm provides the therapist with a cognitive strategy that allows the African American client to redefine himself or herself in a positive way that is culturally congruent to African American heritage and culture. In general, Robinson and Howard-Hamilton's Afrocentric paradigm initiates and promotes psychological health and satisfying relationships for African Americans clients who are in treatment for alcoholism or alcohol-related problems.

Culturally Competent Counseling

"Cultural competence" and "multicultural counselor competence" are phrases that have become increasingly prevalent in the counseling and therapy literature. These terms suggest competence to work effectively with clients from a culture or cultures different from one's own (Harper & Mc-Fadden, 2003). Multicultural counselor competence implies the ability to counsel or therapize across cultures based on the counselor's cultural awareness, culturally accurate knowledge, and culturally appropriate skills as regard to a particular cultural group or groups.

Non–African American and African American counselors and clinicians need to be culturally competent, innovative, and committed to the helping relationship in order to work effectively with African American clients who present alcohol problems or disorders. It cannot be assumed that all African American helping professionals understand the worldview of all African American people. This counseling process includes having an awareness of how the client's African American culture is different from one's own cultural background and how one's cultural worldview can influence the effectiveness of counseling as well as counseling outcomes.

Young (1999) reports that treatment should be rooted in an understanding of, and respect for, the patient's needs, cultural values, and environment. Young goes further to note that culturally competent services are characterized by (a) a treatment staff's knowledge of the native language of the patient, (b) sensitivity to the cultural nuances of the patient population, (c) the use of treatment modalities that reflect the cultural values and needs of the treatment population, and (d) input from the patient population in decision making and policy implementation, so that cultural outsiders do not impose their values. Along this line, James and Johnson (1996) report that cultural sensitivity is an important component in addressing both the personal and public troubles of all people. One report of a national assessment of interracial treatment indicates that African American clientele who perceived White counselors to be effective described them as possessing cultural sensitivity, empathy, rapport, commitment, and effective communication (Harper, 1979).

STRATEGIES AND RECOMMENDATIONS FOR PREVENTION

Prevention should be based on the ethnocultural practices of African Americans as well as the lifestyle or ethnic ways, cultural contexts, city or community ordinances related to alcohol sales and use, and psychosocial reasons or etiology related to African Americans' use of alcohol. Certainly, moderate drinking, preferably when eating, does not usually pose a health problem, risk for alcohol addiction, or basis for psychosocial and health problems. However, some exceptions or precautions to moderate drinking include concerns for alcohol use by pregnant females, persons with certain illnesses, and individuals who tend to become violent after one or two drinks. Nevertheless, prevention strategies should mainly focus on African American subgroups who are at risk for heavy drinking, problem drinking, alcoholism, and inappropriate uses of alcohol regarding time, place, and underage status. Herd (1990) and Dawkins and Harper (1983) note that low-income African Americans in their 30s and 40s are at risk for alcohol problems, while, for White Americans, groups at risk include middle- and upper-class teenagers and young adults in their 20s.

Preventive goals and strategies should focus on (a) changing inappropriate alcohol-related attitudes and practices by the African American families and individuals, (b) countering city ordinances and practices that facilitate heavy drinking and drinking problems in African American communities and neighborhoods, and (c) providing knowledge, attitudes, and skills that will help to prevent alcohol-related illnesses, accidents, violence, interpersonal conflict, family disruption, and sexual offenses (i.e., via schools, higher educational institutions, and public media, such as television and radio).

Although zero-tolerance policies have become popular over the last several years for the prevention of student violations related to alcohol, other drugs, and weapons at schools (Cauchon, 1999), we do not endorse this method of punishment as a broad-brush approach for dissuading inappropriate alcohol behaviors. Zero-tolerance, as a school board policy or state-legislated law, has proven to be inflexible and rigid and thus tends to punish severely model students for minor infractions or inadvertent behavior (Chachon, 1999). If schools are to use zero-tolerance for alcohol-related infractions, we suggest well-defined discipline codes that adequately describe infractions and assign equitable or reasonable punishment for each act.

Community Ordinances and Business Practices

African American professionals and community leaders should oppose racially destructive ordinances, laws, and business practices that result in billboard alcohol advertisements and the location of liquor stores in the midst of African American residential neighborhoods—liquor stores that are often established adjacent to homes, schools, and churches. In order to limit alcohol accessibility, local governments should change or develop ordinances to restrict liquor stores or alcohol outlets to commercial zones such as shopping centers and business districts of a city or community. Furthermore, instead of blatant billboard advertisements in African American residential neighborhoods that negatively impact youth and adults, businesses and corporations of the alcohol industry should take social responsibility aimed at preventing alcohol abuse and alcoholism, for example, by supporting or providing alcohol-free recreational activities, public alcohol information campaigns, and community alcohol education.

Ethnocultural Implications

Prevention should focus on strategies to minimize public drinking by African Americans who are homeless and persistently unemployed. Moreover, university and college personnel should make efforts to minimize the use of alcohol in fraternity and sorority activities (although the practice of binge drinking appears to be less prevalent for African American Greek members as compared to Whites). For African American college athletes, there should be academic tutoring, role model mentoring, and alcohol-free programs as alternatives to group drinking activities. These preventive efforts are especially important for African American athletes who are at risk for alcohol-related problems during the off-season: problems such as alcohol-related road accidents, violence, sexual assault, poor academic study habits, and poor grades. For college students in general, especially at traditionally White universities and colleges, there should be consideration for increased regulation of alcohol use on the campus in terms of restricting time and place of alcohol use, limiting the amount and type of alcohol sold or allowed on campus, and closely monitoring for underage drinking.

Alcohol Education: A Focus on Youth and College Students

There should be efforts toward alcohol education in high-risk or urban schools with majority Black enrollment (K through 12th grade). There should also be public alcohol announcements in the African American community regarding accurate information about the use of alcohol and other drugs by young people and their possible influence on health, violent behavior, accidents, irresponsible behaviors, and sexual assault. Moreover, colleges and universities, especially traditionally White higher educational institutions, need to require some type of course or orientation about alcohol and other drugs for all students, but especially athletes and members of Greek-letter organizations, that is, while giving special attention to the social needs and racial problems of African American students. University counseling must be aware of additional risk for African American students and thus take steps to prevent racial stresses that can lead to problems during the use of alcohol or that may facilitate the use of alcohol by African Americans in order to escape problems on White college campuses such as loneliness, depression, racial indifference, prejudicial decisions, and racist behaviors. In addition, African American churches and other faith-based institutions can play a significant role in providing preventive information and moral education to their youth members and constituencies.

Families and Adults: Health and Social Implications

The following is a list of do's and don'ts for African American families and individual adults who may be at risk for alcoholism and alcohol-related health and social problems. These recommendations may be shared with families and individuals by helping professionals, religious or faith leaders, educational leaders, and community leaders.

- Don't drink alcohol on an empty stomach; eat before or during drinking.
- Don't gulp down alcohol but rather sip and pace drinking—swallowing too much and drinking too fast can lead to inebriation.
- Don't give beer or other alcoholic beverages to babies, for example, to help them go to sleep at night. This is abusive, illegal, and a risk to an infant's health.
- Don't gamble for money (e.g., playing cards) while drinking with family members, friends, fellow employees, or acquaintances. Financial losses and loss of pride can result in anger, arguments, and violence.
- Don't drink heavily as an athlete because of stress, disappointments, off-season time on hand, or as an after-game release from loss or celebration of victory. This recommendation applies to high school, college, and professional African American athletes.
- Don't make binge drinking after work hours a daily habit, whether drinking at home while watching television or drinking at nightclubs or restaurants with binge-drinking friends or drinking partners.
- Don't use alcohol to try to manipulate sexual favors or facilitate sexual abuse (e.g., date rape or sexual attack).
- Don't engage in dare activity while intoxicated (e.g., drinking contests, driving a vehicle at a high rate of speed, playing with guns, or engaging in other risks that can result in bodily harm or even death).
- Don't engage in heavy drinking or drinking at all in cases of pregnancy and chronic health or behavioral problems such as hypertension, diabetes, heart disease, or difficulty in managing anger while drinking.
- Don't drink while using prescribed medication or illicit drugs that can interact with alcohol to create harm to health or a life-threatening situation.
- Don't drink before going to work, and/or don't drink on the job or before engaging in any critical task that requires a sober or attentive state of mind and/or precise perceptual motor skills.
- Don't use alcohol as a pain reliever for painful, chronic symptoms.

CONCLUSIONS

Among African Americans at risk for alcoholism and alcohol problems include African American males, African Americans in their 30s and 40s, homeless drinkers, the chronically unemployed,

African American athletes, and members of Greek-letter organizations on White college campuses. Prevention should target not only these African American subgroups but younger African American males and young African Americans in general before the frustrations of racism, employment problems, and financial problems, later in life, lead to drinking as an escape from, or numbing of, psychological pain and distress. Prevention should also target young African Americans who may drink or party as a cohesive group, such as Greeks in fraternities and sororities, African American athletes, unemployed males, and homeless persons. African American college and professional athletes are especially at risk for alcohol-related problems, especially during the off-season. Moreover, prevention strategies should be aimed at the lifestyle and cultural practices of African American families and individuals as well as the elimination of city ordinances and alcohol business practices that negatively impact African American communities and residents. Intervention or alcoholism treatment should be sensitive to African American culture and should involve outreach counseling and cognitive-behavioral counseling methods, among other ethnoculturally appropriate approaches.

REFERENCES

American Psychiatric Association. (1994). *Diagnostic and statistical manual of mental disorders (DSM-IV)* (4th ed.) Washington, DC: Author.

American Psychological Association. (2001). *Publication manual of the American Psychological Association* (5th ed.). Washington, DC: Author.

Anderson, W., Albrecht, R., McKeag, D., Hough, D., & McGrew, C. (1991). A national survey of alcohol and drug use by college athletes. *The Physician and Sportsmedicine, 19*, 411–427.

Caetano, R., & Clark, C.L. (1998). Trends in alcohol-related problems among Whites, Blacks, and Hispanics: 1984–1995. *Alcoholism: Clinical and Experimental Research, 22*, 534–538.

Cauchon D. (1999). Zero tolerance policies lack flexibility. *USA Today*, April 13.

Cohall, A.T., & Bannister, H.E. (2001). The health status of children and adults. In R. Braithwaite & S.E. Taylor (Eds.), *Health issues in the Black community* (2d ed., pp. 13–43). San Francisco: Jossey-Bass.

Dawkins, M.P., & Harper, F.D. (1983). Alcoholism among women: A comparison of Black and White problem drinkers. *International Journal of the Addictions, 18*, 333–349.

Epstein, J.A., Botvin, G.J., & Diaz, T. (1998). Ethnic and gender differences in alcohol use among a longitudinal sample of inner-city adolescents. *Journal of Gender, Culture, and Health, 3*, 193–207.

Guindon, M.H., & Sobhany, M.S. (2001). Toward cultural competency in diagnosis. *International Journal for the Advancement of Counselling, 23*, 269–282.

Harper, F.D. (1979). *Alcoholism treatment and Black Americans*. Washington, DC: U.S. Government Printing Office (publication #ADM 79–853).

Harper, F.D. (1984). Group strategies with Black alcoholics. *Journal of Specialists for Group Work, 9*, 38–43.

Harper, F.D. (1986). *The Black family and substance abuse*. Detroit: Detroit Urban League.

Harper, F.D. (2001). Alcohol use and misuse. In R. Braithwaite & S.E. Taylor (Eds.), *Health issues in the Black community* (2d ed., pp. 403–418). San Francisco: Jossey-Bass.

Harper, F.D., & McFadden, J. (Eds.). (2003). *Culture and counseling: New approaches*. Boston: Allyn & Bacon.

Harper, F.D., & Saifnoorian, E. (1991). Drinking patterns among African-Americans. In D.J. Pittman & H.R. White (Eds.), *Society, culture, and drinking patterns reexamined* (pp. 327–338). New Brunswick, NJ: Rutgers Center of Alcohol Studies.

Harper, F.D., & Stone, W.O. (1999). Transcendent counseling (TC): A theoretical approach for the year 2000 and beyond. In J. McFadden (Ed.), *Transcultural counseling* (2d ed., pp. 83–108). Alexandria, VA: American Counseling Association Press.

Harper, F.D., & Stone, W.O. (2003). Transcendent counseling: An existential, cognitive-behavioral theory. In F.D. Harper & J. McFadden (Eds.), *Culture and counseling: New approaches* (pp. 233–251). Boston: Allyn & Bacon.

Herd, D. (1990). Subgroup differences in drinking patterns among Black and White men: Results from a national survey. *Journal of Studies on Alcohol, 51*, 221–232.

Herd, D. (1994). Predicting drinking problems among Black and White men: Results from a national survey. *Journal of Studies on Alcohol, 55*, 61–71.

Hildebrand, K.M., Johnson, D.J., & Bogle, K. (2001). Comparison of patterns of alcohol use between high school and college athletes and non-athletes. *College Student Journal, 35*, 358–365.

James, W.H., & Johnson, S.L. (1996). *Doin' drugs: Patterns of African American addiction.* Austin: University of Texas Press.

Jones-Webb, R. (1998). Drinking patterns and problems among African Americans: Recent findings. *Alcohol, Health and Research World, 22*, 260–264.

Lewis, J.A., Dana, R.Q., & Blevins, G.A. (2002). *Substance abuse counseling* (3d ed.). Pacific Grove, CA: Brooks/Cole.

National Collegiate Athletic Association (NCAA). (2001). *NCAA study of substance use habits of college student-athletes.* Retrieved May 8, 2002, from http://www.ncaa.org.

National Institute on Alcohol Abuse and Alcoholism (NIAAA). (1997). *Ninth special report to the U.S. Congress on alcohol and health.* Rockville, MD: Author.

National Institute on Alcohol Abuse & Alcoholism (NIAAA). (2000). *Tenth special report to the U.S. Congress on alcohol and health.* Rockville, MD: Author.

National Institute on Drug Abuse (NIDA). (1995). *Drug use among racial/ethnic minorities.* Washington, DC: U.S. Government Printing Office.

Official Kwanzaa Web site (2002). Retrieved May 16, 2002, from http://www.officialkwanzaawebsite.org/7principles.html.

Presley, C.A., Meilman, P.W., & Leichliter, J.S. (2002). College factors that influence drinking. *Journal of Studies on Alcohol, 62* (Supplement No. 14), 82–90.

Robinson, T., & Howard-Hamilton, M. (1994). An Afrocentric paradigm: Foundation for a healthy self-image and healthy interpersonal relationships. *Journal of Mental Health Counseling, 16*, 327–339.

Robinson, T.L., & Ward, J.V. (1991). A belief in self far greater than anyone's disbelief: Cultivating resistance among African American adolescents. *Women and Therapy, 11*, 87–103.

Selby, R., Weinstein, H.M., & Bird, T.S. (1990). The health of university athletes. *Medicine and Science in Sports and Exercise, 39*, 11–18.

Substance Abuse and Mental Health Services Administration (SAMHSA). (1998). *Prevalence of substance use among racial and ethnic subgroups in the United States, 1991–1993.* Rockville, MD. Author.

Wechsler, H., Davenport, A., Dowdall, G., Moeykens, B., & Castillo, S. (1994). Health and behavioral consequences of binge drinking in college: A national survey of students at 140 campuses. *JAMA, 272*, 1672–1677.

Welsing, F.C. (1991). *The Isis papers.* Chicago: Third World Press.

Williams, J.E., & Newby, R.G. (1993). Assessing the need for alcohol abuse programs for African-American college students. *Journal of Multicultural Counseling and Development, 21*, 155–168.

Young, L. (1999). *Cultural competence: A journey.* Washington, DC: Bureau of Primary Health Care.

CHAPTER 21

Disparate African American and White Infant Mortality Rates in the United States

JANE A. OTADO, CHINUA AKUKWE, AND
JAMES W. COLLINS JR.

INTRODUCTION

Infant mortality rates (IMR) are defined as the number of infant deaths that occur in the first year of life per 1,000 live births. IMR are strong proxy measures of women's health, infant well-being, and access to prenatal and postnatal medical care (U.S. Department of Health and Human Services [USDHHS], 2000; Centers for Disease Control and Prevention [CDC], 1994). As such, high IMR may signify unmet community health needs. Further, in developing countries, IMR is generally seen as a measure or as a major social indicator of the health of a country. In the developed countries, particularly in the Unites States, the IMR is also seen as an indicator of the prevailing socioeconomic conditions and public health practices (USDHHS, 2000), and this may be used as a measure of health disparity between racial/ethnic or other groups (American Academy of Pediatrics, 1986; U.S. Department of Health and Human Services, 2000; Federal Interagency Forum on Child and Family Statistics, 2001).

A major objective of this chapter is to discuss the disparity in infant mortality in the United States between Blacks and Whites and the contribution this disparity makes toward understanding the overall racial disparities in health. Although IMR in the United States declined by approximately 90 percent since the early 1900s (CDC, 1999), this pace has not kept up with that of other industrialized societies. As indicated by the data (Table 21.1), since 1960 the international ranking of the United States in overall IMR declined from 10th to 23d by 1998.

Overall, IMR comprise two major components: the neonatal mortality rate (NMR) (i.e., number of infant deaths in the first 27 days of life per 1,000 live births) and the postneonatal mortality rate (PNMR) (i.e., number of infant deaths between days 28 and 365 per 1,000 live births). In the United States, about two-thirds of all infant deaths occur during the neonatal period where birth defects, disorders related to short gestation, and low birthweight (<2500g, LBW) are the leading causes of mortality. Sudden infant death syndrome (SIDS), birth defects, injuries and homicides are the leading causes of PNMR mortality in the United States.

Race-Specific Infant Mortality Rates

Although infant mortality declined for all racial and ethnic groups in the United States, substantial racial and ethnic disparities have persisted (Table 21.2). Black Americans have more than a twofold

Table 21.1
Infant mortality rates in selected industrialized countries, selected years, 1960–1997

Country[2]	Infant Mortality Rates[3]					International Ranking[1]		Percent Change
	1960	1980	1990	1995	1998	1960	1998	1960-1998
United States	26.0	12.6	9.2	7.6	7.2	10	23	-72.3
Australia	20.2	10.7	8.2	5.7	5.0	4	12	-75.2
Austria	37.5	14.3	7.8	5.4	4.9	20	11	-86.9
Belgium	31.2	12.1	7.9	7.0	5.6	17	18	-82.1
Canada	27.3	10.4	6.8	6.0	5.3	13	14	-80.6
Denmark	21.5	8.4	7.5	5.1	4.7	7	9	-78.1
England &Wales	21.8	12.0	7.9	6.1	5.7	8	20	-73.9
Finland	21.0	7.6	5.6	4.0	4.1	5	5	-80.5
France	27.4	10.0	7.3	4.9	4.6	14	7	-83.2
Germany[4]	35.0	12.4	7.1	5.3	4.6	19	7	-86.9
Hong Kong	41.5	11.2	6.2	4.6	3.2	21	1	-92.3
Ireland	29.3	11.1	8.2	6.3	6.2	15	22	-78.8
Italy	43.9	14.6	8.6	6.2	5.3	23	14	-87.9
Japan	30.4	7.5	4.6	4.3	3.6	16	3	-88.2
Netherlands	17.9	8.6	7.1	5.5	5.2	2	13	-70.9
New Zealand	22.6	12.9	8.3	6.7	5.5	9	16	-75.7
Northern Ireland	27.2	13.4	7.5	7.1	5.6	12	18	-79.4
Norway	18.9	8.1	6.9	4.1	4.0	3	4	-78.8
Scotland	26.4	12.1	7.7	6.2	5.5	11	16	-79.2
Singapore	34.8	21.4	6.7	4.0	4.2	18	6	-87.9
Spain	43.7	12.3	7.6	5.5	5.7	22	20	-87.0
Sweden	16.6	6.9	6.0	4.1	3.5	1	2	-78.9
Switzerland	21.1	9.1	6.8	5.0	4.8	6	10	-77.3

[1]Refers to countries, territories, cities or geographic areas with at least one million populations and with "complete" counts of live births and infant deaths as indicated in the United Nations Demographic Yearbook.
[2]Infant deaths (under 1 year of age) are per 1,000 live births.
[3]Rankings are from the lowest to highest infant mortality rates. Some of the variation in infant mortality rates is due to differences among countries in distinguishing between fetal and infant deaths.
[4]Rates presented for the years prior to the reunification of Germany were calculated by combining information from the Federal Republic of Germany and the German Democratic Republic.

Source: National Center for Health Statistics (2002a). *Health, United States, 2002*. With chartbook on trends in the health of Americans. Abstracted from Table 26, p. 114. Hyattsville, Maryland.

greater IMR than White Americans (Table 21.2 and Figure 21.1). Comparatively speaking, a wide variation exists in infant mortality among other ethnic groups. For instance (data not shown), in 1999 total Hispanic infant mortality rate (IMR) was 5.7 as compared to Whites and Blacks (5.8 and 14.0, respectively) and to total Asians or Pacific Islanders (4.7). The IMR for the Hispanic subgroups were high for infants of Puerto Rican mothers (8.3) and low for Cuban as well as Central and South American mothers (4.7). Rates for infants of Mexican mothers were 5.5. Among the Asian and Pacific Islander subgroups, the IMR were high for Hawaiian (7.2) and low for Japanese (3.0), (Mathews et al., 2002). In a public health achievement report conducted by the CDC (1999), persisting racial and ethnic differences in infant mortality constituted one of the greatest maternal and child health challenges for the 21st century. Thus, the persistence of large ethnic disparities in infant mortality is an important public health problem in the United States.

Table 21.2
Infant mortality rates for Whites and Blacks, United States,
1950–2000

Year	White	Black	Black/White Ratio
1950	26.8	43.9	1.6
1960	22.9	44.3	1.9
1970	17.8	32.6	2.5
1980	10.9	22.2	2.0
1990	7.6	18.0	2.4
1999	5.8	14.6	2.5
2000	5.7	14.1	2.5

Infant Mortality rates are deaths under 1 year per 1,000 live births in specified group. Beginning in 1980, race for live birth is tabulated according to race of mother.

Source: National Center for Health Statistics (2002b).

Figure 21.1
Infant mortality rates for Whites and Blacks, United States, 1950–2000

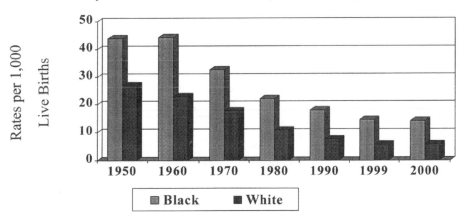

Infant Mortality rates are deaths under 1 year per 1,000 live births in specified group. Beginning in 1980, race for live birth is tabulated according to race of mother.

Source: National Center for Health Statistics (2002b).

Overview of Leading Causes of Infant Death

The rank order of leading causes of infant deaths varies by race of mother (Table 21.3; Figure 21.2). Congenital malformations are the leading cause of death for White infants. Disorders of prematurity/LBW are the leading cause of death for African American infants. African American infants have a twofold greater incidence of SIDS than Whites. Most striking, if the incidence of LBW and

Table 21.3
Five leading cause-specific infant deaths by maternal race among infants born in 1999, United States

Cause-Specific Deaths	Infant Mortality Rates[1]			Black/White Ratio
	All Races	White	Black	
Congenital Anomalies	138.3	134.0	165.3	1.2
Short Gestation and LBW	110.4	75.4	304	4.0
Sudden Infant Death Syndrome (SIDS)	66.7	55.5	129.8	2.3
Maternal Pregnancy Complications	35.0	27.8	76.7	2.8
Respiratory Distress Syndrome	28.4	22.8	61.5	2.7

1. Rates are deaths under 1 year per 100,000 live births in specified group.

Source: National Center for Health Statistics. Linked Birth/Death Data Set for the Period 1999, Hyattsville, MD.

Figure 21.2
Five leading cause-specific infant deaths by maternal race among infants born in 1999, United States

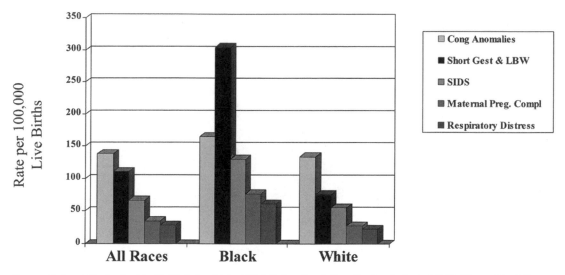

Source: National Center for Health Statistics, Linked Birth/Infant Death Data Set for the Period 1999, Hyattsville, MD.

SIDS among African American infants were reduced to levels observed among non-Hispanic White infants, the racial disparity in IMR would be substantially reduced (Mathews et al., 2002).

Race-Specific Neonatal and Postneonatal Mortality Rates

The data in Table 21.4 show race-specific NMR. Reflecting advances in neonatal medicine, particularly its ability to care for the extremely premature infant, overall NMR declined dramatically among African Americans and Whites. However, the racial disparity has actually widened. The ratio of Black-to-White neonatal mortality rate was 2.0 in 1980; it rose to 2.5 in 1999. This differential reflects the persistent racial disparity in the incidence of preterm-LBW infants.

Table 21.4
Neonatal, postneonatal mortality rates for Whites and Blacks, United States, 1950–2000

Year	Neonatal Mortality Rate[a]			Post Neonatal Mortality Rate[b]		
	White	Black	Back/White Ratio	White	Black	Black/White Ratio
1950	19.4	27.8	1.4	7.4	16.1	2.2
1960	17.2	27.8	1.6	5.7	16.5	2.9
1970	13.8	22.8	1.7	4.0	9.9	2.5
1980	7.4	14.6	2.0	3.5	7.6	2.2
1990	4.8	11.6	2.4	2.8	6.4	2.3
1999	3.9	9.8	2.5	1.9	4.8	2.5
2000	3.8	9.4	2.5	1.9	4.7	2.5

[a]Deaths per 1,000 live births, under 28 days.
[b]Deaths per 1,000 live births, 28 days–11 months.

Source: National Center for Health Statistics (2002b).

The postneonatal mortality rate (deaths to infants' age 28–364 days per 1,000 live births) declined for White infants and Blacks infants since the 1950s (CDC, 1999). However, the decline for Black infants has been slower, contributing to a persistent, large gap in postneonatal mortality rates between Black and White infants. Black infants are more than two times likely to die during the postneonatal period compared to White infants. The postneonatal mortality rate is a reflection of inadequacies in access to care and the social and economic environment in which the mother lives and a child is born (Warner, 1999).

RACIAL DISPARITY IN LOW BIRTH-WEIGHT RATES

Major contributors to the excess mortality among Black infants are the high rates of preterm delivery (those infants born before 37 weeks of completed gestation age) and very low birth weight (less than 1,500 grams) (CDC, 1994, 1999; Collins & David, 1990; National Institute of Child Health and Human Development [NICHD], 2000a). Very low birth-weight (VLBW) infants are at high risk of neurologic disorders, delayed development, learning disabilities, and long-term illness compared with normal birth-weight infants (CDC, 1994, 1999; Eberhardt et al., 2001).

Preterm deliveries occur as a result of several final pathways, including medically indicated early deliveries, spontaneous rupture of membranes, preterm labor, infections, and assisted reproductive technologies. One-third of preterm births may be due to infection/inflammation, with the incidence of bacterial vaginosis at least 2.5 times higher for African American mothers compared with White mothers (NICHD, 2001a). Very low birth-weights are almost all preterm; some are also small for gestational age. Together, VLBW and preterm delivery explain two-thirds of the excess deaths experienced by African Americans infants (CDC, 1994, 1999).

The rate of survival for LBW infants has steadily improved since the late 1960s due to advanced neonatal techniques, while the incidence of low birth weight has declined only slowly. In reviews of infant mortality and low birth weight, it is important to examine two parameters constituting these rates: the birth-weight distribution and the birth-weight specific mortality (CDC, 1994, 1999; Akukwe & Hatcher, 1995; Wilcox & Russel, 1986). Birth-weight distribution, or the risk of VLBW or LBW is often affected by the prevailing socioeconomic and demographic conditions of the mother. This has improved very little, especially for Black mothers in the last few decades. Birth-weight specific

Table 21.5
Percent of live births of low birth weight for Whites and Blacks, United States, 1990–2000

Year	VLBW [c]			LBW [d]		
	White	Black	Black/White Ratio	White	Black	Black/White Ratio
1990	0.95	2.92	3.0	5.7	13.3	2.2
1991	0.96	2.96	3.1	5.8	13.6	2.3
1992	0.96	2.96	3.1	5.8	13.3	2.2
1993	1.01	2.96	3.0	6.0	13.3	2.2
1994	1.02	2.96	3.0	6.1	13.2	2.2
1995	1.06	2.97	2.7	6.2	13.1	2.2
1996	1.09	2.99	2.7	6.3	13.0	2.2
1997	1.13	3.04	2.7	6.5	13.0	1.9
1998	1.15	3.08	2.6	6.5	13.0	1.9
1999	1.15	3.14	2.6	6.6	13.1	1.9
2000	1.14	3.07	2.8	6.5	13.0	1.9

[c]Very Low Birth Weight: Weight less than 1,500 grams (3 lb. 4oz.).
[d]Low Birth Weight: Weight less than 2,500 grams (5 lb. 8oz.).

Source: National Center for Health Statistics (2002b).

mortality is considered a measure of the quality of prenatal and perinatal care and has improved markedly for both Black and White infants (CDC, 1994, 1999; Eberhardt et al., 2001; Kleinman & Kessel, 1987).

As indicated by the data in Table 21.5, the rate of very low birth weight (VLBW) has been increasing for both White and Black infants. The rate of VLBW among births to White mothers has risen over the last two decades, from 0.95 percent in 1990 to 1.14 percent in 2000.

Among births to Black mothers, the rate of VLBW has risen from 2.92 percent in 1990 to 3.1 percent in 2000, almost three times higher than the rate among the White births. Overall low birth weight (LBW) among births to Black mothers declined from 13.3 to 13.0 percent between 1990 and 2000 but remains higher than levels reported for the early and mid-1980s (data not shown). The rate of LBW among births to Whites has been increasing steadily from 5.7 percent in 1990 to 6.5 percent in 2000.

It is evident that the upward trends in VLBW and LBW of recent years have been strongly influenced by the upsurge in the multiple births, particularly among Whites, reflecting their increase in medically assisted pregnancies (Martin & Park, 1999). Additionally, while in the past decade, LBW has increased among White singletons, it has actually decreased among Black singleton infants (Branum & Schoendorf, 2002).

Individual-Level Risk Factors

Race and Ethnicity.   The probability of low birthweight or infant death varies according to the risk factors associated with the mother, the baby, and the index pregnancy (CDC, 1994, 1999). Race and ethnicity are identified risk factors for LBW. However, the exact nature of this risk is still a subject of epidemiological, clinical, and qualitative studies (Pallotto et al., 2000; David & Collins,

1997; O'Campo et al., 1997; Wilcox, 2001; Wilcox & Russel, 1986; Hertz-Picciotto (2001); Pearl et al., 2001; Polednak, 1996).

Poverty.   Poverty is associated with higher risk of low birth weight, especially for African American women. Maternal age is another risk factor, with women greater than 35 years or less than 20 years of age more likely to deliver LBW babies compared to women in their 20s and early 30s (CDC, 1994; Mathews et al., 2002). Infants born to unmarried mothers are also at increased risk of LBW. Maternal smoking increases the incidence of both low birth weight and infant mortality. Tobacco use during pregnancy can restrict the ability of the growing fetus to access oxygen and can lead to LBW and preterm delivery, and ultimately, infant death (Mathews et al., 2002). Low maternal educational attainment (less than high school education), poor maternal nutrition before and during pregnancy, prepregnancy weight and weight gain during pregnancy, and maternal use of alcohol prior and/or during an index pregnancy have been shown to be associated with risk of LBW births. Although Blacks have higher proportions of births to mothers with high-risk sociodemographic characteristics, their traditionally defined sociodemographic status does not account for the racial disparity in reproductive outcome (Berg et al., 2001; Blackmore et al., 1995; Scott-Wright et al., 1998).

Other Risk Factors.   Black women are also more likely to have obstetrical risk factors such as interpregnancy interval less than 12 months, previous history of infant or fetal loss, previous history of LBW, high birth order, inadequate prenatal care, short period of gestation, maternal history of sexually transmitted diseases, especially bacterial vaginosis, low Apgar scores, and poor preconception medical history such as diabetes and heart disease (Federal Interagency Forum on Child and Family Statistics, 2001; Rauh et al., 2001; Mathews et al., 2002; 1997; Akukwe, 1997, 2000). But, similar to the measured sociodemographic characteristics, the increased frequency of obstetrical risk factors among Black females accounts for only a portion of the racial disparity.

Low Birth-Weight Rates of U.S.-born African Americans and Foreign-born African American Women

This persistent disparity in LBW has led some investigators to speculate that genetic factors associated with race influence birth weight. Recently available population-based data from foreign-born women refutes this conceptual model. African American infants of foreign-born mothers have a better birth-weight distribution than African American infants of U.S-born mothers. In 2000, the LBW rate for African American infants of U.S.-born Blacks was 13.4 percent compared to 9.4 percent for African American infants of foreign-born mothers.

The majority of African Americans trace their origins to Western Africa. It is estimated that U.S. Blacks derive about three-quarters of their genetic heritage from West African ancestors and the remainder from Europeans (David & Collins, 1997). Few data have been published on the birth weights of infants born to African-born women in the United States. One study (David & Collins, 1997) found that African American infants of sub-Saharan African-born Black women have a lower LBW rate than African American infants of U.S.-born mothers independent of individual-level sociodemographic characteristics. In support of these findings, Friedman et al. (1993) reported that infants born to Caribbean-born Black mothers had a significantly lower LBW rate than did infants born to U.S.-born Black mothers. Further, a similar study (Pallotto et al., 2000) found that infants born to U.S.-born Black women had a greater LBW rate than do infants born to Caribbean-born Black women even after controlling for sociodemographic and obstetric risk status. These data support the theory that maternal experiences closely related to lifelong minority status contribute to the racial disparity in LBW rates among U.S.-born mothers. Possibilities of such negative psychosocial experiences include unfavorable perception of their residential environment, frequent exposure to stressful life events, and exposure to racial discrimination.

Community-Level Risk Factors

Stress.   The above evidence suggests that sociodemographic and obstetrical risk-related factors do not explain the excess in adverse pregnancy outcomes in Blacks. Additionally, the findings that birth outcomes of the foreign-born Blacks females are substantially more favorable than those of African American females have led to research on the interplay of psychosocial, cultural, and environmental stressors, (Edwards et al., 1994; Blackmore et al., 1993; Murrel, 1996), including racial discrimination factors (Williams et al. 1997; Williams & Williams-Morris, 2000) relative to poor pregnancy outcomes in Black women. For example, it has been suggested that Black women in general are chronically exposed to specific stressors that adversely affect the outcomes of their pregnancies (Collins et al., 2000; Clark et al., 1999; Polednak, 1996; Rauh et al., 2001).

Geronimus (1992) indicated that the cumulative effects of stressors may "weather" African American women, making them more susceptible to adverse pregnancy outcomes, and that a contributing factor to the weathering is a woman's perception of her stressors. Because of the persistency of racial disparities in health outcomes, particularly with regard to the disparity in adverse pregnancy outcomes, some researchers (e.g., Rowley et al., 1993; Clark et al., 1999) argue that research is needed specifically to measure racism and individuals' exposure to racism as a stressor, and, therefore, as a potential contributing factor to racial disparities in adverse pregnancy outcomes.

An emerging area of research is the review of how contextual effects at the neighborhood level contribute to the racial disparity in LBW rates (Pallotto et al., 2000; David & Collins, 1997; O'Campo et al. 1997; Wilcox, 2001; Wilcox & Russel, 1986; Hertz-Picciotto (2001); Pearl et al., 2001; Polednak, 1996; Rauh et al., 2001). Community impoverishment is a strong risk factor for poor obstetric outcome in Black women because of prolonged vulnerabilities to the psychosocial effects of acute and chronic life stressors such as racism and lack of social support before, during, and in between pregnancies (Collins et al., 1998). In addition, the concentration of poverty and lack of social services in impoverished minority neighborhoods are also associated with poor pregnancy outcomes (Polednak, 1996). Pregnancy-related risk factors (such as poor nutrition, less than high school education, smoking, and illicit drug use) can lead to poor obstetric outcomes (Polednak, 1996; Roux, 2001). One study (Pearl et al., 2001) suggests that the combination of adverse individual socioeconomic conditions and residence in a poor neighborhood can have an additive deleterious effect on pregnancy outcomes. A negative perception of a neighborhood of residence by Black women, especially perceived racism, can adversely affect pregnancy outcomes (Collins et al., 1998).

Residential Segregation.   Another area of research inquiry is the effect of persistent Black–White residential segregation or social isolation on pregnancy outcomes. In segregated minority neighborhoods or communities, mostly in urban centers of America, health and socioeconomic indices are poorer than in suburban neighborhoods, and risky behaviors such as smoking and use of illicit drugs are also higher (Polednak, 1996; O'Campo et al., 1997; Roux, 2001). Segregated minority neighborhoods are associated with high rates of low birth weight and infant deaths (Polednak, 1996, 1998; O'Campo et al, 1997; Rauh et al., 2001). Kawachi and Kennedy (1997) indicate that segregated neighborhoods or communities may lack "social connections" regarding emotional support, socioeconomic support (resources), and a sense of well-being, all with deleterious consequences on the overall health status of the individual and the community. Socially isolated individuals with limited community support are less likely to practice healthy behaviors, more likely to smoke or drink, and less likely to have access to regular health care (Kawachi & Kennedy, 1997; Polednak, 1998).

Regarding the relationship between residential segregation and pregnancy outcomes, researchers have focused on whether segregation compounds the effect of poverty and other adverse socioeconomic conditions on pregnancy outcomes; exacerbates the effect of prolonged exposure to chronic life stressors, such as racism and lack of social support; and increases the deleterious effect of risky behaviors, such as smoking and drinking (Polednak, 1996; O'Campo et al, 1997; Pearl et al., 2001; Geronimus, 1992; Collins et al., 1998; Collins et al., 2000; Clark et al., 1999; Edwards et al., 1994; Murrel, 1996).

Policy Implications and Suggestions for Change

The greater LBW rate of African American infants of U.S.-born (compared to foreign-born) women is consistent with a nongenetic conceptual model of population differences in reproductive health; moreover, it implies a social etiology that extends beyond traditionally defined risk factors. Federally funded research initiatives that emphasize a life-course perspective are needed to better delineate the contribution of individual and community-level factors to the reproductive health of U.S.-born African American women. The public and private sectors should reinvigorate the U.S. Department of Health and Human Service's initiative to reduce racial disparities in infant mortality by developing a research infrastructure that is linked with community-based institutions, multidisciplinary in orientation, focused on active community participation, and aggressively committed to the dissemination of research findings to stakeholders in government, the private sector, and community-based organizations.

Further, given that large proportions of African American women reside in or near impoverished neighborhoods associated with stressful social and environmental factors, greater public health attention is needed to improve the quality of life in these heavily blighted areas. Local governments need to work with private enterprises and the business community to revitalize these low-income communities by (a) building and relocating businesses, thereby allowing for greater employment; (b) community leaders/local businesses and community-based organizations working closely with counties/local police to reduce neighborhood crime; and (c) health education seminars through churches and dissemination of health information (e.g., brochures, flyers) of related information to include pregnancy and prenatal care, IMRs, stress and stress management.

RACIAL DISPARITY IN POSTNEONATAL MORTALITY RATES

Nearly half of postneonatal deaths are due to potentially preventable conditions, such as sudden infant death syndrome (SIDS), infections, and unintentional injuries. Unfortunately, African Americans have a twofold greater PNMR than Whites. This disparity persists among non-LBW infants (Scott-Wright et al., 1998; Akukwe & Hatcher, 1995).

Sudden Infant Death Syndrome (SIDS)

The NICHD (2000a) describe the elimination of racial disparities in SIDS rates as one of the most important and challenging maternal and child health problems for the new millennium. Overall, SIDS deaths have declined by more than 40 percent in the last decade. However, SIDS was the third leading cause of infant death for both Whites and Blacks in 1999, and, more importantly, the rates among Black infants are more than double the rate among White infants (see Figure 21.3). The recent rate of decline in SIDS remains greater for Whites compared to African Americans.

Prone sleep position is a strong, but preventable, risk factor for SIDS. The proportion of infants that slept on their stomachs declined from 70 to 17 percent between 1992 and 1998 (NICHD, 2000b) in the general population compared to a much slower decline among African Americans (from 82 percent to 32 percent). Other important risk factors for SIDS include infant low birthweight, impoverishment, low parental education, young maternal age, and environmental tobacco smoke exposure (NICHD, 2000b).

Figure 21.3
Postneonatal mortality by race, sudden infant death syndrome

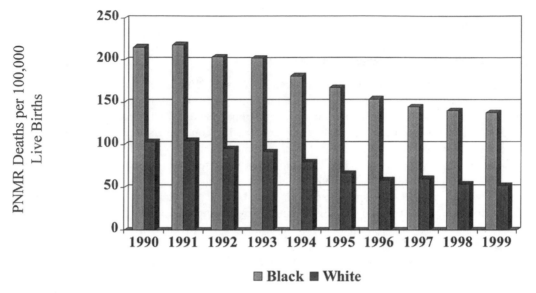

Postneonatal deaths to infants age 28–364 days.

Source: National Center for Health Statistics Compressed Mortality Data Files, 1990–99.

Policy Implications and Suggestions for Change

Postneonatal mortality rates have progressively declined since the 1950s because of steady progress made in improving social economic conditions, improved sanitation, and reduced infections through the use of antibiotics (Scott-Wright et al., 1998; (USDHHS, 2000) 2002; Akukwe & Hatcher, 1995). However, the persisting racial disparities in PNMR reflect the lingering socioeconomic differences among population groups.

Because of the persistence of race-specific differences in the risk factors of SIDS, prevention efforts should be targeted especially to Black infants. Clearly, greater public health attention is needed to facilitate the "back-to-sleep" campaign in African American communities. Further, SIDS evaluation efforts should assess whether race-specific differences are related to variations in the prevalence of preventable risk factors, in methods of diagnosis, or in the effectiveness of prevention messages.

Analysis of population-based data on infant sleeping position for 1996 births by race from ten states participating in Pregnancy Risk Assessment Monitoring System (PRAMS) reported that in most states, respondents usually put their babies to sleep on their sides. In addition, percentage of Black mothers who put their babies to sleep on their stomach was 11 to 54 percent higher than for White mothers (CDC, 1998). This higher rate of stomach sleeping among Blacks than Whites is consistent with the twofold higher rate reported nationally (22 percent versus 43 percent) by Willinger et al. (1998). The back-to-sleep campaign should continue to publicize risk factors for SIDS and ensure that prevention messages reach all segments of the population, especially those at high risk for SIDS.

Accidents (Unintentional Injuries)

Figure 21.4 represents data on mortality rates of unintentional injuries for the last decade. African American infants have more than a twofold greater PNMR from injuries than White infants. Suf-

Figure 21.4
Postneonatal mortality by race accidents (unintentional injuries)

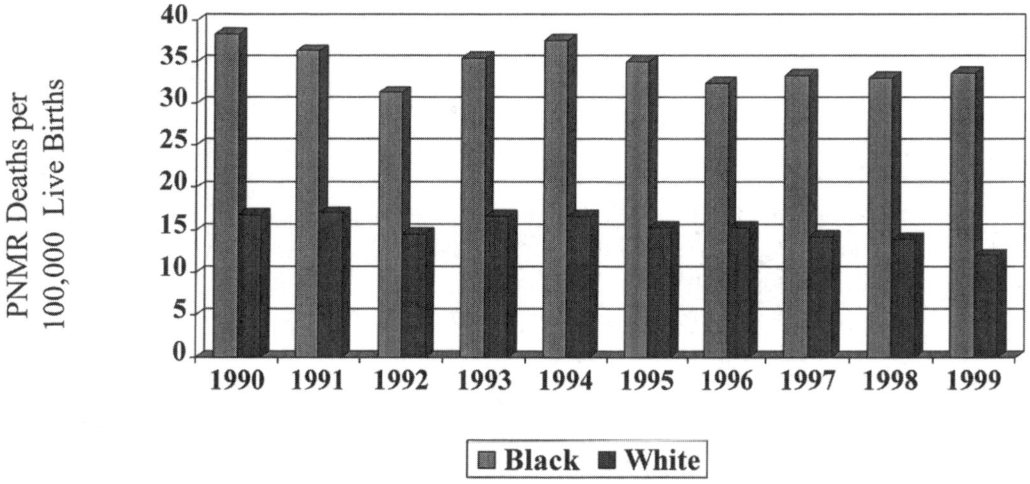

Postneonatal deaths to infants age 28–364 days.

Source: National Center for Health Statistics Compressed Mortality Data Files, 1990–99.

focation is the leading cause of unintentional injuries during the postneonatal period, accounting for almost one-third of all injury cases (Scott-Wright et al., 1998). Motor vehicle accidents represent another common mechanism of fatal injury during the postneonatal period. Infant deaths from motor vehicle crashes are on the decline for both Blacks and Whites, with slower rates of decline for Blacks (Scott-Wright et al., 1998). While suffocation followed by motor vehicle accidents are the leading causes of accidental deaths in the postneonatal period, most of these accidental deaths occur in the home environment (NCHS, 2002). For example, in 1999, 65 percent of the accidental deaths occurred at home, and 9 percent of these accidental deaths occurred in unspecified places (NCHS, 2002).

A breakdown of the 1999 postneonatal deaths indicate the following (data not shown). Deaths due to mechanical suffocation indicate that about 60 percent of these deaths were due to accidental suffocation and strangulation in bed (i.e., bed linen, mother's body, and pillow). Another 11 percent were due to specified threats to breathing, including suffocation on plastic bags. Roughly another 26 percent of suffocation were due to not-otherwise-specified threat to breathing, asphyxiation, aspiration, and unspecified suffocation. The breakdown of motor vehicle-related deaths show that 42 percent of the deaths were specific to the car occupant injured in transport accident. Nontraffic accident of specified type, but victims' mode of transport unknown, accounted for about 36 percent of postneonatal deaths. Further, about 61 percent of postneonatal deaths were due to drowning and submersion while in the bathtub and about 24 percent were due to unspecified drowning and submersion (NCHS, 2002).

Policy Implications and Suggestions for Change

Since most accidental deaths occur in the home environment, and since Black infants are at higher risk than Whites as indicated by the data, it is of crucial importance to identify these groups that are disproportionately affected by various injuries and to address the prevention needs of these groups at risk. The demographic, socioeconomic, and geographic characteristics, including residential/ neighborhood characteristics of the target population, are important considerations in designing a prevention program (NCIPC, 2001). These characteristics shape a person's beliefs, values, preferences, and life experiences. Further, injury prevention counseling is recommended as part of routine pediatric care (NCIPC, 2001). Thus, estimating the proportion of mothers who receive such counseling and assessing their compliance with safety recommendations would be useful in designing and improving age-specific injury prevention programs. Quinlan et al. (1998) reported that a relatively small proportion of children receive injury prevention counseling from their health-care providers.

CONCLUSIONS

Since racial discrimination and African American disadvantage are so pervasive and multilayered in American society, it is not surprising that studies comparing African Americans and Whites can rarely, if ever, truly control for socioeconomic status. Further research into social and environmental risk factors that apply only to the African American population is warranted. Racial disparities in infant birthweight cry out for fresh research initiatives using a life-course conceptual framework. The essence of the new research direction needed is a shift of focus from "race" to "racism." Possible areas for future study include psychophysiological reactions to interpersonal racism, stress-coping mechanisms, social support systems, and environmental factors with demonstrated racial bias.

Since non-LBW African American infants have a twofold greater PNMR than non-LBW white infants, eradication of the racial gap in LBW rates will not singularly eliminate the racial disparity in IMR. Deaths from SIDS, injuries, and infections underlie the African American infant's postneonatal survival disadvantage. As such, broad public policies that address neighborhood discrepancies in infant sleep position, safety, and access to quality medical care are needed to attain the Healthy People 2010 objective call for the elimination of the racial disparity in IMR.

REFERENCES

Akukwe, C. (2000). Maternal and child health services in the twenty-first century: Critical issues, challenges and opportunities. *Health Care for Women International, 21(7)*, 641–653.

Akukwe, C. (1997). Perinatal and infant mortality: A worldwide issue. A commentary. *European Journal of Public Health, 7(2)*, 223–225.

Akukwe, C., & Hatcher, B.H. (1995). *Public Health Initiatives: Reducing Infant Mortality in the District of Columbia*. District of Columbia Commission of Public Health, Washington, DC: Office of Maternal and Child Health.

American Academy of Pediatrics Task Force on Infant Mortality. (1986). Statement on Infant Mortality. *Pediatrics, 78(6)*, 1142–1143.

Berg, C.J., Wilcox, L.S., & D'Almada, P.J. (2001). The prevalence of socioeconomic and behavioral characteristics and their impact on very low birthweight in Black and White infants. *Maternal and Child Health Journal, 5(2)*, 75–84.

Blackmore, C.A., et al. (1993). Is race a factor or a risk marker for preterm delivery? *Ethnicity and Disease, 3*, 372–377.

Blackmore, C.A., Savitz, D.A., Edwards, L.J., Harlow, S.D., & Bowes, W.A. Jr., (1995). Racial differences in patterns of preterm delivery in central North Carolina, United States. *Paediatrics Perinatol Epidemiology, 9(3)*, 281–95.

Branum, A.M., & Schoendorf, K.C. (2002). Changing patterns of low birthweight and preterm birth in the united states, 1981–98. *Paediatric and Perinatal Epidemiology, 16*, 8–15.

Center for Chronic Disease and Health Promotion (CDC). (1999). Achievements in public health, 1990–1999: Healthier mothers and babies. *Morbidity and Mortality Weekly Report, 48* (38), 849–858.

Centers for Disease Control and Prevention (CDC), Division of Reproductive Health, National Center for Chronic Disease and Health Promotion. Pregnancy Risk Assessment Monitoring System Working Group. (1998). Assessment of infant sleeping position—selected states, 1996. *Morbidity and Mortality Weekly Report, 47(41)*, 873–877.

Centers for Disease Control and Prevention (CDC). (1994). From Data to Action: CDC's Public health surveillance for women, infants and children. In L.S., Wilcox, & J.S. Marks, (Ed.), *CDC Monograph*. CDC, Atlanta: U.S. Department of Health and Human Services.

Clark, R., Anderson, N., Clark, V.R., & Williams, D. (1999). Racism as a stressor for African Americans. *American Psychology, 54*, 805–816.

Collins, J.W., Jr., & David, R.J. (1990). The differential effect of traditional risk factors on infant birthweight among Blacks and Whites in Chicago. *American Journal of Public Health, 80*, 679–681.

Collins, J.W., Jr., David, R.J., Symons, R., Handler, A., Wall, S.N., & Andes, S. (1998). African American mothers' perception of their residential environment, stressful life events, and very low birthweight. *Epidemiology, 9*, 286–289.

Collins, J.W., Jr., David, R.J., Symons, R., Handler, A., Wall, S.N., & Dwyer, L. (2000). Low-income African American mothers' perception of exposure to racial discrimination and infant birthweight. *Epidemiology, 11*, 337–339.

David, R.J., & Collins, J.W. Jr., (1997). Differing birth weight among infants of U.S.-born Blacks, African-born, and U.S.-born Whites. *New England Journal of Medicine, 337*(17), 1209–1214.

Eberhardt, M.S., et al. (2001). *Urban and rural health chartbook health, United States.* Hyattsville, MD: National Center for Health Statistics.

Edwards, C.H., et al. (1994). Maternal stress and pregnancy outcomes in a prenatal clinic population. *Journal of Nutrition, 124*, 1006S–1021S.

Federal Interagency Forum on Child and Family Statistics. (2001). *America's children: Key national indicators of well being, 2001.* Washington, DC: Office of Management and Budget, Executive Office of the President.

Friedman, D.J., Cohen, B.B., Mahan, C.M., Lederman, R.I., Vezina, R.J., & Dunn, V.H. (1993). Maternal ethnicity and birthweight among Blacks. *Ethnicity and Disease, 3*, 255–269.

Geronimus, A.T. (1996). African American/White differences in the relationship of maternal age to birthweight: A population-based test of the weathering hypothesis. *Social Science and Medicine, 42*, 589–597.

Geronimus, A.T. (1992). The weathering hypothesis and the health of African American women and infants: Evidence and speculations. *Ethnicity and Disease, 2*, 207–221.

Hertz-Picciotto, I. (2001). Commentary: When brilliant insights lead astray. *International Journal of Epidemiology, 30*, 1243–44

Kawachi, I. & Kennedy, B.P. (1997). Socioeconomic determinants of health: Health and social cohesion: Why care about income inequality? *British Medical Journal, 314*, 1037.

Kleinman, J.C., & Kessel, S.S. (1987). Racial differences in low birthweight trends and risk factors. *New England Journal of Medicine, 317*, 749–753.

Martin, J.A., & Park, M.M. (1999). Trends in twin and triplet births, 1980–97. *National Vital Statistics Reports, 47*(24). Hyattsville, MD: National Center for Health Statistics.

Martin, J.A., Hamilton, B.E., Ventura, S.J., Menacker, F., & Park, M.M. (2002). Births: Final Data for 2000. *National Vital Statistics Reports, 50*(5). Hyattsville, MD: National Center for Health Statistics.

Mathews, T.J., MacDorman, M.F., & Menacker, F. (2002). Infant mortality statistics from the 1999 period linked birth/infant death data set. *National Vital Statistics Reports, 50*(4), 1–28. Hyattsville, MD: National Center for Health Statistics.

Minino, A.M., & Smith, B.L. (2001). Deaths: Preliminary data for 2000. *National Vital Statistics Reports, 49*(12). Hyattsville, MD: National Center for Health Statistics.

Murrel, N.L. (1996). Stress, self-esteem, and racism: Relationship with low birth weight and preterm delivery in African American women. *Journal of Black Nurses Association, 8*(1), 45–53.

National Center for Health Statistics (2002a). *Health, United States, 2002. With chartbook on trends in the health of Americans.* Hyattsville, Maryland.

National Center for Health Statistics (NCHS). (2002b). *National Vital Statistics Reports*, vol. 49(8). Deaths Final Data for 1999, 2001 & Volume 50(15), Deaths Final Data for 2000. NCHS, Hyattsville, MD.

National Center for Injury Prevention and Control (NCIPC). (2001). *Injury fact book—2001–2002.* Atlanta, GA: Centers for Disease Prevention and Control.

National Institute of Child Health and Human Development (NICHD). (2000a). *From cells to selves. Health disparities: Bridging the gap.* Bethesda, MD: Author.

National Institute of Child Health and Human Development (NICHD). (2000b). *From cells to selves. Targeting sudden infant death syndrome (SIDS): A strategic plan.* Bethesda, MD: Author.

O'Campo, P., Xiaonan Xue, Wang, Mei-Cheng, & Caughy, M.O. (1997). Neighborhood risk factors for low birthweight in Baltimore: A multilevel analysis. *American Journal of Public Health, 87,* 1113–1118.

Pallotto, E.K., Collins, J.W., Jr., & David, R.J. (2000). Enigma of maternal race and infant birth weight: A population-based study of U.S.-born Black and Caribbean-born Black women. *American Journal of Epidemiology, 151,* 1080–1085.

Pearl, M., Braveman, P., & Abrams, B. (2001). The relationship of neighborhood socioeconomic characteristics to birthweight among 5 ethnic groups in California. *American Journal of Public Health, 91,* 1808–1814.

Polednak, A. (1998). Mortality among Blacks living in census tracts with public housing projects in Hartford, Connecticut. *Ethnicity and Disease, 8,* 36–42.

Polednak, A. (1996). Trends in U.S. urban Black infant mortality, by degree of residential segregation. *American Journal of Public Health, 86,* 723–726.

Quinlan, K.P., Sacks, J.J., & Kresnow, M. (1998). Exposure to and compliance with pediatric injury prevention counseling—United States, 1994. *Pediatrics, 102(5),* 1–4.

Rauh, V.A., Andrews, H.F., & Garfinkel, R.S. (2001). The contribution of maternal age to racial disparities in birthweight: A multilevel perspective. *American Journal of Public Health, 91(11),* 1815–1824.

Roux, A.V.D. (2001). Investigating neighborhood and area effects on health. *American Journal of Public Health, 91(11),* 1783–1789.

Rowley, D., et al. (1993). Preterm delivery among African American women: A research strategy. *American Journal of Preventive Medicine, 9(SS-6),* 1–6.

Scott-Wright, C.L., Iyasu, S., Rowley, D., & Atrash, H.K. (1998). Postneonatal mortality surveillance—United States, 1980–1994. *Morbidity and Mortality Weekly Report, 47*(SS-2), 15–29.

U.S. Department of Health and Human Services. (2000). *Healthy People 2010* (Conference edition-volume 11). Washington, DC: Author.

Warner, Geoffrey. (1999, Spring). Black infant health: Where to in the 21st century? *The Review of Black Political Economy,* 29–54.

Wilcox, A.J. (2001). Response: Where do we go from here? *International Journal of Epidemiology, 30,* 1245.

Wilcox, A.J., & Russell, L.T. (1986). Birthweight and perinatal mortality III: Towards a new method of analysis. *International Journal of Epidemiology, 15,* 188–96.

Williams, D.R., & Williams-Morris, R. (2000). Racism and mental health: The African American experience. *Ethnicity & Health, 5(3/4),* 243–268.

Williams, D.R., Yu, Y., Jackson, J., & Anderson, N. (1997). Racial differences in physical and mental health: Socioeconomic status, stress, and discrimination. *Journal of Health Psychology, 2,* 335–351.

Willinger, M., et al. (1998). Factors associated with the transition to nonprone sleep positions of infants in the United States: The national infant sleep position study. *Journal of American Medical Association, 280,* 329–39.

CHAPTER 22

Mental Health of African Americans

COLWICK M. WILSON AND
DAVID R. WILLIAMS

Since the mid-1800s, researchers have been interested in the mental health status of African Americans (or Blacks) in the United States (Babcock, 1895; Malzberg, 1944). This search for an understanding of the distribution of mental health problems in the African American population continues to engage the attention of researchers and policymakers, especially in an era of increasing attention to racial disparities in health status. For example, the landmark 1999 report of the surgeon general of the United States on the scientific evidence on mental health status, in part, highlights the importance of racial and ethnic status in mental health problems or disorders. Two years later, a supplemental report was issued that focused explicitly on the role of racial and ethnic minority status in the development of psychiatric illness and in the utilization of mental health services. These reports and others document that important gaps and paradoxes remain in our understanding of African American mental health status and receipt of psychiatric services (Neighbors & Williams, 2001).

This chapter provides an overview of prior research on African American mental health status and places these data in their sociohistorical context. We consider the evidence on the prevalence of multiple indicators of mental health, such as insanity rates, psychological distress, psychiatric disorders, and psychological well-being. Additionally, we highlight a number of important issues that still remain in our attempts to understand African American mental health status in the United States. In so doing, we identify some of the emerging trends in the literature (and recent national studies) that may explicate our search for clarity on racial differences in mental health status.

A BRIEF HISTORY OF BLACK AMERICAN MENTAL HEALTH

Historically, the mental health of African Americans has been examined within the framework of a Black–White comparative paradigm (Neighbors, 1984). As such, most of the available empirical data on African American mental health use Whites as a standard of comparison. To a large extent, the interpretation of these studies reflects the prevailing social ideology of their time. That is, scientific studies were used not only to classify human diversity but also to support the notion that being Black was associated with inferior social standing in American society (Montagu, 1965). In this section, we present a chronological review of the development of these early studies, which were mostly based on treatment samples, together with later studies that used community and national samples.

Census Studies: 1840–1930

In 1840, researchers used the U.S. census data to differentiate the number of residents in mental hospitals by race. The initial report indicated that Blacks had higher rates of insanity than Whites in general and that southern Blacks had lower rates of illness than northern Blacks (Jarvis, 1842a). Moreover, rates of insanity were higher in the North than the South, compelling evidence to the authors that freedom made Blacks crazy! However, subsequent investigation of the 1840 census data uncovered grave errors in the computation of rates of mental illness for Blacks as compared to Whites. For example, the highest proportion (1 in 14) of the mentally ill among Blacks was found in the state of Maine. Careful examination of the data from three towns in Maine revealed the following: (1) there were no colored residents in Limerick, yet four insane Blacks were identified; (2) one Black person was found in Lymington, but there were two Black insane residents listed; and (3) although there were no Blacks in Scarboro, the census data reported six insane residents (Jarvis, 1842b). Despite problems with the evidence, many researchers continued to articulate the view that Blacks were biologically inferior (Lind, 1914) and that slavery had served to protect them from insanity (Babcock, 1895; Witmer, 1891).

In contrast, analysis of census data from 1850 to 1870, which included both the institutionalized and the noninstitutionalized mentally ill, revealed lower rates of mental illness for Blacks compared to Whites (Malzberg, 1944). For the 1880 and 1890 censuses, medical doctors were asked to help in identifying noninstitutionalized mentally ill individuals as a means of securing a more accurate count of this population (Warheit et al., 1975). Nonetheless, the results showed that Whites had higher rates of mental illness than Blacks (Malzberg, 1944; Powell, 1896).

From the next census in 1900 to that of 1920, when first admission rates were used as the measure of the prevalence of mental illness, Blacks again reported lower rates of insanity compared to Whites (Malzberg, 1944). The 1930 census marked a change in the definition of the sample of the mentally ill. Researchers began collecting census data on mental health only from the severely ill in state hospitals. This new definition of mental illness resulted in Blacks reporting higher rates of mental illness than Whites (Warheit et al., 1975; Fischer, 1969). Studies that focus only on the institutionalized mentally ill continue to show higher rates of mental illness for Blacks than Whites (Snowden & Chung, 1990). As was the case in 1930, Blacks are still overrepresented in state mental hospitals, which are the principal source of inpatient care for African Americans (Snowden & Chung, 1990; Mollica et al., 1980). In contrast, Whites are more likely to avoid the stigma associated with state mental hospitals by seeking and obtaining treatment outside these specialized settings, such as general hospitals.

Community and National Studies: 1940 to Present

During World War II, the Selective Service System rejected a significant number of men because they failed the screening test for psychiatric disorders. However, many soldiers who passed the test displayed acute psychiatric reaction to combat. As a result, the military invested enormous resources in the development and use of neuropsychiatric screening and impairment scales (Weissman et al., 1986).

Psychological Distress.   After World War II, researchers modified these measures and began using community-based studies to evaluate the distribution of mental health. The emphasis here was in assessing true prevalence rates in communities rather than in treatment settings by using sophisticated sampling procedures, highly trained lay interviewers, and structured questionnaire design (Gurin et al., 1960; Leighton et al., 1963; Srole et al., 1962). However, the absence of a consensus about a standardized diagnostic instrument for evaluating psychiatric disorders resulted in researchers using measures of psychological distress or depressive symptoms that assess nonspecific emotional symptoms (Crandell & Dohrenwend, 1967; Robins & Regier, 1991; Weissman & Myers, 1978b). Within this framework, mental health status is often conceptualized as a continuum that can be assessed by symptom checklists that typically capture depressed mood, psychological distress, and levels of dysfunction (Link & Dohrenwend, 1980; Vega & Rumbaut, 1991).

Dohrenwend and Dohrenwend's (1969) review of eight of the early community-based studies reveals an inconsistent pattern of findings by race. Four of these studies report higher rates of distress for Blacks (Cohen, Fairbank, & Green, 1939; Hyde & Chisholm, 1944; Leighton et al., 1963; Rosanoff, 1917), while the remaining four reveal higher rates for Whites (Lemkau et al., 1942; Rowntree et al., 1945; Roth & Luton, 1943; Pasamanick et al., 1959). Subsequent community studies conducted during the 1970s and 1980s report higher rates of distress for Whites than Blacks (Antunes et al., 1974; Gaitz & Scott, 1972) or no racial differences at all after adjustments are made for socioeconomic status (Comstock & Helsing, 1976; Mirowsky & Ross, 1980; Schwab et al., 1973; Warheit et al., 1975).

Reviews of the literature on minority mental health find that while some studies report higher levels of distress for Blacks, others reveal lower levels for Blacks as compared to Whites (Vega & Rumbaut, 1991; Williams & Harris Reed, 1999). Some recent studies have also found equivalent rates of distress in Blacks and Whites. For example, a probability sample of the Detroit metropolitan area reported no Black–White difference in psychological distress (Williams et al., 1997). Similarly, a nonsignificant racial difference in psychological distress also emerged in a recent study of a nationally representative sample of adults in the United States (Williams, 2000). Overall, the pattern of findings for racial differences in psychological distress remains unclear. Some studies report higher levels of nonspecific symptoms for Blacks than Whites, while others show lower rates for Blacks or no difference between the two racial groups.

Psychiatric Disorders.   The post–World War II search for diagnostic categories of psychiatric disorder persisted in the face of the increased use of nonspecific measures of distress. This quest for standardization was buttressed by the results of a study of U.S. (New York) and U.K (London) residents, which documented that relatively similar diagnostic rates are possible when common diagnostic and standardized assessment tools are employed (Cooper et al., 1972). This study, together with a confluence of other factors, set the stage for new approaches to addressing the limitations of nonstandardized measures of mental illness.

During the 1970s, significant progress was made in the development of specific diagnostic criteria to obtain standardized information of mental disorder from structured interviews (Endicott & Spitzer, 1978; Spitzer et al., 1978). Among the many instruments that emerged, the Schedule for Affective Disorders and Schizophrenia-Research Diagnostic Criteria (SADS-RDC) received much attention in the research community. This categorical approach of assessing psychiatric symptoms included information on the criterion, subject, occasion, and information variance of 25 discrete psychiatric disorders by employing a structured questionnaire design and operational definitions (Spitzer et al., 1978). It was arguably one of the most developed diagnostic tools available in the United States at the time and was developed in conjunction with the DSM-III (*Diagnostic and Statistical Manual of Mental Disorders*).

One of the first studies to use the SADS-RDC in a community survey was a New Haven study in the late 1970s. In that study, Weissman and Myers (1978a, 1978b) found no significant racial difference for anxiety disorders but higher rates of major depression, minor depression, and depressive personalities for non-Whites (mainly Blacks) than for Whites. Not unlike most studies during this period, a major limitation of this study was the small overall sample size (511) with only 61 non-Whites. Vernon and Roberts (1982) also used SADS-RDC in a study of two southeastern cities ($N = 528$) and found that Blacks, compared to Whites, had higher prevalence of current rates of major and minor depression and lower lifetime rates of these disorders. While this study has a larger number of Blacks (187) than the Weissman and Myers study, Vernon and Roberts (1982) caution that the small overall sample size should be considered when interpreting their results. Weissman and Myers' New Haven study was the precursor for the more expansive and comprehensive National Institute of Mental Health Epidemiologic Catchment Area Study (ECA). Weissman and Myers served as the principal investigators in New Haven, the first (of five) site(s) for the ECA.

The ECA remains the largest mental health study ever conducted in the United States, with 20,000 adults interviewed in five communities from 1980 to 1983 (Robins & Regier, 1991). With an emphasis on the use of highly structured interviews that were administered by lay interviewers and survey sampling techniques that allowed for generalizing the findings to a defined population, the ECA sought to estimate the prevalence of specific psychiatric disorders in community samples of noninstitutionalized persons as well as of institutionalized persons in the defined catchment area (Leaf et al., 1991). These interviews had two standard sections in all of the five sites, a diagnostic section that used the Diagnostic Interview Schedule (DIS) to evaluate the presence or absence of specific diagnostic categories and a Health Services Questionnaire that assessed the utilization of medical and mental health services. The DIS is based on operational criteria and algorithms from the DSM-III and is a fully structured, lay-administered instrument that assesses the presence, severity and duration of symptoms (Boyd et al., 1985; Robins et al., 1981).

Overall, the ECA reports little difference between Blacks and Whites in the prevalence of psychiatric disorders in general (Robins & Reiger, 1991). Specifically, these data reveal that Blacks and Whites were not different in lifetime rates or six-month prevalence of major depression (Robins & Reiger 1991; Somervell et al., 1989). Although not statistically significant, Blacks consistently reported lower rates of major depression than Whites in these data (Weissman et al., 1991). There was also no statistical difference between African Americans and Whites in the overall prevalence of alcohol and drug use or dependence. Further, analysis reveals that these findings may be importantly patterned by age differences. Whites between the ages of 18 and 29 have a rate of alcohol abuse that is twice that of their Black peers, but the lifetime rates of Blacks exceeds that of Whites in all other age groups, with the difference being especially pronounced in the 45–64 category. Additionally, Blacks report higher rates of schizophrenia than Whites, but after adjusting for age, gender, marital status, and socioeconomic (SES) status, this difference disappeared.

Consistent with earlier studies (e.g., Warheit et al., 1986), the ECA data indicate that Blacks had higher one-year prevalence of generalized anxiety compared to Whites (Robins & Regier, 1991). However, African Americans reported higher rates of one-month, one-year, and lifetime prevalence of phobia. In particular, Blacks scored higher than Whites on measures of agoraphobia and simple phobia but not for social phobia. While this pattern of findings persisted for men after controlling for sex, Black women did report higher rates of agoraphobia and simple and social phobia than White women. In addition, Black men and women exceeded their White peers in rates of one-year and lifetime phobia. One exception was that Black and White women aged 30 to 44 reported very similar rates of lifetime phobias (Robins & Regier, 1991).

The first national probability survey to assess psychiatric disorder in the United States was the National Comorbidity Study (NCS), in which over 8,000 adults were interviewed in the early 1990s. Table 22.1 shows the results of the Black–White comparison across four major categories of psychiatric disorders. The first column presents the overall rate for each class of psychiatric disorders. The Black–White ratio is shown in second column where a relative risk greater than 1.0 indicates that Blacks have a higher rate of that particular disorder than Whites. Overall, Blacks do not have higher rates of psychiatric disorders in any of four major classes of disorders than Whites (Kessler

Table 22.1
Overall prevalence and Black–White ratios of psychiatric disorders in a national sample

Psychiatric Disorders	Prevalence in general population (%)	Black/White ratios
Any affective disorder	11.3	0.78
Any anxiety disorder	17.1	0.90
Any substance abuse or dependence	11.3	0.47
Any disorder	29.5	0.70

Source: Adapted from Kessler et al. (1994).

et al., 1994). Lower rates for Blacks than Whites are pronounced for affective disorder (depression) and substance abuse. However, the patterns of findings for some anxiety disorders are different in the NCS than in the ECA. Kessler et al. (1994) report no racial differences in panic disorder, simple phobia, or agoraphobia. Moreover, Magee's (1993) analysis of NCS data suggests that there are complex interactions between race and gender in predicting the levels of phobia. That is, White males tend to report higher current and lifetime rates of agoraphobia, simple phobia, and social phobia than Black men. In contrast, Black women have higher rates of agoraphobia and simple phobia than their White counterparts.

Psychological Well-Being. Researchers have also examined the extent to which membership in socially defined racial groups predicts levels of psychological well-being. This measure is typically viewed as a subjective assessment of positive and negative affect, satisfaction, and the lack of strain that characterizes the quality of life in multiple domains (Andrews & Withey, 1976; Campbell, 1981; Clemente & Williams, 1976). In this regard, Bracy's (1976) review of the literature between 1957 and 1972 revealed that African Americans report significantly lower levels of happiness and life satisfaction than Whites. In addition, Bracy (1976) examined Black-White differences in well-being by using a scale with 11 different domains of life and concluded that Blacks were significantly less satisfied than Whites controlling for family income, education, occupation, northern versus southern residence, household size, and age. Also, low-socioeconomic-status Whites reported higher levels of life satisfaction than Blacks of low socioeconomic status. Moreover, the results of Clemente and Williams' (1976) analysis of the 1973 General Social Survey supported Bracy's findings. They reported that Blacks were less satisfied than Whites with their place of residence, family, friendships, and activities after controlling for demographic and SES characteristics. One recent study using a nationally representative telephone sample of adults noted a marginally significant tendency for Blacks to report higher levels of life satisfaction based on a single-item measure than Whites (Williams, 2000).

Other data suggest that the pattern of lower well-being of Blacks compared to Whites has remained remarkably stable over time. Thomas and Hughes (1986) analyzed General Social Survey (GSS) data for 1972 to 1985 and reported that after controlling for socioeconomic status, age, and marital status, the subjective well-being of Whites was significantly and consistently higher than that of African Americans. Recently, Hughes and Thomas (1998) revisited GSS data from 1972 to 1996 in an effort to examine the extent to which race continues to be significant in levels of subjective well-being. Consistent with their earlier research, Blacks continue to report lower levels than Whites for multiple measures of subjective well-being (Hughes & Thomas, 1998).

In sum, the review of the empirical evidence of Black–White difference across multiple measures of mental health suggests the following. First, Blacks have similar or lower depression rates compared to Whites. For most measures of anxiety disorders (except for social phobias) Blacks report either higher or similar rates to those of Whites. Second, the association between race and depressive symptoms is unclear. Some studies report higher rates for Blacks, others report higher rates for Whites, while still others show no racial differences. Finally, the weight of the evidence over time and from multiple national studies point to lower levels of psychological well-being for Blacks compared to Whites.

PERSISTENT AND EMERGING ISSUES

Despite over 100 years of research evidence documenting mental health status for Blacks in the United States, a number of important issues still remain to be addressed. These unresolved issues may provide additional information that may enhance our understanding of African American mental health over time.

Diversity among African Americans

The focus on a majority/minority comparative paradigm in epidemiological research on racial differences in mental health obscures the heterogeneity of the Black population (Williams & Fenton, 1994). There are variations within racial categories in the United States, and as such it is necessary to consider ethnic and or cultural differences among Blacks when assessing mental health status. Thus, while evaluating differences in mental health status between Blacks and Whites is an important and necessary first step in understanding the psychological and psychiatric status of Blacks in the United States, identification of within-group variations may reveal useful information about the various subgroups that form the African American population. For example, Blacks in the United States include immigrants from the Caribbean region and from the continent of Africa. In 1997, it was estimated that 6 percent of the Black population in the United States was foreign-born and an additional 4 percent of the Black population was of foreign parentage (Schmidley & Gibson, 1999). These 3.5 million Blacks of foreign stock are geographically concentrated in certain regions of the United States and are a substantial proportion of the Black population in some areas such as New York City, Washington, D.C., and South Florida.

Moreover, immigrant Blacks represent very diverse groups. For example, Blacks from the Caribbean region are characterized by different colonial heritages, such as Spanish, French, Dutch, and English. While sharing common cultural norms, these groups are anything but monolithic. Even greater diversity exists among various national origin Black groups from sub-Saharan Africa. Awareness of ethnic differences among Blacks is crucial to understanding both the distribution of mental health problems and the effective targeting of the delivery of mental health services. Future research must assess interactions between mental health and social and psychological resources and stressors across different racial groups, as well as within race, taking ethnicity into account. One national study with a small sample of persons of Caribbean ancestry found that Afro-Caribbeans reported higher levels of stress (especially financial stress), higher levels of psychological distress, and lower levels of life satisfaction than native-born Blacks (Williams, 2000). Future research needs to identify how stressors, migration status, and acculturation combine to affect the mental health of immigrant Blacks. Another neglected dimension of heterogeneity of the Black population is the extent of regional variation in sociodemographic characteristics and health for the native-born Black population.

Some evidence suggests that there are distinctive cultural-ecological regions of residence for the African American population (Williams et al., 1994). However, the associated health consequences linked to residence in these regions have not been clearly identified.

Place and Mental Health

Relatedly, research suggests that the quality of the social environment can affect the mental health status of African Americans. That is, resources and stressors, such as crime rates, quality of educational and health services, neighborhood quality, social cohesion, levels of poverty, and exposure to environmental risks have consequences for mental health status (Dalgard & Tambs, 1997). Consideration of the role of the environment in predicting levels of mental health is heightened when placed within the context of racial and ethnic minorities. The racial residential segregation of American society is a central determinant of racial differences in SES and results in unequal distribution of social and economic resources by race (Williams & Collins, 2001). African Americans live in distinctively different residential environments than Whites, and residence in highly segregated areas is known to adversely affect health (LaVeist, 1993; Williams & Collins, 2001). For example, an initially observed higher rate of cocaine use by Blacks as compared to Whites was reduced to nonsignificance when respondents were grouped into neighborhood clusters as determined by the U.S. census track characteristics (Lille-Blanton et al., 1993).

Comprehensive Measurement of Mental Health Status

Enhancing our understanding of racial differences in mental health requires studies that consider a broad range of endpoints. Most prior research has used one measure of mental health to assess for racial differences. Mental health is a multifaceted phenomenon with multiple indicators, each of which may capture varying aspects of people's lives (Aneshensel & Phelan, 1999). This may be especially salient for comparisons across racial groups. Social groups experience the world in different ways largely due to social inequities that are associated with the relative location and position of minority and majority populations in society. As such, the experiences and interpretations of the circumstances of life may vary across racial groups. This may have important implications for specific measures of mental health outcomes (Coyne & Downey, 1991; Schulberg et al., 1985). Most of the studies of racial differences in mental health are based on single-outcome measures, making it unclear whether the complex pattern of findings reflects differences in study design (Kramer et al., 1973). The use of multiple measures of mental health status within the framework of a specific study will allow for a more complete evaluation of the complexities of mental health for African Americans.

Misdiagnosis

Another important aspect of measurement that is often implicated in differential rates of mental health for Blacks and Whites is misdiagnosis (Neighbors et al., 1989). This is especially pronounced when assessing racial differences in mental health status, especially within the context of psychiatric disorders. For example, Blacks are more likely to be overdiagnosed as schizophrenics and less likely to be diagnosed with mood disorders than Whites (Neighbors et al., 1989; Adebimpe, 1981). The free expression of emotions associated with depression, which is one of the most frequent mood disorders, may be discouraged among Blacks because of existing cultural norms that render such disclosure inappropriate. Indeed, somatization is found to be about twice as prevalent among Blacks than Whites (Heurtin-Roberts et al., 1997; Robins & Regier, 1991).

Some have argued that African Americans are more appropriately characterized as a cultural group (Landrine & Klonoff, 1996). It is therefore possible that given distinctiveness in beliefs and values, minority status may influence both the experience and interpretation of symptoms of mental illness. Misdiagnosis then, gets at the issue of differential rates of disorders across racial groups by suggesting two possible explanations (Neighbors et al., 1989). First, Blacks and Whites express psychiatric symptoms in about the same manner, rendering diagnostic criteria equally applicable to both racial groups. Second, mental illness is experienced and displayed in different ways for Blacks and Whites. Measures of mental health status for Blacks should therefore be approached from the perspective of a careful examination of the items used to assess mental illness. There is growing research attention to the extent to which racial influences can lead to both overdiagnosis and underdiagnosis of mental illness in African Americans (Neighbors & Williams, 2001). However, definitive conclusions to these issues are not currently available. It has also been suggested that researchers should consider unique categories of mental health problems that may reflect the distinctiveness of the Black experience in the United States (Brown, 2003).

Culture and Mental Health

Over the past decade much attention has been given to the ways in which culture impacts the expression, assessment, and interpretation of mental illness (Lopez & Guarnaccia, 2000). Culture has been defined as the values, beliefs, and practices that characterize a particular ethnic group (Betancourt & Lopez, 1993). However, more recent conceptualizations of culture emphasize the importance of exploring and understanding how the larger social context interacts with the individual in a dynamic process that seeks to give meaning to cultural experiences (Lopez & Guarnaccia, 2000). For example, there is a need for mental health professions and related organizations to be aware of the environmental factors that may facilitate the development and legitimacy of stereotypical and prejudicial views of the mental health of ethnocultural groups. In addition, researchers and clinicians may be trained to become aware of their biases and prejudices that may influence the development and interpretation of assessment instruments, data collection methods, analysis, or therapy for specific racial and ethnic groups (Rogler, 1989). A recent Institute of Medicine report documented that Blacks and other racial minorities receive poorer-quality care across a broader range of therapeutic proceedings, including mental health treatment (Smedley et al., 2003). The report suggested that provider bias based on negative stereotypes of clients is a likely contributor to this pattern. Increased awareness of both large social structures and organizations and individuals of cultural biases in the process of defining and treating mental health problems can only serve to clarify some of the present ambiguities around the evidence on racial differences in mental health status in the United States.

The *Diagnostic and Statistical Manual of Mental Disorders*, 4th edition, of the American Psychiatric Association (1994), reveals that some distress idioms or ethnomedical symptoms are more common in specified racial and/or ethnic groups. For example, African Americans are associated with the culturally orientated syndrome referred to as "falling out." This identified "disorder" is "characterized by a sudden collapse, which sometimes occurs without warning but sometimes is preceded by feelings of dizziness or 'swimming' in the head" (p. 846). There is some evidence that ethnomedical symptoms among African Americans overlap with symptoms of DSM III anxiety and other somatization-related psychiatric disorders (Snowden, 1999). Moreover, findings from the ECA indicate that Blacks report significantly higher rates of somatization disorder and syndrome than Whites (Robins & Regier, 1991).

Racism and Mental Health

There is growing research interest in the ways in which racism can affect the health of stigmatized racial and ethnic populations (Krieger, 1999; Harrell et al., 1998; Clark et al., 1999; Rollock & Gordon, 2000). This research suggests that racism operates at multiple levels to affect mental health status (Jones, 2000; Williams & Williams-Morris, 2000). First, institutional mechanisms of racism produce racial differences in socioeconomic mobility and attainment, and SES in turn is a powerful predictor of elevated risk of mental illness. Second, the internalization of the societal stigma of inferiority by at least some African Americans can lead to elevated rates of mental health problems and substance use (e.g., Taylor & Jackson, 1990, 1991).

Third, experiences of racial discrimination are an important type of stressor that has been neglected in the conventional assessment of psychosocial stress. A recent review documented that mental health status has been the most studied health indicator in the burgeoning research on perceived discrimination and health (Williams et al., Neighbors & Jackson 2003). Perceptions of discrimination have been adversely related to psychological distress, psychiatric disorders, and psychological well-being among children and adults for diverse racial/ethnic stigmatized populations in multiple societies. The review concluded that this is a high-priority area for research on racial/ethnic minorities and that the larger literature on stress points to promising new directions for future research.

Access to Mental Health Services

One striking area in which racial disparities exist between Blacks and Whites is that of access to, and use of, mental health services (Freiman et al., 1994). A recent supplement to the first-ever Surgeon General's Report on Mental Health focused on mental health issues related to culture, race, and ethnicity (USDHHS, 2001). This report documents the striking racial/ethnic disparities in mental health care in the United States. Compared to Whites, African Americans and other minorities have less access to, and availability of, mental health services. As noted earlier, when Blacks enter the mental health system, they are also less likely to receive needed services and more likely to receive poorer-quality mental health care. In addition, African Americans are underrepresented as mental health providers and researchers.

The Surgeon General's Report (USDHHS 2001) indicates that these disparities in mental health care impose a greater disability burden on African Americans and other minorities compared to Whites. Accordingly, it calls for improved geographic availability of mental health services, greater integration of mental health care into primary care, greater coordination of care to vulnerable high-need groups, and renewed efforts to reduce barriers to mental health care and to improve the quality of mental health services.

The National Survey of American Life

The National Survey of American Life (NSAL) is a unique new mental health study that offers important new vistas for understanding the mental health of the Black population. Funded by the National Institute of Mental Health and directed by James S. Jackson at the University of Michigan, the study has gathered data from a nationally representative adult sample of about 4,000 native-born Blacks, 2,000 Blacks of non-Hispanic Caribbean ancestry, and 1,000 Whites. Data collection was completed early in 2003.

The study administered a structured diagnostic instrument that uses DSM IV criteria to assess the presence of psychiatric illness. In addition, it included multiple indicators of psychological symptoms, psychological well-being, and impairment linked to mental health problems. The main goals of the study are to examine (1) the nature and distribution of multiple types of stressors among Blacks and other racial groups, (2) the contribution of stressors to psychiatric illness and psychological distress, and (3) how social and psychological resources can shield individuals from the negative effects of stress on mental health and help-seeking.

Two unique features of the study are an adolescent sample and a clinical reinterview. Additional interviews were completed with adolescents aged 13 to 17 in all Black households where an adult was interviewed to yield a national adolescent sample of about 1,500. The adolescent supplement to the NSAL will permit an assessment of a broad range of sociocultural hypotheses about the nature and correlates of mental disorders among African American and Caribbean Black adolescents. A trained clinician also reinterviewed about 10 percent of the adult and adolescent respondents with a semistructured diagnostic instrument and a variety of other assessment scales to allow for a systematic evaluation of the reliability and validity of the broad range of mental disorders assessed with the lay-administered diagnostic interview. No prior study has concurrently assessed rates of psychiatric disorders, nonspecific psychological distress, and psychological well-being along with a broad range of social, psychological, political, and economic contextual risk factors and resources in a large, ethnically diverse national sample of Black Americans.

CONCLUSION

The available evidence of the mental health status of African Americans remains paradoxical and somewhat surprising. The finding of poorer mental health status on some measures of mental health compared to Whites, but similar or even lower rates on other measures, points to the complexities of assessing and delineating existing patterns of mental health status for Blacks. African Americans are disproportionately exposed to adverse social conditions that are often implicated as risk factors for mental illness. Yet, Blacks do not report higher rates of mental illness. Future research on African American mental health needs to better understand the ways in which social and psychological resources, such as social ties, religious participation, and coping can sustain the mental health of African Americans and provide some protection from exposure to a broad range of pathogenic characteristics.

REFERENCES

Adebimpe, V. 1981. Overview: White norms and psychiatric diagnosis of Black patients. *American Journal of Psychiatry, 138*, 279–285.

American Psychiatric Association. 1994. *Diagnostic and statistical manual of mental disorders*, 4th ed. Washington, DC: American Psychiatric Association.

Andrews, F.M., & Withey, S.B. 1976. *Social indicators of well-being.* New York: Plenum Press.

Aneshensel, C.S., & Phelan, J.C. 1999. The sociology of mental health. In C.S. Aneshensel & J.C. Phelan (Eds.). *Handbook of the sociology of mental health* (pp. 3–17). New York: Kluwer Academic Plenum.

Antunes, G., C. Gordon, C.M. Gaitz, & S.J. Scott. 1974. Ethnicity, socioeconomic status and etiology of psychological distress. *Sociology and Social Research, 58*, 361–368.

Babcock, J. 1895. The color insane. *Alienist and Neurologist, 16*, 423–447.

Betancourt, H., & S.R. Lopez. 1983. The study of culture, race and ethnicity in American psychology. *American Psychologists, 48*, 629–637.

Boyd, J.E., et al. 1985. Making diagnosis from DIS data. In *Epidemiologic field methods in psychiatry: The epidemoligic catchment area program.* New York: Academic Press.

Bracy, J.H. 1976. The quality of life experience of Black people. In A. Campbell, P.E. Converse, & W.L. Rodgers (Eds.), *The quality of American life: Perceptions, evaluations, and satisfactions* (pp. 443–69). New York: Russell Sage.

Brown, Tony N. (2003). Critical race theory speaks to the sociology of mental health: Mental health produced by racial stratification. *Journal of Health and Social Behavior, 44(3)*, 292–301.

Campbell, A. 1981. *The sense of well-being in America.* New York: McGraw-Hill.

Clark, Rodney, Norman B. Anderson, Vernessa R. Clark, and David R. Williams. 1999. Racism as a stressor for African Americans: A biopsychosocial model. *American Psychologist, 54(10)*, 805–816.

Clemente, F., & J.S. Williams. 1976. Life satisfaction in the United States. *Social Forces, 54*, 621–631.

Cohen, B.M., R. Fairbank, & E. Green. 1939. Statistical contributions from the Eastern Health District of Baltimore. III. Personality disorder in the Eastern Health District in 1933. *Human Biology, 11*, 112–129.

Comstock, G., & K. Hesling. 1976. Symptoms of depression in two communities. *Psychological Medicine*, 6, 551–63.

Cooper, J.E., R.E. Kendell, B.J. Gurland, L. Sharpe, J.R.M. Copeland, & R. Simon. 1972. *Psychiatric diagnosis in New York and London.* London: Oxford University Press.

Coyne, J.C., & G. Downey. 1991. Social factors and psychopathology: Stress, social support, and coping processes. *Annual Review of Psychology, 42*, 401–425.

Crandell, D.L., & B.P. Dohrenwend. 1967. Some relations among psychiatric symptoms, organic illness, and social class. *American Journal of Psychiatry, 123*, 280–289.

Dalgard, Odd Steffen, & Tambs Kristian. 1997. Urban environment and mental health: A longitudinal study. *British Journal of Psychiatry, 171*, 530–536.

Dohrenwend, B.P. & B.S. Dohrenwend. 1969. *Social status and psychological disorder: A causal inquiry*, New York: Wiley.

Endicott, J., & R.L. Spitzer. 1978. A diagnostic interview: The Schedule for Affective Disorders and Schizophrenia. *Archives of General Psychiatry, 35*, 837–844.

Fischer, J. 1969. Negroes and Whites and rates of mental illness: Reconsideration of a myth. *Psychiatry, 32*, 428–446.

Freiman, M., P. Cunningham, & L. Cornelius. 1994. Use and expenditures for treatment of mental health problems. *Agency for Health Care Quality Research.* Pub # 940085, Rockville, MD.

Gaitz, C., & J. Scott. 1972. Age and measurement of mental health. *Journal of Health and Social Behavior, 13*, 55–67.

Gurin, G.J., J. Veroff, & S. Feld. 1960. *Americans view their mental health.* New York: Basic Books.

Harrell, Jules P., Marcellus M. Merritt, & Jaimalee Kalu. 1998. Racism, stress, and disease. In Reginald L. Jones (Ed.), *African American mental health,* (pp. 247–280). Hampton, VA: Cobb & Henry.

Heurtin-Roberts, S., L. Snowden, & L. Miller. 1997. Expressions of anxiety in African Americans: Ethnography and the epidemiological catchment area studies. *Cultural Medical Psychiatry, 21*, 337–363.

Hughes, M., & M.E. Thomas. 1998. The continuing significance of race revisited: A study of race, class, and quality of life in America, 1972 to 1996. *American Sociological Review, 63*, 785–795.

Hyde, R.W., & R.M. Chisholm. 1944. The relation of mental disorders to race and nationality. *New England Journal of Medicine, 231*, 612–618.

Jarvis, E. 1842a. Statistics in insanity in the United States. *Boston Medical and Surgical Journal, 27*, 116–121.

Jarvis, E. 1842b. Statistics in insanity in the United States. *Boston Medical and Surgical Journal, 27*, 281–282.

Jones, Camara P. 2000. Levels of racism: A theoretical framework and a gardener's tale. *American Journal of Public Health, 90(8)*, 1212–15.

Kessler, R.C., K.A. McGonagle, S. Zhao, C.B. Neslon, M. Hughes, S. Eshleman, H. Wittchen, & K.S. Kendler. 1994. Lifetime and 12-month prevalence of DSM-III-R psychiatric disorders in the United States. *Archives of General Psychiatry, 51*, 8–19.

Kramer, M., B. Rosen, & E. Willis. 1973. Definitions and distributions of mental disorders in a racist society. In C. Willie, M. Kramer, & B. Brown (Eds.), *Racism and mental health* (pp. 353–362). Pittsburgh: University of Pittsburgh Press.

Krieger, Nancy. 1999. Embodying inequality: A review of concepts, measures, and methods for studying health consequences of discrimination. *International Journal of Health Services* 29(2): 295–352.

Landrine, H., & E.A. Klonoff. 1996. *African American acculturation: Deconstructing race and reviving culture.* Newbury Park, CA: Sage.

LaVeist, Thomas A. 1993. Beyond dummy variables and sample selection: What health services researchers ought to know about race as a variable. *Health Services Research, 29*, 1–16.

Leaf, P.J., J.K. Myers, & L.T. McEvoy. 1991. Procedures used in the Epidemiologic Catchment Area Study. In *Psychiatric disorders in America* (pp. 11–32). New York: Free Press.

Leighton, D.C., J.S. Harding, D.B. Macklin, A.M. MacMillan, & A.H. Leighton. 1963. *The character of danger: Stirling County study*, Vol. 3. New York: Basic Books.

Lemkau, P., C. Tietze, & M. Cooper. 1942. Mental hygiene problems in an urban district. *Mental Hygiene, 26*, 100–119.

Lillie-Blanton, Marsha, J.C. Anthony, & C. Schuster. 1993. Probing the meaning of racial or ethnic group comparisons in crack cocaine smoking. *Journal of the American Medical Association, 269*, 993–997.

Lind, J. 1914. The color complex in the Negro. *Psychoanalytic Review, 1*, 404–414.

Link, B., & B.P. Dohrenwend. 1980. Formulation of hypothesis about the true prevalence of demoralization. In B.P. Dohrenwend, B.S. Dohrenwend, M.S. Gould, B. Link, R. Neugebauer, & R. Wunsch-Hitzig (Eds.), *Mental illness in the United States: Epidemiological estimates* (pp. 114–132). New York: Praeger.

Lopez, R.S., & P.J.J. Gaurnaccia. 2000. Cultural psychopathology: Uncovering the social world of mental illness. *Annual Review of Psychology, 51*, 571–598.

Magee, W.J. 1993. Psychological predictors of agoraphobia, simple phobia, and social phobia onset in a U.S. national sample. Ann Arbor: University of Michigan Press.

Malzberg, B. 1944. Mental disease among American Negroes: A statistical analysis. In O. Klineberg (Ed.), *Characteristics of the American Negro* (pp. 373–402). New York: Harper.

Mirowsky, J., & C.E. Ross. 1980. Minority status, ethnic culture and distress: A comparison of Blacks, Whites, Mexicans and Mexican Americans. *American Journal of Sociology, 86*, 479–495.

Mollica, R.F., J.D. Blum, & F. Redlich. 1980. Equity and the psychiatric care of the Black patient. *Journal of Nervous and Mental Disease, 168*, 279–285.

Montagu, A. 1965. *The concept of race*. New York: Free Press.

Neighbors, H.W. 1984. The distribution of psychiatric morbidity in Black Americans. *Community Mental Health Journal, 20*, 169–81.

Neighbors, H.W., J.S. Jackson, L. Campbell, & D. Williams. 1989. The influence of racial factors on psychiatric diagnosis: A review and suggestions for research. *Community Mental Health Journal, 25*, 301–311.

Neighbors, H.W. & D.R. Williams. 2001. The epidemiology of mental disorder 1985 to 2000. In R.L. Braithwaite & S. Taylor (Eds.), *Health issues in the Black community, Second Edition*, 99–128. San Francisco: Jossey-Bass.

Pasamanick, B., D.W. Roberts, P.W. Lemkau, & D.B. Kreuger. 1959. A survey of mental disease in an urban population: Prevalence by race and income. In B. Pasamanick (Ed.), *Epidemiology of mental disorder* (pp. 353–462). Washington, DC: American Association for the Advancement of Science.

Powell, T.O. 1896. The increase of insanity and tuberculosis in southern Negro since 1860, and its alliances and some supposed causes. *Journal of the American Medical Association, 27*, 1185–1188.

Robins, L., & D.A. Reiger. 1991. *Psychiatric disorders in America: The Epidemiologic Catchment Area Study*. New York: Free Press.

Robins, L.N., J.E. Helzer, J.L. Croughhan, & K.L. Ratcliff. 1981. National Institute of Mental Health Diagnostic Interview Schedule: Its history, characteristics and validity. *Archives of General Psychiatry, 38*, 381–389.

Rogler, L.H. 1989. The meaning of culturally sensitive research in mental health. *American Journal of Psychiatry, 146*, 296–303.

Rollock, David, and Edmund W. Gordon. 2000. Racism and mental health into the 21st century: Perspectives and parameters. *American Journal of Orthopsychiatry* 70(1): 5–13.

Rosanoff, A.J. 1917. Survey of mental disorders in Nassau County, New York, July–October, 1916. *Psychiatric Bulletin, 2*, 109–231.

Roth, W.F., & F.B. Luton. 1943. The mental hygiene program in Tennessee. *American Journal of Psychiatry, 99*, 662–675.

Rowntree, L.G., K.H. McGill, & L.P. Hellman. 1945. Mental and personality disorders in Selective Service registrants. *Journal of the American Medical Association, 128*, 1084–1087.

Schmidley, A.D. & Campbell Gibson. 1999. *U.S. Census Bureau, Current Population Reports, Series P23–195, profile of the foreign-born population in the United States: 1997*. Washington, DC: U.S. Government Printing Office.

Schulberg, H.C., M. Saul, M. McClelland, M. Ganguli, W. Christy, & R. Frank. 1985. Assessing depression in primary medical and psychiatric practices. *Archives of General Psychology, 24*, 1164–1170.

Schwab, J., N. McGinnis, & G. Warheit. 1973. Social psychiatric impairment: Racial comparisons. *American Journal of Psychiatry, 130*, 183–87.

Smedley, Brian D., Adrienne Y. Stith, & Alan R. Nelson (Eds.). 2003. *Unequal treatment: Confronting racial and ethnic disparities in health care*. Institute of Medicine. Washington, DC: National Academies Press.

Snowden, L.R. 1999. African American folk idiom and mental health services use. *Cultural Diversity and Ethnic Minority Psychology, 5*, 364–369.

Snowden, L.R., & F.K. Chung. 1990. Use of inpatient mental health services by members of ethnic minority groups. *American Psychologist, 45*, 347–355.

Somervell, P., D. Philip, J. Leaf, M. Weissman, D.G. Blazer, & M.L. Bruce. 1989. The prevalence of major depression in Black and White adults in five United States communities. *American Journal of Epidemiology, 130(4)*, 725–735.

Spitzer, R.L., J. Endicott, & E. Robins. 1978. Research diagnostic criteria: Rationale and reliability. *Archives of General Psychiatry, 35*, 773–782.

Srole, L., T.S. Langner, S.T. Michael, M.D. Opler & T.C. Rennie. 1962. *Mental health in the metropolis: The Midtown Manhattan Study*. Vol. 1. New York: McGraw-Hill.

Taylor, J., & B. Jackson. 1990. Factors affecting alcohol consumption in Black women, part II. *International Journal of Addictions 25(12)*, 1415–1427.

Taylor, Jerome, & B.B. Jackson. 1991. Evaluation of a holistic model of mental health symptoms in African American women. *Journal of Black Psychology, 18*, 19–45.

Thomas, M.E., & M. Hughes. 1986. The continuing significance of race: A study of race, class, and quality of life in America, 1972–1985. *American Sociological Review, 51*, 830–41.

U.S. Department of Health and Human Services (USDHHS). 2001. *Mental health: Culture, race, and ethnicity— A supplement to mental health: A Report of the Surgeon General-Executive Summary*. Rockville, MD: USDHHS, Public Health Service, Office of the Surgeon General.

Vega, W.A., & R.G. Rumbaut. 1991. Ethnic minorities and mental health. *Annual Review of Sociology, 17*, 351–383.

Vernon, S.W., & R. Roberts. 1982. Use of SADS-RDC in a tri-ethnic community survey. *Archives of General Psychiatry, 39*, 47–52.

Warheit, G., Holzer, C., & Arey, S. 1975. Race and mental illness: An epidemiological update. *Journal of Health and Social Behavior, 16*, 243–56.

Warheit, G.J., R.A. Bell, J.J. Schwab, & J.M. Buhl. 1986. An epidemiologic assessment of mental health problems in southeastern United States. In M.M. Weissman, J.K. Myers, & C.E. Ross (Eds.), *Community surveys of psychiatric disorders* (pp. 191–208). New Brunswick, NJ: Rutgers University Press.

Weissman, M.M., M.L. Bruce, P.J. Leaf, L.P. Florio, & C. Holzer. 1991. Affective disorders. In L.N. Robins & D. Reiger (Eds.), *Psychiatric disorders in America: Epidemiologic catchment Area Study*, (pp. 53–80). New York: Free Press.

Weissman, M.M., & J.K. Myers. 1978a. Affective disorders in a U.S. urban community: The use of research diagnostic criteria in an epidemiological survey. *Archives of General Psychiatry, 35*, 1304–1311.

Weissman, M.M., & J.K. Myers. 1978b. Rates and risks of depressive symptoms in a United States urban community. *Acta Psychiatrica Scandinavica, 57*, 219–231.

Weissman, M.M., J.K. Myers, & C.E. Ross. 1986. Community surveys of psychiatric epidemiology: An introduction. In M.M. Weissman, J.K. Myers, & C.E. Ross (Eds.), *Community surveys of psychiatric disorders*, (pp. 33–45). New Brunswick, NJ: Rutgers University Press.

Williams, D.R. 2000. Race, stress, and mental health: Findings from the Commonwealth Minority Health Survey. In C. Hogue, M. Hargraves, & K. Scott-Collins (Eds.), *Minority health*, (pp. 209–243). Baltimore,: Johns Hopkins University Press.

Williams, David R., & Chiquita A. Collins. 2001. Racial residential segregation: A fundamental cause of racial disparities in health. *Public Health Reports, 116*, 404–415.

Williams, D.R., & B.T. Fenton. 1994. The mental health of African Americans: Findings, questions, and directions. In Ivor L. Livingston (Ed.), *Handbook of Black American health: The mosaic of conditions, issues, policies, and prospects*. Westport, CT: Greenwood Press.

Williams, David R., & Michelle Harris-Reid. 1999. Race and mental health: Emerging patterns and promising approaches. In Allan V. Horwitz & Teresa L. Scheid (Eds.), *A handbook for the study of mental health: Social contexts, theories, and systems* (pp. 295–314). New York: Cambridge University Press.

Williams, David R., Risa Lavizzo-Mourey, & Rueben C. Warren. 1994. The concept of race and health status in America. *Public Health Reports, 109(1)*, 26–41.

Williams, David R., & Harold W. Neighbors. 2001. Racism, discrimination and hypertension: Evidence and needed research. *Ethnicity & Disease, 11*, 800–816.

Williams, David R., Harold W. Neighbors, & James S. Jackson. 2003. Racial/ethnic discrimination and health: Findings from community Studies. *American Journal of Public Health, 93(2)*, 200–208.

Williams, David R., & Ruth Williams-Morris. 2000. Racism and mental health: The African American experience. *Ethnicity & Health, 5*, 243–68.

Williams, D.R., Y. Yu, J. Jackson, & N. Anderson. (1997). Racial differences in physical and mental health: Socioeconomic status, stress, and discrimination. *Journal of Health Psychology, 2*, 335–351.

Witmer, A.H. 1891. Insanity in the colored race in the United States. *Alienist and Neurologist, 12*, 19–30.

CHAPTER 23

Vulnerability of African Americans to Adverse Health: The Importance of Social Status and Stress

IVOR LENSWORTH LIVINGSTON, ROBERT M. BROWN III,
AND SHAFFIRAN LIVINGSTON

INTRODUCTION

> In the realm of ideas everything depends on enthusiasm; in the real world, all rest on perseverance.
> —Johann Wolfgang von Goethe

While good health is a desirable and attainable goal for millions of people, for a vast number of poor and minority populations, although it may be desirable, it has been beyond their reach. "Improving the quality of care all Americans receive will require the elimination of racial disparities in health" (Bierman et al., 2002, p. 91). As the United States is increasingly becoming diverse (U.S. Bureau of the Census, 2000), achieving racial and ethnic equality in health has become even more important.

Minority groups, especially African Americans (or Blacks as they will sometimes be called), experience a poorer overall health status and lower levels of access to health care than White Americans and experience a disproportionate burden of chronic and infectious illness. "This higher burden of disease and mortality among minorities has profound implications for all Americans, as it results in a less healthy nation and higher costs for health and rehabilitative care. All members of a community are affected by the poor status of its least healthy members" (Smedley et al., 2003, p. 31). For this reason the Healthy People 2010 initiative has established a far-reaching goal of eliminating health disparities, noting that "the health of the individual is almost inseparable from the health of the larger community, and . . . the Nation" (USDHHS, 2000, p. 15).

Generally speaking, life expectances have increased across racial and gender lines, where White females live the longest and Black males live the shortest. For example, the following life expectancies at birth by race and gender for 1999 and 2000 are: White females (79.9, 80.0) and males (74.6, 74.8) and Black females (74.7, 75.0) and males (67.8, 68.3). In terms of infant mortality (death before reaching 1 year), which is correlated with low socioeconomic status, there was a slight decrease for both races. Again, between the years 1999 and 2000, the rates vary in Blacks (14.6, 14.0) and Whites (5.8 to 5.7) (Minino & Smith, 2001).

This chapter focuses on how vulnerable African Americans are to experience adverse health outcomes, especially those who are poor and experiencing stress. It has been said that increased vulnerability to adverse health among African Americans may be mediated by several environmental factors and experiences that influence behavioral choices, affect availability of services, and may directly impact physiologic function. Health care factors probably play an important role in creating and sustaining health disparities, but these factors exist downstream from the non-health-care forces that create disease in the first place. All of these factors act together to create racial and ethnic health disparities, and they should be measured and addressed more holistically. (Hogan et al., 2001, p. 136)

While these authors are in agreement that a holistic approach is needed to successfully address racial and ethnic health disparities, the emphasis is on selected environmental, or exogamous, factors and individual, or endogamous, factors that affect African Americans' behavioral choices, which in time may lead to adverse health outcomes.

An antecedent environmental factor discussed in the chapter is social status, which is determined largely by one's socioeconomic status, or SES. One's SES influences one's vulnerability to experience/perceive a variety of stressors, which in turn leads to stress. Stress is viewed as having a preeminent role in the overall life and health conditions of African Americans (see Livingston, 1985a, 1985b, 1988a, 1991). Therefore, the premise conveyed in this chapter is that African Americans, especially those who are vulnerable because of their low SES, are more likely to experience stress and, therefore, over time, increased ill-health outcomes. To meaningfully understand the social status–stress–health relationship among any group, especially African Americans, it is important to have a conceptual model as a guiding framework. This being the case, a generic, process-oriented, sociopsychophysiological model (or SPPM) of the stress process is presented. Using the SPPM allows for the successful achievement of the following goals:

a. To conceptualize how African Americans perceive stress;
b. To ascertain the relative positioning and integrating of variables associated with the multifaceted and dynamic social status–stress–health relationship;
c. To better understand how individuals' bodies react to stress;
d. To discuss the various dysfunctional outcomes that are likely to occur, especially as a result of chronic exposure to stressful experiences; and
e. To discuss possible ways to intervene along the designated stress-health continuum.

Because of space and other limitations, the chapter addresses some, but not all, of these conditions. These discussions demonstrate that understanding and reducing stress among African Americans will, in turn, contribute important information that ultimately helps to eliminate racial and ethnic disparities in health.

DISTRIBUTION AND HETEROGENEITY OF BLACKS IN THE UNITED STATES

Geographic Distribution

What is the distribution pattern of African Americans in the United States? If a discussion is about the social status and related stress associated with African Americans, it is prudent to first speak about their location and distribution in the U.S. population. It is also prudent to speak about the growing, yet not sufficiently recognized, diversity in the Black U.S. population.

As of April 1, 2000, the U.S. population was 281.4 million. Of the total, 36.4 million, or 12.9 percent, reported as Black or African Americans. This number includes 34.7 million people, or 12.3 percent, who reported only Blacks in addition to 1.8 million people, or 0.6 percent, who reported

Figure 23.1
Percent Black or African American alone or in combination, 2000

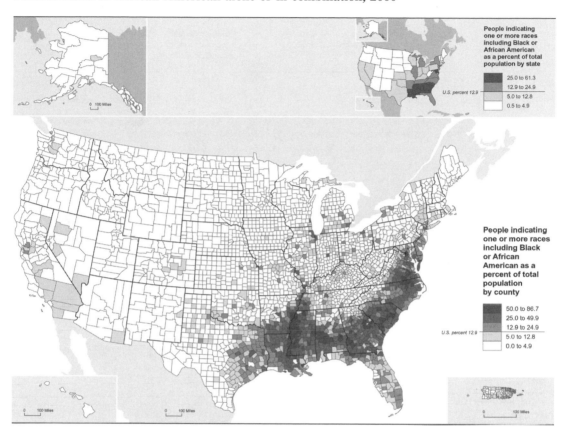

Blacks as well as one of the other races (McKinnon, 2001[1]). As seen in Figure 23.1, the majority of African Americans are located in the eastern and southeastern parts of the United States. Of all the respondents who reported Black, 54 percent lived in the South, 19 percent lived in the Midwest, 18 percent lived in the Northeast, and 10 percent lived in the West (McKinnon, 2001).

In terms of the cities with the largest African American populations, Table 23.1 presents information on the ten largest places in total population and in Black American population in 2000 (McKinnon, 2001). Using the designation of Black or African American in combination, leading the numbers in these cities are New York (26.6 percent, or 2,2274.049); Chicago (37.4 percent, or 1,084,221); Detroit (82.8 percent, or 787,687); Philadelphia (44.3 percent, or 672,162); and Houston (25.9 percent, or 505,101), to mention the first five. Among places of 100,000 or more population, the highest proportion of Blacks was in Gary, Indiana, with 85 percent, followed by Detroit with 83 percent (McKinnon, 2001).

The Heterogeneity of the Black U.S. Population

It should be noted that based on the U.S. census, the term "Black or African American" refers to people having origins in any of the Black race groups of Africa. It includes people who reported "Black, African American, or Negro" or wrote in entries such as African American, Afro American,

Table 23.1
Ten largest places in total population and in Black or African American population, 2000

Place	Total Population		Black or African American Alone		Black or African American Alone or in Combination		Percent of Total Population	
	Rank	Number	Rank	Number	Rank	Number	Black or African American Alone	Black or African American Alone or in Combination
New York, NY	1	8,008,278	1	2,129,762	1	2,274,049	26.6	28.4
Los Angeles, CA	2	3,694,820	7	415,195	6	444,635	11.2	12.0
Chicago, IL	3	2,896,016	2	1,065,009	2	1,084,221	36.8	37.4
Houston, TX	4	1,953,631	5	494,496	5	505,101	25.3	25.9
Philadelphia, PA	5	1,517,550	4	655,824	4	672,162	43.2	44.3
Phoenix, AZ	6	1,321,045	60	67,416	53	76,065	5.1	5.8
San Diego, CA	7	1,223,400	36	96,216	32	109,470	7.9	8.9
Dallas, TX	8	1,188,580	11	307,957	11	314,678	25.9	26.5
San Antonio, TX	9	1,144,646	48	78,120	45	84,250	6.8	7.4
Detroit, MI	10	951,270	3	775,772	3	787,687	81.6	82.8
Baltimore, MD	17	651,154	6	418,951	7	424,449	64.3	65.2
Memphis, TN	18	650,100	8	399,208	8	402,367	61.4	61.9
Washington, DC	21	572,059	9	343,312	9	350,455	60.0	61.3
New Orleans, LA	31	484,674	10	325,947	10	329,171	67.3	67.9

Source: U.S. Census Bureau, census 2000 redistricting Data (Public Law 94–171) Summary File, Table PL-1.

Nigerian, or Haitian (McKinnon, 2001). Again, as mentioned before, based on the vast cultural differences between these Black groups, the overall Black data need to be disaggregated to reflect the major groups of ethnic, foreign-born immigrants.

Although the terms African American and Blacks are used interchangeably throughout this chapter, in some respects the former implies the existence of a homogeneous group. As a matter of fact, while the latter is seen as less desirable to be used because of its possible negative connotations, by its generic label it is the umbrella term under which a variety of non-American Blacks, foreign-born Blacks, or immigrant Blacks can be identified. While it was customary for the majority of foreign-born Blacks to come from the Caribbean (formerly referred to as the West Indies), in recent years the numbers of immigrants from Africa have been increasing (USINS, 2002). By 2000, 2.2 million Blacks in the United States (6.3 percent) were born outside the United States, and another 1.4 million Blacks (3.9 percent) had at least one parent who was foreign-born (Kington & Lucas, 2003).

The need to disaggregate racial and ethnic data, or information that are collected on or about African Americans, is important given the heterogeneity of the Black population in the United States. It has been said (Williams, 2000) that the revised schema of the Office of Management and Budget (OMB) does not adequately take into account the diversity of the Black population. Foreign-born Blacks (e.g., from the Caribbean and Africa) are likely to have different beliefs, behaviors, and physical functioning. These differences, in turn, may be able to predict important diversity in health status (Williams, 2000). For example, one study showed that U.S.-born Black women and Haitian women had higher rates of cervical cancer than English-speaking Caribbean women, but both English-speaking Caribbean women and Haitian immigrant women had lower rates of breast cancer than U.S.-born Black women (Fruchter et al., 1990). However, when subsequent reference is made to African Americans in this chapter, the assumption is that this reference consists of both U.S.-born Blacks as well as foreign-born Blacks.

SOCIAL STATUS AND THE HEALTH OF AFRICAN AMERICANS

It is argued that the health of African Americans is, to a great extent, associated with their social status (or SES) in the United States and that this (negative or lower) status, in turn, contributes to their vulnerability to experience stress. Furthermore, over time, if they continue to experience (chronic) stress, their vulnerability to a variety of adverse health outcomes will increase. Although social status is influenced by many factors, it is also argued in this chapter that the main contributing factor is socioeconomic status (or SES). It is further argued that African Americans who are most vulnerable to ill health, disease, and destructive lifestyle behaviors are the ones who are relatively poor and, therefore, more likely to experience (chronic) stress.

Socioeconomic Status

The most basic causes of health disparities are SES disparities (Link & Phelan, 1995). SES has traditionally been defined by education, income, and occupation. However, education is perhaps the most basic SES component since it shapes future occupational opportunities and earning potential. Better-educated persons gain more ready access to information and resources to promote health (Ross & Wu, 1995). "While SES is clearly linked to morbidity and mortality, the mechanisms responsible for the association are not well understood" (Adler & Newman, 2002, p. 61).

Whatever the means used to assess SES, it has been reliably associated with a wide range of health problems, including low birth weight, cardiovascular disease, hypertension, arthritis, diabetes, and cancer (Pamuk, 1998; Livingston et al., 2003), all of which are disproportionately seen in the African American population. SES has been conceptualized and measured in a variety of ways. For a comprehensive review of the measurement issues related to social class in general and for implications related to health, see Krieger et al. (1997).

In the United States there is a strong association between SES and race, and it is suggested that the higher prevalence of hypertension (which is a major risk factor for cardiovascular disease) and cardiovascular disease (CVD) in Blacks may be attributed to psychosocial factors, including those associated with SES. It is further stated that the possible pathways through which SES affects CVD include the effects of chronic stress mediated by the brain (which is the main position to be discussed later in the chapter), differences in lifestyles and behavior patterns, and access to health care (Pickering, 1999).

The Poverty Guidelines. Each year the U.S. Department of Health and Human Services (USDHHS) issues poverty guidelines. These guidelines, which are issued each year in the *Federal Register*, are a simplification of the poverty thresholds, and they are used primarily for administrative purposes—for instance, determining financial eligibility for certain federal programs. Sometimes the poverty guidelines are loosely referred to as the Federal Poverty Level (FPL). Also, the poverty guidelines are calculated in terms of size of family unit (SFU). The 2003 HHS poverty guidelines as per size of family unit is as follows: $8,980 (SFU = 1); $12,120 (SFU = 2); $15,260 (SFU = 3); $18,400 (SFU = 4); $21,540 (SFU = 5); $24,680 (SFU = 6); $27,820 (SFU = 7); $30,960 (SFU = 8) (2003 HHS Poverty Guidelines, 2003).

The number of poor African Americans dropped by 600,000 to 9.1 million between 1996 and 1997, while their poverty rate fell from 28.4 percent to 26.5 percent. For Hispanics, who may be of any race, the number in poverty declined from 8.7 million to 8.3 million, and their poverty rate dropped from 29.4 percent to 27.1 percent. In both years, the poverty rate for Hispanics did not

Figure 23.2
Percentage of Blacks living below the poverty line by state, 1999

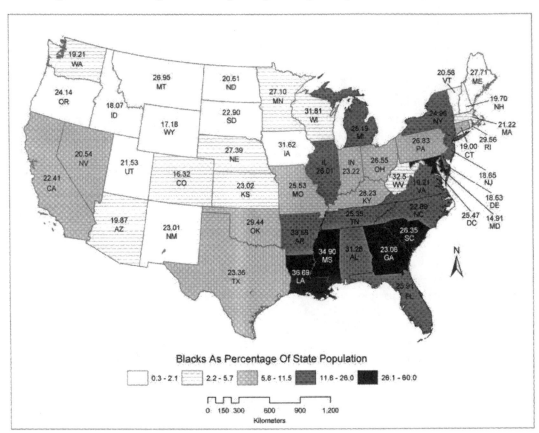

Source: Data calculated using Census 2000, Table P159B (http://factfinder.census.govs/).

differ statistically from that of African Americans. Although the poverty rates dropped for African Americans and Hispanics, they remained significantly higher than the rates for Caucasians (11.0 percent) and for Asians and Pacific Islanders (14.0 percent) (U.S. Census Bureau, 1997). A clearer picture of the distribution of Blacks below the povery level on a state basis is seen in Figure 23.2. The states and districts with the five largest percentages on Blacks below the poverty level are Louisiana (37 percent), Mississippi (35 percent), Arkansas (34 percent), West Virginia (33 percent), and Iowa and Wisconsin (both at approximately 32 percent). The relationship between race and SES was aptly stated by Williams (2000): "Although there is a strong relationship between race and SES, they are not equivalent. For example, the rate of poverty is three times higher for Blacks than for Whites, but two-thirds of Blacks are not poor, and two-thirds of all poor Americans are White" (p. 98).

A Select Focus on Socioeconomic Status-Related Health Outcomes

As far back as the twelfth century investigators have known that SES is inversely related to poor health; that is, as SES levels increase, rates of physical morbidity and mortality decrease (for reviews, see Adler et al., 1994; Williams & Collins, 1995). Research suggests that SES differences between

Figure 23.3
The relationship between social status, stress, and health using selected conditions

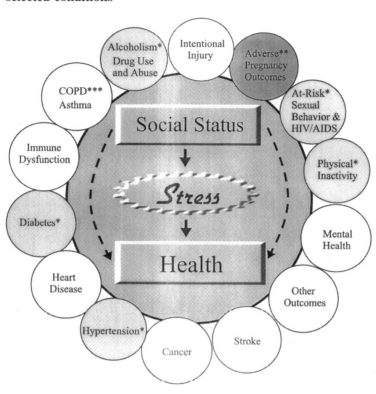

Source: Original model (© 2004) designed for this chapter by Ivor L. Livingston.

* A select number of health conditions influenced by stress, and to be elaborated on when the stress model is later discussed.
** A more specific discussion is made of the stress-health relationship with the stress model using adverse pregnancy outcomes as an example.
*** Chronic Obstructive Pulmonary disease.

races account for the majority of racial differences in health. Adjusting racial (Black–White) disparities in health for SES sometimes eliminates, but always substantially reduces, these differences (Williams & Collins, 1995; Lillie-Blanton et al., 1996). However, race often has an impact on health independently of SES: within levels of SES, Blacks still have an inferior health status than Whites (House & Williams, 2001). See Figure 23.3 for an example of selected health conditions that are either directly or indirectly influenced by the social status–stress relationship.

African American Children and Young Adults

In childhood, the best indicator of the relationship between poverty and health is infant mortality. Poor pregnancy outcomes, including prematurity, birth defects, low birth weight, and infant death are associated with low income, low educational level, low occupational status, and other conditions related to being socially and economically disadvantaged (Smedley et al., 2003). In 1997, the infant mortality rate (IMR) among African American infants was 2.3 times that of Caucasian infants.

Although IMRs have declined for both racial groups, the proportional discrepancy between African Americans and Caucasians remains largely unchanged (Hoyert et al., 1999). Low birth weight (LBW) for African Americans remains twice as high as that of Caucasians—13 percent in 1998 (Ventura et al., 2000).

Disproportionate traumatic death and developmental limitations are also associated with children who are poor. For example, iron deficiency is more than twice as common in low-income children, aged 1 and 2, than among other children of similar ages in the wider population (USDHHS, 2000). Growth retardation affects 16 percent of low-income children younger than 6 years of age, and in the mid-1980s, an estimated three million children, virtually all of whom were from low-income families, had blood lead levels that exceeded 15 ug/dL. This lead level was sufficient to place them at risk for impaired mental and physical development (USDHHS, 2000).

Homicide is the second leading cause of death for young persons aged 15–24 years and the leading cause of death for African Americans in this age group (Singh et al., 1996). In 1998, physical assault victimization among adolescents took place twice as often as in the general population of persons 12 years and older. While the total assaults were similar across racial and ethnic groups, aggravated assault was higher for Blacks than Whites (11.9 vs. 7.0 per 1,000). Rates of assault victimization decreased from 54.2 per 1,000 persons in households with annual incomes of less than $7,500 to less than 30 per 1,000 persons in households with annual incomes greater than $35,000 (DOJ, 1999).

African American Adults

The work on SES and health has raised important empirical questions regarding the relative importance of SES for different racial groups (e.g., see Anderson & Armstead, 1995). SES appears to confer fewer health benefits for members of ethnic minorities in the United States (e.g., Ren & Amick, 1996), while other research suggests that "marginal increases in socioeconomic status generally have larger positive effects on the health of Blacks than on the health of Whites" (Schoenbaum & Waidmann, 1997, p. 71). The distribution of risk factors and resources is influenced by the conditions under which people live and work. Given the interaction between social status and risk factors, it has been reported that comparable stressful events have stronger negative effects on low-SES persons than those of higher status (Kessler, 1979).

There may also be interesting race, class, and gender interactions as well involving mental health outcomes. For example, Williams et al. (1992) found that SES was inversely related to psychiatric disorders among both Whites and Blacks. However, the relationship was stronger among White males than among Black males, because lower-SES White males had higher rates of psychiatric disorders than their Black counterparts. For women the situation was somewhat different. For example, lower-SES Black women had higher rates of substance abuse than lower-SES White women. Therefore, it was suggested that "the interaction between race and SES in mental health outcomes may depend on whether distress or psychiatric disorders are being considered and may also vary across gender and type of disorder" (Ostrove et al., 1999, p. 453).

With respect to older ages, the pattern of increased vulnerability to injury, disease, and death continues with segments of the population defined as having low incomes or being poor. Poverty appears to be a predisposing factor associated with a greater risk for murder of acquaintances and family members, as well as robbery-motivated killings of strangers (USDHHS, 2000). Activity limitations are four times more common among people with 8 years of education than among individuals with 16 years or more. It has also been reported that bed disability days increase as income decreases (National Institute on Disability and Rehabilitation Research, 1989).

PREVALENCE OF RACIAL DIFFERENCES ON SELECTED STRESS-RELATED CONDITIONS: AN OVERVIEW

There is a void of information on the national level that shows racial differences, if any, on survey questions relating specifically to stress. However, some reports (i.e., prevalence data) exist on information from a national sample of respondents on mental health characteristics. One such report is the National Health Interview Survey (NHIS) conducted by the National Center for Health Statistics (NCHS). In an early release of selected estimates based on data from the January–September 2002 NHIS (which was released March 19, 2003), six psychological distress questions were asked. The questions asked how often a respondent experienced certain symptoms of psychological distress during the last 30 days. The age-sex-adjusted prevalence of serious psychological distress was 3.6 percent for Hispanic or Latino persons, 2.8 percent of White non-Hispanic persons, and a 3.3 percent for Black or African non-Hispanic persons. While Whites reported fewer psychological distress, next by African Americas and lastly by Hispanics or Latinos, the differences were not statistically significant (NCHS, 2003).

In the case of more analytical studies, it has been reported that racial differences in distress tend to disappear when controlled for socioeconomic status (SES) (Williams, 1986). The higher rates of distress in Blacks, versus their White counterparts, have been attributed to characteristics of their social situation, such as a greater number of life stressors (Kessler, 1979 and higher levels of alienation and powerlessness (Mirowsky & Ross, 1989). The interaction between race and SES has also been addressed. For example, Kessler and Neighbors (1986) reanalyzed data from eight epidemio logic surveys and reported that although controlling for SES reduced the association between race and psychological distress, low-SES Blacks had higher rates of distress than low-SES Whites. In a similar manner, Ulbrich et al. (1989) reported higher levels of psychological distress in Blacks with low income and occupational levels compared to their White counterparts.

SOCIAL STATUS, STRESS, AND HEALTH: A CONCEPTUAL MODEL

The relationship between social status (i.e., SES), stress, and the health in the general population and in the African American population in particular is fundamental to the position taken in this chapter. As seen in the conceptual and process-oriented sociopsychophysiological model (SPPM) of stress (Figure 23.4), the premise, which has empirical support, is that a person's sociodemographic background, in this case primarily race and social status (largely determined by SES) contributes to increased vulnerability to experience exaggerated psychological and physiological (chronic) stress, over time. In addition to a person's sociodemographic characteristics, the initiation as well as the response to stress are influenced by constitutional factors, psychological and behavioral factors, and coping responses over time. Some of the stress-related health outcomes, seen in Figure 23.3, are discussed later in the chapter. Because these relationships are as important as they are complex and dynamic, an attempt is made to explain them in the context of a sociopsychophysiological model (or SPPM) of stress.

How is Stress Viewed?

Although there is no universally accepted definition of stress, a dominant view is that it clearly involves a "person–environment" interaction (or transaction) (Lazarus & Folkman, 1984) 1980; Livingston, 1988b). While stress is an internal reaction that involves various physiologic processes, for purposes of this chapter the main concerns are with the sociopsychological factors, or stressors, that

Figure 23.4

A sociopsychophysiological model of the stress process

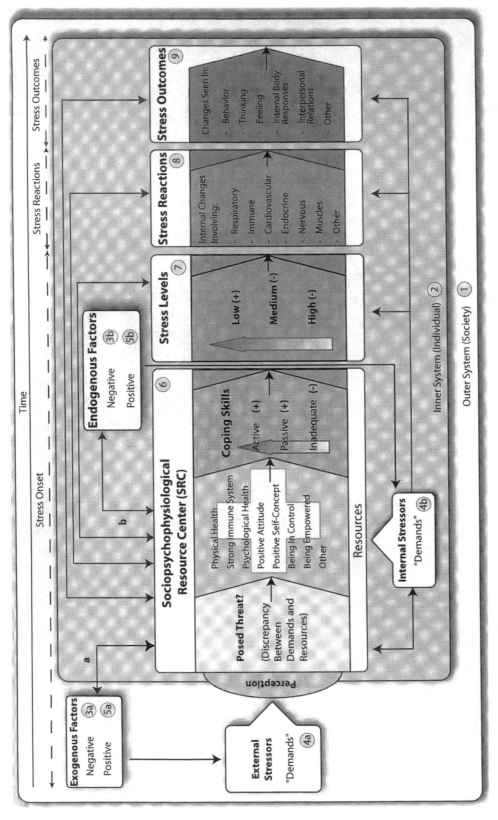

This model is a further modified version that last appeared in the following publication: Livingston, I.L. "Social Status, Stress and Health: Black Americans at Risk." In I.L. Livingston (Ed.), *Handbook of Black American Health* (pp. 236–252) (Westport, CT: Greenwood Press, 1994).

[a] External conditions in society contributing to the functioning of the SRC.
[b] Internal factors within the individual contributing to the functioning of the SRC.
↔ Bidirectional arrows reflect the reciprocal nature of designated elements of the model.

initiate the stress process and the need to maintain balance, or homeostasis/allostasis to relieve the stress (McEwen, 2002).

The Conceptual Importance of the SPPM

Given the multidisciplinary and multidimensional aspects of the SPPM (which is evidenced in its label), it is not surprising that various theories from different disciplines are applicable to the SPPM. For example, from sociology and organizational psychology, systems theory posits a hierarchical ordering of social, psychological, and biological levels, or systems, each of which has its own resources, needs, and limitations. Also, these systems are interrelated in such a manner that a change at one level invariably impacts behavior at other levels. Consistent with a systems perspective, the SPPM suggests that an individual's experience of stress may be the result of, as well as a contributor to, the stressors and changes within society as a whole.

An Overview of the SPPM

Although a brief explanation of the SPPM is provided in this chapter in the context of how it can facilitate the understanding of the stress–APO relationship, a more in-depth description and explanation of the SPPM can be found elsewhere (Livingston, 1994). As seen in Figure 23.4, the following features should be noted about the SPPM:

a) it is a *generic* interactive model (see bidirectional arrows);

b) it has three basic stages (i.e., **onset, reaction** and **outcomes**); and

c) these three stages comprise nine basic components. Of importance to the SPPM is the fact that the wider *society*, or *outer system (1)*, subsumes the *individual*, or *inner system* (e.g., African Americans) *(2)*. With the exception of exogenous factors *(3a* and *5a)* and external stressors *(4a)*, all other components (i.e., endogenous factors: *(3b, 5b)*; internal stressors: *(4b)*; SRC *(6)*; stress levels *(7)*; stress reactions *(8)*; and stress outcomes *(9)* are subsumed under the inner system *(2)*, or basically within the individual. Also, there is an ongoing interaction, over time, between both systems. The inclusion of time is very important in that it allows for chronic experiences and exposures to stressors and, subsequently, to related levels of stress *(7)*, stress reactions *(8)* and dysfunctional stress (health) outcomes *(9)*.

The SPPM (see Figure 23.4) explicitly shows that at onset stage, or first stage of the stress process, a sociopsychological or interactionist perspective is the dominant characteristic of the model. Therefore, stress occurs as a result of a complex *perceived* transaction, that is, involving *external (1) demands (4a)* (e.g., discrimination, Clarke et al., 1999) and individual *(2) resources (6)* (e.g., having support and adequate coping skills). This reservoir of resident resources, which if adequately endowed is literally the "epicenter" or "core center" of individuals' resources, is referred to as the *sociopsychophysiological resource center* or *SRC* (Livingston et al., 2003). The SRC is defined as *"The mind body enduring capacity that individuals have that filters, mediates, neutralizes, and subsequently serves to stabilize all entering noxious and other stimuli or stressors"* (Livingston, 1994).

As indicated by the positive (+) sign in the SRC, the resident resources should include the ideal factors, related to less stress and better health over time (e.g., higher levels of a sense of control or self-efficacy, Henry, 2001; Taylor & Seeman, 1999; lower levels of depression, pessimism, salience of weaknesses (Stansfeld et al., 1998); and persistence as a desirable quality in pursuit of good health (Henry, 1998). Most of these resource-related qualities are associated with middle and upper SES positions. For example, Henry and Craig-Leas (1995) found that the salience of negative events and of personal weaknesses was much stronger among lower-class individuals. Additionally, Henry (2000), found that higher-class individuals held a greater sense of possibilities and that this provided an empowering perception. This was associated with the individual being more likely to embrace change and see change as an opportunity for growth. This basic transactional view of stress is consistent with how stress has been viewed by others in the past (Lazarus & Folkman, 1984; Livingston, 1988a). Based on this perceived transaction, stress is subjective; that is, an individual's perception or view of the demands, or stressors (which can be both internal and external), determines whether stress literally occurs (Livingston, 1992, 1994; Lazarus & Folkman, 1984).

While the transactional view of stress emphasizes *external stressors* or *demands (4a)*, there are also *internal stressors (4b)* (e.g., psychological deficits, health conditions) that may or may not be conscious to individuals and are therefore not mediated by their "perceptual apparatus." However, these stressors are still very real and important and impact all aspects of the stress process, especially their own *SRCs (6)*.

The SPPM also shows that outside, or exogenous, factors impact both external stressors *(4a)* (e.g., crowded and unsanitary housing, air and water pollution, poor working conditions, and other such deficits that disproportionately affect those in the lower SES strata, IOM, 2001) as well as the SRC *(6)*. This impacting process occurs through various negative factors *(3a)* (e.g., racism, Clarke et al., 1999; low SES, Forman 1997; ethnicity, Williams & Collins, 1995) and positive factors *(5a)* (e.g., social support, McNeilly et al., 1996; religious participation, Jones, 1997). In a similar manner for endogenous factors, both negative *(3b)* (e.g., maladaptive coping responses that do not attenuate stress responses, Burchfield, 1985) and positive *(5b)* (e.g., more general coping responses as "John Henryism," James et al., 1983; empowerment, Henry, 2001) factors impact the SRC *(6)*.

Depending on the nature of the exogenous and endogenous factors, as well as how they impact the dominant social status–stress–health relationship, or simply the stress–health relationship, they may be either labeled as *moderating* or *mediating* factors. Consistent with the work of Baron and Kenny (1986), *moderator* variables are viewed as factors that influence the direction or magnitude of the relationship between predictor (social status and/or stress) and criterion variable (e.g., health outcome). Conversely, *mediator* variables are seen as factors that account for the relationship between the predictor and criterion variables. Based on the SPPM, if either the *moderator* or *mediator* variables are external to the individual, and they *contribute* to an increase in the stress–health relationship (i.e., having a *moderating* effect by influencing the direction of the relationship or having a *mediating* effect by simply making the relationship possible in the first place), they are considered negative *(3a)*. However, if these factors contribute to a decrease in the dominant *stress–health* relationship, they are considered positive *(5a)*. In a similar manner, if the variables are internal to the individual, and they *contribute* to an increase in the stress–health relationship, they are considered negative *(3b)*, and if they contribute to a decrease in the stress–health relationship, they are considered positive *(5b)*.

In progressing from left to right in the SPPM, the last segment of the *stress onset* phase of the stress process is the box dealing with stress levels *(7)*. This point in the model shows the actual, "internal" level of stress the individual is experiencing based on the dynamic transactions that have taken place. At this point, both the kind and level of stress experienced have important implications for subsequent stages in the stress process, that is, stress reactions *(8)* and stress outcomes *(9)*. The combined effects of chronic and acute perceptions of stressors have the potential to contribute to psychological and physiological sequelae that could be especially toxic for African Americans. As seen in the SPPM, if the accumulated stress is not reduced, for example, by contributions from positive *endogenous factors (5b)* and/or contributions from the *SRC (6)*, for example, via adaptive coping skills (Burchfield, 1985) over time, chronic stress or "allostatic load" (McEwen, 2000, 2002) builds to destructive levels.

Increasing unmitigated stress then, in turn, leads to the second stage of the stress process—*stress reaction (8)*, which in turn leads to the last stage—stress outcomes *(9)*. The following statements are consistent with the tenets of the SPPM. "Over time, chronic perceptions of racism *[(4a)]* coupled with more passive coping responses *[(3b)* and *(7)]* may lead to frequent increases in and prolonged activation of sympathetic functioning *[(8)]* resulting in higher resting systolic blood pressure levels *[(9)]*" (Clark et al., 1999, p. 811). Various authors have proposed that such chronic stress-induced sympathetic activation may be among the factors that contribute to hypertension (for a review, see Manuck et al., 1990).

A Selected Focus of the SPPM on Adverse Pregnancy Outcomes for African American Women

Although an overview was given of the SPPM in the previous section, in an effort to describe the utility of the SPPM in better understanding a defined stress–health outcome relationship, a selected focus is taken of the stress–adverse pregnancy outcome (APO) relationship as it applies to at-risk (i.e., low social status or SES) African American women. Because of space limitations, a more thorough discussion can be seen elsewhere (Livingston et al., 2003).

Why the Focus on the Stress–APO Relationship?   African Americans continue to trail their Caucasian counterparts in having proportionately higher rates of maternal mortality (Koonin et al., 1997) and infant mortality (NCHS, 2001), both of which contribute to racial and ethnic disparities in health. Important contributors to APO are low birth weight (LBW), very low birth weight (VLBW), and premature births (Livingston et al., 2003). Infants born weighing less than 1,500 grams, or very low birth weight (VLBW), due to early delivery with or without slow fetal growth, are at significantly increased risk of mortality and morbidity. In the United States, among Black mothers, the VLBW rate is three times higher than among White mothers (NCHS, 2001).

In the case of premature births, preterm labor is a clinical syndrome characterized by uterine contractility, cervical ripening, and/or membrane rupture occurring before 37 weeks of gestation (Romero et al., 1990). Preterm is generally defined as a delivery before 37 weeks' gestation (with very preterm being before 32 weeks of gestation). There is a twofold increase in preterm birth in African American women compared with virtually any other U.S. population, with an even greater discrepancy in very early preterm birth (Goldenberg et al., 1996). No satisfactory explanation for these differences has been advanced (Goldenberg et al., 2002).

There is growing evidence that women who experience high levels of social and psychological stress during pregnancy are at a significantly increased risk for conditions related to APOs, such as shorter gestation, earlier onset of spontaneous labor, and preterm delivery. These risks still exist even after adjustments are made for the effects of other established biomedical, sociodemographic, and behavioral risk factors (Wadhwa, 1998).

In an attempt to explain the stress–APO relationship, Geronimus (1992) indicated that the cumulative effects of stressors may "weather" African American women, making them more susceptible to APOs. In a related manner, it was also said that a contributing factor to weathering is a woman's perception of her stressors. Collins et al. (1997), in analyzing birth weight, ethnicity, place of residence (by census tract), and adequacy of prenatal care, reported that residence in very low-income (median annual family income less than $10,000), or impoverished neighborhoods, was associated with a 60 percent greater LBW rate for African American women who received prenatal care. These findings confirm, in part, that unmeasured factors closely related with African Americans' race and poverty also affect APOs, even in the presence of adequate prenatal care utilization. These findings also support the "weathering" experiences of African American women mentioned before (Geronimus, 1992).

Stress Onset

It is reasoned in this chapter that a contributing factor to the stress–health relationship for African Americans is their perception of, and negative experiences with, the daily realities of both positive *(5a)* (for example, social support [McNeilly et al., 1996]) and negative exogenous factors *(3a)* (e.g., racism, discrimination, and/or low SES conditions or poverty-related experiences [Clarke et al., 1998], or low SES [Forman et al., 1997]).

Exogenous Factors, External Stressors, and the SRC.   As is illustrated in the SPPM (see Figure 23.3), if African American women are predisposed to experience a host of negative (i.e., *adverse*), exogenous factors *(3a)*—for example, poverty, racism, undesirable life events—these factors could contribute to related stressors or demands *(4a)*, for example, including crowding, crime, noise pollution, discrimination, and other hazards or stressors (Baum et al., 1999). In the absence of more positive (i.e., *moderating*) exogenous factors *(5a)* (e.g., social support [McNeilly et al., 1996]) the perceived-stressors could lead to perceived threat in their SRCs *(6)*. It is important to note that given the dynamic nature of the SPPM, an initially predisposing negative, exogenous condition *(3a)* (e.g., racism, low socioeconomic status, Clark et al., 1999) may itself be perceived as a stressor *(4a)* (e.g., discrimination, as seen in denial of certain needs involving housing, hospitalization, and work, Baum et al., 1999). It has been said that a woman's perception that she resides in a 'bad' ["posed threat"] neighborhood may be a chronic stressor that disproportionately affects the reproductive outcome of African Americans (Collins et al., 1998).

Another example of a possible negative exogenous condition has to do with the disproportionately large percentage of African Americans who live in impoverished urban communities infiltrated with violence and illicit drug traffic (McCord & Freeman, 1990). Again, depending on the capabilities of the women's SRCs *(6)*, as well as various other factors (e.g., the availability of moderating, positive exogenous factors *[5a]*), they may or may not perceive these factors as external stressors *(4a)*. Only recently have researchers started to suspect that such a residential pattern of "difficult" living contributes to the unexplained threefold greater incidence of very-low-birthweight (VLBW < 1,500 gm) infants among African Americans compared with Caucasians (Collins et al., 1997; Polednak, 1996).

It is the cumulatively challenged, or chronic exposure to adverse SES conditions *(3a)* that may have the largest impact on health *(9)*. Additionally, low-socioeconomic pregnant women experience more stressful life events *(4a)* during their pregnancy (Rutter & Quine, 1990) (i.e., versus the less obvious and more difficult to measure internal stressors—*[4b]*). Furthermore, chronic stressors are embedded within, and accrue from, the environment of low-socioeconomic women *(3a)*. Therefore, the threat caused by financial insecurity *(3a)* can lead to (i.e., be perceived as) various related external stressors *(4a)*, such as poor and crowded housing conditions, domestic violence, and stressful working conditions.

Reports also indicate that a high frequency of stressors (e.g., undesirable life events or stressful life events—SLEs conditions) during pregnancy are associated with an increased risk of low birth weight, preterm delivery, and spontaneous abortion (Neugebauer et al., 1996). This being the case, experiencing these SLEs *(3a)* may lead to acute stressors *(4a)* that can contribute to the elevated VLBW rate among African American women (Collins et al., 1998).

Endogenous Factors, Internal Stressors, and the SRC.   The SRC *(6)* plays a very important mediating role in African American women experiencing internal eliciting stressors *(4b*—e.g., infection, trauma. Depending on the individual makeup and constitution of women, these stressors can result from negative endogamous factors *(3b)*, for example, poor physical health, inadequate nutrition, inadequate sleep (Frankish et al., 1998). Again, focusing on the dynamic nature of the SPPM and how stress is defined in the model, negative endogenous factors are not the only risk factors that can contribute to internal stressors, depending on the "disposition" or the SRCs of the women involved. Additionally, and as seen in Figure 23.1 (note the bidirectional arrows), based on the perceived experiences women have with exogenous factors (*3a* and *5a*) and external stressors *(4a)*, these factors can indirectly affect their internal stressors *(4b)* through the functioning of their SRCs, and vice versa. Also, endogenous factors can directly impact their internal stressors, or there may be an indirect pathway through their SRCs, again as illustrated by the arrows shown in the SPPM.

Factors that are potential buffers, or moderators, in the stress–APO relationship are positive endogamous factors *(5b)*, such as having strong personality characteristics like a "hardy personality" (Major et al., 1998). These factors are also likely to reduce the effects of stressors, both external *(4a)* and, to a lesser extent, internal stressors *(4b)* by moderating their effects and, ultimately, as moderating variables (Baron & Kenny, 1986), decrease the overall strength of the stress–APO relationship. Again, because of the dynamic nature of the SPPM, the moderating effect may be in an indirect manner, where these *positive endogamous factors (5b)* can increase the personal resiliency of women's SRCs, thereby reducing the perceived threat of external stressors *(4a)*. Alternatively, they can act directly through a pathway to internal stressors, thereby reducing the latter's potential negative effect. Contributing factors to personal resiliency include self-esteem, optimism, and mastery beliefs of being in control of life's activities (Kramer et al., 2001).

According to Henry (2001), empowered individuals are more likely to take proactive steps in terms of personal health, while disempowered individuals are more likely to take a fatalistic approach. It was found that high-SES individuals held a greater sense of possibilities and that this provided an empowering perception (Henry, 2001). Also, this was associated with the individual being more likely to embrace change (e.g., in the form of exogenous and/or external stressors) and to see change as an opportunity for growth. Conversely, lower-SES individuals were found to be more likely to exhibit preferences for stability in their lives. Another manifestation of weaker self-confidence *(3b)*, which is very relevant to the stress–APO relationship for African American women implied in the SPPM, is the preference among lower-SES groups to avoid stressful, challenging tasks in their lives (Hobel et al., 1999). Such activities run counter to the assumption that, in some cases, stressful circumstances must and should be addressed, rather than avoided.

Other more physiologic factors can exist that serve as possible examples of negative endogamous factors *(3b)*. A very important factor in elucidating the behavioral and/or biological influences moderating the effects of prenatal stress on gestational outcomes is the role of the corticotropin-releasing hormone (CRH). Basically, the CRH, as a hypothalamic neuropeptide, plays a central role in regulating the activity of the hypothalamic-pituitary-adrenal HPA axis and in the physiological response to stress. Recent reports suggest that the effects of psychosocial stressors *(4a)* may be mediated by cortisol-induced positive feedback increases in placenta secretion of CRH (Hobel et al., 1999; Lockwood, 1999). Additionally, overwhelming evidence indicates that women in preterm labor have significantly elevated levels of CRH compared with gestational age-matched control women and that these elevations of CRH precede the onset of preterm labor, in some cases by several weeks (Hobel et al., 1999; Wadhwa, 1998).

It has been reported (Petraglia et al., 1995) that neuroendocrine stress responses, including epinephrine, norepinephrine, and cortisol, provoke CRH release from placental tissue in vitro. In a related manner it is said "that maternal psychological stress may precipitate surges in neuroendocrine stress responses that stimulate placental CRH production, priming the placental-fetal feed-forward loop to hasten delivery from a stressed environment" (Rich-Edwards, 2001, p. 126). Therefore, given the mediating role of CRH, it qualifies as a dynamic example of a negative endogenous factor *(3b)* in the SPPM that could impact the stress-APOs of African American women. It is important to note that because the relationship between endogenous factors (e.g., *3b*) and internal stressors *(4b)* is usually at the subliminal level and, therefore, beneath women's perceptual/appraisal mechanisms, any ensuing affecting relationships between these conditions (e.g., CRH and internal stressors) are possibly beyond any conscious awareness. Again, for these reasons it is more difficult to intervene, especially when the relationships involve endogenous factors and internal stressors.

Stress Reaction

This second phase *(8)* may be experienced, depending on the functional state of African American women's SRCs *(6)*, which in turn contributes to their stress levels *(7)*. When activated, especially for a protracted period of time, this stage involves a complex series of measurable neuroendocrinologic reactions and changes. As seen in Figure 23.1, the host of possible internal stress reactions can be manifested through a variety of changes involving hormones, organs, and internal body systems.

Acute stress increases immune function and also enhances the formation of potentially dangerous events. However, failure to shut off the stress response when it is no longer needed results in the suppression of immune function and remodeling of brain cells in the hippocampus. According to McEwen (2000, 2002), such an occurrence is captured in the concepts of allostasis and allostatic load. The concept of "allostasis" (active responding of biological mediators that maintain homeostasis) leads to the concept of "allostatic load" (the wear and tear of the body due to overuse of allostasis by repeated stress regulation of the mediators—failure to shut them off when no longer needed).

It has been theorized that frequently stressful experiences, whether they are concurrent, feared, and/or remembered, increase allostatic load. Therefore, women's experience of negative exogenous factors *(3a)* (e.g., racism), which can lead to, or be perceived as, external stressors *(4a)* (e.g., feeling of being discriminated against), creates an allostatic load that imprints itself upon their HPA axis prior to conception. It is also reasoned that this alters the endocrine milieu in which the placenta is established, thereby potentially affecting the hormonal interaction between fetus, placenta, and mother (Rich-Edwards et al., 2001). Based on the SPPM seen in Figure 23.1, chronic stress levels *(7)*, without any ameliorative moderation from the SRC *(6)*, are likely to contribute to allostatic load *(8)* (McEwen, 2000), which in turn can lead to a variety of stress–health outcomes *(9)* (e.g., APOs for African American women).

In a prevalence study of maternal stress and bacteria vaginosis (BV) involving a sample of pregnant women (less than 20 weeks of gestation) who were enrolled at health centers in an urban setting, it was reported that BV (positive) women had a significantly higher mean chronic stress score than BV (negative) women. Also, African American women were 2.5 times more likely to have BV than non-African American women. Furthermore, even after controlling for sociodemographic and behavioral risk factors, moderate to high levels of chronic stress remained not only significant but also substantially associated with BV status. These authors concluded that at least part of the variation in susceptibility to this infectious syndrome may be attributed to physiologic changes caused by high maternal levels of chronic stress (Culhane et al., 2001).

Stress Outcomes

Adverse Pregnancy Outcomes.   Although the focus of this chapter has been on the stress–APO relationship, mentioned earlier, various other factors (e.g., prenatal care, nutritional factors) have to be taken into account, along with stress, in any comprehensive attempt to improve our understanding of APOs, especially among at-risk African American women. However, it has been said (Wadhwa, 1998) that the importance of stress is increasingly being recognized.

In an attempt to show the relationship between stress and other health outcomes, what follows is a brief overview of selected health conditions that are increasingly being recognized as having a stress component to them. These selected conditions were earlier highlighted in Figure 23.3. These conditions are discussed under this last phase of the stress process because it is here where they would be recognized.

Alcoholism.   When compared with the general U.S. population, African Americans have the same or lower rates of alcohol use (SAMHSA, 1998). However, despite these relatively lower rates, African Americans tend to have higher rates of alcohol-related social and health problems versus a national sample of U.S. residents (NIAAA, 2000a). For example, African American males have higher rates of cirrhosis of the liver, and SES predictors place African American women at greater risk for fetal alcohol syndrome (NIAAA, 2000b).

Epidemiologic studies (e.g., Klatsky, 1995) and other reports (e.g., Livingston, 1985a) support the hypothesis that regular alcohol use above a defined threshold is related to elevated blood pressure (or HBP). Other studies suggest that (psychological) stress affects hormones that are associated with elevated BP (Henry, Liu & Meehan, 1995). Researchers believe "that people increase their alcohol use to relieve tension or depression caused by exposure to stress and to things that cause stress (i.e., stressors)" (Russell et al., 1999, p. 299).

Asthma.   Morbidity and mortality due to asthma are increasing in the United States, especially among African Americans (Bailey et al., 1994). Minority groups, especially those living in poverty *(3a)*, are more likely to die of asthma and to require emergency care for exacerbations of asthma than Caucasian persons not living in poverty (Strunk et al., 2002). High levels of stress *(7)* have been shown to predict the onset of asthma in children genetically at risk and to correlate with higher asthma morbidity (Sandberg et al., 2000).

Coronary Heart Disease.   African Americans experience a disproportionate incidence of morbidity and mortality from coronary heart disease (CHD) compared to their Caucasian counterparts (Jones et al., 2002). SES is inversely related to CHD and often remains predictive independently of other risk factors. Persons with atherosclerosis and increased reactivity to laboratory-induced mental stress demonstrate a generalized exaggerated response to everyday life stresses (stressors—*4a*) (Fredrikson et al., 1990) and be at greater risk for myocardial ischemia (MI) and CHD events (Kral et al., 1997).

Physical Inactivity and Other CHD Risk Factors.   Although there are many risk factors for CHD, a salient condition is physical inactivity (Fletcher et al., 1996). Regular aerobic physical activity increases exercise capacity *(5b & 7)* and plays a role in both primary and secondary prevention of cardiovascular disease (CVD) (Miller et al., 1997). Exercise also improves self-confidence and self-esteem (Folkins & Sime, 1981) and attenuates cardiovascular and neurohumoral responses to mental stress (stressors *3b*) (Blumenthal et al., 1990). Studies reveal that compared with sedentary individuals, active persons *(5b)* exhibit reduced cardiovascular responses to stress (Crews & Launders, 1987).

Diabetes.   African Americans have higher rates of diabetes and suffer disproportionately due to complications of the disease compared with Caucasian Americans (USDHHS, 2000; Livingston, 1993a). The number of persons with diabetes in the African American, Hispanic, and Native American communities is 1–5 times greater than in Caucasian communities (Flegal et al., 1991). Deaths from diabetes are 2 times higher for African Americans than Caucasian Americans, and diabetes-related renal failure is 2.5 times higher in the African American population than in the Hispanic population (Clark, 1998).

While various factors are associated with its etiology, diabetic stress *(7)* is increasingly recognized as both a possible antecedent and consequent associated with diabetes. It has been said that for people who have diabetes, the fight-or-flight (stress) response (see a discussion in Livingston & Ackah (1992) does not work well. Because insulin is not always able to allow the extra energy into cells (which is a by-product of the stress reaction *(8)*), glucose piles up into the blood resulting in a lack of glycemic control (Peyrot & McMurry, 1992). Blood glucose (BG) elevations, which is secondary to the stress hormone release, have been an accepted component of the stress response.

Drug Use and Abuse.   Given the socioeconomic disparities among racial/ethnic subgroups, it is not surprising that many minority subgroups have a greater prevalence of substance abuse than individuals in the total U.S. population (NIDA, 1995). Living in relatively unhealthful situations, as evidenced by high levels of poverty and illiteracy *(3a)*, substantially increases vulnerability to substance abuse *(9)*. The prevalence of substance abuse is also generally higher in urban areas *(1)* than in suburban or rural areas (SAMHSA, 1995). Studies have reported that individuals exposed to stress are more likely to abuse drugs and other stimulants or undergo relapse (e.g., Jacobsen et al., 2000).

HIV Infection, AIDS, and Immune Dysfunctions.   Stress plays a crucial role in HIV infection and AIDS. On a behavioral level, stress may contribute to HIV/AIDS for African Americans (as well as for others) because of intravenous (IV) drug use and unsafe sexual practices. It was reported (Sanders, 1983), for example, that risky sexual behavior of having three or more partners during the prior month was related to self-reports of having sex to relieve tension. These suggestions are very important for African Americans given that HIV infection and AIDS are disproportionately distributed in the Black population.

Stress-produced corticosteriods tend to have an adverse effect on important elements of the immunological apparatus (Rabin, 1999). Therefore, it has been suggested that stress may play a role in the onset of infectious diseases (e.g., AIDS) by further suppressing the body's immune system (Livingston, 1988b) through, for example, the shrinkage of the thymus gland and reduction in the number of lymphocytes (T cells) in the blood (Elliott & Eisdorfer, 1982).

It has also been recently reported that stress weakens the immune system and, therefore, increases vulnerability to catching a cold. Furthermore, chronic stress could place individuals at greater risk for conditions that involve excessive inflammation, such as allergic reactions, autoimmune disease (like systemic lupus erythematosus or SLE, which disproportionately affects African American women, McCarty et al., 1995), and infectious and rheumatologic illnesses (Senay, 2002).

Hypertension.   African Americans are at increased risk for hypertension, with incidence and prevalence studies suggesting a risk approximately two to three times higher than that in Caucasians (Vargas et al., 2000). African American men and women have double the hypertension prevalence rate of their Caucasian counterparts by age 25 (Ogden et al., 2001). Established risk factors for hypertension, such as parental history, physical activity, or age, do not fully explain this increased risk (Vargas et al., 2000).

Although various factors have been associated with the etiology of hypertension, two that have importance and are germane to the position taken in this chapter are stress *(4a, 4b, 7)* (Livingston, 1985a, 1985b, 1987, 1991; James et al., 1987) and SES (low *3a*) (Smith & Kington, 1997). Overt acts of discrimination *(4a)* constraints on opportunities for self-fulfillment and achievement *(4a)* resulting from institutional racism *(3a)*, may interact with other stressors *(4a, 4b)*, coping resources, or responses in explaining higher prevalence on morbidity among African Americans (David & Collins, 1991; Krieger et al., 1993). Physiological stress responses resulting from the inability to attain valued goals have been implicated in the development of hypertension among African American men (Dressler, 1990).

Summary of Other Health Outcomes.   As seen in Figure 23.3, as well as from reading the evidence in the literature, stress impacts (directly and/or indirectly) a great deal more health outcomes than what is listed, and certainly more than space allows to be discussed. By way of some summary statements, stress has also been linked to depression (Kendler et al., 1995); the healing process (e.g., surgical wounds) (Kiecolt-Glaser et al., 1995); breast cancer survival (Spiegel et al., 1989); chronic obstructive pulmonary disease (COPD) (Narsavage & Weaver, 1994); and stroke (Nielsen et al., 2003).

REDUCING STRESS AND DECREASING RACIAL AND ETHNIC HEALTH DISPARITIES

Any meaningful attempt at successfully reducing racial and ethnic health disparities involving African Americans, which include all other Blacks living in the United States who claim ancestry from Africa, will have to be deliberate, comprehensive, multileveled, and multidisciplined. Because there are relatively few "process-oriented" models to follow, it is recommended that the SPPM discussed in the chapter be used as a conceptual guide as efforts are made to reduce the stress low SES African Americans experience on a daily basis. As discussed in the chapter, this stress (along with other contributing factors), over time, contributes to racial and ethnic disparities in health.

Because macro-level conditions have to be essentially addressed at the societal and institutional levels *(1)*, such as issues dealing with *institutional racism* (Clarke et al., 1999), *poverty (3a)* (House & Williams, 2001), and/or having access to quality health care *(3a)*, they require more protracted and long-term societal efforts. For these reasons, macro-level changes, though extremely important, are not addressed in the remainder of the chapter. These issues are sufficiently important to be discussed separately elsewhere. Additionally, the health education efforts that are suggested are more amenable to the micro-level approach. These latter approaches are basically within the scope of African Americans *(2)* and essentially involve lifestyle changes or modifications. It has been said (USDHHS, 1985), that health behaviors and lifestyle account for more of the variation in health than medical care and genetic factors combined.

The conceptual framework presented with the SPPM has important implications for health education research and practice. In health education practice, the SPPM suggests that any comprehensive approach should include interventions aimed at multiple factors depicted in the model. Intervention programs can be more effective if they focus on reducing sources of stress (i.e., ultimately external *[4a]* and internal stressors *[4b]*), in addition to teaching individuals how to cope with stress-related situations (e.g., racism). Additionally, health education interventions can be directed at strengthening the moderating factors (e.g., positive exogenous factors *[5a]* like social support and positive endogenous factors *[5b]* like self-efficacy and control). If these conditions occur, they contribute to the strengthening of the reducing stress *(7)* and stress reactions *(8)* and, ultimately, improving the overall health *(9)*, especially of relatively poor, at-risk African Americans.

Micro-level Approach

As seen in the SPPM in Figure 23.4, although intervention efforts are directed at the micro-level, versus the macro-level, because of the dynamic interaction between both levels, a change in the micro-level can initiate a "perceptual" change in the macro level. Because of these constraints, it is suggested that present and future intervention efforts should, therefore, be more directed at emphasizing the importance and presence of positive, moderating (both exogenous *(5a)* and endogenous *(5b)* factors, especially those that are more accessible, controllable, and modifiable when the resources of at-risk African Americans are taken into consideration.

Positive Exogenous Factors.   As an example of a positive, exogenous, moderating factor, social support (Hoffman & Hatch, 1996) is usually the most frequently cited in the literature. In the case of African American women, care should be taken to include the number of persons in their social network who can be relied upon for the five main functions of support: instrumental, emotional, informative, normative, and companionship (Kramer et al., 2001). As discussed before, these experiences are valuable in buffering or moderating the stressful experiences that African Americans may perceive. But perhaps more importantly of all, whatever efforts are used, the overall emphasis of these efforts should be directed to increasing the resiliency of the African Americans' SRCs *(6)*.

Positive Endogenous Factors.   These factors can include a variety of factors, including psychosocial conditions and behavioral factors. It has been said that self-efficacy *(5b, 6)* seems to be at the core of a variety of class-distinctive modes of thought (Henry, 2001). It was reported that higher-class (vs. lower-class—*3a*) individuals had a greater sense of possibilities and that this provided an empowering perception (or feelings of greater self-efficacy—*5b, 6*) (Henry, 2001). Stansfeld et al.

(1998) found that lower-class status was associated with greater depression and lower sense of well-being, together with greater salience of negative events, all of which had a negative impact on self-efficacy.

Issues to Address.   Although the main focus of any health education appeal to the African American population is to increase the functional strength and resiliency of their SRCs, the success of these efforts will, in part, be determined by answers to the following questions: (a) How, where, and by whom will the message be directed to at-risk Blacks as a group? (e.g., using Black media, billboards, and videos with culturally appropriate expressions and messages articulated by "known" personalities in the Black community; information presented in schools, at work environments, at community meeting places and on public transportation); and (b) What are the specific messages contained in the educational directives to Blacks? (e.g., information pertaining to "enabling" factors that will serve to strengthen the SRCs of African Americans) (see Livingston, Otado & Warren, 2003).

Because there is an inverse relationship between socioeconomic status (SES), or poverty, and stress, the content and medium used to educate poor, at-risk Black Americans about stress and stress management have to be innovative, yet culturally specific, appropriate, and relevant (Resnicow & Braithwaite, 2001). For example, popular, easy-to-read, humorous, informative, attractive and culturally-relevant and appropriate "comic-styled" readers with a "continuous story" can and should be made available (i.e., free and placed at convenient locations) to residents in low-income neighborhoods. They should also be readily available at highly frequented locations and establishments (e.g., beauty parlors, barber shops, churches) by African Americans, especially those who are relative poor. One such comic styled-reader can be called *"StressReducto,"* where, because of its presentation and content matter, residents are eager to read the next copy that is published.

Whatever stress management intervention approach is adopted (e.g., biofeedback training [Romano, 1988]; progressive relaxation [Jacobson, 1938]; rezeroing [Livingston, 1992]), it should be culturally specific and sensitive to the "needs" of the at-risk Black population. Given the importance of relaxation in stress management, the method chosen should teach Blacks about the value of relaxation and how best to relax.

Following the suggestion of Romano (1988), the adopted method will be more successful if it includes the following eight factors: (1) *education* as to the nature of stress; (2) *self-awareness*, where individuals are sensitive to the presence of stressors and stress associated with themselves; (3) *presentation, demonstration, and practice of intervention*, where individuals have to literally practice and experience the effectiveness of designated interventions (e.g., breathing techniques); (4) *lifestyle management*, where individuals determine what aspects of their lifestyle are contributing to stress; (5) *goal setting and stress management strategy*, where the individual sets his or her own goals and develops a strategy to meet these goals; (6) *implementation of the strategy*, where after the strategy is decided for its appropriateness, it is then carried out; (7) *follow-up and evaluation*, where the individual periodically evaluates if the strategy is accomplishing its stated goals; and (8) *continuation*, where the old strategy or a variation of it is continued after evaluation. According to Romano (1988), with this last factor individuals (i.e., at-risk African Americans) develop a plan through which they can better prepare for, and manage, the stressors (see Figure 23.4, *4a* and *4b*) in their lives.

CONCLUSION

There is no justifiable reason that African Americans, especially those relegated by a combination of poverty and racism to low SES positions, should experience approximately 60,000 more deaths (i.e., due to higher rates in heart disease, cancers, stroke, infant mortality, homicides) a year than their Caucasian counterparts. There is no compelling reason that life expectancy for African Americans has lagged behind that of the total population throughout the twenty-first century. Lastly, there is no compelling reason that over one-third of African Americans live in poverty, which is three times that of Caucasians; over half live in urban areas inundated with poverty, crowded and substandard housing, poor schools, unemployment and underemployment, pervasive drug culture, excessive street violence, and generally high levels of stress.

The SPPM of the stress process mentioned in this chapter (see Figure 23.4) offers a practical and functional guide for (a) stress management interventions alluded to before, (b) theory building, and (c) research. In terms of theory building and research, more empirical (and, hopefully, longitudinal) studies are needed with a "holistic" health orientation that focus on *intra*racial differences in perception of stressors, effective coping strategies (i.e., knowing the formula for building a strong and resilient sociopsychophysiological resource center, or SRC) and physiological reactions and effects of stress. Because of the heterogeneous composition of African Americans living in America, these studies should, for example, focus on Black immigrants and differences between them and Blacks born in America, i.e., essentially these should be an *intra*racial focus.

In order to facilitate these suggested and other research activities, block grants and other resource allocations (e.g., by the federal government) should be offered on a competitive basis for research and other institutions to conduct these comprehensive studies on stress and coping mechanisms. These studies would help to establish important Black intraracial patterns of variations and, if possible, causal patterns that contribute to sustained, positive health outcomes. The contributions of these and other similar research endeavors will, in the long run, offer important solutions to interracial and intraracial disparities in health that many believe are further embedded in a complex series of stress–ethnicity–status relationships and disparities.

NOTE

1. This report discusses data for 50 states and the District of Columbia, but not Puerto Rico. The Census 2000 Redistricting Data (Public Law 94-171). Summary File was released on a state-by-state basis in March 2001.

REFERENCES

Adler, N.E., & Newman, K. (2002). Socioeconomic disparities in health: Pathways and policies. *Health Affairs, 21(2)*, 60–76.

Adler, N.E., et al. (1994). Socioeconomic status and health: The challenge of the gradient. *American Psychologist, 49*, 15–24.

Anderson, N.B., & Armstead, C.A. (1995). Toward understanding the association of socioeconomic status and health: A new challenge for the biopsychosocial approach. *Psychosomatic Medicine, 57*, 213–225.

Bailey, W.C., Wilson, S.R., Weiss, K.B., Windsor, R.A., & Wolfe, J.M. (1994). Measures for use in asthma clinicl research: Overview of the NIH workshop. *American Journal of Critical Care Medicine, 149 (pt. 2)*, S1–8.

Baron, R.M., & Kenny, D.A. (1986). The moderator-mediator variable distinction in social psychological research: Conceptual, strategic and statistical considerations. *Journal of Personlaity and Social Psychology, 51*, 1173–1182.

Baum, A., Garofalo, J.P., & Yali, A.M. (1999). Socioeconomic status and chronic stress: Does stress account for SES effects on health? *Annals of the New York Academy of Sciences, 896*, 131–144.

Bierman, A.S., Collins, L.N., & Eisenberg, J.M. (2002). Addressing racial and ethnic barriers to effective health care: The need for better data. *Health Affairs, 21(3)*, 91–102.

Blumenthal, J.A., et al. (1990). Aerobic exercise reduces levels of cardiovascular and sympathoadrenal responses to mental stress in subjects without prior evidence of myocardial ischemia. *American Journal of Cardiology, 65*, 93–98.

Burchfield, S.R. (1985). Stress: An integrative framework. In S.R. Burchfield (Ed.), *Stress: Psychological and physiological interactions* (pp. 381–394). New York: Hemisphere.

Cassel, J. (1976). The contribution of the social environment to host resistance. *American Journal of Epidemiology, 104*, 107–124.

Clark, C. (1998). How should we respond to the worldwide diabetes epidemic? *Diabetes Care, 21*, 475–476.

Clarke, R., Anderson, Clark V.R., & Williams, D.R. (1999). Racism as a stressor for African Americans. *American Psychologist, 54(10)*, 805–816.

Collins, J.W., Wall, S.N., & David, R.J. (1997). Adequacy of prenatal care utilization, maternal ethnicity, and infant birthweight in Chicago. *Journal of the National Medical Association, 89(3)*, 198–203.

Collins J., Herman A., & David, R. (1997). Prevalence of very low birthweight in relation to income-incongruity among African-American and White parents in Chicago. *American Journal of Public Health, 87*, 414–417.

Collins, J.W., Jr, David, R.J., Symons, R., Handler, A., Wall, S., & Andes, S. (1998). African American mothers' perception of their residential environment, stressful life events and very low birthweight. *Epidemiology, 9*, 286–289.

Crews, D.J., & Launders, D.M. (1987). A meta-analytic review of aerobic fitness and reactivity to psychosocial stressors. *Medicine and Science in Sports and Exercise, 19*, S114–S120.

Culhane, J.F., Rauh, V., McCollum, K.F., Hogan, V.K., Agnew, K., & Wadhwa, P.D. (2001). Maternal stress is associated with bacterial vaginosis in human pregnancy. *Maternal and Child Health Journal, 5(2)*, 127–134.

David, R.J., & Collins, J.W. (1991). Bad outcomes in Black babies: Race or racism? *Ethnicity and Disease, 1*, 236–244.

Department of Justice (DOJ). (1999). Criminal victimization 1998: Changes 1997–98 with trends, 1993–98. Pub. No. NCJ-176353. Washington, DC: DOJ.

Dressler, W.W. (1990). Lifestyle, stress and blood pressure in a southern Black community. *Psychosomatic Medicine, 52*, 182–198.

Dressler, W.W., & Bindon, J. (2000). The health consequences of cultural consonance: Cultural dimensions of lifestyle, support, and arterial blood pressure in an African American community. *American Anthrolopogist, 10(2)*, 244–260.

Dunkel-Schetter, C., Gurung, R., Lobel, M., & Wadhwa, P.D. (2000). Stress processes in pregnancy and birth: Psychological, biological and sociocultural influences. In A. Baum, A. Ravenson, & T. Singer (Eds.), *Handbook of health psychology* (pp. 495–518). Hillsdale, NJ: Erlbaum, 2000.

Elliott, G.R., & Eisdorfer, C. (Eds.). (1982). *Stress and human health*. New York: Springer.

Flegal, K., et al. (1991). Prevalence of diabetes in Mexican Americans, Cubans and Puerto Ricans from the Hispanic and Nutrition Examination Survey, 1982–1984. *Diabetes Care, 14*, 628–638.

Fletcher, G.F., et al. (1996). Statement on exercise: Benefits and recommendations for physical activity programs for all Americans. *Circulation, 94*, 857–862.

Folkins, C.H., & Sime, W.E. (1981). Physical fitness training and mental health. *American Journal of Psychology, 36*, 373–389.

Forman, T.A., Williams, D.R., & Jackson, J.S. (1997). Race, place and discrimination. *Perspectives on Social Problems, 9*, 231–261.

Frankish, C.J., Milligan, C.D., & Reid, C. (1998). A review of relationships between active living and determinants of health. *Social Science and Medicine, 47*, 287–301.

Fredrikson, M., Tuomisto, M., & Melin, B. (1990). Blood pressure in healthy men and women under laboratory and naturalistic conditions. *Journal of Psychosomatic Research, 34*, 675–686.

Fruchter, R.G., et al. (1990). Cervix and breast cancer incidence in immigrant Caribbean women. *American Journal of Public Health, 80*, 722–724.

Gary, L.E. (1983). The impact of alcohol and drug use on homicidal violence. In T.D. Watts & R. Wright (Eds.), *Black alcoholism: Toward a comprehensive understanding* (pp. 136–151). Springfield, IL: Charles C. Thomas.

Geronimus, A.T. (1992). The weathering hypothesis and the health of African American women and infants: Evidence and speculations. *Ethnicity and Disease, 2*, 207–21.

Glaser, R. (1996). The effects of stress on the immune system: Implications for health. Science Writers Briefing, Sponsored by Office of Behavioral and Social Sciences Research and the American Psychological Association, NIH.

Goldenberg, R.L., Andrews, W.W., & Hauth, J.C. (2002). Choriodecidual infection and preterm birth. *Nutrition Reviews, 60(5)*, S19–S25.

Goldenberg, R.L., Klebanoff, M.A., Nugent, R., Krohn, M.A., Hillier, S., & Andrews, W.W. (1996). Bacterial colonization of the vagina during pregnancy in four ethnic group. Vaginal Infections and Prematurity Study Group. *American Journal of Obstetrics & Gynecology, 174*, 168–121.

Halford, W.K., & Cuddihy, S. (1990). Psychological stress and blood glucose regulation in type I diabetic patients. *Health Psychology, 9(5)*, 516–528.

He, J, Ogden, L.G., Bazzano, L.A., Vupputuri, S., Loria, C., Whelton, P.K. (2001). Risk factors for congestive heart failure in US men and women: NHANES I epidemiologic follow-up study. *Archives of Internal Medicine, 161(7)*, 996–1002.

Henry, P. (1998). An examination of subculture characteristics of social class groups in contemporary society. Doctoral dissertation, Marketing Department, University of New South Wales.

Henry, P. (2000). Modes of thought that vary systematically with both social class and age. *Psychology and Marketing, 17(5)*, 421–440.

Henry, P. (2001). An examination of the pathways through which social class impacts health outcomes. *Academy of Marketing review (Online), 01 03*. Available at: http://www.amsrev/theory/henry03-01.html

Henry, P. & Craig-Leas, M. (1995). Distinctive world views of social classes. In K. Grant & I. Walker (Eds.), Volume 1, *Proceedings of the Seventh Bi-Annual World Marketing Congress* College Station, TX: Academy of Marketing Science.

Henry, P., Liu, J., & Meehan, W.P. (1995). Psychological stress and hypertension. In J.H. Laragh and B.M. Brenner (Eds.), *Hypertension: Path physiology, diagnosis and management* (2d ed.) (pp. 905–921). New York: Raven Press.

Hobel, C.J., Dunkel-Schetter, C., Roesch, S.C., Castro, L.C., & Arora, C.P. (1999). Maternal plasma corticotropin-releasing hormone associated with stress at 20 week's gestation in pregnancies ending in preterm delivery. *American Jounal of Obstetrics and Gynecology, 180*, S257–S263.

Hoffman, S., & Hatch, M.C. (1996). Stress, social support and pregnancy outcome: A reassessment based on recent research. *Paedeiatric and Perinatal Epidemiology, 10*, 380–405.

Hogan, V.K., Njoroge, T., Durant, T.M., & Ferre, C.D. (2001). Eliminating disparities in perinatal outcomes—lessons learned. *Maternal and Child Health Journal, 5(2), 135–140.*

House, J.S., & Williams, D.R. (2001). Understanding and reducing socioeconomic and racial/ethnic disparities in health. In B.D. Smedley, A.Y. Stith, & A.R. Nelson (Eds.), Unequal treatment: Confronting racial and ethnic disparities in health care. Washington, DC: National Academy Press.

Hoyert, D.L., Kockanck, K.D., & Murph, S.L. (1999). Final data for 1997. *National Vital Statistics Report, 47*, 19.

Institute of Medicine (IOM). (2001). *Health and behavior.* Committee on Health and Behavior. IOM, Washington, DC: National Academy Press.

Jackson, L.E. (1993). Understanding, eliciting and negotiating clients' multicultural health beliefs. *Nurse Practitioner, 8(4)*, 30–43.

Jacobsen, L.K., Southwick, S.M., & Kosten, T.R. (2001). Substance use disorders in patients with posttraumatic disorder: A review of the literature. *American Journal of Psychiatry, 158(8)*, 1184–1190.

Jacobson, E. (1938). *Progressive relaxation* (2d ed.). Chicago: University of Chicago Press.

James, S.A., Hartnett, S.A., & Kalsbeek, W.D. (1983). John Henryism and blood pressure differences among Black men. *Journal of Behavioral Medicine, 6*, 259–278.

James, S.A., Strogatz, D.S., Wing, S.B., & Ramsey, D.L. (1987). Socioeconomic status, John Henryism and high blood pressure in Blacks and Whites. *American Journal of Epidemiology, 126*, 664–773.

Jones, D.W., et al. (2002). Risk factors for coronary heart disease in African Americans: The Atherosclerosis Risk in Communities Study, 1987–1997. *Archives of Internal Medicine, 162*, 2565–2572.

Jones, J.M. (1997). *Prejudice and racism* (2d ed.). New York: McGraw-Hill.

Kendler, K.S., et al. (1995). Stressful life events, genetic liability and onset of an episode of major depression in women. *American Journal of Psychiatry, 152,* 833–842.

Kessler, R.C. (1979). Stress, social status and psychological distress. *Journal of Health and Social Behavior, 20,* 259–273.

Kessler, R.R., & Neighbors, H. (1986). A new perspective on the relationships among race, social class and psychological distress. *Journal of Health and Social Behavior, 27,* 107–115.

Kiecolt-Glaser, J.K., Dura, J.R., Speicher, C.E., Trask, O.J., & Glaser, R. (1995). Spousal caregivers of dementia victims: Longitudinal changes in immunity and health. *Psychosomatic Medicine, 53,* 345–362.

Kingston, R., & Lucas, J. (2003). The health status, health insurance, and health care utilization patterns of immigrant Black men. *American Journal of Public Health* (in press).

Klatsky, A.L. (1995). Blood pressure and alcohol intake. In J.H. Laragh and B.M. Brenner (Eds.), *Hypertension: Path physiology, diagnosis and management,* 2d ed. (pp. 2649–2681). New York: Raven Press.

Koonin, L.M., Mackay, A.P., Berg, C.J., Atrash, H.K., & Smith, J.C. (1997). Pregnancy-related mortality surveillance, United States, 1987–1990. *MMWR (Morbidity Mortality Weekly Report), 46(SS 4),* 17–36.

Kral, B.G., Beckey, L.C., Blumenthal, R.S., Aversand, T., Fleisher, L.A., Yook, R.M., & Becker, D.M. (1997). Exaggerated reactivity to mental stress is associated with exercise-induced myocardial ischemia in an asymptomatic high-risk population. *Circulation, 96,* 4246–4253.

Kramer, M.S., Goulet, L., Lydon, J., Seguin, L., McNamara, H., Dassa, C., & Platt, W. (2001). Socio-economic disparities in preterm birth: Causal pathways and mechanisms. *Paediatric and Prenatal Epidemiology,15 (Suppl. 2),* 104–123.

Krieger, N. (2000). Discrimination and health. In Berkfman, L.F., & Kawachi, I. (Eds.), *Social epidemiology* (pp. 36–75). New York: Oxford University Press.

Krieger, N., Rowley, D.L., Herman, A.A., Avery, B., & Phillips, M.T. (1993). Racism, sexism and socials class: Implications for studies of health health, disease and well-being. *American Journal of Preventive Medicine, 9 (Suppl. 6),* 82–122.

Krieger, N., Williams, D.R., & Moss, N.E. (1997). Measuring social class in U.S. public health research: Concepts, methodologies and guidelines. *Annual Review of Public Health, 18,* 341–378.

Lazarus, R.S., & Folkman, S. (1984). Stress, appraisal and coping. New York: Springer.

Lillie-Blanton, M., Parsons, P.E., Gayle, H., & Dievler, A. (1996). Racial differences in health: Not just Black and White, but shades of gray. *Annual Review of Public Health, 17,* 411–448.

Link, B.G., & Phelan, J. (1995). Social conditions as fundamental causes of disease. *Journal of Health and Social Behavior, Spec. No,* 80–94.

Livingston, I.L. (1985a). Alcohol consumption and hypertension: A review with suggested implications. *Journal of the National Medical Association, 77,* 129–135.

Livingston, I.L. (1985b). The importance of stress in the interpretation of the race–hypertension association. *Humanity and Society, 9(2),* 168–181.

Livingston, I.L. (1986/1987). Blacks, lifestyle and hypertension: The importance of health education. *The Humboldt Journal of Social Relations, 14,* 195–213.

Livingston, I.L. (1988a). Co-factors, host susceptibility, and AIDS: An argument for stress. *Journal of the National Medical Association, 80,* 49–59.

Livingston, I.L. (1988b). Stress and health dysfunctions: The importance of health education. *Stress and Medicine, 4(3),* 155–161.

Livingston, I.L. (1991). Stress, hypertension and renal disease in Black Americans: A review with implications. *National Journal of Sociology, 5(2),* 143–181.

Livingston, I.L. (1992). *The ABC's of stress management—taking control of your life.* Salt Lake City, UT: Northwest.

Livingston, I.L. (1993a). Renal disease and Black Americans: Selected Issues. *Social Science and Medicine, 37(5),* 613–621.

Livingston, I.L. (1993b). Stress, hypertension and young Black Americans: The importance of counseling. *Journal of Multicultural Counseling, 2(3),* 132–142.

Livingston, I.L., & Ackah, S. (1992). Hypertension, end-stage renal disease and rehabilitation: A look at Black Americans. *The Western Journal of Black Studies, 16*, 103–112.

Livingston, I.L., Levine, D.M., Moore, R. (1991). Social integration and Black intraracial blood pressure variation. *Ethnicity and Disease, 1(2)*, 135–149.

Livingston, I.L. (1994). Social status, stress and health: Black Americans at risk. In I.L. Livingston (Ed.), *Handbook of Black American health* (pp. 236–252). Westport, CT: Greenwood Press.

Livingston, I.L., Otado, J. & Warren, C. (2003). Stress, adverse pregnancy outcomes and African American females: Assessing the implications using a conceptual model. *Journal of the National Medical Association, 95(11)*, 1103–1109.

Lobel, M., Dunkel-Schetter, C., and Scrimshaw, S.C.M. (1992). Prenatal maternal stress and prematurity: A prospective study of socioeconomically disadvantaged women. *Health Psychology, 11*, 32–40.

Lockwood, C.J. (1999). Stress-associated preterm delivery: The role of corticotropin-releasing hormone. *American Journal of Obstetrics and Gynecology, 180*, S264–S266.

Major, B., Richards, C., Cooper, M.L., Cozzarelli, C., & Zubek, J. (1998). Personal resilience, cognitive appraisals, and coping: An integrative model of adjustment to abortion. *Journal of Personality and Social Psychology, 74*, 735–752.

Manuck, S., Kasprowicz, A., & Muldoon, M. (1990). Behaviorally-evoked cardiovascular reactivity and hypertension: Conceptual issues and potentional associations. *Annals of Behavioral Medicine, 12*, 17–29.

Marmot, M.G., Fuhrer, R., Ettner, S.L., Marks, N.F., Bumpass, L.L., & Ryff, C.D. (1998). Contribution of psychosocial factors to socioeconomic differences in health. *Milbank Quarterly, 76*, 403–448.

McCarty, D.J., et al. (1995). Incidence of systemic lupus erythematosus, race and gender differences. *Arthritis Rheumatism, 38(9)*, 1260–1270.

McCord, C., & Freeman, H.P. (1990). Excess mortality in Harlem. *New England Journal of Medicine, 322*, 173–177.

McEwen, B.S. (2000). The neurobiology of stress: from serendipity to clinical relevance. *Brain Research, 886*, 172–189.

McEwen, B.S. (2002). *The end of stress as we know it*. Washington, DC: Joseph Henry Press.

McKinnon, J. (2001). The Black population: 2000. Census 2000 Brief. U.S. Census Bureau. U.S. Department of Commerce, Economics and Statistics Administration.

McNeilly, M., et al. (1996). The convergent, discriminant, and concurrent criterion validity of the perceived racism scale: A multidimensional assessment of White racism among African Americans. In R.L. Jones (Ed.), *Handbook of tests and measurements for Black Americans*, vol. 2 (pp. 359–374). Hampton, VA: Cobb and Henry.

Miller, T., et al. (1997). Exercise and its role in the prevention and rehabilitation of cardiovascular disease. *Annals of Behavioral Medicine, 3*, 220–229.

Minino, A.M., & Smith, B.L. (2001). Deaths: Preliminary data for 2000. National Center for Health Statistics, *National Vital Statistics Reports, 49(12)*.

Minority Programs. (1992). Fact finding team recommendations. Presented to the N.I.H. Associate Director for Minority Programs, National Institutes of Health, Office of Minority Programs (OMP).

Mirowsky, J., & Ross, C.E. (1989). *Causes of psychological distress*. New York: Aldine de Gruyter.

Moore, E.K. (1990). *Status of African American children Twentieth Anniversary Report 1970–1990*. Washington, DC: National Black Child Development Institute.

Myers, H. (1982). Stress, ethnicity and social class: A model for research with Black populations. In E.E. Jones (Ed.), *Minority mental health* (pp. 118–148). New York: Praeger.

Narsavage, G.L., & Weaver, T.E. (1994). Physiologic status, coping and hardiness as predictors of outcomes in chronic obstructive pulmonary disease. *Nursing Research, 43*, 90–94.

National Center for Health Statistics (NCHS). (1992). Advance report on final mortality statistics, 1989. Monthly vital statistics report, Vol. 40, No. 8, Suppl. 2. Hyattsville, MD: Public Health Service.

National Center for Health Statistics (NCHS). (2001). Births: Final data for 1999. *National Vital Statistics Report, 49(1)*, Hyattsville, MD.

National Center for Health Statistics (NCHS). (2003). Early release of selected estimates based on data from the January–September 2002 National Health Interview Survey (Released 3/19/03). Hyattsville, MD.

National Institute on Alcohol Abuse & Alcoholism (NIAAA). (2000a). *Ninth special report to the U.S. Congress on alcohol and health*. Rockville, MD: Author.

National Institute on Alcohol Abuse & Alcoholism (NIAAA). (2000b). *Tenth special report to the U.S. Congress on alcohol and health*. Rockville, MD: Author.

National Institute of Diabetes and Digestive and Kidney Diseases. (2002). Diabetes in African Americans. Publication No. 02-3266. Bethesda, MD.

National Institute on Disability and Rehabilitation Research. (1989). Chartbook on disability in the United States. Washington, DC: The Institute.

National Institute on Drug Abuse (NIDA). (1995). *Drug use among racial/ethnic minorities*, NIH Pub. No. 95-3888, Rockville, MD: NIDA.

Navarro, V. (November 17, 1990). Race or class versus race and class: Mortality differentials in the United States. *The Lancet*, 1238–1240.

Neugebauer, R., Kline, J., Stein, Z., Shrout, P., Warburton, D., & Susser, M. (1996). Association of stressful life events and chromosomally normal spontaneous abortions. *American Journal of Epidemiology, 143*, 588–596.

Nielsen, N., Boysen, G., & Gronbaek, M. (March 14, 2003). Self-reported stress linked to fatal stroke: Unhealthy habits may be factor. *Stroke Journal Report*, American Heart Association.

Office on Smoking and Health. (1987). Unpublished data from the National Health Interview Survey.

Ostrove, J.M., Feldman, P., & Adler, N.E. (1999). Relations among socioeconomic status indicators and health for Americans and Whites. *Journal of Health Psychology, 4(4)*, 451–463.

Otten, M.W., Teutsch, S.M., Williamson, D.F., & Marks, J. (1990). The effect of known risk factors on the excess mortality of Black adults in the United States. *Journal of the American Medical Association, 263*, 845–850.

Pamuk, E. (1998). Socioeconomic status and health chartbook: Health United States, 1998. Hyattsville, MD: National Center for Health Statistics.

Pearlin, L.T., Lieberman, M.A., Menaghan, E.G., and Mullan, J.T. (1981). The stress process. *Journal of Health and Social Behavior, 22*, 337–356.

Petraglia, F., et al. (1995). Maternal plasma and placental immunoreactive corticotropin-releasing factor concentrations in infection-associated term and pre-term delivery. *Placenta, 8*, 541–556.

Peyrot, M.F., & McMurry, J.F. (1992). Stress buffering and glycemic control: The role of coping styles. *Diabetes Care, 15(7)*, 842–846.

Pickering, T. (1999). Cardiovascular pathways: Socioeconomic status and stress effects on hypertension and cardiovascular function. *Annals New York Academy of Sciences, 896*, 262–277.

Pleis, J.R., & Coles, R. (2002). Summary health statistics for U.S. adults: National Health Interview Survey, 1998. National Center for Health Statistics. *Vital Health Statistics, 10(209)*.

Polednak, A. (1996). Trends in U.S. urban Black infant mortality, by degree of residential segregation. *American Journal of Public Health, 86*, 723–726.

Public Health Service. (1988). The Surgeon's Report on Nutrition and Health. Washington, DC: U.S. Department of Health and Human Services.

Rabin, B.S. (1999). Stress, immune function and health: The connection. New York: John Wiley and Sons.

Ren, X.S., & Amick, B.C. (1996). Racial and ethnic disparities in self-assessed health status: Evidence from the National Survey of Families and Households. *Ethnicity and Disease, 1*, 293–303.

Resnicow, K., & Braithwaite, R.L. (2001). Cultural sensitivity in public health. In R.L. Braithwaite & S.E. Taylor (Eds.), *Health issues in the black community* (2d) (pp. 516–542). San Francisco, CA: Jossey-Bass Publishers.

Rich-Edwards, J., Krieger, N., Majzoub, J., Zierler, S., Lieberman, E., & Gillman, M. (2001). Maternal experiences of racism and violence as predictors of preterm birth: Rationale and study design. *Paediatric and Perinatal Epidemiology, 15 (Suppl. 2)*, 124–135.

Romano, J.L. (1988). Stress management counseling: From crisis to prevention. *Counseling Psychology Quarterly, 1*, 211–219.

Romero, E., Avilia, C., Santhanam, U., & Sehgal, P.B. (1990). Amniotic fluid interleukin-6 in preterm labor: Association with infection. *Abstract. Journal of Clinical Investigation, 85*, 1392–400.

Ross, C.E., & Wu, C. (1995, October). The links between education and health. *American Sociological Review*, 719–745.

Russell, M., Cooper, L., Frone, M.R., & Peirce, R.S. (1999). A longitudinal study of stress, alcohol, and blood pressure in community-based samples of Blacks and non-Blacks. *Alcohol Research and Health, 23(4)*, 299–306.

Rutter, D.R., & Quine, L. (1990). Inequalities in pregnancy outcomes: A review of psychosocial and behavioral mediators. *Social Science in Medicine, 38*, 553–568.

Sandberg, S., et al. (2000). The role of acute and chronic stress in asthma attacks in children. *The Lancet, 356*, 982–987.

Sanders, L. (1983). *The seduction of Peter S.* New York: Putnam.

Saunders, E. (1991). *Cardiovascular disease in Blacks*. Philadelphia: F.A. Davis.

Schoenbaum, M., & Waidmann, T. (1997). Race, socioeconomic status and health: Accounting for race differences in health. *Journal of Gerontology, 52B*, 61–73.

Seligman, M.E.P. (1975). *Helplessness: On depression, development and death*. San Francisco: W.H. Freeman.

Selik, R.M., Castro, K.G., & Papaionnou, M. (1988). Racial/ethnic differences in the risk of AIDS in the United States. *American Journal of Public Health, 78*, 1539–1544.

Selye, H. (1976). *The stress of life*. New York: McGraw-Hill.

Senay, E. (November 4, 2002). Stress: Hazardous for your life. *The Early Show*.

Singh, G.K., Kochanek, K.D., & MacDorman, M.F. (1996). Advance report of final mortality ststistics, 1994. *Mortality Vital Statistics Report, 45*, 3S.

Sinha, R., Fuse, T., Aubin, L.R., & O'Malley, S.S. (2000). Psychological stress, drug-related cues, and cocaine craving. *Psychopharmacology, 152*, 140–148.

Smedley, B.D., Stith, A.Y., & Nelson, A.R. (Eds.). (2003). Unequal treatment: confronting racial and ethnic disparities in health care. Washington, DC: Institute of Medicine, National Academies Press.

Smith, J.P., & Kington, R.S. (1997). Race, socioeconomic status and health in late life. In L.G. Matin & B.J. Soldo (Eds.), *Racial and ethnic differences in the health of older Americans* (pp. 106–162). Washington, DC: National Academy Press.

Sobel, D.S. (Ed.). (1979). *Ways of health*. New York: Harcourt Brace Jovanovich.

Spiegel, D., Bloom, H.C., Kraemer, J.R., & Gotthcil, E. (1989). Effect of psychosocial treatment on survival of patients with metastatic cancer. *The Lancet, 2*, 888–901.

Stansfeld, S.A., Head, J., & Marmot, M.G. (1998). Explaining social class differences in depression and well-being. *Social Psychiatry and Psychiatric Epidemiology, 33(1)*, 1–9.

Strunk, R.C., Ford, J.G., & Taggart, V. (2002). Reducing disparities in asthma care: Priorities for research—National Heart, Lung, and Blood Institute Workshop Report. *Journal of Allergy Clinical Immunology, 109(2)*, 229–237.

Substance Abuse and Mental Health Services Administration (SAMHSA). (1995). Annual Medical Examiner Data, 1993. Data from the Drug Abuse Warning Network. DHHS Publication Number (SMA) 95-3019.

Substance Abuse and Mental Health Services Administration (SAMHSA). (1998). *Prevalance of substance abuse among racial and ethnic subgroups in the United States, 1991–1993*. Rockville, MD: Author.

Taylor, S., & Seeman, T. (1999). Psychosocial resources and the SES-relationship. In N. Adler, M. Marmot, B. McEwen, & J. Stewart (Eds.), *Socioeconomic status in industrial nations: Social psychological and biological pathways* (pp. 210–225). New York: New York Academy of Sciences.

The 2003 HHS Povert Guidelines. (2003). *Federal Register, 68(2)*, 6456–6458.

Ulbrich, P., Warheit, G., & Zimmerman, R. (1989). Race, socioeconomic status and psychological distress. *Journal of Health and Social Behavior, 30*, 131–146.

U.S. Census Bureau. (1997). United States Department of Commerce News. Available at http://www.census.gov/Press-Release/cb98-175.html (Accessed March 15, 2003).

U.S. Census Bureau. (2000). Available at http://www.census.gov (Accessed March 15, 2003).

U.S. Department of Health and Human Services (USDHHS). (1985). Report of the Secretary's Task Force on Black and Minority Health. Volume I: Executive Summary. Washington, DC: U.S. Government Printing Office.

U.S. Department of Health and Human Services (USDHHS). (2000). Healthy People 2010. Understanding and improving health (2d ed.). Washington, DC: U.S. Government Printing Office.

U.S. Immigration and Naturalization Service (USINS). (2002). Statistical yearbook of the Immigration and Naturalization Service. Washington, DC: U.S. Government Printing Office.

Ventura, S.J., et al. (2000). Births: Final data for 1997. *National Vital Statistics Report, 48*, 3.

Wadhwa, P.D. (1998). Prenatal stress and life-span development. In H. Friedman (Ed.), *Encyclopedia of mental health* (pp. 265–280). San Diego: Academic Press.

Whaley, A.L. (1992). A culturally sensitive approach to the prevention of interpersonal violence among urban Black youth. *Journal of the National Medical Association, 84*, 585–588.

Williams, D.R. (1986). The epidemiology of mental illness in Afro-Americans. *Hospital and Community Psychiatry, 77(1)*, 42–49.

Williams, D.R. (1995). African American mental health: Persisting questions and paradoxical findings. African American Research Perspectives, 2, 1, 8–16.

Williams, D.R. (2000). Race/ethnicity and the 2000 Census: Recommendations for African American and other Black populations in the United States. *American Journal of Public Health, 90(11)*, 1728–1730.

Williams, D.R., & Collins, C. (1995). Socioeconomic and racial differences in health: Patterns and explanations. *Annual Review of Sociology, 21*, 349–386.

Williams, D.R., Lavizzo-Mourey, R., & Warren, R. (1994). The concept of race and health status in America. *Public Health Reports, 109*, 1, 26–41.

Williams, D.R., Takeuchi, D.T., & Adair, R.K. (1992). Socioeconomic status and psychiatric disorder among Blacks and Whites. *Social Forces, 71*, 179–194.

Vargas, C.M., Ingram, D.D., & Gillum, R.F. (2000). Incidence of hypertension and educational attainment: the NHANES I epidemiologic follow-up study. First National Health and Nutrition Examination Survey. *American Journal of Epidemiology, 152(3)*, 272–278.

CHAPTER 24

Nutrition Concerns of Black Americans

DEBORAH BLOCKER AND
IVIS T. FORRESTER-ANDERSON

INTRODUCTION

Good nutrition is crucial to the maintenance of health, and dietary factors contribute substantially to preventable chronic illness and premature death. Preliminary data from the Centers for Disease Control (2001) identify the ten leading causes of death in the United States in 2000. Of the ten, five are associated directly or indirectly with diet (heart disease, some types of cancer, cerebrovascular disease, diabetes mellitus, and kidney diseases). Chronic diseases such as these disproportionately affect Black Americans and thus are the focus of this chapter. These complex disorders are of multifactorial etiology involving interactions of environmental, behavioral, social, and genetic factors. Racial disparities in health are associated with poverty, inadequate access to health care, discrimination, and other risk factors (Feldman & Fulwood, 1999). Moreover, the diet consumed by Black Americans is associated with the etiology and pathogenesis of several chronic diseases, which predisposes Blacks to an excess chronic disease burden and is thus a major contributor to racial health disparities.

Although overnutrition is clearly the major nutrition concern of the majority of Black Americans, it is difficult to characterize the Black American diet because of the high degree of diversity in terms of socioeconomic status, geography, and ethnicity. However, it is possible to make some generalizations. According to Luke et al. (2001) the nutritional status in the African diaspora forms a continuum from predominantly undernutrition in Africa, to coexisting under- and overnutrition in the Caribbean, to predominantly overnutrition and its attendant chronic diseases in the United States and the United Kingdom. Analysis of the U.S. Department of Agriculture's 1994–1996 Healthy Eating Index scores shows that African Americans had poorer diets than Whites (Nutrition Insights Number 6, 1998). Kayrooz et al. (1998) found that nearly 81 percent of urban African American women studied had a high fat intake, and Patterson et al. (1995) reported that Blacks ate a diet with less variety than Whites and consumed more high-fat and fried food. Among Blacks in the United States, those born in the South have the highest death rate from chronic diseases (Greenberg & Schneider, 1991; Fang et al., 1996), and southern-born Blacks are more likely to consume diets associated with increased chronic disease risk (Greenberg et al., 1998). Kumanyika (1993) has described the Black diet as being high in fat and salt and low in fruits, vegetables, fiber, and calcium.

In general, Black Americans living at or near poverty consume diets that are marginal in vitamins A, D, E, B-complex, vitamin C, calcium, magnesium, iron, and zinc. Black Americans also tend to consume a greater percentage of calories from animal protein (meat) than do Whites. The diets of many Black Americans are low in foods that are good sources of complex carbohydrates and dietary fiber, namely, whole-grain products, and fresh fruits and vegetables. Additionally, 60–95 percent of adult Black Americans are lactose-intolerant, and many of these individuals habitually avoid milk and milk products. Dairy products are the best source of calcium in the U.S. diet (Kumanyika & Helitzer, 1985; Kittler & Sucher, 2001). While acknowledging the nonmonolithic nature of the Black American community, this chapter describes the major diet-related chronic diseases affecting Black Americans followed by recommendations for dietary and lifestyle modifications to prevent and/or ameliorate these disorders and suggestions for public health policy/interventions.

DIET-RELATED CHRONIC DISEASES DISPROPORTIONATELY AFFECTING BLACK AMERICANS

Coronary Heart Disease

Coronary heart disease (CHD) is the most common form of cardiovascular disease in the United States, affecting approximately 12 to 13 million Americans. Despite a declining trend since the 1960s, CHD claims about 500,000 lives each year (National Heart, Lung & Blood Institute, 1993). The age-adjusted death rate for CHD between 1987 and 1996 declined by 22.2 percent, and according to the results of the State Economic Areas Surrounding the ARIC Study Communities survey, the five-year annual CHD mortality rate declined differentially by gender and race. White men and women declined at a rate of 2.6 percent. For Black men and women, the rate of decline was 1.6 percent and 2.2 percent, respectively (Williams et al., 1999). Data from the Framingham Heart Study show estimated lifetime risk for developing coronary artery disease to be one out of every two men and one out of every three women age 40 and older. At age 70, the risk is one out of every three men and one out of every four women in their remaining years of life (National Institutes of Health, 1999).

CHD is characterized by narrowing of the inner walls of the coronary arteries resulting in reduced supply of oxygen-rich blood and nutrients to the heart (ischemia). This is almost always due to atherosclerosis, which in turn is strongly associated with elevated serum cholesterol and elevated levels of low-density lipoprotein cholesterol. The disease may lead to chest pain (angina), heart attacks (myocardial infarction), and sudden death as a result of disturbances in cardiac rhythm (Krantz & McCeney, 2002).

Sempos et al. (1993) reported that more than 50 million Americans have blood cholesterol that require medical intervention, and more than 90 million have blood cholesterol values that are not desirable. Despite these figures, average total cholesterol declined from 213 mg/dl in 1976–1980 to 203 in 1988–1994. Similarly, the prevalence of high blood cholesterol declined from 26 percent to 19 percent during this time period (Healthy People 2000 Review, 1998–1999). Blood cholesterol values of ≤199 mg/dl are desirable and are associated with reduced risk for CHD. Compared to Whites, serum cholesterol levels seem to be more favorable among African Americans. Wilson et al. (1983) examined a sample of 100 highly educated African Americans and found significantly lower total cholesterol levels than in a comparable White sample. Analysis of the National Health and Nutrition Examination Survey II data (NHANES II) of 1976–1980 by Sempos et al. (1989), and the NHANES III of 1988–1994 by Allison et al. (1999) showed no racial differences in serum/blood cholesterol. Mean blood cholesterol values for Blacks and Whites, 20 years of age and older, were 204 and 206, respectively, in 1988–1994 (Healthy People 2010, 2000a).

Risk factors for CHD include diabetes, obesity, hypertension, smoking and elevated levels of total cholesterol, low-density lipoprotein, triglyceride, and homocysteine. Also, low levels of high-density lipoprotein, physical inactivity, and reduced sensitivity to insulin are known risk factors for CHD (Lee et al., 2001; Slawta et al., 2002; Katzmarzyk et al., 2001; Welch & Losculzo, 1998). Controlling risk factors remains the key to preventing illnesses and deaths from CHD. A review of the NHANES III data by Becker et al. (1998) shows the prevalence of high blood pressure ($\geq$140/90 mm Hg) to be higher among non-Hispanic and non-Latino Blacks (40 percent) than among Whites (27 percent). Further, racial and gender breakdown shows the prevalence among African American women and men to be 27 and 34 percent, respectively, and among Caucasian women and men to be 18 and 26 percent, respectively.

Diabetes is a major predisposing factor to the development of CHD and is 1.4 to 2.2 times more prevalent in African Americans compared to Whites (Carter et al., 1996). Other factors such as smoking account for the increased CVD risk among African Americans. Becker et al. (1998) reported that more Black men (35.1 percent) than White men (27.4 percent) are smokers; however, both White men and women smoke more packs of cigarettes per day than their Black counterparts. Data from the Centers for Disease Control and Prevention, National Health Interview Survey for 1999, show that smoking among Black males 18 years of age and older is 28.7 percent, and it is 25.4 percent among White males, while among White and Black females it is 22.1 and 20.8 percent, respectively (Health, United States, 2001).

Race is strongly associated with CHD morbidity and mortality. Results of the HERITAGE heart study show that White men have a significantly higher coronary heart disease risk index than Black men (2.3 vs. 1.5, respectively, while among women, the risk is higher in Whites (−4.0) than in Blacks (−4.6) but the difference is not significant (Katzmarzyk et al., 2001). Mortality rate for CHD is higher in African Americans than in Whites. In 1998, coronary heart disease deaths among non-Hispanic or non-Latino Blacks and Whites were 262 and 216 per 100,000 population, respectively. The age-adjusted death rate for CHD was 42 percent higher in African Americans males than in White males, 65 percent higher in African American females than in White females, and almost twice as high in males than in females (Mosca, 2002; American Heart Association, 2001; Healthy People 2010, 2000a). Prevention of coronary heat disease in women is especially important because women perceive themselves as being at low risk, and because women are less likely than men to be referred for evaluation and treatment once coronary heart disease symptoms appear (Bickell et al., 1992; Shaw et al., 1994; Steingart et al., 1991).

The major nutrition-related risk factors for CHD are dietary fats and obesity (Stamler & Shekelle, 1988). Obesity is discussed later in this chapter. For dietary fat, there is strong and consistent clinical, epidemiologic, and experimental animal evidence that high intakes of saturated fats increase serum total and low-density lipoprotein cholesterol (LDL-C), which increase the risk for coronary artery disease. Dietary cholesterol intake has a less significant effect on serum cholesterol levels than does saturated fat intake (Committee on Diet & Health, 1989). Dietary factors shown to reduce serum cholesterol levels include monounsaturated fatty acids and polyunsaturated fatty acids, soluble fiber, and vegetarian diets (Kris-Etherton et al., 1988; Committee on Diet & Health, 1989). The traditional Black American diet, which stresses the consumption of meat (particularly pork), fried foods, and eggs, would imply that there is a higher intake of cholesterol and saturated fats among Blacks (Kittler & Sucher, 1989). However, results of the NHANES III survey show no difference between mean blood serum values for Blacks and Whites. More research is needed to elucidate the factors responsible for the disparity in coronary heart disease incidence between Blacks, Whites, and people of other ethnic backgrounds.

Hypertension

The prevalence of high blood pressure rises with increasing age. Lifestyle factors predisposing to increased risk of hypertension include a high sodium chloride intake, excessive consumption of calories, physical inactivity, excessive alcohol consumption, and deficient intake of potassium. Estimates based on the 1988–1991 National Health and Nutrition Examination Survey (NHANES III) indicate that approximately 50 million, or one in every four, adults in the United States have hypertension or high blood pressure, that is, greater than 140/90 (Joint National Committee on Detection, Evaluation and Treatment of High Blood Pressure, 1993). The most recent report by the National High Blood Pressure Education Program states the following:

In those older than age 50, systolic blood pressure (BP) of greater than 140 mm Hg is a more important cardiovascular disease (CVD) risk factor than diastolic BP; beginning at 115/75 mm Hg, CVD risk doubles for each increment of 20/10 mm Hg; those who are normotensive at 55 years of age will have a 90% lifetime risk of developing hypertension; prehypertensive individuals (systolic BP 120–139 mm Hg or diastolic BP 80-89 mm Hg) require health-promoting lifestyle modifications to prevent the progressive rise in blood pressure and CVD; for uncomplicated hypertension, thiazide diuretic should be used in drug treatment for most, either alone or combined with drugs from other classes. . . . (Chobanian et al., 2004, p. 1)

Hypertension (HTN) disproportionately affects Black Americans. In fact, the Intersalt Cooperative Research Group (Intersalt) (1988) reports that the highest rates of hypertension worldwide occur in Black Americans. HTN is associated with an increased risk of developing coronary heart disease, stroke, congestive heart failure, renal insufficiency, and peripheral vascular disease (MacMahon et al. 1990).

The major dietary correlates of HTN are obesity and salt (sodium) intake. Research studies (both cross-sectional and prospective observational) identify a strong relationship between body weight and blood pressure, and clinical trials in hypertensive and normotensive persons have documented that losing excess weight reduces blood pressure. The magnitude of blood pressure reduction is directly related to the extent of weight that is lost; however, even modest reductions in weight can produce a favorable lowering of blood pressure (Stamler, 1991).

A considerable body of evidence documents a positive relationship between sodium intake and blood pressure (Elliott, 1991; Frost et al., 1991; Cutler et al., 1991; Intersalt, 1988). This susceptibility to sodium- or salt-induced HTN is probably genetically determined. The concept of salt or sodium sensitivity means that these individuals will have increased blood pressure in response to high sodium intake. One-third of the U.S. population is thought to be salt-sensitive; however, this subgroup cannot yet be reliably identified. Freis et al. (1988) report there is a greater frequency of salt-sensitive hypertension in Black Americans, and according to Blaustein and Grim (1991), this suggests that decreasing dietary sodium intake can be beneficial in lowering blood pressure in this salt-sensitive subgroup. The dietary recommendation is to limit total salt intake to less than 6 g/day (Sacks et al. 1995). In the general population, decreasing salt intake should not cause any detrimental effects because there is no known benefit from consuming large amounts of salt.

Reduced alcohol consumption is effective in lowering blood pressure in hypertensives (Puddey, 1987). The INTERSALT (1988) study identified an inverse relationship between blood pressure and potassium status, including dietary intake of potassium and serum, urine, and total body potassium. A lower sodium:potassium ratio has been shown to be associated with an increased risk of hypertension. The diets of many Black Americans are low in fresh fruits and vegetables, which contribute potassium (Kumanyika, 1993; Kittler & Sucher, 2001). Research studies have reported evidence that consumption of omega-3 polyunsaturated fatty acids (n-3 PUFA), from either fish oil supplements or certain high-fat fish may reduce blood pressure (Knapp & FitzGerald, 1989).

Epidemiologic and clinical evidence also suggests an inverse, albeit inconsistent, association between dietary calcium intake and blood pressure. This further suggests that a deficiency of dietary calcium may have implications for increased hypertension risk. Blacks may be at particular risk because most adult Black Americans are lactose-intolerant and therefore tend to avoid milk and milk products rich in calcium (Kumanyika & Helitzer; 1985; Kittler & Sucher, 2001). There may also be positive effects of increased intakes of magnesium, omega 6 and omega 3 PUFA, and dietary fiber on blood pressure. Psychosocial stressors are likely also greater among Blacks than Whites. In reviewing research on psychosocial factors predisposing Blacks to higher CHD risk, Kumanyika and Adams-Campbell (1991) report that several psychosocial factors have been associated, but not in a consistent fashion with blood pressure and hypertension in Blacks.

In summary, the most effective dietary approaches for the prevention and treatment of HTN are weight loss, reduction in sodium intake, and avoidance of excessive alcohol consumption. The evidence regarding the role of increased potassium intake on lowering blood pressure is not as strong as that for reducing sodium; however, the increased consumption of potassium-rich fruits and vegetables is highly recommended. The evidence for the effectiveness of calcium, magnesium, omega 3 PUFA and fish oils, and fiber on blood pressure is not as convincing. Among nondietary methods to lower blood pressure, the most effective approach is to increase physical activity, while the evidence is not as strong for the efficacy of stress management.

Diabetes Mellitus

Diabetes mellitus is an endocrine disorder characterized by an insufficient and/or ineffective secretion of insulin, which is accompanied by an elevation in plasma glucose levels as well as abnormalities in lipoprotein and amino acid metabolism (American Diabetes Association, 1997). The prevalence of diabetes in the United States is estimated at over 16 million (National Diabetes Information Clearinghouse, 2002). There are two major types of diabetes, Type I, or insulin-dependent diabetes mellitus (IDDM), and Type II, or noninsulin-dependent diabetes mellitus (NIDDM). NIDDM represents approximately 95 percent of all cases of diabetes. The prevalence of Type II diabetes has tripled in the last 30 years, and much of the increase is attributed to the stunning increases in obesity. Excessive abdominal fat poses an especially high risk for developing the disease. Obese people (BMI of 30 or greater) have a five-times greater risk of diabetes than people with a normal BMI of 25 or less (Harris et al., 1998). Other risk factors for NIDDM include physical inactivity, family history of diabetes, and racial or ethnic background. Compared to Whites, Black adults have a 60 percent higher rate of Type II diabetes (Tull & Roseman, 1995).

IDDM is the predominant form of the disease in children, adolescents, and young adults. In IDDM, the onset of diabetic symptoms tends to be rapid. These symptoms are the result of insufficient insulin secretion, and therefore patients require exogenous insulin injections to control the disease. NIDDM, on the other hand, appears most commonly after the age of 40 and is strongly associated with obesity. The onset of diabetic symptoms is gradual, often evolving over a span of several years. The primary cause of hyperglycemia in NIDDM is apparently reduced insulin sensitivity of peripheral tissues (insulin resistance) as opposed to decreased insulin secretion. NIDDM is most often controlled by diet, weight reduction, the use of oral hypoglycemic agents, and sometimes insulin injections (Harris et al., 1998).

In diabetes, the absence or ineffectiveness of insulin and the resultant hyperglycemia engender numerous metabolic aberrations affecting many body systems. The prevalence of IDDM is 1.5 times higher among Whites than Blacks (Harris et al., 1998; Tull & Roseman, 1995). However, the reverse is true of NIDDM. The statistics on NIDDM in Black Americans are startling and sobering. According to the National Diabetes Information Clearinghouse (2002), 2.8 million Black Americans have diabetes, that is, approximately 13 percent of all Black Americans. Black Americans are twice as likely to have diabetes as White Americans of similar age, and Black Americans with the disease are more likely to develop diabetic complications and experience greater disability from those complications, including diabetic atherosclerosis, diabetic retinopathy, diabetic neuropathy, and diabetic nephropathy. Black women are more seriously affected by these complications than are Black men. Death rates for people with diabetes are 27 percent higher for Black Americans compared with Whites. One of the most alarming trends in diabetes prevalence involves children. While Black American children seem to have lower rates of Type I diabetes than White children, there is an increasing prevalence of Type II diabetes in children, especially in Black Americans, Native Americans, and Hispanics (Ludwig & Ebbeling, 2001).

Pi-Sunyer (1990) points out that both genetic predisposition and environment are likely involved in the pathogenesis of obesity and diabetes and that more research is needed to clarify this interrelationship in Blacks. Hyperinsulinemia and insulin resistance may be a common pathogenic mechanism relating NIDDM, obesity, and hypertension, all of which have a higher prevalence rate in Blacks (Douglas, 1990).

Diet is a major environmental factor in the pathogenesis of diabetes because it is a major determinant of obesity. Obesity is the only factor that has been consistently related to the prevalence of NIDDM. Diets with high total caloric intake, high percentage of calories from fat, and low percentage of calories from complex carbohydrates are positively associated with diabetes prevalence (Tull & Roseman, 1995).

Obesity

An estimated 97 million adults in the United States are either overweight or obese (Kuczmarski et al., 1997). Data from the 1988–1994 NHANES survey show a 25 percent increase in overweight, from 44.8 to 56.0 percent, and a 75 percent increase in obesity, from 13.3 to 23.3 percent, over 1960–1962 data (Health, United States, 2001). In general, a higher proportion of men are overweight than women, but a higher proportion of women are obese than men. In women, overweight and obesity are more prevalent among racial and ethnic minorities than in Whites. Black non-Hispanic females have a higher prevalence of overweight and obesity than black non-Hispanic males, White non-Hispanic males, or White non-Hispanic females. People from lower socioeconomic status experience a higher prevalence of overweight and obesity than those from higher socioeconomic status (Health, United States, 2001; Healthy People 2010b). However, a higher proportion of men from lower socioeconomic status compared to those of higher socioeconomic status are at a healthy weight.

Overweight and obesity contribute to high rates of morbidity and mortality, with obesity-related deaths in the United States reaching an estimated 300,000 each year. The conditions are risk factors for a number of diseases, including non-insulin-dependent diabetes mellitus (Ford et al., 1997; Lipton et al., 1993), hypertension (Dyer & Elliott, 1989), sleep apnea and respiratory problems (Young et al., 1993), gallbladder disease (Stampfer et al., 1992), osteoarthritis (Hochberg et al., 1995), coronary artery disease and stroke (Rexrode et al., 1997; Hubert et al., 1983), and cancers such as those of the endometrium, breast, gallbladder, ovaries and cervix in women, and colorectal and prostate in men (Chute et al., 1991). Rodriquez et al. (2002) and Becker et al. (1998) reported that overweight and obesity also are risk factors for cardiovascular diseases, elevated total and low-density lipoprotein cholesterol, reduced levels of high-density lipoprotein cholesterol, and hypertriglyceridemia. Additionally, obese and overweight individuals may suffer from social stigmatization, discrimination, and lowered self-esteem (Healthy People 2010b).

For adults, overweight is defined as a body mass index (BMI) of ≥ 25 kg/m^2, and obesity as a BMI of ≥ 30 kg/m^2 (Health, United States, 2001; Healthy People 2010b). Body mass index is weight in kilograms divided by height in meters. According to the NHANES III report, only 34 percent of African Americans are of desirable BMI (18.5-<25), while 43 percent of Whites are of desirable BMI. A higher proportion of White women (47 percent) have desirable BMI compared to Black women (34 percent), while 40 percent of Black men have desirable BMI compared to 38 percent of White men (Healthy People 2010). The data further show that morbidity at BMI of ≥30, compared to BMI of < 25, results in an increased prevalence in health conditions such as hypertension, total blood cholesterol, and high-density lipoprotein in both men and women.

Body mass index serves as an important surrogate of body fat. While BMI gives weight-to-height relationship and serves as an important predictor of several chronic diseases, fat distribution, particularly abdominal fat (waist circumference), is another independent predictor of chronic diseases (Tchernof et al., 1996; Okosun et al., 2000). Waist circumference is gaining acceptance over the popularly used waist-to-hip ratio as the best anthropometric measurement for determining abdominal adiposity. Problems inherent in the waist-to-hip ratio include difficulty to interpret, since obese and lean individuals can have similar ratios. Waist circumference of ≥ 120 cm for men, and ≥ 88 cm for women are associated with increased risk for stroke, Type II diabetes, insulin resistance, myocardial infarction, hypertension, and breast cancer. Generally, waist-to-hip ratios above 0.9 in males, and 1.0 in females suggest increased risk for chronic diseases. Waist-to-hip circumference ratios are higher in Black women than in White women, especially in middle age (Gillum, 1987b). In Black and White males, the ratio is similar before age 65. After age 65, Black males have, on average, lower waist-to-hip circumference ratios than do White Males (Gillum, 1987a).

The number of overweight children in the United States has grown considerably since the conduct of NHANES II. Yip et al. (1992) defined overweight in children as age- and sex-specific body mass index (BMI) percentile ranking of 95 percent or above. During 1988–1994, 11 percent of children age 6–11 and 10.5 percent of adolescents 12–19 years of age were overweight (NHANES III). A higher proportion (15 percent) of African American children, 6–19 years of age, are obese or overweight compared to 10 percent of White children. Further, 15 percent of African American children 6–11 years old and 13 percent of the 12–19-year-olds are either overweight or obese. Data from the Pediatric Nutrition Surveillance System (PedNSS), show a high prevalence (11.3 percent) of overweight among children less than 2 years of age, and 8.6 percent among those less than 5 years of age. The prevalence of overweight was highest among Hispanic children and lowest among White children (Centers for Disease Control and Prevention, 1998). Further, data from the National Longitudinal Survey of Youths also show an increase in overweight and obesity among children and that race/ethnicity and geographic location strongly influence the prevalence of overweight in children (Strauss & Pollack, 2001). For example, compared to 1986, overweight prevalence in 1998 was 120 percent higher in African American and Hispanic children and 50 percent higher in Whites. This represents an overall prevalence of overweight of 12.3 percent in White children, 21.5 percent in African Americans, and 21.8 in Hispanics. African American and Hispanic children living in the southern states are more likely to be overweight than non-Hispanic White children or children in other regions of the country (Strauss & Pollack, 2001).

Health problems associated with overweight in childhood include high blood pressure (Gutin et al., 1990), high blood cholesterol (Freedman et al., 1992), orthopedic disorders (Dietz et al., 1982), and psychosocial disorders (Dietz, 1985). The high prevalence of childhood obesity is particularly disturbing because several studies, including the Newcastle Thousand Families Study, have shown that obesity in childhood contributes to overweight in adulthood (Wright et al., 2001; Dietz, 1998; Whitaker et al., 1997).

Obesity occurs when more energy is consumed than is expended. Its development is associated with genetic, metabolic, and physiological factors that are not modifiable and with a number of modifiable factors such as nutritional, social, cultural, and environmental. Dietary factors contribute significantly to the burden of morbidity and mortality associated with overweight and obesity. The overconsumption of total and saturated fats and the limited consumption of vegetables, fruits, whole grains high in complex carbohydrates, and dietary fiber are major concerns. Current recommendations for total and saturated fat consumption are 30 and 10 percent or less of total calories, respectively.

The 1994–1996 Continuing Survey of Food Intake of Individuals (CSFII) and the report of Allison et al. (1999) show total dietary fat accounts for approximately 33 percent, saturated fats 11 percent, and trans-fatty acids 2.6 percent of calories in the U.S. diet. Only 26 percent of African Americans consume 30 percent of calories or less from total fat, and 31 percent consume the recommended 10 percent or less from saturated fats compared to 33 percent and 35 percent, respectively, for Whites (USDHHS 2000b).

Interestingly, mean food energy intake for non-Hispanic Whites (2,029 kilocalories) is 100 kilocalories higher than for Mexican Americans, other Hispanics and non-Hispanic Blacks (Moshfegh et al., 1999). Blacks compared to Whites consume less than the recommended servings of fruits and vegetables, including dark green and deep yellow vegetables; and grain products including whole grains. For example, among Blacks 2 years of age and older who are not Hispanic or Latino, only 24 percent consume the recommended servings of fruits, compared to 27 percent among non-Hispanic or Latino Whites. Vegetable and grain consumption among Blacks and Whites show that 43 percent of Blacks who are not Hispanic or Latino consumed three or more daily servings of vegetables, and 40 percent consumed 6 or more servings of grains compared to 50 and 54 percent, respectively, for Whites (USDHHS 2000b).

American children are consuming more sugar drinks, and the increased consumption is correlated with BMI and the odds of becoming obese (USDA, 1999). In addition, a considerable amount of fats and sugars are contributed to the American diet by baked products such as cookies, cakes, and doughnuts (Morton & Guthrie, 1998). The CSFII data show that African American children consume more potato chips and French fries than other Americans. Further, African American children consume as much as 20 percent of daily calories from snacks (USDA, 1999). This risk of obesity is further exacerbated by the growing trend in eating away from home, which explains why much of the family food budget (40 percent) accounts for restaurant and carry-out meals (Healthy People 2010b). These foods are generally higher in fats, cholesterol, and sodium and are lower in fiber and calcium and contribute toward the problem of obesity and other diet-related diseases. In contrast, people who consume "produce-rich" diets are likely substituting fruits and vegetables for fats and sugars, thus helping to reduce obesity.

While the diet is a major contributor to the prevalence of overweight and obesity, physical inactivity, especially among children, is on the rise and has contributed to the escalation in the prevalence of obesity (USDHHS 2000b). Less activity at home and at school and more time spent watching television and on the computer have been implicated. In addition to facilitating weight control, physical activity, especially among the elderly, improves muscular strength, muscle flexibility, and endurance. Only 15 percent of adults engaged in 30 minutes of physical activity five or more days per week. Among non-Hispanic or non-Latino Blacks and Whites, 10 and 16 percent, respectively, engaged in physical activity lasting 30 minutes, five or more days per week (Healthy People 2010b). Recommendations for weight reduction or control must include diet, physical activity, and behavior modifications.

Certain Cancers

Cancer is the second leading cause of death in the United States, causing over 500,000 deaths/ year. Cancer is not one but many diseases with multifactorial etiologies and associated with a variety of risk factors (USDHHS 2000a). Incidence rates of many cancers are substantially higher for Black Americans, including esosphageal, multiple myeloma, liver, cervical, stomach, larynx, prostate, oral cavity and pharynx, pancreas, and lung compared to Whites. However, Blacks have a lower incidence of the following cancers: melanoma, endometrial, thyroid, breast, bladder, leukemia, lymphoma, ovary, testis, and brain (Zahm, & Fraumeni, 1995). In general, Black Americans, other racial/ethnic minorities, and those with low incomes have poorer cancer survival rates than White and middle- and upper-income Americans (Bradley et al., 2001). For example, the incidence rate of breast cancer is higher for White women; however, the mortality rate from the disease is higher for Black women (Baquet & Commiskey, 2000). Black American women are more likely to die of breast and colon cancers than are women of any other racial and ethnic group, in part, because cancer is diagnosed at later stages in Black American females (USDHHS 2000a). Black American men are more likely to present with clinically advanced-stage prostate cancer than Whites. This increased likelihood cannot be fully explained by socioeconomic, clinical, or pathologic factors (Hoffman et al., 2001).

Boring et al., (1992) point out that despite the fact that cancer mortality rates were comparable for all races 30 years ago, cancer mortality since then has increased for Black men and women, 66 and 10 percent, respectively. Much of this cancer burden can be attributed to cigarette smoking. There is a higher prevalence of cigarette smoking among Blacks; however, smoking among Blacks now appears to be on the decline, especially in the adolescent age group. There is also encouraging evidence that Blacks are participating more fully in cancer early detection initiatives. In fact, Black American women receive more frequent Pap tests than women of other racial/ethnic groups (Harlan et al., 1991). Despite these positive trends, Black men experience an increased risk of cancer versus non-Black males with a 25 percent higher risk of all cancers and a 45 percent higher incidence of lung cancer, and only 39 percent of Blacks with cancer survive five years after diagnosis, compared to 50 percent of Whites (USDHHS 2000a).

Although it is impossible to quantify the percentage of human cancer attributable to diet, at least one-third of all cancer mortality is thought to be related to nutrition. The role of dietary factors in the pathogenesis of various types of cancer were summarized in Healthy People 2010. Dietary fat intake (via epidemiologic and experimental animal evidence) is associated with increasing the risk of certain cancers (e.g., breast, colon, rectum, endometrium, prostate). Research has linked increased consumption of fat from animal sources to increased risk of prostate cancer among Black men (Hayes et al., 1999; Clinton & Giovannucci, 1998). Overweight and lack of physical activity have been associated with increased risk of colon, breast, and endometrial cancers. This relationship is most likely hormonally mediated (Bianchini et al., 2002).

Increased intake of fruits and vegetables is associated with a lower risk of several cancers, most notably mouth, bladder, colon, lung, and stomach. Dietary fiber may have a beneficial effect especially on colon cancer. Vitamin A has been reported to protect against epithelial cancers, apparently by promoting normal cellular differentiation. B-carotene also exerts a protective effect, presumably due to its role as an antioxidant. Nutrient antioxidants (like B-carotene, vitamins E and C, and selenium) can quench free radicals and their oxidative products and may minimize carcinogenesis. B-carotene has also been reported to enhance several aspects of immune function. There is also encouraging recent evidence that several water-soluble vitamins, including riboflavin, folic acid, and vitamin B12, may block the initiation or promotion of cancer. The National Cancer Institute (NCI) developed the five a Day for Better Health Program in 1991, a national program that promotes the consumption of five or more servings of vegetables and fruit daily for better health, recognizing that a diet rich in vegetables and fruit reduces the risk of cancer and other chronic diseases. Vegetables and fruit are important sources of several essential nutrients, including vitamin C, folate and other B vitamins, pro-vitamin A and other carotenoids, potassium, calcium, iron, and dietary fiber (Monograph: 5 A Day for Better Health Program, 2001).

The evidence was most conclusive for vegetables and fruit and cancers of the mouth and pharynx, esophagus, lung, and stomach and for vegetables alone and cancers of the colon and rectum. The association of vegetables and fruit with cancer incidence was judged to be strong, particularly for vegetables, with about a halving of risk overall found to be associated with consuming at least five servings of vegetables and fruit per day as compared to only one or two servings. Relevant substances

Table 24.1
Recommendations for dietary and lifestyle modifications

Cardiovascular Disease	Decrease saturated fat, total fat and cholesterol intake; increase dietary fiber intake by consuming less meat and greater amounts of whole grains and fresh fruits and vegetables. Decrease the prevalence of obesity by increasing physical activity.
Hypertension	Decrease the consumption of foods that are high in sodium chloride and calories and increase the intake of foods that are higher in calcium and potassium content. Increase physical activity and consume alcohol in moderation.
Diabetes Mellitus	Weight reduction facilitated by consumption of a diet that is low in fat, moderate in protein, and high in complex carbohydrates as well as an increase in physical activity.
Obesity	Weight reduction involving a holistic approach combining diet, increasing physical activity, and behavior modification. Implementation of nutrition education initiatives designed within the cultural context of the Black community and specifically targeting the Black family.
Certain Cancers	Decrease the prevalence of obesity by modifying food intake and increasing physical activity. Dietary recommendations include: increasing consumption of fresh fruits and vegetables and whole grains, while decreasing dietary fat, especially saturated fat intake. The diet should include a wide variety of fruits, vegetables, whole grains, and legumes. Three to five servings of vegetables and two to four servings of fruits per day are recommended, and alcohol consumption should be limited.

in vegetables and fruit include phytochemicals such as dithiolthiones, flavonoids, glucosinolates, and allium compounds, as well as carotenoids, other antioxidants, vitamins, folate, and minerals such as selenium and calcium (World Cancer Research Fund and the American Institute for Cancer Research, 1997). Frequent consumption of lycopene-rich tomato products is associated with a lower risk of prostate cancer (Giovannucci et al., 2002).

In summary, the major dietary associations for cancers that have the highest prevalence in the Black community can also be identified. For lung cancer, the predominant cause is exposure to tobacco smoke. Breast cancer is still more common among White women than Black, but rates are increasing among Black women. There is evidence that breast cancer mortality is positively correlated with total caloric intake, dietary fat, especially animal fats, and negatively correlated with intake of complex carbohydrates and dietary fiber. Obesity, which is twice as prevalent for Black women than for White, is also positively associated with breast cancer risk. Prostate cancer rates are especially high in Black males. Several studies show a positive correlation between this type of cancer and total dietary fat intake. Data on diet and colorectal cancer are inconsistent; however, many studies report that high meat intake, low vegetable intake, high saturated fat intake, and low dietary fiber intake are all positively correlated with colorectal cancer risk. Research must provide increased

Table 24.2
Recommendations for public health policy/interventions

Individual Level	Interventions should help Black Americans find culturally acceptable and specific ways of integrating healthy diet and physical activity into their daily lives. The most effective education programs will advocate and support gradual modifications in diet and lifestyle that enable Black Americans to enjoy and celebrate many of the foods in their traditional diet prepared in more healthful ways.
Community Level	Public health professionals and community organizations can create programs to encourage healthier food choices and make available safe and affordable places to exercise. Nutrition education aimed at Black Americans must take into account Black dietary patterns, specifically targeting weight control, reducing the percentage of calories from fat, lowering salt intake, increasing fruit and vegetable intake, and increasing the intake of complex carbohydrates and dietary fiber. These efforts must be designed and implemented within the context of Black culture and with the full participation of members of the Black American community at every stage of the process. Nutrition intervention programs should be coordinated with activities and programs existing in schools, community centers, and churches.
Public Policy Level	Encourage the food industry to make the components of a healthy diet, especially fresh fruits and vegetables and other complex carbohydrates and low-fat foods, more affordable, accessible, and attractive in Black American communities. National, state, and local governments should find new ways to support culturally appropriate and relevant nutrition education, and to set and enforce standards for responsible food advertising. Second, policies should be developed and implemented to increase the accessibility and affordability of physical activity in Black American communities by making parks, recreational facilities, and fitness centers safer and more available. Increased funds must be made available to finance existing and new nutrition research and education initiatives; increase the numbers of Black nutrition professionals; and increase nutritional surveillance and longitudinal prospective studies with large sample sizes, reflecting the socioeconomic, geographic, and cultural diversity in the Black American community.

evidence of different diet and cancer interactions, and we must increase nutrition education in diet modification (e.g., increased green and yellow vegetable intake).

RECOMMENDATIONS

Recommendations for dietary and lifestyle modifications for the prevention of diet-related chronic diseases are shown in Table 24.1. These recommendations are consistent with those proposed by the

American Dietetic Association (Stark, 2002), American Heart Association (American Heart Association, 2004), the American Cancer Society (Glade, 1999), the American Diabetes Association (American Diabetes Association, 2004), and Healthy People 2010 (2000). Recommendations for public health policy/interventions follow in Table 24.2 (Blocker & Freudenberg, 2001). In addition to diet, lifestyle, and public policy changes, in order to truly reduce racial/ethnic disparities in health, this country must also aggressively address the societal correlates of poor health status among Blacks, namely, persistent institutional racism, poverty, and inadequate access to quality health care. This will require a major and unwavering commitment of resources and a reorganization of our national priorities.

REFERENCES

Allison, D.B., Egan, S.K., Barraj, L.M., Caughman, C., Infante, M., & Heimbach, J.T. (1999). Estimated intake of trans fatty and other fatty acids in the U.S. population. *Journal American Dietetic Association, 99*, 166–174.

American Diabetes Association. (2004). Nutrition principles and recommendations in diabetes. *Diabetes Care, 27*, S36.

American Diabetes Association. (1997). Report of the expert committee on the diagnosis and Classification of Diabetes Mellitus. *Diabetes Care, 20*, 1183–1197.

American Heart Association (2004). Dietary Guidelines. Available at http://www.americanheart.org/presenter. jhtml?identifier=1330. Accessed January 28, 2004.

American Heart Association. (2001). Heart and stroke statistical update. Dallas: American Heart Association, 2000. Retrieved July 2001 from http://www.americanheart.org/statistical/pdf/HSSTATS2001_1.0.pdf

Baquet, C.R. & Commiskey, P. (2000). Socioeconomic factors and breast carcinoma in multicultural women. *Cancer, 88*, 1256–1264.

Becker, D.M., Yook, R.M., May, T.F., Blumenthal, R.S., & Becker, L.C. (1998). Markedly high prevalence of coronary risk factors in apparently healthy African-Americans with premature coronary artery disease. *American Journal Cardiology*, 1046–1051.

Bianchini, F., Kaaks, R., & Vainio, H. (2002) Weight control and physical activity in cancer prevention. *Obesity Reviews, 3*, 5–8.

Bickell, N.A., Pieper, K.S., Lee, K.L., Mark, D.B., Glower, D.D., & Pryor, D.B. (1992). Referral pattern for coronary artery disease treatment: Gender bias or good clinical judgment? *Annals of Internal Medicine, 116*, 791–797.

Blaustein, M.P., & Grim, C.E. (1991). The pathogenesis of hypertension: Black–white differences. *Cardiovascular Clinics, 21(3)*, 97–114.

Blocker, D.E., & Freudenberg, N. (2001) Developing Comprehensive Approaches to Prevention and Control of Obesity Among Low-Income, Urban, African-American Women. *Journal of the American Medical Women's Association, 56*, 59–64.

Boring, C.C., Squires, T.S., & Heath, C.W. (1992). Cancer statistics for African Americans. *CA-A Cancer Journal for Clinicians, 42(1)*, 7–17.

Bradley, C.J., Given, C.W., & Roberts, C. (2001). Disparities in Cancer Diagnosis and Survival. *Cancer 91*, 178–188.

Carter, J.S., Pugh, J.A., & Monterossa, A. (1996). Non-insulin dependent diabetes mellitus in minorities in the United States. *Annals of Internal Medicine, 125*, 221–232.

Centers for Disease Control and Prevention. (1998). *Pediatric nutrition surveillance, 1977. Full report.* Atlanta: U.S. Department of Health and Human Services, Centers for Disease Control and Prevention.

Chobanian, A.V., Bakris, G.L., Black, H.R., Cushman, W.C., Green, L.A., Izzo, J.L., Jr., Jones, D.W., Materson, B.J., Oparil, S., Wright, J.T. Jr., & Roccella, E.J. (2004). Seventh report of the Joint National Committee on Prevention, Detection, Evaluation, and Treatment of High Blood Pressure. *Hypertension, 43(1)*, 1–3.

Chute, C.G., Willett, W.C., & Colditz, G.A. (1991). A prospective study of body mass, height, and smoking on the risk of colorectal cancer in women. *Cancer Causes and Control, 2*, 117–124.

Clinton, S.K., & Giovannucci, E. (1998). Diet, Nutrition, and Prostate Cancer. *Annual Review of Nutrition, 18,* 413–440.

Committee on Diet and Health. (1989). Diet and health: implications for reducing chronic disease risk. Food and Nutrition Board. Commission on Life Sciences. National Research Council. Washington: National Academy Press.

Cutler, J.A., Follmann, D., Elliott, P., & Suh, I. (1991). An overview of randomized trials of sodium reduction and blood pressure. *Hypertension, 17(Suppl I),* I-27–I-33.

Dietz, W.H. (1985). Implications and treatment of adolescent obesity. *Clinical Nutrition, 4,* 103–108.

Dietz, W.H. (1998). Health consequences of obesity in youth: Childhood predictors of adult disease. *Pediatrics, 101,* 518–525.

Dietz, W.J., Gross, W.C., & Kirkpatrick, J.A. (1982). Blount disease (tibia vara): Another skeletal disorder associated with childhood obesity. *Journal of Pediatrics, 101,* 735–737.

Douglas, J.G. (1990). Hypertension and diabetes in Blacks. *Diabetes Care, 13 (11, Suppl. 4),* 1191–1195.

Dyer, A.R., & Elliott, P. (1989). The INTERSALT study: Relations of body mass index to blood pressure, INTERSALT Co-operative Research Group. *Journal Human Hypertension, 3,* 299–308.

Elliott, P. (1991). Observational studies of salt and blood pressure. *Hypertension 17(Suppl I),* I-3-I-8.

Fang, J., Madhavan, S., & Alderman, M. (1996). The association between birthplace and mortality from cardiovascular causes among Black and White residents of New York City. *New England Journal of Medicine, 335,* 1545–1551.

Feldman, R.H., & Fulwood, R. (1999). The three leading causes of death in African Americans: Barriers to reducing excess disparity and to improving health behaviors. *Journal of Health Care for the Poor and Underserved, 10(1),* 45–71.

Ford, E.S., Williamson, D.F., & Liu, S. (1997). Weight change and diabetes incidence: Findings from a national cohort of U.S. adults. *American Journal Epidemiology, 146,* 214–222.

Freedman, D.S., Lee, S.L., Byers, T., Kuester, S., & Sell, K.I. (1992). Serum cholesterol levels in a multiracial sample of 7,439 preschool children from Arizona. *Preventive Medicine, 21,* 162–176.

Freis, E.D., Reda, D.J., & Materson, B.J. (1988). Volume (weight) loss and blood pressure following thiazide diuretics. *Hypertension, 12(3),* 244–250.

Frost, C.D., Law, M.R., & Wald, N.J. (1991). By how much does dietary salt reduction lower blood pressure? II analysis of observational data within populations. *British Medical Journal, 302,* 815–818.

Gillum, R.F. (1987a). The association of body fat distribution with hypertension, hypertensive heart disease, coronary heart disease, diabetes and cardiovascular risk factor in men and women aged 18–79 years. *Journal of Chronic Diseases, 40,* 421–428.

Gillum, R.F. (1987b). Overweight and obesity in Black women: A review of published data from the National Center for Health Statistics. *Journal of the National Medical Association, 79,* 865–871.

Giovannucci E., Rimm E.B., Liu Y., Stampfer M.J., & Willett W.C. (2002). A prospective study of tomato products, lycopene, and prostate cancer risk. *Journal of the National Cancer Institute, 94(5),* 391–398.

Glade, M.J. (1999). Food, nutrition, and the prevention of cancer: A global perspective. American Institute for Cancer Research/World Cancer Research Fund, American Institute for Cancer Research, 1997. *Nutrition, 15(6),* 523–6.

Greenberg, M., Schneider, D. (1991). Region of birth and mortality of Blacks in the United States. *International Journal of Epidemiology, 21,* 324–328.

Greenberg, M.R., Schneider, D., Northridge, M.E., & Ganz, M.L. (1998). Region of birth and Black diets: The Harlem household survey. *American Journal of Public Health, 88(8),* 1199–1202.

Gutin, B., Basch, C., Shea, S., Contento, I., DeLozier, M., Rips, J., Irigoyen, M., & Zybert, P. (1990). Blood pressure, fitness, and fatness in 5- and 6-year-old children. *Journal of the American Medical Association, 264,* 1123–1127.

Harlan, L.C., Bernstein, A.B., & Kessler, L.G. (1991). Cervical cancer screening: Who is not screened and why? *American Journal of Public Health, 81,* 885–890.

Harris, M.I., et al. (1998). Prevalence of diabetes, impaired fasting glucose, and impaired glucose tolerance in U.S. adults: The Third National Health and Nutrition Examination Survey, 1988–94. *Diabetes Care, 21,* 518–524.

Hayes, R.B., Ziegler, R.G., Gridley, G., Swanson, C., Greenberg, R.S., Swanson, G.M., Schoenberg, J.B.,

Silverman, D.T., Brown, L.M., Pottern, L.M., Liff, J., Schwartz, A.G., Fraumeni, J.F., Hoover, R.N. (1999). Dietary factors and risks for prostate cancer among Blacks and Whites in the United States. *Cancer Epidemiology, Biomarkers & Prevention, 8*, 25–34.

Health, United States, (2001). With Urban and Rural Health Chart Book, Department of Health and Human Services, Centers for Disease Control and Prevention, National Center for Health Statistics. Hyattsville, MD.

Hochberg, M.C., Lethbridge-Cejku, M., Scott, W.W., Reichle, R., Plato, C.C., & Tobin, J.D. (1995). The association of body weight, body fatness and body fat distribution with osteoarthritis of the knee: Data from the Baltimore Longitudinal Study of Aging. *Journal of Rheumatology, 22*, 488–493.

Hoffman, R.M., Gilliland, F.D., Eley, W., Harlan, L.C., Stephenson, R.A., Stanford, J.L., Albertson, P.C., Hamilton, A.S., Hunt, W.C., & Potosky, A.L. (2001). Racial and ethnic differences in advanced-stage prostate cancer: The prostate cancer outcomes study. *Journal of the National Cancer Institute, 93*, 388–395. http://www.nal.usda.gov/ttic/tektran/data/000010/39/0000103944.html.

Hubert, H.B., Feinleib, M., McNamara, P.M., & Castelli, W.P. (1983). Obesity as an independent risk factor for cardiovascular disease: A 26-year follow-up of participants in the Framingham Heart Study. *Circulation, 67*, 968–977.

Intersalt Cooperative Research Group (1988). Intersalt: An international study of electrolyte excretion and blood pressure. Results for 24 hour urinary sodium and potassium excretion. *British Medical Journal, 297*, 319–328.

Joint National Committee on Detection, Evaluation and Treatment of High Blood Pressure. (1993). The fifth report of the Joint National Committee on Detection, Evaluation and Treatment of High Blood Pressure. *Archives of Internal Medicine, 153*, 154–183.

Katzmarzyk, P.T., Gagnon, J.L., & Leon, A.S. (2001). Fitness, fatness and estimated coronary heart disease risk: The HERITAGE family study. *Medicine and Science in Sports and Exercise, 33*, 585–590.

Kayrooz K., Moy, T.F., Yanek, L.R., & Becker, D.M. (1998). Dietary fat patterns in urban African American women. *Journal of Community Health, 23*, 453–469.

Kittler, P.G., & Sucher, K. (1989). *Food and Culture in America*. New York: Van Nostrand Reinhold.

Kittler, P.G., & Sucher, K. (2001). *Food and Culture*. Third Edition. Belmont, CA: Wadsworth/Thomson Learning.

Knapp, H.R., & Fitzgerald, G.A. (1989). The antihypertensive effects of fish oil. A controlled study of polyunsaturated fatty acid supplements in essential hypertension. *New England Journal of Medicine, 320*, 1037–1043.

Krantz, D.S., & McCeney, M.K. (2002). Effects of psychological and social factors on organic disease: A critical assessment of research on coronary heart disease. *Annual Review of Psychology, 53*, 341–69.

Kris-Etherton, P.M., Krummel, D., Dreon, D., Mackey, S., & Wood, P.D. (1988). The effect of diet on plasma lipids, lipoproteins, and coronary heart disease. *Journal of the American Dietetic Association, 88*, 1373–1400.

Kuczmarski, R.J., Carol, M.D., Flegal, K.M., & Troiano, R.P. (1997). Varying body mass cutoff points to describe overweight prevalence among U.S. adults. NHANES III (1988 to 1994). *Obesity Research, 5*, 542–548.

Kumanyika, S. (1993). Diet and Nutrition as Influences on the Morbidity/Mortality Gap. *Annals of Epidemiology, 3*, 154–158.

Kumanyika, S., & Adams-Campbell, L.L. (1991). Obesity, diet, and psychosocial factors contributing to ardiovascular disease in blacks. *Cardiovascular Clinics, 21(3)*, 47–73.

Kumanyika, S., & Helitzer, D.L. (1985). Nutritional status and dietary pattern of racial minorities in the United States. In: Report of the Secretary's Task Force on Black and Minority Health, Vol. II. Washington, DC: U.S. Dept. of Health and Human Services, U.S. Government Printing Office.

Larsson, B., Bjorntorp, P., & Tibblin, G. (1981). The health consequences of moderate obesity. *International Journal of Obesity, 5*, 97–116.

Lee, C.D., Folsom, A.R., Nieto, F.J., Chambless, L.E., Shahar, E., & Wolfe, D.A. (2001). White blood cell count and incidence of coronary heart disease and ischemic stroke and mortality from cardiovascular disease in African American and White men and women: Atherosclerosis risk in communities study. *American Journal of Epidemiology, 154*, 758–764.

Lipton, R.D., Liao, Y., Cao, G., Cooper, R.S., & McGee, D. (1993). Determinants of incidence of non-insulin-dependent diabetes mellitus among Blacks and Whites in a national sample. The NHANES I Epidemiologic Follow-up Study. *American Journal of Epidemiology, 138*, 826–839.

Ludwig, D.S., & Ebbeling, C.B. (2001). Type 2 diabetes mellitus in children. *Journal of the American Medical Association, 286*, 1427–1430.

Luke, A., Cooper, R.S., Prewitt, T.E., Adeyemo, A.A., & Forrester, T.E. (2001). Nutritional consequences of the African diaspora. *Annual Review of Nutrition, 21*, 47–71.

MacMahon, S., Peto, R., Cutler, J., et al. (1990). Blood pressure, stroke, and coronary heart disease. Part 1, prolonged differences in blood pressure: prospective observational studies corrected for the regression dilution bias. *Lancet, 335*, 765–774.

Monograph: 5 A Day for Better Health Program. (2001). National Institutes of Health. National Cancer Institute. Available at http://www.5aday.gov/pdf/masimaxmonograph.pdf. Accessed October 19, 2002.

Morton, J.F., & Guthrie, J.F. (1998). Changes in children's total fat intake and their food sources of fat 1989–1991 versus 1994–1995: Implications for diet quality. *Family Economics and Nutrition Review, 11*, 44–57.

Mosca, L.J. (2002). Optimal management of cholesterol levels and the prevention of coronary heart disease in women. *American Family Physician, 65*, 217–226.

Moshfegh, A., Tippett, K.S., Borrud, L.G., & Perloff, B.P. (1999). Food and nutrient intakes by individuals in the United States, by Hispanic origin and race, 1994–96. From the National Diabetes Information Clearinghouse. (2002). National diabetes statistics. NIH publication 02-3892. Fact sheet. Available at: www.niddk.nih.gov/health/diabetes/pubs/dmstats/dmstats.htm. Accessed October 12, 2002.

National Diabetes Information Clearinghouse. (2002). National diabetes statistics. NIH publication 02-3892. Fact sheet. Available at: www.niddk.nih.gov/health/diabetes/pubs/dmstats/dmstats.htm. Accessed October 12, 2002.

National Heart, Lung and Blood Institute. (1993, July). *Facts about Coronary Heart Disease*. Bethesda, MD: National Institutes of Health, Public Health Service, National Heart, Lung and Blood Institute.

National Heart, Lung and Blood Institute. (1998, October). *Morbidity and mortality: 1998 Chart book on Cardiovascular, lung, and blood diseases*. Bethesda, MD: National Institutes of Health, Public Health Service, National Heart, Lung and Blood Institute.

National Institutes of Health. (1999). *First estimates of lifetime risk for developing coronary heart disease*. Bethesda, MD: National Institutes of Health, Public Health Service, National Heart, Lung and Blood Institute.

Okosun, I.S., Liao, Y., Rotimi, C.N., Choi, S., & Cooper, R.S. (2000). Predictive values of waist circumference for dyslipidemia, type 2 diabetes, hypertension in overweight White, Black, and Hispanic Americans. *Journal Clinical Epidemiology, 53*, 401–408.

Pi-Sunyer, F.X. (1990). Obesity in blacks. *Diabetes Care, 13(11)*, 1144–1149.

Puddey, I.B., Beilin, L.J., Vandongen, R. (1987). Regular alcohol use raises blood pressure in treated hypertensive subjects. *Lancet, 1*, 647–651.

Rexrode, K.M., et al. (1997). A prospective study of body mass index, weight change, and risk of stroke in women. *Journal of the American Medical Association, 277*, 1539–1545.

Rodriquez, C., Pablos-Mendez, A., Palmas, W., Lantigua, R., Mayeux, R., & Berglund, L. (2002). Comparison of modifiable determinants of lipids and lipoprotein levels among African-Americans, Hispanics, and non-Hispanic Caucasians > 65 years of age living in New York City. *American Journal of Cardiology, 89*, 178–183.

Sacks, F.M., et al. (1995). Rationale and design of the dietary approaches to stop hypertension trial (DASH). A multicenter controlled-feeding study of dietary patterns to lower blood pressure. *Annals of Epidemiology, 5(2)*, 108–18.

Sempos, C.T., et al. (1993). Prevalence of high blood cholesterol among U.S. adults: An update based on guidelines from the second part of the National Cholesterol Education Program Treatment panel. *Journal of the American Medical Association, 269*, 3009–3014.

Sempos, C., et al. (1989). The prevalence of high blood cholesterol levels among adults in the United States. *Journal of the American Medical Association, 262*, 45–62.

Shaw, L.J., Miller, D.D., Romeis, J.C., Kargl, D., Younis, L.T., & Chaitman, B.R. (1994). Gender differences in the non-invasive evaluation and management of people with suspected coronary artery disease. *Annals of Internal Medicine, 12*, 559–566.

Slawta, J.N., McCubbin, J.A., & Wilcox, A.R. (2002). Coronary heart disease risk between active and inactive women with multiple sclerosis. *Medicine and Science in Sports and Exercise, 34*, 905–912.

Stamler, J. (1991). Epidemiologic findings on body mass and blood pressure in adults. *Annals of Epidemiology, 1*, 347–362.

Stamler, J., & Shekelle, R. (1988). Dietary cholesterol and human coronary heart disease. *Arch Pathol Lab Med., 112*, 1032–1040.

Stampfer, M.J., Maclure, K.M., Colditz, G.A., Manson, J.E., & Willett, W.C. (1992). Risk of symptomatic gallstones in women with severe obesity. *American Journal of Clinical Nutrition, 55*, 652–658.

Stark, C. (2002). Position of the American Dietetic Association: Weight management. *Journal of the American Dietetic Association, 102(8)*, 1144–1155.

Steingart, R.M., Packer, M., Hamm, P., Coglianese, M.E., Gersh, B., & Geltman, E.M. (1991). Sex differences in the management of coronary artery disease. Survival and ventricular enlargement investigators. *New England Journal of Medicine, 325*, 226–230.

Strauss, R.S., & Pollack, H.A. (2001). Epidemic increase in childhood overweight. 1986–1998. *Journal of the American Medical Association, 286*, 845–2848.

Tchernof, A., LaMarche, B., & Prud'Homme, D. (1996). The dense LDL phenotype: Association with plasma lipoprotein levels, visceral obesity, and hyperinsulinemia in men. *Diabetes Care, 19*, 629–637.

Tull, E.S., & Roseman, J.M. (1995). Diabetes in African Americans. Chapter 31 in Diabetes in America. 2d ed. NIH Publication No. 95-1468, pp. 613–630. Bethesda, MD: National Institute of Diabetes and Digestive and Kidney Diseases, National Institutes of Health.

U.S. Department of Agriculture (USDA), Agricultural Research Service. (1999, February). *Data Tables: Food and nutrient intakes by Hispanic origin and race, 1994–1996*. Online. ARS Food Surveys Research Group, available on the "Products" page at http://www.barc.usda.gov/bhnrc/foodsurvey/home.htm February, 1999.

U.S. Department of Health and Human Services. (2000). Healthy People 2000 Review. (1998–1999). Centers for Disease Control and Prevention, National Center for Health Statistics. Hyattsville, MD.

U.S. Department of Health and Human Services. (2000a). Healthy People 2010. Volume 1, with Understanding and Improving Health. Washington, DC: U.S. Government Printing Office.

U.S. Department of Health and Human Services. (2000b). Healthy People 2010, 2d ed. Volume II. with Understanding and Improving Health. Washington, DC: U.S. Government Printing Office.

Welch, G.N., & Losculzo, J. (1998). Homocystine and atherosclerosis. *New England Journal of Medicine, 338*, 1042–1050.

Whitaker, R.C., Wright, J.A., Pepe, M.S., Seidel, K.D., & Dietz, W.H. (1997). Predicting obesity in young adults from childhood and parental obesity. *New England Journal of Medicine, 337*, 869–873.

Williams, J.E., Massing, M., Rosamond, W.D., Sorlie, P.D., & Tyroler, H.A. (1999). Racial Disparities in CHD mortality from 1968–1992 in the state economic areas surrounding the ARIC Study Communities. *Annals of Epidemiology, 9*, 472–480.

Wilson, P.W., Savage, D.D., Castelli, W.P., Garrison, R.J., Donahue, R.P., & Feinleib, M. (1983). HDL-cholesterol in a sample of Black adults. *Metabolism, 32*, 328–332.

World Cancer Research Fund and the American Institute for Cancer Research. (1997). Food, nutrition and the prevention of cancer: a global perspective. Washington, DC: American Institute for Cancer Research.

Wright, C.M., Parker, L., & Lamont, D. (2001). Implications for childhood obesity for adult health, findings from thousand families cohort study. *British Medical Journal, 323*, 1280–1284.

Yip, R., Parvanta, I., Scanlon, K., Borland, E.W., Russell, C.M., & Trowbridge, F.L. (1992). Pediatric Nutrition Surveillance System—United States, 1980–1991. *Morbidity and Mortality Weekly Report, 41(SS-7)*, 1–24.

Young, T., Palta, M., Dempsey, J., Skatrud, J., Weber, S., & Badr, S. (1993). The occurrence of sleep-disordered breathing among middle-aged adults. *New England Journal of Medicine, 328*, 1230–1235.

Zahm, S.H. & Fraumeni, J.F. (1995). Racial, ethnic, and gender variations in cancer risk: Considerations for future epidemiologic research. *Environment Health Perspectives, 103 (Suppl 8)*, 283–286.

CHAPTER 25

Physical Activity in Black America

CARLOS J. CRESPO AND ROSS E. ANDERSEN

INTRODUCTION

The U.S. Department of Health and Human Services has identified ten leading health indicators for the nation as part of its Healthy People 2010 National Health Objectives. The overarching goals of this initiative are to help individuals of all ages increase life expectancy and improve their quality of life and to eliminate health disparities among different segments of the population. The leading health indicators are used to measure the health of the nation over the next ten years. As a group, the leading health indicators reflect the major health concerns in the United States at the beginning of the twenty-first century. These leading health indicators were selected on the basis of their ability to motivate action, the availability of data to measure progress, and their importance as public health issues.

The leading health indicators are:

1. Physical Activity
2. Overweight and Obesity
3. Tobacco Use
4. Substance Abuse
5. Responsible Sexual Behavior
6. Mental Health
7. Injury and Violence
8. Environmental Quality
9. Immunization
10. Access to Health Care

In this chapter we discuss how these health indicators impact the African American community. This chapter highlights the public health significance of physical activity as an important determinant of health in Black America. Eliminating health disparities among different segments of the population includes closing the gaps that exist by gender, race or ethnicity, education or income, disability, living in rural localities, or sexual orientation. This chapter provides information on the prevalence of physical inactivity in Black America within the context of the Healthy People 2010 and provides a descriptive epidemiological characterization of the disparities in physical inactivity between non-Hispanic Whites and Black Americans.

The information presented comes from national representative samples of non-Hispanic Blacks, a term used to refer to Black Americans not of Hispanic origin. The Centers for Disease Control and Prevention, which includes the National Center for Health Statistics, have been monitoring health promotion practices of racial and ethnic minorities in the United States for more than 30 years. Unfortunately, sedentary lifestyles were not monitored by the federal government until 1985 as part of the National Health Interview Survey. This chapter presents data from the 1991, 1995, 1997 and 2002 National Health Interview Survey, the 1996–1998 Behavioral Risk Factor Surveillance System, and the Third National Health and Nutrition Examination Survey conducted between 1988 and 1994. The latter was designed to oversample Blacks and Mexican Americans in order to produce reliable estimates when studying ethnic groups in smaller groups (e.g., age groups, education, income, and occupation). Other corollary information comes from peer review scientific articles that specifically discuss physical activity in Black Americans.

DEFINITIONS OF FITNESS TERMINOLOGY

Physical activity refers to any bodily movement, produced by contraction of skeletal muscle that substantially increases energy expenditure. Within this broad definition there are other forms of physical activity that are not mutually exclusive of each other. One of the most common forms of physical activity studied in the epidemiological literature is "leisure-time physical activity" in reference to activities conducted outside of work or for transportation. Occupational physical activity represents energy expenditure through participation in work-related endeavors. Transportation physical activity refers to activities designed to take a person from one place to another. Exercise, on the other hand, is defined as a planned, structured, and repetitive bodily movement done to improve or maintain one or more components of physical fitness. Some types of physical activities such as bicycling and walking can easily fit into more than one category. This creates some problems when assessing total physical activity in the population and in population subgroups such as women, children, and minorities. Physical fitness is defined as the ability to carry out daily tasks with vigor and alertness, without undue fatigue, and with ample energy to enjoy leisure-time pursuits and to meet unforeseen emergencies. Thus, fitness is a set of attributes that relates to the ability to perform physical activities and can be health-related or skill-related (U.S. Department of Health and Human Services, 1996a).

Major health-related components of fitness are cardiorespiratory endurance, muscular strength, muscular endurance, flexibility, and body composition. Cardiorespiratory endurance relates to the ability of the circulatory and respiratory system to supply oxygen during sustained physical activity. Muscular endurance is the ability of the muscle to continue to perform without fatigue, whereas muscular strength is the ability of the muscle to exert force. Flexibility is another health-related component based on the range of motion available at a joint. Body composition is the relative amounts of muscle, fat, bone, and other vital parts of the body. An example of a component of body composition is percent of body fat. The above health-related components of fitness are categorized as such because they are associated with the prevention of specific diseases or conditions, such as coronary heart disease, osteoporosis, fractures from falls, diabetes, obesity, and high blood pressure among others (Nieman, 1999).

Skill-related fitness components have specific benefits to performance-related endeavors and are not necessarily related to disease prevention or health promotion. Broadly, these include agility, coordination, speed, reaction time, and power. Agility relates to the ability to rapidly change position;

coordination is the ability to use the senses such as sight and hearing together with body parts in performing motor tasks smoothly and accurately; speed refers to performing movements within a short period of time; reaction power relates to the time elapsed between stimulation and the beginning of the reaction to it; and power is the rate at which one can perform work. Balance is a skill-related component of fitness but can be classified as a health-related component because of its importance in the prevention of falls and fractures. Balance relates to the maintenance of equilibrium while stationary or moving (Nieman, 1999; U.S. Department of Health and Human Services, 1996a).

The public health emphasis is in the development of health-related fitness, not skill-related fitness. Lifetime participation in physical activity such as walking, jogging, and bicycling do promote health-related fitness, whereas participation in organized sports requires the contribution and development of both skill- and health-related fitness components. Participation in organized sports without the appropriate training and development of health-related fitness components such as aerobic endurance, muscular strength and endurance, flexibility and proper body weight may result in an increased risk of musculoskeletal injury. Thus, constant maintenance of an appropriate age-specific fitness level is of public health importance, especially among minority populations who prefer to take part in team sports such as basketball or football.

NATIONAL PUBLIC HEALTH INITIATIVES TO INCREASE PHYSICAL ACTIVITY

In 1996, the surgeon general published a document titled "The Surgeon General Report on Physical Activity and Health" to examine the most up-to-date information on the benefits of physical activity (U.S. Department of Health and Human Services, 1996a). This publication underscored the need to provide some guidelines to the public about the amount and quality of physical activity necessary for optimal health. Recommendations on the amount and type of physical activity needed had been proposed by the American College and Sports Medicine and the Centers for Disease Control and Prevention (Pate et al., 1995) and the National Institutes of Health (NIH, 1996).

The NIH Consensus Development Conference in recognition of the diverse attitudes toward exercise and the epidemic of physical inactivity (Crespo et al., 1996) recommended that the appropriate type of activity is best determined by the individual's preference and what will be sustained. Specifically, the report states that people who are not active should accumulate at least 30 minutes of moderate-intensity physical activity daily by adding a few minutes each day until reaching their personal goal. The defined levels of efforts depend on individual characteristics such as baseline fitness and health status. The 30 minutes of moderate-intensity physical activity, such as brisk walking, can be initially met in three bouts of 10 minutes of physical activity throughout the day (NIH, 1996). This recommendation was similar to that of the American College of Sports Medicine and the Centers for Disease Control and Prevention guidelines that all adults perform 30 or more minutes of moderate-intensity physical activity on most, and preferably all, days—either in a single session or accumulated in multiple bouts, each lasting at least 8–10 minutes (Pate et al., 1995).

The new recommendations to accumulate 30 minutes of moderate-intensity physical activity (50 percent of a person's maximal oxygen uptake or VO_2 max on healthy adults, and 40 percent VO_2 max on persons with low fitness levels) is different from earlier recommendations to participate for 20–45 continuous minutes in vigorous-intensity physical activity (60 percent of a person's VO_2 max). It is also different in that the weekly frequency of exercise sessions increased from three times a week to five to seven days a week. This new recommendation takes into account the difference between exercising for fitness compared with exercising for health in general. This change has important public health implications, because now people who did not have the time or resources to take aside 45–60 minutes to engage in vigorous-intensity physical activity can now accumulate 30 minutes throughout the day. It is a public health message to stimulate the starting of an exercise program by segments of the population who have traditionally reported low levels of physical activity participation such as race/ethnic minorities and women (Crespo et al., 1999; Crespo et al., 2000; Crespo et al., 1996). This new physical activity public health message was incorporated into the most recent National Health Objectives, also known as Healthy People 2010.

The 2010 objectives reflect the scientific advances that have taken place over the past 20 years and have one single, overarching purpose: promoting health and preventing illness, disability, and premature death with the central goals of increasing the quality and years of healthy life and eliminating health disparities. Reducing disparities did not eliminate disparities.

The physical activity and fitness area of the Healthy People 2010 contains 15 objectives that deal exclusively with participation in physical activity. Of all the objectives and focus areas, the Healthy People 2010 have identified ten leading health indicators, and physical activity is one of these leading health indicators. This categorization shows that physical activity remains at the top of the public health agenda and underscores the need to allocate valuable resources to *eliminate the gap* between those who are active and those who are not. In 1991, 24 percent of Whites in the United States were physically inactive, while 28 percent of African Americans were inactive during leisure-time. Inactivity has since increased in all segments of the population, but the percent increase in African Americans is considerably much greater than the percent increase observed among Whites (52 percent compared with 36 percent, respectively) (see Table 25.1).

Differences in race/ethnicity show that minorities suffer disproportionately from chronic diseases that are more commonly observed among persons who are physically inactive (U.S. Department of Health and Human Services, 1996; Kington & Smith, 1997; Crespo et al., 2000; Centers for Disease Control and Prevention, 1998). For example, Blacks suffer disproportionately from higher rates of heart disease, stroke, and certain cancers than Whites, while Hispanics (especially Mexican Americans and Puerto Ricans) and American Indians have very high rates of Type II diabetes. While information about biological and genetic predispositions could explain some of these health disparities, it is the interaction between societal and other environmental factors that can provide better clues on how to prevent diseases and reduce the levels of physical inactivity observed in minority populations (Kington & Smith, 1997; Crespo et al., 1999; Power et al., 1999; Fraser et al., 1997; Montgomery & Carter-Pokras, 1993; Adams-Campbell et al., 2000; Brownson et al., 2001).

SOCIAL DETERMINANTS OF PHYSICAL INACTIVITY AMONG AFRICAN AMERICANS

Physical inactivity during leisure-time or no leisure-time physical activity (no LTPA) has been assessed in several national surveys such as the National Health Interview Survey, Behavioral Risk Factor Surveillance System, and the National Health and Nutrition Examination Survey. Participants were asked to specify from a list of activities what their participation level was. These surveys also allowed for persons to report any activity not previously mentioned. If persons answered that they did not participate in any activity, then these participants are classified as physically inactive during leisure time or persons who engage in "no LTPA." To assess and report levels of physical inactivity are relatively easier to do than to quantify how physically active a person is. Inactive means no participation in physical activities during leisure time, whereas physically active individuals may be minimally active for less than 30 minutes a week to three to four hours per week. Among African Americans, however, limiting the assessment of physical to only leisure-time physical activity may misclassify persons who engage in transportation or occupational physical activities (Young et al., 1998). In an urban population of African Americans in Baltimore, researchers found that participation in leisure-time physical activity was 18 percent for men and 16 percent for women, but when other forms of physical activity were included such as walking at or to work, physical activity participation

Table 25.1
Prevalence of no leisure-time physical activity in U.S. adults 18 years and older and target goals for the Healthy People 2000 and 2010

	Healthy People 2000			Healthy People 2010*	
No LTPA	Baseline, 1991	1995	Target	Baseline, 1997	Target
Non-Hispanic Whites[#]	24 percent	23 percent	15 percent	36 percent	20 percent
Non-Hispanic Blacks	28 percent	28 percent	20 percent	52 percent	20 percent
Hispanics	34 percent	31 percent	25 percent	54 percent	20 percent
American Indian/Alaska Native	29 percent	23 percent	21 percent	46 percent	20 percent
Asian Pacific Islanders	-	-	-	42 percent	20 percent

*During 1997 the questions used to assess participation in vigorous and light-to-moderate physical activity changed from those used in previous NHIS 1985–1995.
#Baseline for non-Hispanic Whites was established using the 1985 National Health Interview Survey; prevalence estimates for 1985 and 1991 were both 24 percent.

Source: The updated healthy people 2010 government website: http://www.healthypeople.gov/Document/HTML/Volume2/22Physical.htm.

increased to 41 percent and 38 percent in African American men and women, respectively (Young et al., 1998).

Thus, given the major challenges involved in accurately assessing varied levels of participation in physical activity and the lack of a national survey that assesses cardiorespiratory fitness or maximal aerobic capacity in all segments of society, we will use physical inactivity, or no LTPA, as the main health indicator to eliminate the disproportionate number of racial and ethnic minorities who are inactive when compared with Whites. Also, physical *inactivity* is the primary risk factor that has been recognized as an independent major risk factor for heart disease and other chronic conditions highly prevalent in African Americans. The major strategy of public health officials and health-care professionals is to move people who are predominantly in the inactive category to people who participate in some kind of physical activity most days of the week (see Figures 25.1 and 25.2).

Regional Differences

Regional differences show that, on average, physical inactivity is highest in Southeast, followed by the Northeast and Southwest and lowest in Northeast states (see Figure 25.1). Coincidentally, it

Figure 25.1
Percent of adults physically inactive in leisure-time

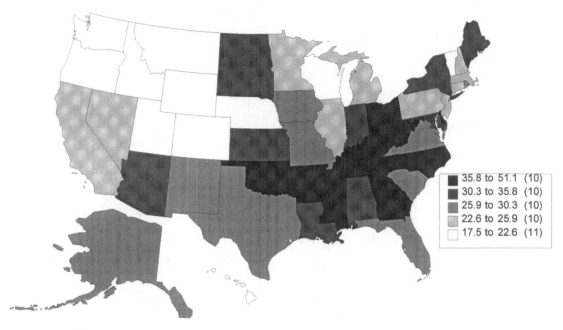

35.8 to 51.1 (10)
30.3 to 35.8 (10)
25.9 to 30.3 (10)
22.6 to 25.9 (10)
17.5 to 22.6 (11)

Behavioral Risk Factor Surveillance System, 1996.

Figure 25.2
Prevalence of no leisure-time physical activity by race/ethnicity in U.S. adults, 20 years and older

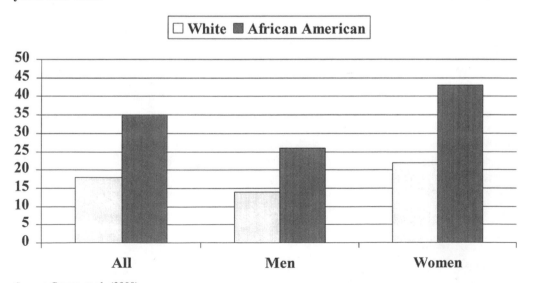

□ White ■ African American

Source: Crespo et al. (2000).

Table 25.2
Age-adjusted prevalence and ranking (per 100) of the ten
most frequently reported leisure-time physical activities
of the U.S. adult population aged 20 years and older,
1988 through 1991

| | Rank (percent) | | | |
| | White | | African American | |
Activity	Men	Women	Men	Women
Walking	2 (52)	1 (52)	1 (54)	1 (43)
Gardening or yard work	1 (65)	2 (47)	2 (44)	3 (24)
Calisthenics	3 (22)	3 (24)	3 (27)	4 (19)
Cycling	3 (22)	4 (23)	7 (20)	5 (14)
Jogging or running	6 (17)	8 (8)	5 (23)	7 (8)
Weight Lifting	7 (16)	8 (8)	6 (22)	8 (5)
Swimming	5 (18)	6 (15)	9 (5)	9 (3)
Other dancing*	8 (14)	5 (18)	4 (24)	2 (26)
Aerobics or aerobic dancing	- - -	7 (13)	- - -	6 (13)
Basketball	- - -	- - -	8 (18)	- - -
Tennis	- - -	10 (2)	- - -	- - -
Football	- - -	- - -	10 (4)	- - -
Softball or baseball	10 (6)	- - -	10 (4)	- - -
Golfing	9 (11)	- - -	- - -	- - -
Bowling	- - -	- - -	- - -	10 (2)

*Other dancing represents any types of dancing activity outside aerobic exercises or aerobic dancing

Source: Adapted from Crespo et al. (1996).

is noticeable that the percent of the population that is Black is highest in the southeast states followed by the northeast states. One of the few studies that have purposely oversampled African Americans is the Third National Health and Nutrition Examination Survey (NHANES III). The NHANES III oversampled minorities to more clearly characterize the prevalence of risk factors and health conditions in selected minority groups when examining age, sex, and race specific prevalence. NHANES III was designed to obtain a national representative sample of Blacks and Mexican Americans and found that the highest prevalence of physical inactivity was observed among African Americans and Mexican Americans (Figure 25.2) (Crespo et al., 2000).

Popular Activities

Among men, inactivity was somewhat comparable until 39 years of age. After age 40, African American men were twice as likely to report being physically inactive when compared with their

Figure 25.3
Age-specific prevalence of no leisure-time physical activity by race/ethnicity in men

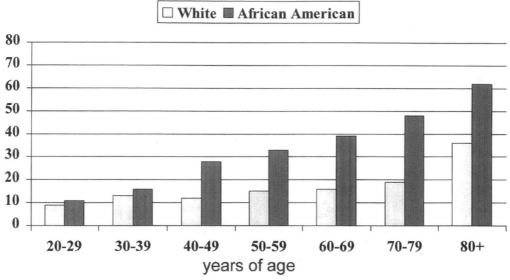

Source: Crespo et al. (2000).

White counterparts. Physical inactivity estimates among African American women were higher in every age group when compared with White women. Some of the similarities in the prevalence of physical activity observed between African American and White men aged 20–39 years may be due higher participation in team sports (e.g., basketball and football) among African American men. After 40 years of age, participation in these sports declined due to injury or not enough persons to create teams of same age-peers. On the other hand, White men may be engaging in sports or activities that can be maintained throughout their life. Walking and gardening are consistently popular activities among African Americans and Whites, but basketball and football were not in the top ten most popular activities among White men, whereas golf, swimming, and tennis were more popular among White men (see Table 25.2 and Figures 25.3 and 25.4).

Socioeconomic Class

Differences in social class are hypothesized to be one of the main reasons that health disparities exist in minorities populations (Winkleby et al., 1998). Measurement of social class and its relation to health indicators is complex. Education is mostly related to health behaviors such as physical activity; income is mostly associated with the things we can buy such as health insurance, prescription medication, and access to health care; and occupation is related to exposures to chemicals, among others (Liberatos et al., 1988). Table 25.2 shows that regardless of educational attainment or household earnings, African Americans were more physically inactive than Whites. One hypothesis is that African Americans may be employed in manual and hard-labor occupations that require higher energy expenditure than Whites, even when both have the same education and income levels (MMWR, 1993).

Figure 25.4
Age-specific prevalence of no leisure-time physical activity by race/ethnicity in women

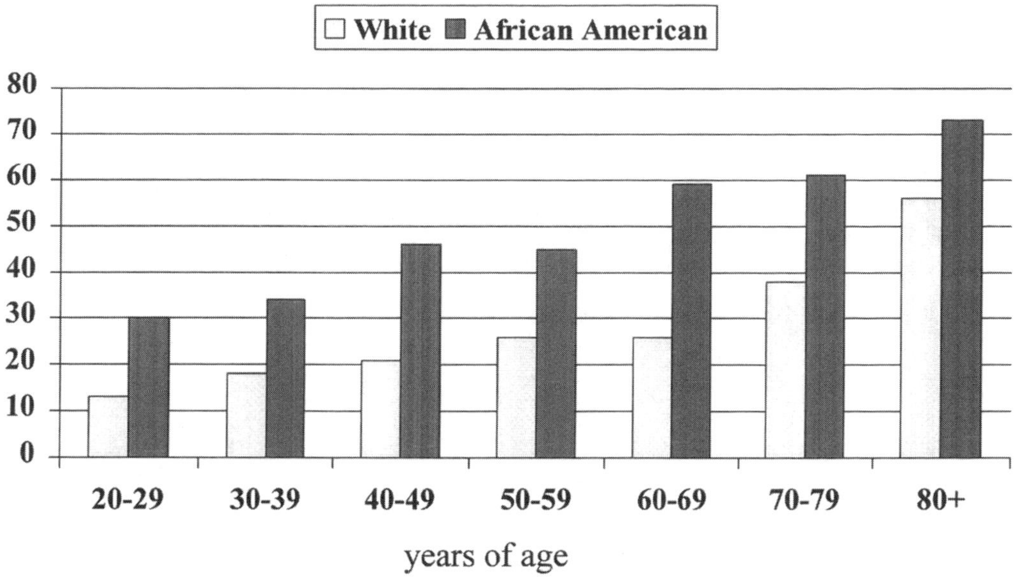

□ White   ■ African American

years of age

Source: Crespo et al. (2000).

Employment Status

A recent report using data from the 1990 National Health Interview Survey studied the percent of employed adults reporting participation in leisure-time physical activity and also hard occupational physical activity by race/ethnicity (MMWR Morbidity and Mortality and Weekly Report, 2000). Table 25.3 shows that White adults have the lowest levels of physical inactivity during leisure-time and the highest percentage of adults meeting the recommended guidelines of moderate-intensity physical activity for 30 minutes five or more days a week, and they also have the lowest percentages of employed adults who engage in heavy work for five or more hours a day. On the other hand, while 30.1 percent of African Americans are employed in jobs that required hard occupational activity five or more hours a week, only 21.9 percent of Whites engaged in hard labor for five or more hours a day (see Tables 25.3 and 25.4).

Occupational Status

We examined the prevalence of no leisure-time physical activity by different categories of occupation using the U.S. Census Occupational Classification Codes provided by NCHS and by information on retirement status and on being a homemaker (Crespo et al., 2000). We divided NHANES III participants into six occupational classifications: white-collar professionals; white-collar other, which includes those working in technical jobs and in offices; blue-collar workers who engage in mostly manual labors, farming, and unskilled jobs; those who reported being retired; homemakers; and other pursuits such as students or unemployed. Our results indicate that regardless of their occupational status, the prevalence of physical inactivity continued to be higher among African Americans than among Whites. For men, however, those who work in the "White-collar other"

Table 25.3
Percent of employed White, Black, and Hispanic adults who reported being sedentary during leisure-time, moderately active for 30 minutes, five or more days a week, and who reported hard occupational physical activity

	Leisure-time and occupational physical activity patterns		
	No leisure-time physical activity	Moderate leisure-time physical activity (30 min, 5 d/wk)	5+ hours of hard occupational activity
Non-Hispanic Whites	22.3 (20.9-23.7)	32.3 (31.2-33.4)	21.9 (20.9-22.9)
Non-Hispanic Blacks	28.8 (25.9-31.7)	30.3 (28.2-32.4)	30.1 (27.6-32.7)
Hispanics	33.9 (30.4-37.4)	26.6 (23.3-32.5)	33.0 (30.1-33.6)

Centers for Disease Control and Prevention (2000). Prevalence of Leisure-Time and Occupational Physical Activity Among Employed Adults—United States, 1990. *Morbidity Mortality Weekly Report, 49(19)*, 420–424.

category (mostly nonprofessional office workers) had physical inactivity levels that were similar between Whites and African Americans.

Among those who reported being in the "white-collar professionals" (e.g., doctors, lawyers, professors, managers), African American men had twice the age-adjusted rate of inactivity than those observed among Whites, and this was true for both men and women. Blue-collar workers' prevalence of physical inactivity was lowest among White men followed by African American men, and highest among African American women. Retired White men and both African American men and women were consistently the group with the highest levels of physical inactivity during leisure-time; this may be due to higher prevalence of chronic diseases in older ages (McGee et al., 1996); however, this was not evident among White women. Although homemakers are not viewed as employees, in our occupational classification system we were able to separate this group from other occupational categories. The sample size of White men who reported being a homemaker was too small to provide meaningful estimates, but we were able to compare levels of leisure-time inactivity among women who reported being homemakers as their main occupation. African American women had twice the levels of inactivity when compared with White women homemakers (see Tables 25.5 and 25.6).

PHYSICAL ACTIVITY THROUGH THE LIFESPAN

Physical Activity in African American Children

There have been very few studies examining the prevalence and determinants of physical activity in African American children. The Bogalusa Heart Study is the longest and most detailed study of Black and White children in the world. The focus is on understanding the early natural history of coronary artery disease and essential hypertension. Since 1972, this study, designed to be representative of the southeastern United States, was part of four National Institutes of Health-sponsored

Table 25.4
Age-adjusted prevalence of no leisure-time physical activity among non-Hispanic White, non-Hispanic Black, and Mexican American men and women aged 20 years and older according to social class indicator

Social Class Indicator	Whites		African Americans	
Men	N	mean $\pm$ SE	N	mean $\pm$ SE
Education$^\square$				
<12 y	1192	22 $\pm$ 2.1	913	33 $\pm$ 2.4***
12 y	1062	15 $\pm$ 1.3	765	22 $\pm$ 2.3*
13-15 y	624	13 $\pm$ 1.6	394	21 $\pm$ 3.2
16+ y	821	7 $\pm$ 1.1	193	14 $\pm$ 2.7**
Income†				
<$10,000	282	22 $\pm$ 4.5	423	40 $\pm$ 3.4***
$10,000-$19,999	887	21 $\pm$ 2.0	691	27 $\pm$ 2.3
$20,000-$34,999	906	15 $\pm$ 1.6	490	20 $\pm$ 2.6
$35,000-$49,999	594	10 $\pm$ 1.4	280	20 $\pm$ 2.7*
$50,000+	1065	10 $\pm$ 1.1	416	20 $\pm$ 2.4***
Women				
Education$^\square$				
<12 y	1295	36 $\pm$ 3.1	990	51 $\pm$ 2.4***
12 y	1559	25 $\pm$ 1.4	1018	45 $\pm$ 2.3***
13-15 y	804	15 $\pm$ 1.5	482	32 $\pm$ 3.1***
16+ y	709	14 $\pm$ 1.5	260	30 $\pm$ 3.2***
Income†				
<$10,000	566	30 $\pm$ 3.1	675	46 $\pm$ 3.9***
$10,000-$19,999	1025	27 $\pm$ 2.0	786	47 $\pm$ 2.2***
$20,000-$34,999	949	22 $\pm$ 2.0	531	38 $\pm$ 2.2***
$35,000-$49,999	622	16 $\pm$ 1.8	264	32 $\pm$ 3.2***
$50,000+	1250	20 $\pm$ 1.5	515	43 $\pm$ 2.8***

$\square$ Based on years of school completed.
$\dagger$ Based on total annual household income.
* $p < 0.05$; ** $p < 0.01$; *** $p < 0.001$; different from non-Hispanic whites.

Source: Crespo et al. (2000).

Figure 25.5
Occupation and prevalence of no leisure-time physical activity by race/ethnicity in men

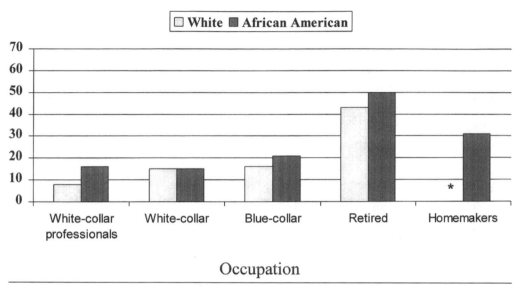

*Sample size too small to calculate prevalence estimates.

Source: Crespo et al. (2000).

Figure 25.6
Occupation and prevalence of no leisure-time physical activity by race/ethnicity in women

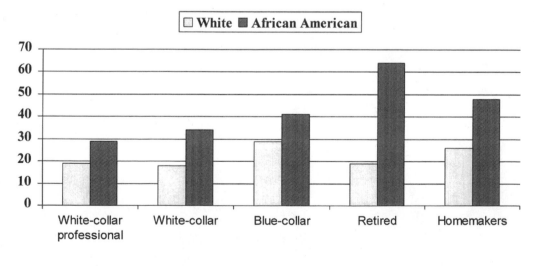

Source: Crespo et al. (2000).

Specialized Centers of Research (SCOR) at Louisiana State University Medical Center. Substudies from the Bogalusa Heart study have included investigating the relationship of socioeconomic status, blood pressure, lipids, genetics, exercise, heart murmurs, diabetes, and cardiovascular health. Currently, there is the post–high school study, which carries the children up to the age of 38, as well as a precursor study of children with/without parental history of myocardial infarction.

Multiple publications have described cross-sectional and longitudinal observations on more than 14,000 children and young adults in Bogalusa, Louisiana. Results from the Bogalusa Heart Study give a clear picture of the early natural history of C-V risk factors, early coronary artery disease, and essential hypertension in a total biracial population. Researchers at the University at Buffalo examined physical and sedentary activity in schoolchildren (Epstein et al., 1996). During this study a Self-Administered Physical Activity Checklist (SAPAC) was used to monitor sedentary and physical activity behaviors during the previous 24 hours among White and Black children. The checklist consisted of 21 physical activities, and spaces for four "other" activities were also provided. Additionally, television/video viewing and video/computer game playing (categorized as sedentary activity) were also monitored. Other information included physical education classes, recess time, and any other activities outside of school.

The importance of Epstein findings using the SAPAC is that it not only investigated the amount of physical activity and sedentary behaviors in a biracial group of children and adolescents but also reported the type of activity and the temporal structuring of the activity. Children spent an average of 168 minutes of physical activity per day. As expected, boys were more physically active than girls, regardless of race. White children were more likely to report outdoor play than Black children, as well as football and gymnastics, and they performed these activities for longer periods. On the other hand, more Black children participated in basketball, dance, and jump rope, and they spent more time in these activities than White children. Black children also spent more time doing selected sedentary activities than White children, both in total minutes and in percent of total reported activity. Interestingly, the study found a positive and significant relationship between reported minutes of physical activity and minutes of sedentary activity in both White and Black children. Thus, the more active the children, the more likely they are to engage in sedentary activities. Both physical and sedentary activities were more likely to occur outside of school hours. Not surprisingly, children who did not attend physical education classes had less total physical activity than those who did. Additionally, children did not compensate for lack of physical education classes by being more active outside of school hours.

We assessed the prevalence of television (TV) viewing using a national representative of White and African American children aged 8–16 years using the average of two questions that assessed hours of TV watching the previous day (see Figure 25.7). The two questions were asked about three to five weeks apart. Marked differences were noted between the percent of White and African American children who reported watching four or more hours of TV a day. Almost 40 percent of African American children watched four or more hours a day of television for both boys and girls, compared with 16 percent and 12 percent of White boys and girls, respectively (Crespo et al., 2001; Andersen et al., 1998).

The increasing amount of time that minority children spent watching television is of public health concerns because of alarming and disproportionate prevalence of obesity in minority children (Ogden et al., 2002). Investigators have attempted to manipulate the choice of sedentary behaviors with physical activity and food intake (Epstein et al., 2002; Goldfield et al., 2001; Epstein, 1996). They have found that allowing children to freely negotiate and choose the time spent in sedentary pursuits and in physical activities of their choice can have significant implications in adopting a more active lifestyle.

The majority of the research aimed at reducing sedentary behaviors and increasing healthful eating and physical activity has been conducted in White children (Robinson, 1999). Ford et al. (2002)

Figure 25.7
Prevalence (per 100) of daily television watching habits among White and African American children aged 8 to 16 years

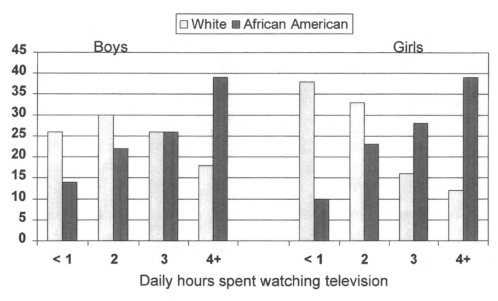

Source: NHANES III, 1988 to 1994.

conducted a randomized, controlled pilot study among 28 families with African American children between the ages of 7 and 12 years who received primary care at an urban community clinic. The main aim of the study was to use a primary care setting to reduce hours of children's television, videotape, and video game use in African American children. All families (intervention and control groups) received a brief 5 to 10 minutes of counseling followed by a prepared script. The behavioral intervention received an additional 15- to 20-minute discussion about setting television budgets, and parents received a brochure about parental guidance in lowering children's TV viewing. An electronic television time manager would control power to the television, videotapes, and video games. This device would lock the power plug to these appliances and allow for monitoring and budgeting viewing time for each member of the household through the use of a four-digit personal identification number. The intervention group reported reduced time watching television, videotapes, or video games compared with the control group. More importantly in this feasibility study, they found a significant increase in weekly hours of organized physical activity in the behavioral intervention group compared to the control (counseling-only) group (Kimm et al., 2002).

Determinants of physical activity among African American children have been studied with regard to the psychological, environmental, and sociocultural influences (Trost et al., 1999; Lindquist et al., 1997; Pate et al., 2002). Trost et al. (1999) assessed psychosocial and environmental variables and their impact in influencing physical activity in a group of 119 African American sixth graders from four public middle schools in South Carolina. The psychosocial variables measured self-efficacy, social influences, and belief outcomes. The environmental variables included perceived physical activity behaviors of parents and peers, access to sporting and/or fitness equipment at home, involvement in community physical activity organizations, participation in community sports teams over the preceding six months, and self-reported hours spent watching television or playing video games. The results showed that active African American boys exhibited higher levels of self-efficacy about physical activity and also reported greater involvement in community-based, physical activity organizations than low-active boys. Active African American girls were more likely to have higher levels of physical activity and self-efficacy and higher scores on the beliefs regarding physical activity outcomes (e.g., keep me in shape, make me more attractive, be more fun than less active African American girls). Self-efficacy—the belief that a person possesses the ability to perform a particular behavior—has been consistently an important predictor of physical activity in children and adults regardless of race.

Another study in Alabama included 120 healthy African American and White children followed for 5 years, ages 6–13 years. Sociocultural and physiological variables included sex, race, age, single-two-parent home, pubertal development, and social class. The researchers found single-parent home status to be significantly related to higher sedentary behavior such as time spent watching television independent of race. On average, children of single-parent homes watched 30 more minutes of television per day than children of two-parent homes (Lindquist et al., 1997).

Because of the alarming trend in obesity, researchers have been interested in learning more about physical activity changes of children and adolescents (Kimm et al., 2002; Trost et al., 1999; Lindquist et al., 1999; Gordon-Larsen et al., 1999; Desmond et al., 1990; Crespo et al., 2001; Kimm et al., 2002). A prospective cohort of 1,213 Black girls and 1,166 White girls enrolled in the National Heart, Lung, and Blood Institute Growth and Health Study was monitored from ages 9–10 years until ages 18–19 years. Physical activity was reported in Metabolic Equivalents or METs. One MET is equal to 3.5 ml/Oxygen per minute per kilogram of body weight and is the equivalent of energy expenditure of a person at rest. Different activities have different energy expenditures or METs; the higher the METs, the greater the energy expenditure (Ainsworth et al., 2000). For example, brisk walking has an MET value of approximately 3.5 while running has an MET value of 7–10+ depending on the intensity. Using this method of physical activity assessment during leisure-time, Kimm et al. (2002), found that by the age of 16–17 years, 56 percent of Black girls and 31 percent of White girls reported no habitual leisure-time physical activity. A significant deterrent of physical activity among Black girls was pregnancy, while cigarette smoking was significantly associated with a decline in physical activity among White girls. Higher body mass index (BMI = wt/h^2) was associated with greater decline in activity among both Black and White girls.

Physical Activity in African American Adolescents

The information presented on children demonstrates higher levels of sedentary behaviors (e.g., television viewing) and lower levels of physical activity participation among African American children than among White children. To what extent these behaviors track into adolescence is of public health importance. Kimm et al. (2002) showed a significantly higher decline in Black girls' physical activity into adolescence than White girls (Kimm et al., 2002). We have also reported substantial decline in physical activity levels among African American girls, as well as among White girls (Andersen et al., 1998; Crespo et al., 2001), while boys tend to stay equally active or increase physical activity levels as they go from childhood into adolescence. The National Longitudinal Study of Adolescent Health was designed to determine the extent to which health behavior patterns, such as physical activity, vary by ethnicity among subpopulations of U.S. adolescents. This is nationally representative data with more than 14,000 U.S. adolescents, including 3,135 non-Hispanic Blacks, 2,446 Hispanics, and 976 Asians. Again, physical inactivity—assessed as time spent watching television or playing video or computer games—was greater among Black adolescents than White adolescents. Participation in five or more bouts of moderate to vigorous-intensity physical activity of 5–8 METs were lowest among female and minority adolescents. With the exception of Asian females, minorities were more inactive than their White counterparts. While the levels of physical activity between White and Black adolescents were not drastically different, the levels of physical inactivity were significantly higher in Black adolescents. These findings persisted after controlling for sex, age, urban residence, socioeconomic status, in-school status, and month of interview (Gordon-Larsen et al., 1999).

Physical fitness and perception of exercise were measured in urban Black and White adolescents in 24 Black and 20 White students. Using the Health Belief Model—where a person's health-related behavior is believed to be dependent on the perception of four critical areas: severity of a potential illness, person's susceptibility to that illness, benefit of taking a preventive action, and barriers to taking action—a standardized Harvard Step Test was used to assess physical fitness, and the adolescents were also asked to assess their own perception of their level of fitness. Black adolescents were more successful at self-classification than White students with regard to their own fitness levels. Of interest was that 38 percent of Black and 27 percent of White adolescents in good physical fitness condition stated that they did not engage in regular aerobic exercise. One hypothesis is that these adolescents may be active but do not perceive their activity as aerobic exercise but as games they play with their friends. Both Black and White adolescents had several serious misperceptions about exercise. For example, there was wide agreement with the concept of "no pain, no gain"; how fast you run is more important than how far you run; and wearing extra layers of clothes while exercising will help the body rid itself of body fat. These misperceptions should be addressed in health education and physical education classes in schools (Desmond et al., 1990). Other studies have found participation in organized sports, friend support, and nurture from biological fathers to be significantly associated with higher physical activity among African American adolescents (Bungum & Vincent, 1997).

In summary, physical inactivity is consistently higher among African American children and adolescents than among their White counterparts. It is also apparent that inactive children become inactive adolescents, and more importantly the percent of physically active African American girls who become less active as they grow into adolescence is of clinical and public health significance given the associated diseases associated with physical inactivity (e.g., high blood pressure, Type II diabetes, and obesity). Strategies to increase participation in physical activity among minority children should take advantage of well-developed interventions among White children such as budgeting of TV time, negotiating sedentary time, providing safe environments for play and games, and improving curricula that teach lifetime skills to engage in exercise programs and physical activity pursuits (Bungum & Vincent, 1997).

LTPA in College-Aged African Americans

Few studies have described physical activity patterns of African American college students. Emerging evidence has demonstrated an epidemic of physical inactivity among African American children and adolescents and also the disproportionate levels of sedentary lifestyles in minority adults (Crespo et al., 1996; Crespo et al., 2001; Andersen et al., 1998; Crespo et al., 2000; Kimm et al., 2002). College-aged students are at a unique point in life where for the first time they are living outside of their homes and are now more responsible for making independent decisions in how they manage their time. Most institutions of higher education offer safe and suitable environments for students to participate in exercise training programs.

Kelley et al. (1998) investigated physical activity habits of African American college students attending a historically Black college and confirmed the alarming levels of physical inactivity among African American female students when compared with their male counterparts. Whereas 42 percent of male college-students were classified as low or very low-active, 65 percent of African American female college students reported being in the same category. Of those who reported being in the high to moderately active category, the most common forms of physical activity for males were moving heavy objects, weightlifting, shoveling snow, and strenuous sports such as basketball, football, skating or skiing. Other less strenuous, but popular, activities for male students included softball, shooting baskets, volleyball, Ping-Pong, leisurely jogging, swimming, and walking or hiking. The most popular high-intensity physical activity included running or jogging and exercise dancing, while the most common moderate-intensity activities were walking and hiking and home exercises. There is a clear gender difference in the amount and variety of physical activities practiced (Kelley et al., 1998). Adderley-Kelly assessed health behaviors of undergraduate African American female nursing students and found that although these students practice healthy behaviors with regard to smoking, substance abuse, nutrition, and stress control, a high percent of students had low levels of exercise and fitness behaviors. Only 16 percent of these African American nursing students reported having an excellent score in their health and fitness category. This is of concern because these undergraduate (junior class) nursing students will be the future health professionals who will teach health promotion and disease promotion in predominantly African American communities (Adderley-Kelly & Green, 2000).

Physical Activity in African American Women

As previously observed in Table 25.4, physical inactivity is greater among women, but certain distinctive patterns are observed among African American women. For example, the prevalence of physical inactivity is highest among African American women with low household annual income (<$20,000), but it is also unexpectedly high among African American women in the highest annual household income bracket ($50,000 or more) when compared with their White counterparts. One possible explanation is that African American women who live in a household with an annual income of $50,000 may need to spend more time at work in order to be in that income bracket (Crespo et al., 1999, 2000; Sweeney, 1999).

In 1995, 64,524 African American women aged 21 to 69 years were enrolled in the Black's Women Health Study. A questionnaire collected information on time spent walking for exercise, in moderate activities such as housework and gardening, and in strenuous physical activities such as running, aerobics, basketball, and swimming. Fifty-seven percent reported an hour or less per week walking for exercise, while 18 percent reported engaging in moderate activities and 61 percent in strenuous activities. Lack of participation in walking for exercise was 19 percent, 2 percent for moderate activities, and 34 percent reported engaging in no strenuous activities (Kumanyika et al., 1999).

The Coronary Artery Risk Development in Young Adults study (CARDIA) recruited a large sample of Black and White women aged 18 to 30 years. Physical activity patterns were assessed in a large sample of Black and White women (N = 1,408 and N = 1,250, respectively) and found that on average African American women were less physically active during the past year but more physically active before high school when compared with White women. The most common activities among African American women were walking, dancing, and home exercises, and the least common were swimming and racket sports. The largest race difference in participation rates (with White women doing more) were observed for swimming, followed by biking and leisure sports. Being married was negatively related to physical activity scores in White women, but no association in between marital status and physical activity was observed in African American women. Married, divorced, and never-married African American women, however, had significantly lower physical activity scores than their White counterparts. Similar findings were observed when the number of children being parented was taken into account (Bild et al., 1993).

In an attempt to better understand which predictors are most important in influencing high rates

Figure 25.8
Marital status and prevalence of no leisure-time physical activity by race/ethnicity in men

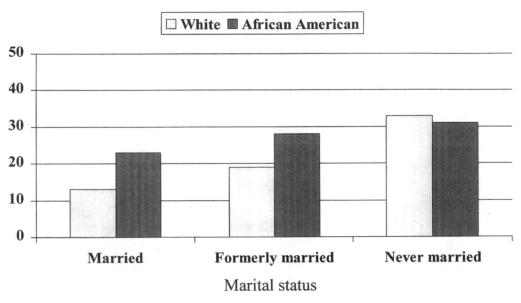

Source: Crespo et al. (2000).

of participation in leisure-time physical activity among urban White, African American, and Mexican American women, Ransdell and Wells (1998) found that the only variable that was a significant predictor of high physical activity participation in White women was education. Among minority women, the only significant predictor of physical activity was marital status (Ransdell & Wells, 1998).

We examined if marital status was related to physical inactivity during leisure-time (Crespo et al., 2000). Our results illustrate that married men, especially White and Black men, have the lowest age-adjusted prevalence of no LTPA when compared to the formerly married and never married men. For women, however, the prevalence of physical inactivity was not related to marital status. Prevalence estimates for non-Hispanic White and Black women and Mexican American women did not change substantially whether they were married or not. Thus, married men may be at an advantage with regard to participation in leisure-time physical activity, partially because they may have more free time to engage in recreational pursuits. Working mothers are working more hours in order to earn the same salary as men, subtracting valuable time from the little free time available to exercise. While the number of hours that husbands spent at work has not changed in the past 25 years, the number of hours that women spent at work has increased (see Figures 25.8–25.10).

Brownson et al. (2000) studied the patterns and correlates of physical activity in a multiracial group of U.S. women 40 years and older (Brownson et al., 2000). The findings confirmed high levels of physical inactivity among African American and American Indian/Alaskan Native women while participation in vigorous-intensity physical activity was the lowest among the same race/ethnic groups. Women living in rural regions were also more likely than urban inhabitants to be completely inactive during leisure-time. In a study of a rural African American community, Malone (1997) found seasonal variations in participation rates in physical activity with higher levels in the spring and the summer. In this rural community there was less physical activity associated with work in

Figure 25.9
Marital status and prevalence of no leisure-time physical activity by race/ethnicity in women

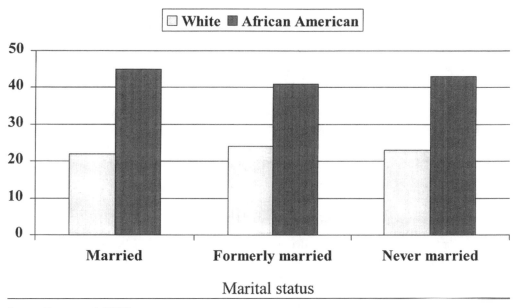

Source: Crespo et al. (2000).

Figure 25.10
The time crunch, families, and the labor market, 1969–1996

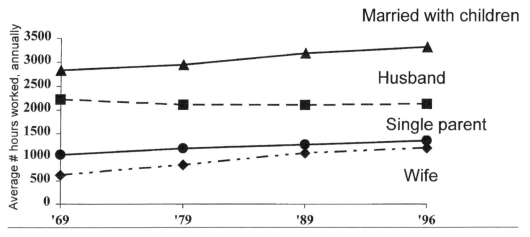

Families with at least one child under age 18 years.

Source: The Washington Post, May 25, 1999, Report from Council of Economic Advisers.

winter as compared to summer. No significant differences in activity levels between smoker and nonsmokers were observed. One important finding from this study is that the quantity of physical activity performed might not be adequately assessed by routine questions related to activity levels of urban populations. In fact, the residents in this study spent approximately 1,500 minutes per week in moderate-intensity physical activity, which is 12 times more than the minimal recommendation of approximately 90 to 120 minutes. Thus, it is important to take into account the different types of activities of rural population and the seasonal variations involved in considering not only leisure-time physical activities but also occupational and transportation physical activities in a rural African American community (Malone, 1997).

One study found that older women may be more fearful of engaging in leisure-time physical activity if they perceived that the crime in their neighborhood was high (MMWR, 1999). This barrier was less significant among men. Since minorities tend to live in areas with high poverty, the interaction between poverty-area residences and changes in physical activity in minority populations is of research interest. Findings from the Alameda County Study suggest that these two are linked and deserve further validation in other communities (Yen & Kaplan, 1998).

Physical Activity in Older African Americans

It is not clear if lack of exercise in older African Americans is primarily due to lack of lifetime habits to participate in exercise programs or if the concomitant increase in chronic diseases that disproportionately affect African Americans are partially responsible for the lack of physical activity observed in older African American men and women. In a study of cardiovascular risk factors of older U.S. adults, age 65–84 years, Sundquist et al. (2001) reported increased levels of Type II diabetes, physical inactivity, abdominal obesity, and hypertension among African American women when compared with White women. African American men had higher levels of Type II diabetes, physical inactivity, and hypertension than their White counterparts. No significant differences were observed for smoking habits or blood cholesterol. In this national sample of older women and men, African American men demonstrated the higher prevalence of cardiovascular disease risk factors even after taking into account age and socioeconomic status (Sundquist et al., 2001).

We have presented data that support the notion that among retired African American men and women, lack of leisure-time physical activity is very high (see Figures 25.3 and 25.4) (Crespo et al., 2000). The Atherosclerosis Risk in Communities Study (ARIC) investigated prospectively the influence of retirement on leisure-time physical activity and found participation in exercise or sports increased significantly for retirees over the six-year period in African American and White men and women. Researchers investigated whether work activity was replaced with sport and leisure activities and found no differences in sport activities after retirement for African American and White women; however, for African American men sport scores declined significantly across all occupational categories. When retired persons were compared with those who continued to work, retirement was associated with a significant increase in sports and exercise participation, as well as television watching over a six-year period. Among those physically active at baseline, retirement was associated with maintaining their physical activity participation when compared with those who continued to work. Among those who were sedentary at baseline, however, retirement was associated with adoption of physical activity when compared with those who continued to work. Walking, gardening, yard work, and mowing were the most commonly adopted activities. Race-gender differences show the largest gain in sport participation occurring among those with the lowest work scores (e.g., the least active at work) reaching significance for African American and White men only. This study highlights the importance of knowing more about interactions of retirement, employment, and physical activity among minorities, especially as they enter a new stage in their life where work activity is significantly reduced.

One study examined the effect of exercise and dietary behavior in African American elders through the "stages of change" model. The stages of change model suggests that individuals move through five stages of change: (1) precontemplation—no intention to change; (2) contemplation—aware that a problem exists; (3) preparation—plan to take new action soon; (4) action—modification of behavior is initiated; and (5) maintenance—consistently engaging in new behavior (Prochaska et al., 1988). Thirty-seven African American elders with hypertension age 55–87 years and predominantly female (70.3 percent) were interviewed regarding their diet and exercise behaviors as part of a pilot study. As a group, these elders scored higher on the contemplation, action, and maintenance stages in regard to exercise than on the precontemplation stage. These findings suggest that African American elders are not necessarily resistant to change and can be motivated to adopt new healthy behaviors and are not "set in their ways." These results also highlight the need to tailor intervention programs to match elders' current stage of change, rather than assuming that they are all at the same stage. For example, elders in the precontemplation stage need more educational and attitudinal intervention about exercise, while elders in the maintenance stage need continued access to activities and locations where they can continue to exercise (Davis, 2000).

FUTURE RESEARCH AND POSSIBLE OBSTACLES IN MINORITY PHYSICAL ACTIVITY

We need more research to understand the social and environmental barriers that interfere with racial and ethnic minorities to freely exercise in their neighborhood. Other promising areas of research to increase participation in physical activity among women and minorities may include access to affordable fitness facilities, child care, crime prevention, and culturally appropriate social marketing.

As a public health measure, increasing the amount of physical activity in the school, either by enforcing the current physical education requirements or by requiring more school-based physical education, could have a significant impact on the overall physical activity of children.

Healthy People 2000 recognized the importance of clinicians' counseling about physical activity; unfortunately, fewer than 15 percent of all clinicians formulated an exercise plan for their patients. Only 25 percent of internists did so; all estimates were well below the goal of 50 percent. *Healthy People 2010* does not include an objective to track the percent of physicians who advise their patients about exercise. Yet, it is clear that for racial and ethnic minorities the advice of a clinician to adopt an active lifestyle is important. Moreover, it is imperative that clinicians take into account the different environments that surround the life of minorities. Culturally appropriate advice may include empathic suggestions that take into account the preferred activities rather than "telling" patients to exercise.

Racial and ethnic minorities hold in high esteem family relationships, faith-based organizations, social gatherings, and respect for authority. Clinicians, health educators, and fitness specialists should use these social and cultural institutions as frameworks in planning exercise programs for the different race/ethnic groups they come in contact with. More over, those planning interventions aimed at female adolescents and minorities should consider using unique strategies for specific ethnic group and age subgroups. There are also ample opportunities for physicians to have an impact on the physical activity of minorities by using their community standing to influence school policies and to counsel patients individually during office visits (Bungum et al., 1997; Ford et al., 2002).

SUMMARY

In summary, we describe disparities in physical inactivity among minority populations and the need to understand specific barriers affecting racial and ethnic minorities. The prevalence of physical inactivity is higher in women than in men, but it is highest among minority women. We know that the types of physical activities in which racial and ethnic minorities prefer to participate are different from those of Whites. For example, social dancing consistently was one of the top five physical activities reported among African American men and women and also among White women. White men reported golf as one of their top ten activities, whereas African American men reported basketball and football as popular activities. Walking and gardening consistently ranked in the "top three" list for all groups. However, the advice to go for a walk cannot be generalized to all segments of society since certain neighborhoods may be perceived as less safe than others.

The national health objectives for the year 2010 provide an excellent opportunity for clinicians to intervene at the individual as well as the community level. All the physical activity objectives provide target goals to increase physical activity among all race/ethnic, gender, and age groups. Children are advised to engage in fewer sedentary pursuits such as less time watching television. There are objectives for communities to support and facilitate walking and bicycling trips and for schools to increase the number and quality of physical education classes. In contrast to previous national health objectives, the target goal for each objective will be the same for all racial/ethnic groups. Thus, the benefit of an active lifestyle will be a major priority for all segments of society. Finally, as opposed to other public health interventions that may prove costly, an active lifestyle will benefit everyone. Physical activity is today's best buy in public health because it is free, simple, safe, and effective in preventing heart disease, diabetes, certain cancers, stroke, obesity, stress, depression, and other diseases.

REFERENCES

Adams-Campbell, L.L., Rosenberg, L., Washburn, R.A., Rao, R.S., Kim, K.S., & Palmer, J. (2000). Descriptive epidemiology of physical activity in African-American women. *Preventive Medicine, 30*, 43–50.

Adderley-Kelly, B. & Green, P.M. (2000). Health behaviors of undergraduate African American nursing students. *Association of Black Nursing Faculty Journal, 11*, 7–12.

Ainsworth, B.E., Haskell, W.L., Whitt, M.C., Irwin, M.L., Swartz, A.M., Strath, S.J., O'Brien, W.L., Bassett, D.R., Jr., Schmitz, K.H., Emplaincourt, P.O., Jacobs, D.R., Jr., & Leon, A.S. (2000). Compendium of physical activities: an update of activity codes and MET intensities. *Medicine and Science in Sports and Exercise, 32*, S498–S504.

Andersen, R.E., Crespo, C.J., Bartlett, S.J., Cheskin, L.J., & Pratt, M. (1998). Relationship of physical activity and television watching with body weight and level of fatness among children: results from the Third National Health and Nutrition Examination Survey. *Journal of the American Medical Association, 279*, 938–942.

Bild, D.E., Jacobs, D.R., Jr., Sidney, S., Haskell, W.L., Anderssen, N., & Oberman, A. (1993). Physical activity in young Black and White women. The CARDIA Study. *Annals of Epidemiology, 3*, 636–644.

Brownson, R.C., Baker, E.A., Housemann, R.A., Brennan, L.K., & Bacak, S.J. (2001). Environmental and policy determinants of physical activity in the United States. *American Journal of Public Health, 91*, 1995–2003.

Brownson, R.C., Eyler, A.A., King, A.C., Brown, D.R., Shyu, Y.L., & Sallis, J.F. (2000). Patterns and correlates of physical activity among U.S. women 40 years and older. *American Journal of Public Health, 90*, 264–270.

Bungum, T.J., & Vincent, M.L. (1997). Determinants of physical activity among female adolescents. *American Journal of Preventive Medicine, 13*, 115–122.

Centers for Disease Control and Prevention. (1998). Forecasted state-specific estimates of self-reported asthma prevalence—United States, 1998. *Morbidity and Mortality Weekly Report, 47*, 1022–1025.

Crespo, C.J., Ainsworth, B.E., Keteyian, S.J., Heath, G.W., & Smit, E. (1999). Prevalence of physical inactivity and its relation to social class in U.S. adults: Results from the Third National Health and Nutrition Examination Survey, 1988–1994. *Medicine and Science in Sports and Exercise, 31*, 1821–1827.

Crespo, C.J., Keteyian, S.J., Heath, G.W., & Sempos, C.T. (1996). Leisure-time physical activity among U.S. adults. Results from the Third National Health and Nutrition Examination Survey. *Archives Internal Medicine, 156,* 93–98.

Crespo, C.J., Smit, E., Andersen, R.E., Carter-Pokras, O., & Ainsworth, B.E. (2000). Race/ethnicity, social class and their relation to physical inactivity during leisure time: Results from the Third National Health and Nutrition Examination Survey, 1988–1994. *American Journal Preventive Medicine, 18,* 46–53.

Crespo, C.J., Smit, E., Troiano, R.P., Bartlett, S.J., Macera, C.A., & Andersen, R.E. (2001). Television watching, energy intake, and obesity in U.S. children: Results from the third National Health and Nutrition Examination Survey, 1988–1994. *Archives of Pediatric Adolescent Medicine, 155,* 360–365.

Davis, L. (2000). Exercise and dietary behaviors in African American elders: Stages of change in efficacy expectancies. *Journal of the Association of Black Nursing Faculty, 11,* 56–58.

Desmond, S.M., Price, J.H., Lock, R.S., Smith, D., & Stewart, P.W. (1990). Urban Black and White adolescents' physical fitness status and perceptions of exercise. *Journal School Health, 60,* 220–226.

Epstein, L.H. (1996). Family-based behavioural intervention for obese children. *International Journal of Obesity, 20 Suppl 1,* S14–S21.

Epstein, L.H., Coleman, K.J., & Myers, M.D. (1996). Exercise in treating obesity in children and adolescents. *Medicine and Science in Sports and Exercise, 28,* 428–435.

Epstein, L.H., Paluch, R.A., Consalvi, A., Riordan, K., & Scholl, T. (2002). Effects of manipulating sedentary behavior on physical activity and food intake. *Journal of Pediatrics, 140,* 334–339.

Ford, B.S., McDonald, T.E., Owens, A.S., & Robinson, T.N. (2002). Primary care interventions to reduce television viewing in African-American children. *American Journal of Preventive Medicine, 22,* 106–109.

Fraser, G.E., Sumburcru, D., Pribis, P., Neil, R.L., & Frankson, M.A. (1997). Association among health habits, risk factors, and all-cause mortality in a Black California population. *Epidemiology, 8,* 168–174.

Goldfield, G.S., Epstein, L.H., Kilanowski, C.K., Paluch, R.A., & Kogut-Bossler, B. (2001). Cost-effectiveness of group and mixed family-based treatment for childhood obesity. *International Journal of Obesity and Related Metabolic Disorders, 25,* 1843–1849.

Gordon-Larsen, P., McMurray, R.G., & Popkin, B.M. (1999). Adolescent physical activity and inactivity vary by ethnicity: The National Longitudinal Study of Adolescent Health. *J Pediatr, 135,* 301–306.

Kelley, G.A., Lowing, L., & Kelley, K. (1998). Psychological readiness of Black college students to be physically active. *Journal American College Health, 47,* 83–87.

Kimm, S.Y., Glynn, N.W., Kriska, A.M., Barton, B.A., Kronsberg, S.S., Daniels, S.R., Crawford, P.B., Sabry, Z.I., & Liu, K. (2002). Decline in physical activity in Black girls and White girls during adolescence. *New England Journal of Medicine, 347,* 709–715.

Kington, R.S. & Smith, J.P. (1997). Socioeconomic status and racial and ethnic differences in functional status associated with chronic diseases. *AJPH, 87,* 805–810.

Kumanyika, S.K., Adams-Campbell, L., Van Horn, B., Ten Have, T.R., Treu, J.A., Askov, E., Williams, J., Achterberg, C., Zaghloul, S., Monsegu, D., Bright, M., Stoy, D.B., Malone-Jackson, M., Mooney, D., Deiling, S., & Caulfield, J. (1999). Outcomes of a cardiovascular nutrition counseling program in African-Americans with elevated blood pressure or cholesterol level. *Journal of the American Dietary Association, 99,* 1380–1391.

Liberatos, P., Link, B.G., & Kelsey, J.L. (1988). The measurement of social class in epidemiology. *Epidemiol Review, 10,* 87–121.

Lindquist, C.H., Reynolds, K.D., & Goran, M.I. (1999). Sociocultural determinants of physical activity among children. *Preventive Medicine, 29,* 305–312.

Lindquist, T.L., Beilin, L.J., & Knuiman, M.W. (1997). Influence of lifestyle, coping, and job stress on blood pressure in men and women. *Hypertension, 29,* 1–7.

Malone, C.M. (1997). The prevalence of physical activity or inactivity in a rural African American community. *Journal of National Black Nurses Association, 9,* 58–65.

McGee, D., Cooper, R., Liao, Y., & Durazo-Arvizu, R. (1996). Patterns of comorbidity and mortality risk in Blacks and Whites. *Annals of Epidemiology, 6,* 381–385.

MMWR (1993). Prevalence of sedentary lifestyle—Behavioral Risk Factor Surveillance System, United States, 1991. *Morbidity and Mortality Weekly Report, 42*, 576–579.

MMWR (1999). Neighborhood safety and the prevalence of physical inactivity—selected states, 1996. *Morbidity and Mortality Weekly Report, 48*, 143–146.

MMWR (2000). Prevalence of leisure-time and occupational physical activity among employed adults, United States, 1990. *Morbidity and Mortality Weekly Report*, 420–424.

Montgomery, L.E. & Carter-Pokras, O. (1993). Health status by social class and/or minority status: Implications for environmental equity research. *Toxicology and Industrial Health, 9*, 729–773.

National Institutes of Health. (1996). Physical activity and cardiovascular health. NIH Consensus Development Panel on Physical Activity and Cardiovascular Health. *JAMA, 276*, 241–246.

Nieman, D.C. (1999). *Exercise testing and prescription: A health related approach*. Mountain View, CA: Mayfield.

Ogden, C.L., Flegal, K.M., Carroll, M.D., & Johnson, C.L. (2002). Prevalence and trends in overweight among U.S. children and adolescents, 1999–2000. *Journal of the American Medical Association, 288*, 1728–1732.

Pate, R.R., Freedson, P.S., Sallis, J.F., Taylor, W.C., Sirard, J., Trost, S.G., & Dowda, M. (2002). Compliance with physical activity guidelines: Prevalence in a population of children and youth. *Annals of Epidemiology, 12*, 303–308.

Pate, R.R., Pratt, M., Blair, S.N., Haskell, W.L., Macera, C.A., Bouchard, C., Buchner, D., Ettinger, W., Heath, G.W., & King, A.C. (1995). Physical activity and public health. A recommendation from the Centers for Disease Control and Prevention and the American College of Sports Medicine. *Journal of the American Medical Association, 273*, 402–407.

Power, M.L., Heaney, R.P., Kalkwarf, H.J., Pitkin, R.M., Repke, J.T., Tsang, R.C., & Schulkin, J. (1999). The role of calcium in health and disease. *American Journal Obstetrics Gynecology, 181*, 1560–1569.

Prochaska, J.O., Velicer, W.F., Diclemente, C.C., & Fava, J. (1988). Measuring processes of change: Applications to the cessation of smoking. *Journal Consulting Clinical Psychology, 56*, 520–528.

Ransdell, L.B., & Wells, C.L. (1998). Physical activity in urban White, African-American, and Mexican-American women. *Med Sci Sports Exerc, 30*, 1608–1615.

Robinson, T.N. (1999). Reducing children's television viewing to prevent obesity: A randomized controlled trial. *JAMA, 282*, 1561–1567.

Sundquist, J., Winkleby, M.A., & Pudaric, S. (2001). Cardiovascular disease risk factors among older Black, Mexican-American, and White women and men: An analysis of NHANES III, 1988–1994. Third National Health and Nutrition Examination Survey. *Journal of the American Geriatric Society, 49*, 109–116.

Sweeney, M.M. (1999). Gender, race, and changing families: The shifting economic foundations of marriage [abstract]. *Dissertation Abstracts International, 59*, 3663.

Trost, S.G., Pate, R.R., Ward, D.S., Saunders, R., & Riner, W. (1999). Determinants of physical activity in active and low-active, sixth grade African-American youth. *Journal of School Health, 69*, 29–34.

U.S. Department of Health and Human Services (USDHHS). (1996a). From the Centers for Disease Control and Prevention/National Center for Health Statistics—Health Status Indicator Reports—"State of the Art". *Healthy People 2000*, 8.

U.S. Department of Health and Human Services (USDHHS). (1996b). The surgeon general's report on physical activity and health. U.S. Department of Health and Human Services, Public Health Services, Centers for Disease Control and Prevention, National Center for Chronic Disease Prevention and Health Promotion.

Winkleby, M.A., Kraemer, H.C., Ahn, D.K., & Varady, A.N. (1998). Ethnic and socioeconomic differences in cardiovascular disease risk factors: Findings for women from the Third National Health and Nutrition Examination Survey, 1988–1994. *Journal of the American Medical Association, 280*, 356–362.

Yen, I.H. & Kaplan, G.A. (1998). Poverty area residence and changes in physical activity level: Evidence from the Alameda County Study. *American Journal of Public Health, 88*, 1709–1712.

Young, D.R., Miller, K.W., Wilder, L.B., Yanek, L.R., & Becker, D.M. (1998). Physical activity patterns of urban African Americans. *Journal of Community Health, 23*, 99–112.

CHAPTER 26

Reproductive Health Disparities among African American Women

DIANE L. ROWLEY AND YVONNE W. FRY

INTRODUCTION

Reproductive health focuses on maintaining health and wellness from menarche to menopause and includes a woman's ability to control her fertility, a woman's need to have good health and healthy children, and a woman's lifetime care for her reproductive organs. The health of a woman during her reproductive years also influences her risk for chronic diseases after menopause. For example, the risk of diabetes and hypertension, diseases that tend to appear after menopause, are higher among women who experienced gestational diabetes or pregnancy-induced hypertension. Therefore, protection of health and prevention of poor health are paramount for good reproductive outcomes. For women in the reproductive years, the two overarching goals of *Healthy People 2010*, the health prevention agenda for the nation, are intertwined. These two goals are first, to help individuals of all ages increase life expectancy *and* improve their quality of life and, second, to eliminate health disparities.

Quality of life reflects a general sense of happiness and satisfaction with life. It includes all aspects of life, including health, recreation, culture, rights, values, beliefs, aspirations, and the conditions that support a life containing these elements. *Health-related quality of life* reflects a personal sense of physical and mental health and the ability to react to factors in the physical and social environments. Surveys in which one rates his/her health as "poor," "fair," "good," "very good," or "excellent," can be reliable indicators of one's perceived health. In 1996, 90 percent of people in the United States reported their health as good, very good, or excellent (http://www.healthypeople.gov/document/html/uih/uih_2.htm, accessed 4/24/2003). Reproductive-age women who report their health-related quality of life as very good or excellent are less likely to experience frequent activity limitation, physical impairment, mental distress, depression, and stress or anxiety than women in fair or poor health (Ahluwalia et al., 2003). Sixty-two percent of women in the United States report their general health as very good or excellent. However, African American women are more likely to report being in poor or good health, whereas White women are more likely to report being in very good health (Office of Research on Women's Health, 2002). African American women 18 to 44 years of age are more likely to report more than 14 days per month of physical health impairment, depression, and stress or anxiety (Ahluwalia et al., 2003).

SOME ISSUES CONTRIBUTING TO HEALTH DISPARITIES

For African American women disparities exist in both health care and health outcomes. Women's reproductive health-care needs include family planning services, preconception and prenatal care, and general preventive care. Family planning services refer to receiving a birth control method or prescription for a method, a checkup or medical test related to using a birth control method, counseling about birth control methods, a sterilizing operation, or counseling about getting sterilized (Abma et al., 1997).

Birth Control Measures

African American women are only slightly less likely to report using some form of birth control compared to White women. Condom use is similar for African American and White women, and condom use for protection against sexually transmitted diseases actually is higher among unmarried African American women than unmarried White women (Anderson et al., 1996).

Other types of birth control methods also vary by race. Implant and injectable birth control is more common among African American women than White women; 13 percent of African American women in their early 20s, as compared to 8 percent of Whites, use one of these methods. Interestingly, African American adolescent women are more likely to use implant and injectable contraceptives versus White adolescents, who more commonly use oral contraceptives (Santelli et al., 2000). African American adolescent women, especially those whose parents are high school- or college-educated, more commonly use condoms. Unfortunately, use of the implant or injectable contraceptives is associated with greatly reduced use of condoms, which are still needed for protection from sexually transmitted diseases.

Sterilization

Sterilization rates have always been higher for African American women compared to White women, and the disparity seems to be increasing. In 1982, 22 percent of White women reported being sterilized, compared to 30 percent of African American women (Piccinino & Mosher, 1998). By 1995, 25 percent of White women and 40 percent of African American women reported having undergone an operation that resulted in sterilization (Piccinino & Mosher, 1998). In 1997, the same proportion of African American and White women reported receiving family planning services, but African American women were almost two times more likely to receive sterilization operations. As expected, sterilization rates increase with age, but African American women in every age category have higher sterilization rates in 1995; 36 percent of White women age 35–39 and 63 percent of African American women of the same age reported being sterilized (Abma et al., 1997). Unfortunately, while survey data can give accurate estimates of the percent of women who use these birth control methods, the surveys do not indicate whether women are satisfied with the birth control methods they have chosen.

Preconception Care

Preconception care provides early and continuing assessment of risks prior to pregnancy and includes nutritional status (over- or underweight, BMI, dietary habits—vegetarianism), medical risk factors (diabetes, hypertension, sickle-cell disease or trait, lupus, epilepsy), medication or drug, cigarette or alcohol use, domestic violence issues, infectious disease transmission prevention (HIV, syphilis, herpes, gonorrhea, hepatitis, etc.), counseling and referral resources (lack of support, finan-

Figure 26.1
Percent of mothers receiving late or no prenatal care, by race and age, United States, 2000

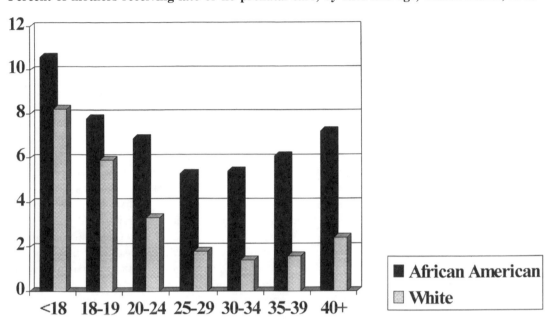

cial resources), and, of course, family planning services (contraception, recommended spacing intervals for optimal pregnancy outcomes) (Bernstein & Sanghvi, 1999; Jack et al., 1998; Gregory & Davidson, 1999). Although not proven through studies, health providers suspect that early intervention before conception could decrease the risk for preterm births and low birth weight, outcomes that are more common among African American women. However, access to care may limit the opportunity for preconception care for African American women.

Prenatal Care

Prenatal care services improve birth outcomes, and beginning prenatal care early in pregnancy is important, yet African American women of all ages are more likely to start care late during pregnancy (Figure 26.1). Poverty, low income, and low education are associated with receiving late or no prenatal care. Nearly one-third of all Black women lived in poverty in 1999 (Office of Research on Women's Health, 2002). Low-income women who receive health-care coverage only after their pregnancy begin, those who report physical violence, and those who report being "too tired" to go to care are more likely to receive late care (Gazmararian et al., 1999; Egerter et al., 2002). Among women with insurance coverage, high rates of unintended pregnancy and lack of a regular source of care prevent some from getting into care early (Braveman et al., 2000). Although a disparity in prenatal care use by African American women continues, the disparity in use of prenatal care between African American and White women steadily declined in the 1980s and 1990s. This reduction in the size of the disparity is partly due to a decline in the proportion of births to African American women who are less than 18 years or who have less than a high school education (Alexander et al., 2002).

The results of several studies have suggested that the content of prenatal care might differ for African American women and White women. Furthermore, even though more intensive monitoring is recommended during late pregnancy (i.e., the eighth and ninth months of gestation), African

American women make fewer prenatal-care visits during this time period than do White women. Researchers have determined that African American women, in comparison with White women, often receive fewer services and insufficient health-promotion education during their prenatal visits. Other factors, such as quality of prenatal care, delivery care and postpartum care, and interaction between health-seeking behaviors and satisfaction with care may explain part of this difference.

Access to Quality Care

African American women face problems with access to care and with the quality of health care they receive for all types of health-care needs. There are many hindrances to access to care for women of color that may or may not be perceived or experienced by White women. A major barrier is repeatedly reported as cultural incompetence or insensitivity or lack of respect for cultural diversity (Kriteck et al., 2002). Women feel neither respected nor empowered and in some cases are simply unfamiliar with what is required or expected of them in their health-seeking behaviors.

There are limitations in the communication of health information due to differences in language, inappropriate use of medical vocabulary, traditions and family beliefs, and values and culture. Additional issues include funding and lack of resources, with changes in Medicaid, more uninsured persons with increased job layoffs, and the working poor who are either uninsured or underinsured, unserved or underserved by the health system. Even when financial resources are available, they are not necessarily appropriately accessed for preventive and primary care. For example, State-CHIP programs have been in place for several years, yet all who are qualified to receive these services for their children have not or are not yet signed up. This can be an issue of lack of advertising or communication of the process or too many other stressors in the lives of the persons for whom these services are to be made available.

Access to a primary care physician benefits all patients, with those women of color having a primary physician being twice as likely as those without to receive preventive care (Cornelius et al., 2002). The use of preventive services by all women differs significantly with health insurance coverage (OWHR, NIH). The actual nature, quality, and quantity of this preventive care are also of question. All providers do not consistently comply with standards of care, best practices, and evidenced-based guidelines that suggest the frequency and timing of preventive diagnostic activities such as regular blood pressure screenings, mammograms, Pap smears, cholesterol and height and weight checks, and diabetes screenings. Differences may exist based on the payment source(s) of visits made by women of color, while other differences have been documented as gender-specific (lack of evaluation for coronary events/ lack of suspicion of cardiovascular compromise, etc.).

Finally, there are issues of access with respect to rural versus urban availability of primary care providers. All of these issues need consideration for policies and evaluation of existing health service strategies with an eye to implementing new, community-driven recommendations to address disparities.

ADOLESCENT REPRODUCTIVE HEALTH

Adolescents constitute 16 percent of all African American females (OWHR, NIH), and health disparities among adolescents are an important problem. Unprotected sexual intercourse and multiple sex partners place young people at risk for HIV infection, other STDs, and pregnancy. Each year, approximately three million cases of sexually transmitted diseases (STDs) occur among teenagers, and approximately 860,000 teenagers become pregnant. In 2001, 46 percent of high school students had ever had sexual intercourse; 53 percent of African American, and 41 percent of White high school females reported having had sex at least once in their lifetimes (Table 26.1) (Brener et al., 2002).

Sexual behaviors that contribute to unintended pregnancy and STDs, including HIV infection,

Table 26.1
Percent of high school female students who engage in sexual behaviors by race/ethnicity, United States, Youth Risk Behavior Survey, 2001

Category	White	Black	Hispanic
Ever had sexual intercourse	41%	53%	44%
First sexual intercourse before age 13 years	3%	8%	4%
Currently sexually active+	32%	39%	34%
Responsible sexual behavior*	84%	85%	82%

+Had sexual intercourse in the three months prior to the survey
*This includes students who had never had sexual intercourse, had had sexual intercourse, but not during the three months prior to the survey, or had used a condom the last time they had sexual intercourse in the three months prior to the survey.

Figure 26.2
Teen pregnancy rates, age 15–17, by race/ethnicity, United States, 1991, 1996, and 2000

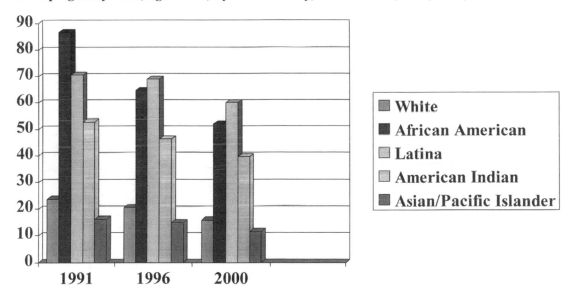

White
African American
Latina
American Indian
Asian/Pacific Islander

were not necessarily higher among African American teen women compared to White teen women. In 2001, African American teen women as compared to White teens were more likely to report using a condom during last sexual intercourse (61 percent vs. 51 percent), but far less likely to report using a birth control pill (8 percent vs. 27 percent). African American female students (12 percent) were significantly more likely than Latina and White female students (6.2 percent and 4 percent, respectively) to have been pregnant.

Teen pregnancy rates include the number of live births, legally induced abortions, and estimated spontaneous abortions. The rate of teen births has steadily declined over the past decade (Figure 26.2). Rates vary substantially from state to state, with states having more racial/ethnic minority teens having higher birthrates. In 2000 rates for teenagers 15–19 years ranged from 23.4 per 1,000 in New Hampshire to 72.0 in Mississippi. A significant decrease in birthrates to teens, especially to those 15–17 years old and to those who are African American (23 percent decline) versus White (7 percent decline), occurred from 1991 to 1996. Over the same years abortion rates for teenagers continued to decrease.

Despite the declines in both pregnancies and abortions, there continues to be a disparity in the rates of pregnancies in African American and Latina teenagers versus Whites (Figure 26.2). Birthrates for African American adolescents 15–17 years of age still are 3.2 times higher than that of Whites (Santelli et al., 2000). Some contributors to this situation include high neighborhood unemployment, single-parent household, poverty (birthrate approximately ten times higher than that of high-income teens), peer pressure, lack of knowledge of how to negotiate contraceptive usage (especially condoms), lack of access to health services or lack of knowledge of its availability, physical or sexual abuse, exposure to domestic violence, intimate partner violence, substance abuse, poor school performance or experience, fear of lack of confidentiality in seeking birth control services.

PREGNANCY OUTCOMES

Disturbing disparities are present for both pregnancy-related deaths and pregnancy complications. Pregnancy-related deaths in the United States decreased dramatically in the 50 years prior to 1987, but since that time no improvements have occurred (Berg et al., 1996). National statistics indicate that since 1987 the overall disparity in pregnancy-related deaths has increased. African American women are now four times more likely to die than White women (Koonin et al., 1997). This fourfold increased risk for maternal death among African American women as compared to White women is one of the largest racial disparities among major public health indicators.

Risk factors for pregnancy-related deaths are older maternal age, low educational attainment, high parity, and no prenatal care. Surprisingly, the disparity exists mainly among women at low risk for maternal death (women who have few deliveries and who deliver normal birth-weight babies) while no disparity has been found among African American and White women who are high risk (have a high number of deliveries and who deliver low birth-weight babies) (Saftlas et al., 2000). Disparity in pregnancy-related mortality is higher for African American women than for White women at all ages, and the disparity between African American women and White women widens with increasingly older maternal age. Mortality for African American women increases sharply with age, beginning with women aged 25–29 years. For women who are pregnant at age 35 or greater, African American women are at least six times more likely to die than White women (Figure 26.3).

African American women have a higher risk than White women of dying from every pregnancy-related cause of death reported, including the three leading causes of pregnancy-related deaths in the United States: hemorrhage, embolism, and hypertensive disorders of pregnancy (Berg et al., 1996). African American women are 3 times more likely to die from hemorrhage and 2.5 times more likely to die from a pulmonary embolism and have a 3 to 4 times higher risk of death from hypertensive disorders of pregnancy (Chang et al., 2002; Chichakli et al., Franks et al., 1990). For the next two most frequent causes of pregnancy-related death, cardiomyopathy and complications of anesthesia, the risk is 6 to 7 times greater for African American women than for White women (Chang et al., 2002; Chichkali et al., 1999). Higher levels of education are associated with decreased pregnancy-related mortality among White women; however, the risk for pregnancy-related death does not decline with higher educational level among African American women. Prenatal care reduces the risk of pregnancy-related death; however, for African American women death rates are higher at all levels of prenatal care compared to White women (Table 26.2).

Abortion-related deaths are defined as "deaths resulting from a direct complication of an abortion,

Figure 26.3
Pregnancy-related mortality ratios,* by age and race, United States, 1991–1999

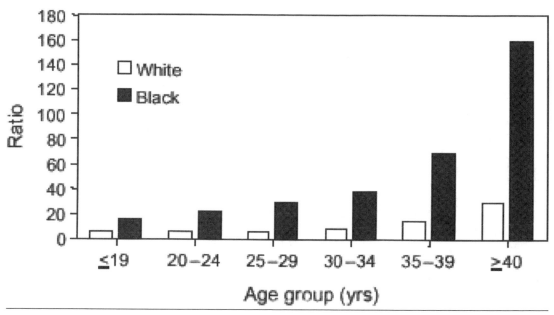

*Deaths per 100,000 live births.

from an indirect complication caused by the chain of events initiated by an abortion, or from the aggravation of a preexisting condition by the physiologic or psychological effects of an abortion" (Lawson et al., 1994). A spontaneous abortion occurs when a pregnancy spontaneously terminates before 20 completed weeks of gestation (Saraiya et al., 1999). Both of these outcomes are associated with disparities. Women of color (African American and other races) have a 3.8-fold increased risk of dying after a spontaneous abortion versus White women (Saraiya et al., 1999). The major contributors to these spontaneous abortion deaths were, in order, infection (59 percent), hemorrhage (18 percent), embolism (13 percent), complication of anesthesia (5 percent), and other (5 percent). When deaths from legal abortions were reviewed, women of color had a 2.5-increased risk of death versus White women.

Similar to the spontaneous abortion, legal abortions occurring after 12 weeks are associated with significantly increased risk of death. From 1972 to 1987, the disparity in deaths from legal abortions decreased by 20 percent; however, despite these advances, the case-fatality rate of legal abortion-related deaths remains at twice the level of that of White women. African American women and other women of color may be more likely to seek these services later in the pregnancy, thus immediately increasing their likelihood of a bad outcome. Issues of access, finances, and social stressors also must be considered. Continued access to late abortions may be important to women of color because they lack access to appropriate preconception care health education and contraceptives. In addition, they face economic and geographic barriers to earlier, safer abortions (Grimes, 1998).

Severe complications during pregnancy are more common than most people think. Maternal complications are the fifth leading cause of death for infants. For every 100 live births, 22 women are hospitalized for conditions not related to delivery. African American women are 40–60 percent more likely to be hospitalized for a pregnancy complication and once hospitalized have a longer length of stay compared to White women (Franks et al., 1992). Yet, African American women are 400 percent

Table 26.2
Race-specific pregnancy-related mortality ratios* by
trimester of prenatal care initiation, United States,
1991–1999

Prenatal care[+] by Trimester	White	Black	All Deaths
First	3.6	13.1	5.0
Second	4.4	12.7	6.6
Third	3.7	10.9	5.8
No Care	14.9	29.1	19.8

*Pregnancy-related deaths among women who delivered a live-born infant
per 100,000 live births.
[+]Trimester prenatal car began

Source: Chang et al. (2002).

more likely to die of a pregnancy complication. This discrepancy suggests that African American women may not be getting appropriate care for their conditions. Preterm labor, urinary tract infections, pregnancy-induced hypertension, and placental hemorrhage are the most important reasons for hospitalization (Scott et al., 1997). Preterm labor is a significant cause of infant mortality because it can lead to a preterm birth, defined as delivery of a baby before 37 completed weeks of gestation.

African American families are more than twice as likely to suffer the loss of a baby because of a preterm birth. Infants born between 20 and 32 weeks gestation are at very high risk of death and, if they survive, are more likely to have disabilities compared to babies born at term. The risk of death for all babies born before 32 weeks gestation is 50 times greater than for infants born at term (Mathews et al., 2002), and African American families are almost three times more likely to have a baby born before 32 weeks gestation. Socioeconomic (SES) factors should influence the preterm delivery rate in African American women. But while high SES is associated with a reduction in the rate of preterm/low birth-weight babies among White women, the same is not true for African American women. A hypothesis that is currently being examined is that social factors like stress and racism may influence adverse pregnancy outcomes among African American women.

African American women are at greater risk of antepartum hemorrhage, a condition that is caused by abruptio placenta (defined as the premature separation of a normally implanted placenta), placenta previa (defined as improper implantation of the placenta so that it is over the cervix), and bleeding associated with coagulation defects. The risk for abruptio placenta is higher for African American women. Women with abruptio placenta are at higher risk for preterm labor, preterm delivery, and stillbirth. Over the 1970s and 1980s, the rate of placenta previa increased for African American and other racial/ethnic minority women but remained stable for White women (Iysau et al., 1993).

Hypertensive disorders of pregnancy are classified as pregnancy-induced hypertension and chronic hypertension. Pregnancy-induced hypertension is elevated blood pressure during the pregnancy but not prior to pregnancy. Chronic hypertension refers to elevated blood pressure that is present and documented before pregnancy. The presence of chronic hypertension among women of childbearing age who are not pregnant is higher for African American women compared to White women. Not surprising, hospitalizations for chronic hypertension during pregnancy are 2.5 times higher among African American women versus White women. Chronic hypertension increases with age, and African American women age 30–39 have almost a four times higher rate of chronic hypertension during pregnancy compared to other women. The higher rate of maternal hypertension, particularly chronic hypertension, experienced by African American women may contribute to the disparity in outcomes observed between African American and other women (Samadi et al., 1996). All women with chronic hypertension are over four times more likely to experience inadequate fetal growth and two times more likely to have a preterm delivery (Samadi et al., 1996).

Maternal hypertension also increases the risk for antepartum hemorrhage. Compared to African American pregnant women with normal blood pressure, those with maternal hypertension are over three times more likely to experience antepartum hemorrhage. Both pregnancy-induced hypertension and chronic hypertension during pregnancy can progress to preeclampsia and eclampsia. Preeclampsia consists of hypertension with protein in urine and edema. When preeclampsia progresses to a convulsive phase, it is called eclampsia. Because African American women have higher rates of chronic hypertension, they also have higher rates of preeclampsia. Other risk factors for preeclampsia include obesity, a condition more common in African American women, sickle-cell trait, and work-related stress (Dekker, 1999). Additionally, African American women are 3.1 times more likely to die from preeclampsia or eclampsia than White women (MacKay et al., 2001).

Between 1970 and 1989 the rate of ectopic pregnancies increased, and although they still accounted for less than 2 percent of all reported pregnancies, they were associated with 13 percent of all pregnancy-related deaths (Goldner et al., 1993). The risk of ectopic pregnancy and death from its complications is consistently higher for African American and other racial/ethnic minority women than for White women. Ectopic pregnancy is associated with vaginal douching, a practice that is more common among African American women (Kendrick et al., 1997). African American women douche at twice the rate of White women (55 percent vs. 21 percent), and in one study 6 percent of African American women douched during pregnancy, with only 1 percent of White women doing so (Fiscella et al., 2002).

Women who douche are two times more likely to have bacterial vaginosis (BV) (Ness et al., 2002). BV is caused by a replacement of the normal vaginal flora (hydrogen-peroxide producing lactobacilli that are protective of the vaginal environment) by an overgrowth of bacteria such as Gardnerella vaginalis, Mycoplasma hominis. Multiple undesired outcomes are associated with douching, including acquisition of HIV, preterm labor and delivery, PID, and other sexually transmitted diseases (Ness et al., 2002). Thus, the finding that douching is more prevalent in African American women than White women may be partially responsible for the Black–White differences in pregnancy outcomes.

COMMON HEALTH PROBLEMS

Nutrition and Obesity

Micronutrients and anemia during pregnancy are important for both the mother's and the baby's health. The two most important micronutrients are iron and folate. Iron deficiency is the most common cause of anemia, and maternal iron deficiency anemia might cause low birth weight and preterm delivery (MMWR, 2002b). Iron deficiency anemia among women of color 12 to 45 years old is three times greater than the 2010 health objective for the nation (MMWR, 2002b). Folic acid supplementation during the preconception period reduces the occurrence and recurrence of neural tube defects. In 1992, the U.S. Public Health Service recommended that all women of childbearing age take 400 µg of folic acid. Since 1998, folate has been added to cereal grain products. Although all women of childbearing age have demonstrated an increase in folate status, African American and Mexican

American women had lower folate levels prior to 1998 and still do not have levels similar to those of White women (MMWR, 2002a).

Since 1976, there has been a worrisome increase in the proportion of people in the United States who are overweight or obese. Obesity is defined as an excessively high amount of body fat in relation to lean body mass and is based on having a body mass index (BMI) of 25 or more. BMI is calculated by dividing a person's weight in kilograms by her height in meters squared (Garrow & Webster, 1985). Individuals with a BMI of 25 to 29.9 are considered overweight, while individuals with a BMI of 30 or more are considered obese. Overweight may or may not be due to increases in body fat. It may also be due to an increase in lean muscle. For example, professional athletes may be very lean and muscular, with very little body fat, yet they may weigh more than others of the same height. While they may qualify as "overweight" due to their large muscle mass, they are not necessarily "over fat," regardless of BMI (http://www.cdc.gov/nccdphp/dnpa/obesity/defining.htm#BMI). African American women sometimes refer to themselves as "thick" or "big-boned" and, therefore, consider themselves to be naturally heavier than women of other ethnic groups, but it is not easy to determine whether overweight or obesity is due to lots of muscle and bigger bone structure or more fat. Moderate to severe obesity is mainly due to excess fat.

For men the proportion of overweight and obesity tends to be similar across race/ethnic groups, but for women, obesity is higher for African American and Mexican American women than for White women. Especially disturbing is that the percent of African American women who are extremely obese in early adult life is much higher than for White women. Among women in their 20s, 5 percent of White women, 11 percent of African American women, and 8 percent of Mexican American women are considered moderately to severely obese. Severe obesity increases for women in their 30s to 8 percent of White women, 19 percent of African American women, and 15 percent of Mexican American women. By their fourth decade, 1 out of 10 White women and almost 1 out of 4 African American women are moderately to severely obese (Flegal et al., 1998).

Overweight and obesity during the reproductive years are link to menstrual irregularities, infertility, and irregular ovulation. During pregnancy obesity puts pregnant women at risk for gestational diabetes, pregnancy hypertension and preeclampsia, a slightly higher rate of urinary tract infections, and being more likely to deliver by cesarean section. During the reproductive years and during pregnancy, foods that contribute most to nutrient and fiber intake may differ for African American and White women. During pregnancy, low-income African American women consume more calories and fewer nutrients than low-income White women (Siega-Riz et al., 2002). More work needs to focus on understanding the social and environmental factors that may play a role in obesity, such as the easy availability of energy-dense, high-fat foods and the opportunities for physical activity at work and in other aspects of life (Kumanyika, 1998).

Hysterectomy, Uterine Fibroids, and Endometriosis

Hysterectomy is the second most frequently performed surgery among reproductive-age women in the United States, exceeded only by cesarean section. Hysterectomy rates for women 35 to 44 years of age are significantly higher for African American women compared to White women (Keshavarz et al., 2002). Uterine fibroids (uterine leiomyomas) are the most frequent reason for hysterectomy in the United States and the most common, noncancerous tumors in women of childbearing age (Table 26.3).

The rate of fibroids (16.9 per 1,000) is two times greater for African American women compared to White women (8.2 per 1,000). (Kjerulff et al., 1996). Rates for fibroids peak earlier for African American women (35–39 years of age vs. 40–44 years). African American women may be at higher risk because the risk of fibroids increases with BMI, and at least one group has suggested that the

Table 26.3

Estimated rates of hysterectomy, by race of women who obtained the procedure and primary discharge diagnosis, United States, 1994–1999

	Race											
	White			Black			Other[†]			All races		
Diagnosis	Rate	SE[§]	No.	Rate	SE	No.	Rate	SE	No.	Rate	SE	No.
Endometrial hyperplasia	0.2	0.02	108,486	0.1	0.02	8,615	0.2	0.04	4,550[¶]	0.2	0.01	121,651
Endometriosis	1.1	0.08	564,191	0.6	0.09	46,806	0.7	0.10	19,837	1.0	0.06	630,834
Uterine leiomyoma	1.8	0.10	954,166	4.2	0.29	332,786	2.6	0.33	74,834	2.1	0.08	1,361,786
Uterine prolapse	1.0	0.08	547,933	0.3	0.04	19,792	0.9	0.15	25,894	0.9	0.05	593,619
Other	0.7	0.06	391,112	0.6	0.05	44,662	0.8	0.13	21,376	0.7	0.04	457,150
Total	5.3	0.32	2,868,666	6.2	0.36	489,165	5.9	0.67	167,406	5.5	0.22	3,525,237

*Per 1,000 female, civilian residents aged $\geq$ 15 years in each diagnosis and race category. Rates by race were adjusted by redistributing the number of women for whom race was unknown according to the known distribution of race in the National Hospital Discharge Survey. Rates were calculated by applying population weights to the sum of the numbers of hysterectomies obtained each year, and dividing this value by the sum of the population estimates for each year. Population estimates were obtained from the U.S. Department of Commerce. U.S. Bureau of the Census.

[†]Includes Asian, Pacific Islander, American Indian, Alaskan Native, and other races.

[§]Standard error.

[¶]Based on 30–59 women in the sample; number was unreliable.

Source: Keshavarz et al. (2002).

tendency to keloid may be a risk factor (Schwartz, 2001). Fibroids are associated with an increased risk of pregnancy complications, including preterm labor, placental abruption, cesarean section, and breech presentation.

Women who report symptoms such as excessive bleeding, pelvic pain, pressure, and problems with bladder control are more likely to be treated for fibroids. African American women appear to have larger and more numerous fibroids at diagnosis, are more likely to be anemic than White women (56 percent vs. 38 percent), and are more likely to complain of severe pelvic pain. Management of symptomatic fibroids ranges from surgery (hysterectomy or myomectomy), to hormonal therapy, and more recently, to uterine artery embolization.

Surgical treatment with hysterectomy results in sterility. Myomectomy may also reduce fertility. African American women tend to undergo surgical treatment at younger ages than White women and, after surgery, are more likely to have in-hospital complications. Hormonal therapy, treatment with gonadotrophin-releasing hormone agonists, has been used for a number of years but has draw-backs that include the discomfort of menopausal-like symptoms, loss of bone mineral density, and substantial regrowth of the fibroids immediately after therapy is stopped (Floridon et al., 2001). Uterine artery embolization, a recently developed procedure, has minimized the complications of therapy and has protected childbearing. This new procedure is available even to women considered high-risk because of obesity or heart or lung disease and is associated with high patient satisfaction (Floridon et al., 2001). Over the next decade, the need for surgical and hormonal treatment should decline.

Endometriosis is the third leading cause of hospitalization for gynecologic illnesses. It is defined as the presence of endometrial tissue (tissue from the womb) in places external to the womb. Symptoms are caused by bleeding of the endometrial tissue into the surrounding area, which leads to inflammation, scarring, and adhesions. Women can experience painful menstrual periods, pelvic pain not related to menses, painful intercourse, painful urination, and painful bowel movements (Missmer & Cramer, 2003). Little is known about the occurrence of this condition among African American women because African American women are often misdiagnosed as having pelvic inflammatory disease rather than endometriosis (Missmer & Cramer 2003). The effects of misdiagnosis can be physically and mentally debilitating.

Urinary Tract Infections

There is up to an 8 percent incidence of urinary tract infection in pregnancy. It is possible to miss the diagnosis of UTI in a pregnant woman, as it is asymptomatic in 2–10 percent of pregnant women. This can result in intrauterine growth retardation (IUGR), preterm delivery (PTD), and low birth weight (LBW). Acute (symptomatic) cystitis occurs in 30 percent of untreated asymptomatic bacteriuria. Pyelonephritis occurs in 20–50 percent of pregnant women with untreated asymptomatic bacteriuria, which can lead to preterm delivery. Higher rates of bacteriuria among Black women may account for roughly 5 percent of the disparity in preterm delivery experienced by African American women (Fiscella, 1996).

REPRODUCTIVE CANCERS

The two most common reproductive-related cancers among women in the United States are breast cancer and cervical. Racial differences exist in the incidence, mortality, and survival rates for these cancers. Breast cancer is the most common cancer among African American women and the second leading cause of death among African American women; only lung cancer causes more deaths (American Cancer Society, 2002). Although African American women are less likely to have breast cancer than White women, they are more likely to die from breast cancer than White women. The five-year survival rate for African Americans is 71 percent compared to 86 percent for White Americans. When 1992–1997 survival within each stage of cancer (localized, regional, or distant) was examined, African American women were 17 percent less likely than White women to survive five years past diagnosis and 1.8 times more likely to be diagnosed at the most advanced stage (Krieger, 2002). This disparity in breast cancer deaths increased in the 1990s because the death rate for White women declined while the death rate for African American women showed little change.

African American women now use mammography screening at similar rates as White women, but they are more likely to have advanced-stage disease when diagnosed and to have biologically high-grade tumors, estrogen receptor negative tumors compared to White women. African American women probably don't receive the same treatment as White women. Treatment differences may be related to being low-income, uninsured, or publicly insured by Medicaid or Medicare. Even after taking into account the stage of diagnosis, African American women who are underinsured or uninsured are less likely to receive surgical treatment that White women (Bradley et al., 2002).

In 1990, the U.S. government passed the Breast and Cervical Cancer Mortality Prevention Act with the goal of increasing access to cancer-screening services for low-income and uninsured women. Women of color, especially African American women, should benefit from the program because low-income and uninsured status is more common; however, only 12–15 percent of eligible women have used the early detection services because of insufficient funds to provide services to all eligible women (Benard et al., 2001). To eliminate this disparity, appropriate treatment for stage and pathology of disease needs to be given to all women, regardless of insurance status and economic status. Focused research in populations of color will be important for improving breast cancer rates and outcomes (Haynes & Smedley 1999), and African Americans need to be involved in setting cancer priorities.

African Americans are twice as likely to be diagnosed with cervical cancer and two to three times more likely to die from cervical cancer. Cervical cancer is one of the most preventable cancers because precancerous lesions can be identified through the Pap (Papanicolaou) screening and treatment during the precancerous phase. Compared to White women, African American women are more likely to be diagnosed at an older age and more likely to have a late stage at the time of diagnosis and to have tumors that are poorly differentiated or have a more severe prognosis. Although the disparities in rates between African Americans and Whites have declined since 1990, differences in rates persist. This persistent disparity has been attributed to several factors, including differences in the prevalence of risk factors for cervical cancer; differences in screening, diagnostic evaluation, and treatment; and differences in the stage of disease at diagnosis (Lawson et al., 2000).

Race-specific differences in incidence and death rates for cervical cancer also varied by age. During 1992–1996, among women age <35 years, the rate of invasive cervical cancer among African American women was lower than the rate among White women. However, in older age groups, incidence rates among White women fluctuated between 13 and 15 per 100,000 women, whereas rates among African women tended to increase with age to approximately 32 per 100,000 for those age ≥75 years. Death rates for cervical cancer increased with advancing age; however, rates were substantially higher for African American women age >40 years than for White women the same age. Regardless of race, most cervical cancer deaths occur among women age ≥50 years. For women in whom invasive, but localized (i.e., Stage I), cervical cancer has been diagnosed, the five-year relative survival rate is approximately 90 percent. In contrast, for women with advanced invasive cervical cancer (beyond the cervix and pelvis [i.e., Stage III and IV, respectively]), the five-year relative survival rate is approximately 12 percent. Moreover, five-year relative survival rates for local and regional stages are lower for Blacks than for Whites (Lawson et al., 2000).

Cervical cancer is associated with certain types of human papilloma viruses (HPV), type 16 being the most common. The association between HPV infection and cervical neoplasia appears to be stronger than the association between smoking and lung cancer, cervical cancers, HPV type 16 being the most common. HPV detection is important to identify those patients who may be at high risk for the development of cervical neoplasia (Einstein & Goldberg, 2002), yet no information on the distribution of HPV infections by race/ethnicity is readily available.

EMERGING FACTORS RELATED TO REPRODUCTIVE HEALTH DISPARITIES

Violence

Intimate partner violence (IPV) is any type of violence between couples and includes throwing items, pushing, shoving, slapping, punching, kicking, biting, burning, choking, forcing sex, or threatening with a knife, gun, or other instrument/ available tool. It can occur in either direction, female-to-male partner violence (FMPV), or male-to-female partner violence (MFPV). The occurrence of IPV varies by study, with some studies suggesting a similarity between urban and rural locations and between African American and White women in the actual lifetime incidence of IPV (Lee et al., 2002). Other studies that include couples still together show much variation by race, with MFPV 23 percent for African Americans, 17 percent for Hispanics, and 12 percent for Whites. Conversely and perhaps surprisingly, the FMPV rates in the same study were 30 percent for African Americans, 21 percent for Hispanics, and 16 percent among Whites (Caetano et al., 2001).

Studies within the U.S. Army (1989–1997) corroborate that there is a difference in the occurrence of IPV in African American versus White couples, with the former having a higher incidence. Although rates of aggression between men and women in the military were described as similar, the injuries sustained by women exceeded those of men (McCarroll et al., 1999). Of significance is the fact that the army designates only these occurrences between partners as spousal abuse and only between married persons.

The numerous contributors to the behaviors of IPV, with respect to both the perpetrator and the victim, include alcohol (4–41 percent) or other drug intake, low socioeconomic status, and male or female approval of aggression. Alcohol dependence contributes more to IPV among African Americans than for Whites and Hispanics (Caetano et al., 2001). Among the military spouses, housing, medical care, screening for drug and alcohol use, and completion of high school education are less important factors than in the general population, but military families have stressors associated with the potential for deployment in wartime, moving from base to base, and separation.

Of those impacted by IPV, African American and Native American women more frequently suffer severe injuries, especially due to increased use of weapons against them. Latina and African American women report more emotional or mental health sequelae. Cultural competence and sensitivity of the health-care providers are paramount in handling issues of IPV and rape, as the health-seeking behaviors vary greatly among women depending on their race or ethnicity. White women are much more likely to report rape and seek psychological counseling than African American women. Asian women may be submitting to cultural expectations of good behavior and tolerating abuse without perceiving the availability of any resource for relief. Latina and Native American women tend to wait for direct inquiry by the health-care provider before sharing information on IPV (Lee et al., 2002).

Intimate partner homicides (IPH) are more common in African American families than White families, and this may contribute to the discrepancy in life expectancy between the two groups. There are a 6.4-year difference for African American men and 4.4 years for African American women (MMWR, 2001). Intimate partner homicides were high among African American men and women (knives being the women's weapon of choice), and the lowest rates among Whites, and Asian or Pacific Islanders. Fifty percent of these homicides occur between spouses, and 33 percent between boy/girlfriends (Paulozzi et al., 2001). Studies show that despite an overall decline in the IPV over the last 20 years, African American women have a higher occurrence of intimate partner *homicide* than White women (Lee et al., 2002). There is an increase in the occurrence of IPH with increased difference in age of the male perpetrator versus the female victim (Paulozzi et al., 2001).

Pregnancy is not even protected from abuse. Actually, abuse during pregnancy is not uncommon, with prevalence rates reported to be 3.9–8.3 percent (McFarlane et al., 1999). Not surprising, the same authors found increased association of complications of pregnancy with abuse of pregnant women, including those related to health disparities, such as low prenatal weight gain, low birthweight deliveries, anemia, infections, bleeding in the first and second trimesters, use of nonprescription drugs, alcohol, and tobacco, and maternal depression and/or suicidal ideation/ attempts (McFarlane et al., 1999; McFarlane et al., 2002). The very serious take-home message from these studies is that women who are abused during pregnancy were usually also abused prior to the pregnancy. Not only is their abuse ongoing, but it is more severe, with major implications for their pregnancy and birth outcomes. This also flags an area of health opportunity; clinicians can take an active role in assessing pregnant women to rule out abuse, at a time where they are more likely to consistently seek care. Offering intervention at this time in the reproductive course of women promises to impact the outcomes for a major subset of the population.

Racism and Stress as Causes of Racial/Ethnic Health Disparities

Many factors affecting these disparities are not well understood. For example, the disparities in the infant mortality rate and the maternal mortality rate in African Americans compared to White Americans have remained around the same despite tremendous advances in medical and technological developments. The lack of progress in reducing the disparities indicate that factors that lead to an overall population decline in disease rates are not the same as the fundamental causes of the disparity. Important emerging factors for the disparity are its social and psychological causes. Social position (the interplay between race, gender, and social class) and the effects of living in a race-conscious society (i.e., institutional racism, individual exposure to racism, and internalized racism) influence health disparities (Krieger et al., 1993; Jones, 2000).

Racism, gender discrimination, and stress may have independent and overlapping pathways to poor reproductive health outcomes. Racism and psychological stress may intervene on reproductive health independently of each other or together to cause health disparities (Hogue et al., 2001; Wadhwa et al., 2001). Psychosocial models that explain discrimination, perceived racism, institutional and intrapersonal racism, and their effects on health have been published recently. A body of work has reported relationships between psychological stress, physiological stress, structural/contextual stress and bacterial vaginosis, low birth weight, and preterm birth (Collins et al., 2000; Culhane et al., 2002; Culhane et al., 2001; Dole et al., 2003; Jackson et al., 2001; Rich-Edwards et al., 2001). More research in this area will help in the design of interventions that will reduce the disparity. The new research must be infused with attention to community participatory models that incorporate the knowledge women of color have about their lives and that report findings back to women (Jackson, 2002). Solutions to health disparities may rest on broad strategies that improve the entire community and that alter the structural policies.

REFERENCES

Abma, J.C., Chandra, A., Mosher, W.D., Peterson, L.S., & Piccinino, L.J. (1997). Fertility, family planning and women's health: New data from the 1995 National Survey of Family Growth. *Vital and Health Statistics, Series 23, No. 19.*

Ahluwalia, I.B., Holtzman, D., Mack, K.A., & Mokdad, A. (2003). Health-related quality of life among women of reproductive age: Behavioral Risk Factor Surveillance System (BRFSS), 1998–2001. *Journal of Women's Health, 12(1),* 5–9.

Alexander, G.R., Kogan, M.D., & Nabukera, S. (2002). Racial differences in prenatal care use in the United States: Are disparities decreasing? *American Journal of Public Health, 92(2),* 1970–1975.

American Cancer Society. (2002) *Cancer Facts and Figures.* American Cancer Society, Inc. Atlanta, GA.

Anderson, J.E., Brackbill, R., & Mosher, W.D. (1996). Condom use for disease prevention among unmarried U.S. women. *Family Planning Perspectives, 28(1),* 25–28.

Benard, V.B., Lee, N.C., Piper, M., & Richardson, L. (2001). Race-specific results of Papanicolaou testing and the rate of cervical neoplasia in the National Breast and Cervical Cancer Early Detection Program, 1991–1998 (United States). *Cancer Causes Control, 2(1),* 61–68.

Berg, C.J., Atrash, H.K., Koonin, L.M., & Tucker, M. (1996). Pregnancy-related mortality in the United States, 1987–1990. *Obstetrics & Gynecology, 88(2),* 161–167.

Bernstein, P.S., & Sanghvi, T. (1999). Improving preconception care. *American Journal of Obstetrics and Gynecology, 180(1S-II) Supplement,* 79S.

Bradley, C.J., Givens, C.W., & Roberts, C. (2002). Race, socioeconomic status, and breast cancer treatment and survival. *Journal National Cancer Institute, 94(7),* 490–496.

Braveman, P., Marchi, K., Egerter, S., Pearl, M., & Neuhaus, J. (2000). Barriers to timely prenatal care among women with insurance: The importance of prepregnancy factors. *Obstetrics and Gynecology, 95(6 Pt 1),* 874–880.

Brener, N., Lowry, R., Kann, L., et al. (2002). Trends in sexual behaviors among high school students—United States, 1991–2001. *Monthly Morbidity Weekly Report, 51(38),* 856–859.

Caetano R., Nelson S., & Cunradi, C. (2001). Intimate partner violence, dependence symptoms and social consequences from drinking among White, Black and Hispanic couples in the United States. *Am J Addict, 10 Suppl,* 60–69.

Chang, J., Elam-Evans, L.D., Berg, C.J., Herndon, J., Flowers L., Seed, K.A., & Syverson, K.J. (2002). Pregnancy-Related Mortality Surveillance—United States, 1991–1999. *Mortality and Morbidity Surveillance Summaries* 52 (SS02), 1–8.

Chichakli, L.O., Atrash, H.K., & MacKay, A.P., Musani, A.S., & Berg, C.J. (1999). Pregnancy-related mortality in the United States due to hemorrhage: 1979–1992. *Obstetrics & Gynecology, 94(5 Pt 1),* 721–725.

Collins, J.W., Jr., David, R.J., Symons, R., Handler, A., Wall, S.N., & Dwyer, L. (2000). Low-income African-American mothers' perception of exposure to racial discrimination and infant birth weight. *Epidemiology, 11(3)*, 337–339.

Cornelius, L.J., Smith, P.L., & Simpson, G.M. (2002). What factors hinder women of color from obtaining preventive health care? *American Journal of Public Health, 292(4)*, 535–538.

Culhane J.F., Rauh, V., McCollum, K.F., Elo, I.T, & Hogan, V. (2002). Exposure to chronic stress and ethnic differences in rates of bacterial vaginosis among pregnant women. *American Journal of Obstetrics and Gynecology, 187(5)*, 1272–1276.

Culhane, J.F., Rauh, V., McCollum, K.F., Hogan, V.K., Agnew, K., & Wadhwa, P.D. (2001). Maternal stress is associated with bacterial vaginosis in human pregnancy. *Maternal and Child Health Journal, 5(2)*,127–134.

Dekker, G.A. (1999). Risk factors for preeclampsia. *Clinical Obstetrics and Gynecology, 42(3)*, 422–447.

Diabetes in America, 2d ed. (1995). National Diabetes Data Group. National Institutes of Health. National Institute of Diabetes and Digestive and Kidney Diseases. NIH Publication No. 95–1468.

Dole, N., Savitz, D.A., Hertz-Picciotto, I., Siega-Riz, A.M., & McMahon, M.J. (2003). Maternal stress and preterm birth. *American Journal of Epidemiology, 157(1)*, 14–24.

Egerter, S., Braveman, P., & Marchi, K. (2002). Timing of insurance coverage and use of prenatal care among low-income women. *American Journal of Public Health, 92(3)*, 423–427.

Einstein, M.H., & Goldberg, G.L. (2002). Human papilloma virus and cervical neoplasia. *Cancer Investigations, 20(7–8)*, 1080–1085.

Fiscella, K. (1996). Racial disparities in preterm births: The role of urogenital infections. *Public Health Report, 111*, 104–113.

Fiscella, K., Franks, P., Kendrick, J.S., Meldrum, S., & Kieke, B.A., Jr. (2002). Risk of preterm birth that is associated with vaginal douching. *American Journal of Obstetrics and Gynecology, 186(6)*,1345–1350.

Flegal, K.M., Carroll, M.D., & Kuczmarski, R.J., & Johnson, C.L. (1998). Overweight and obesity in the United States: Prevalence and trends, 1960–1994. *International Journal of Obesity, 22*, 39–47.

Floridon, C., Lund, N., & Thomsen, S.G. (2001). Alternative treatment for symptomatic fibroids. *Current Opinion in Obstetrics and Gynecology, 13*, 491–495.

Franks, A.L., Atrash, H.K., & Lawson, H.W. (1990). Obstetrical pulmonary embolism mortality, United States, 1970–1985. *American Journal of Obstetrics and Gynecology, 80(6)*, 720–722.

Franks, A.L., Kendrick, J.S., & Olson, D.R. (1992). Hospitalizations for pregnancy complications, United States, 1986–1987. *American Journal of Obstetrics and Gynecology, 166(5)*, 1339–1344.

Galtire-Dereure, F., Boegner, C., & Bringer, J. (2000). Obesity and pregnancy: Complications and cost. *American Journal of Clinical Nutrition, 71*, 1242s–1248s.

Garrow, J.S., & Webster, J. (1985). Quetelet's index (W/H²) as a measure of fatness. *International Journal of Obesity, 9*, 147–153.

Gazmararian, J.A., Arrington, T.L., Bailey, C.M., Schwarz, K.S., & Koplan, J.P. (1999). Prenatal care for low-income women enrolled in a managed-care organization. *Obstetrics and Gynecology, 94(2)*,177–184.

Goldner, T.E., Lawson, H.W., & Xia, Z., Atrash, H.K. (1993). Surveillance for ectopic pregnancy—United States, 1970–1989. *Morbidity Mortality Weekly Report CDC Surveillance Summary, 42(SS-6)*, 79–85.

Gregory, K.D., & Davidson, E. (1999). Prenatal care: Who needs it and why? *Clinical Obstetrics and Gynecology.* 42(4): 725–736.

Grimes, D.A. (1994). The role of hormonal contraceptives: The morbidity and mortality of pregnancy: Still risky business. *American Journal of Obstetrics and Gynecology, 170(5S) Supplement*, 1489–1494.

Grimes, D.A. (1998). The continuing need for late abortions. *JAMA, 280(8)*, 747–750.

Grunbaum, J., et al. (2002). Youth Risk Behavior Surveillance—United States. *Morbidity and Mortality Weekly Report Surveillance Summaries, 28,2002 51(SS04)*, 1–64.

Haynes, M.A., and Smedley, B.D. (Eds.). (1999). Committee on Cancer Research among Minorities and the Medically Underserved, Institute of Medicine, *The Unequal Burden of Cancer: An Assessment of NIH Research and Programs for Ethnic Minorities and the Medically Underserved.* Washington, DC: National Academy Press.

Hogue, C.J.R., Hoffman, S., & Hatch, M.C. (2001). Stress and preterm delivery: A conceptual framework. *Paediatric and Perinatal Epidemiology, 15(s2)*, 30–39.

http://www.cdc.gov/nccdphp/dnpa/obesity/defining.htm#BMI, retrieved March 22, 2003.

http://www.healthypeople.gov/document/html/uih/uih_2.htm, retrieved April 4/24/2003.

Iyasu, S., Saftlas, A.K., Rowley, D.L., Koonin, L.M., Lawson, H.W., & Atrash, H.K. (1993). The epidemiology of placenta previa in the United States, 1979 through 1987. *American Journal of Obstetrics and Gynecology, 168(5)*, 1424–1429.

Jack, B.W., Culpepper, L, Babcock, J., Kogan, M.D., & Weismiller, D. (1998). Addressing preconception risks identified at the time of a negative pregnancy test: A randomized trial. *The Journal of Family Practice, 47(1)*, 33–38.

Jackson, F.M. (2002). Considerations for community-based research with African American women. *American Journal of Public Health, 92(2)*, 561–564.

Jackson, F.M., Phillips, M.T., Hogue, C.J, & Curry-Owens, T.Y. (2001). Examining the burdens of gendered racism: Implications for pregnancy outcomes among college-educated African American women. *Maternal and Child Health Journal, 5(2)*, 95–107.

Jones, C.P. (2000). Levels of racism: A theoretic framework and a gardener's tale. *American Journal of Public Health, 90(8)*, 1212–1215.

Kendrick, J.S., Atrash, H.K., & Strauss, L.T. (1997). Vaginal douching and the risk of ectopic pregnancy among Black women. *American Journal of Obstetrics and Gynecology, 176(5)*, 991–997.

Keshavarz, H., Hillis, S.D., Kieke, B.A., & Marchbanks, P.A. (2002). Hysterectomy surveillance—United States, 1994–1999. *Mortality and Morbidity Weekly Report Surveillance Summary, 51(SS05)*, 1–8.

Kjerulff, K.H., Erickson, B.A., & Langenberg, P.W. (1996). Chronic gynecologic conditions reported by U.S. women: Findings from the National Health Interview Survey, 1984–1992. *American Journal of Public Health, 86*, 195–199.

Klerman, L.V., Ramey, S.L., Goldenberg, R.L., Marbury, S., Hou, J., & Cliver, S.P. (2001). A randomized trial of augmented prenatal care for multiple-risk, Medicaid-eligible African American women. *American Journal of Public Health, 91(1)*, 105–111.

Klerman, L.V., & Reynolds, D.W. (1994). Interconception care: A new role for the pediatrician. *Pediatrics, 93(2)*, 327–329.

Koonin, L.M., Atrash, H.K., & Lawson, H.W. (1991). Maternal mortality surveillance, United States, 1979–1986. *Morbidity Mortality Weekly Report CDC Surveillance Summary, 40(2)*, 1–13.

Koonin, L.M., Ellerbrock, T.D., & Atrash, H.K. (1989). Pregnancy-associated deaths due to AIDS in the United States. *Journal of the American Medical Association, 261(9)*, 1306–1309.

Koonin, L.M., MacKay, A.P., & Berg, C.J., Atrash H.K., & Smith, J.C. (1997). Pregnancy-related mortality surveillance, United States, 1987–1990. *Morbidity Mortality Weekly Report CDC Surveillance Summary, 46(4)*, 17–36.

Krieger, N. (2002). Is breast cancer a disease of affluence, poverty, or both? The case of African American women. *American Journal of Public Health, 92(4)*, 611–613.

Krieger, N., Rowley, D.L., Herman, A.A., Avery, B., & Phillips, M.T. (1993). Racism, sexism, and social class: Implications for studies of health, disease, and well-being. *American Journal of Preventive Medicine, 9(6 Suppl)*, 82–122.

Kritek, P.B., et al. (2002). Eliminating health disparities among minority women: A report on conference workshop process and outcomes. Public Health Matters. *American Journal of Public Health, 92(4)*, 580–587.

Kumanyika, S.K. (1998). Obesity in African Americans: Biobehavioral consequences of culture. *Ethnicity and Disease, Winter, 8(1)*, 93–96.

Lawson, H.W., & Atrash, H.K., Saftlas, A.F. & Linch, E.L. (1989). Ectopic pregnancy in the United States, 1970–1986. *Morbidity and Mortality Weekly Report CDC Surveillance Summary, 38(2)*, 1–10.

Lawson, H.W., Frye, A., Atrash, H.K., Smith, J.C., Shulman, H.B., & Ramick, M. (1994). Abortion mortality, United States, 1972 through 1987. *American Journal of Obstetrics and Gynecolology, 171(5)*, 1365–1372.

Lawson, H.W., Henson, R., Bobo, J.K., & Kaeser, M.K. (2000) Implementing recommendations for the early detection of breast and cervical cancer among low-income women *Morbidity and Mortality Weekly Reports Recommendations and Reports, 49, No. RR02*, 35–55.

Lee, R.K., Thompson, V.L., & Mechanic, M.B. (2002). Intimate partner violence and women of color: A call for innovations. *American Journal of Public Health, 92(4)*, 530–534.

Liff, J.M., et al. (Eds.). (1996). Racial/ethnic patterns of cancer in the United States 1998–1992, National Cancer Institute. NIH Pub. No. 96–4104. Bethesda, MD.

MacKay, A.P., Berg, C.J., & Atrash, H.K. (2001). Pregnancy-related mortality from preeclampsia and eclampsia. *Obstetrics and Gynecology, 97(4)*, 533–538.

Mathews, T.J., Menacker, F., & MacDorman, M. (2002). Infant mortality statistics from the 2000 period linked birth/infant death data set. *National Vital Statistics Reports, 50(12)*.

McCarroll, J.E., Newby, J.H., Thayer, L.E., Norwood, A.E., Fullerton, C.S., & Ursano, R.J. (1999). Reports of spouse abuse in the U.S. Army Central Registry (1989–1997). *Military Medicine, 164(2)*, 77–84.

McFarlane, J., Campbell, J.C., Sharps, P., & Watson K. (2002). Abuse during pregnancy and femicide: Urgent implications for women's health. *Obstetrics and Gynecology, 100(1)*, 27–36.

McFarlane, J., Parker, B., Soeken, K., Silva, C., & Reed, S. (1999). Severity of abuse before and during pregnancy for African American, Hispanic, and Anglo women. *Journal of Nurse Midwifery, 44(2)*, 139–144.

Missmer, S.A., & Cramer, D.W. (2003). The epidemiology of endometriosis. *Obstetrics and Gynecology Clinics, 30(1)*, 1–15.

Morbidity Mortality Weekly Report. CDC Surveillance Summary, 38(ss-2), 1–10.

Morbidity Mortality Weekly Report (1999). Preterm singleton birth—United States, 1989–1996, *48(09)*, 185–189.

Morbidity and Mortality Weekly Report. (2001). Influence of homicide on racial disparity in life expectancy—United States, 1998, *50(36)*, 780–783.

Morbidity and Mortality Weekly Report. (2002a). Folate status in women of childbearing age, by race/ethnicity—United States. *Morbidity and Mortality Weekly Report, 51(36)*, 808–810.

Morbidity and Mortality Weekly Report. (2002b). Iron deficiency—United States, 1999–2000. *Morbidity and Mortality Weekly Report, 51(40)*, 897–899.

Ness, R.B., et al. (2002). Douching in relation to bacterial vaginosis, lactobacilli, and facultative bacteria in the vagina. *Obstetrics and Gynecology, 100(4)*, 765–772.

Office of Research on Womens's Health (2002). *Women of Color Health Data Book* (2d Edition). Bethesda, Maryland, National Institutes of Health.

Panting-Kemp, A., Geller, S.E., & Nguyen, T. (2000). Maternal deaths in an urban perinatal network, 1992–1998. *American Journal of Obstetrics and Gynecology, 183(5)*, 1207–1212.

Paulozzi, L.J., Saltzman, L.E., Thompson, M.P., & Holmgreen, P. (2001). Surveillance for homicide among intimate partners—United States, 1981–1998. *Morbidity and Mortality Weekly Report CDC Surveillance Summary, 12,50(3)*, 1–15.

Piccinino, L.J. & Mosher, W.D. (1998). Trends in contraceptive use in the United States: 1982–1995. *Family Planning Perspectives, 30(1)*, 4–10 & 46.

Rich-Edwards, J., Krieger, N., Majzoub, J., Zierler, S., Lieberman, E., & Gillman, M. (2001). Maternal experiences of racism and violence as predictors of preterm birth: Rationale and study design. *Paediatric and Perinatal Epidemiology, 15(s2)*, 124–135.

Rowley, D.L., Hogue, C.J., Blackmore, C.A., Ferre, C.D., Hatfield-Timajchy, K., Branch, P., & Atrash, H.K. (1993). Preterm delivery among African-American women: A research strategy. *American Journal of Preventive Medicine, 9(6 Suppl)*, 1–6.

Saftlas, A.F., Koonin, L.M., & Atrash, H.K. (2000). Racial disparity in pregnancy-related mortality associated with livebirth: Can established risk factors explain it? *American Journal of Epidemiology, 152(5)*, 413–419.

Saftlas, A.F., Olson, D.R., Atrash, H.K., Rochat, R., & Rowley, D. (1991). National trends in the incidence of abruptio placentae, 1979–1987. *Obstetrics & Gynecology, 78(6)*, 1081–1086.

Saftlas, A.F., Olson, D.R., Franks, A.L., Atrash, H.K. Pokras, R. (1990). Epidemiology of preeclampsia and eclampsia in the United States, 1979–1986. *Obstetrics & Gynecology,163(2)*, 460–465.

Samadi, A.R. & Mayberry, R.M. (1998). Maternal hypertension and spontaneous preterm births among Black women. *Obstetrics & Gynecology, 91(6)*, 899–904.

Samadi, A.R., Mayberry, R.M., Zaidi, A.A., Pleasant, J.C., McGhee, N., Jr., & Rice, R.J. (1996). Maternal hypertension and associated pregnancy complications among African-American and other women in the United States. *Obstetrics & Gynecology, 87(4)*, 557–563.

Santelli, J.S., Lowry, R., Brener, N.D., & Robin, L. (2000). The association of sexual behaviors with socioeconomic status, family structure, and race/ethnicity among U.S. adolescents. *American Journal of Public Health, 90(10)*,1582–1588.

Saraiya, M., Green, C.A., Berg, C.J., Hopkins, F.W., Koonin, L.M., & Atrash, H.K. (1999). Spontaneous abortion-related deaths among women in the United States—1981–1991. *Obstetrics and Gynecology, 94(2)*, 172–176.

Schwartz, S.M. (2001). Epidemiology of uterine leiomyomata. *Clinical Obstetrics and Gynecology, 44(2)*, 316–326.

Scott, C.L., Chavez, G.F., Atrash, H.K., Taylor, D.J., Shah, R.S., & Rowley D. (1997). Hospitalizations for severe complications of pregnancy, 1987–1992. *Obstetrics & Gynecology*, (90), 225–229.

Siega-Riz, A.M., Bodnar, L., & Savitz, D.A. (2002). What are pregnant women eating? Nutrient and food group differences by race. *American Journal of Obstetrics and Gynecology, 186(3)*, 480–486.

Wadhwa, P.D., et al. (2001). Stress, infection, and preterm birth: A biobehavioural perspective. *Paediatric and Perinatal Epidemiology, 15(s2)*,17–29.

Women of Color Health Data Book. (2000). Bethesda, MD: Office of Research on Women's Health. National Institutes of Health.